AF745987

Handbook of Experimental Pharmacology

Volume 290

Editor-in-Chief

Martin C. Michel, Department of Pharmacology, Johannes Gutenberg Universität, Mainz, Germany

Editorial Board Members

James E. Barrett, Center for Substance Abuse Research, Lewis Katz School of Medicine at Temple University, Philadelphia, USA

David Centurión, Department of Pharmacobiology, Center for Research and Advanced Studies, Mexico City, Mexico

Veit Flockerzi, Institute for Experimental and Clinical Pharmacology and Toxicology, Saarland University, Homburg, Germany

Kathryn Elaine Meier, Department of Pharmaceutical Sciences, Washington State University Spokane, Spokane, WA, USA

Clive P. Page, SIPP, Kings College London, Waterloo Campus, London, UK

Roland Seifert, Institute of Pharmacology, Hannover Medical School, Hannover, Germany

KeWei Wang, School of Pharmacy, Qingdao University, Qingdao, China

The *Handbook of Experimental Pharmacology* is one of the most authoritative and influential book series in pharmacology. It provides critical and comprehensive discussions of the most significant areas of pharmacological research, written by leading international authorities. Each volume in the series represents the most informative and contemporary account of its subject available, making it an unrivalled reference source.

HEP is indexed in PubMed and Scopus.

Zijian Li • Kunhong Xiao
Editors

Pharmacology of GPCRs Biased Signaling and Agonists

Springer

Editors
Zijian Li
Institute of Vascular Medicine
Peking University Third Hospital
Beijing, China

Kunhong Xiao
Allegheny Health Network Cancer Institute
Pittsburgh, PA, USA

ISSN 0171-2004 ISSN 1865-0325 (electronic)
Handbook of Experimental Pharmacology
ISBN 978-3-032-13228-4 ISBN 978-3-032-13229-1 (eBook)
https://doi.org/10.1007/978-3-032-13229-1

© The Editor(s) (if applicable) and The Author(s), under exclusive license to Springer Nature Switzerland AG 2026

This work is subject to copyright. All rights are solely and exclusively licensed by the Publisher, whether the whole or part of the material is concerned, specifically the rights of translation, reprinting, reuse of illustrations, recitation, broadcasting, reproduction on microfilms or in any other physical way, and transmission or information storage and retrieval, electronic adaptation, computer software, or by similar or dissimilar methodology now known or hereafter developed.
The use of general descriptive names, registered names, trademarks, service marks, etc. in this publication does not imply, even in the absence of a specific statement, that such names are exempt from the relevant protective laws and regulations and therefore free for general use.
The publisher, the authors and the editors are safe to assume that the advice and information in this book are believed to be true and accurate at the date of publication. Neither the publisher nor the authors or the editors give a warranty, expressed or implied, with respect to the material contained herein or for any errors or omissions that may have been made. The publisher remains neutral with regard to jurisdictional claims in published maps and institutional affiliations.

This Springer imprint is published by the registered company Springer Nature Switzerland AG
The registered company address is: Gewerbestrasse 11, 6330 Cham, Switzerland

If disposing of this product, please recycle the paper.

Foreword

One of the most basic tenets of classical pharmacological theory has been that the relative efficacy of receptor ligands remains consistent regardless of the signal being measured. This was an obvious consequence of the idea that receptors existed in only two conformations, inactive and active, with all downstream signaling being a direct function of the concentration of active receptors. But with the modern understanding that multiple active conformations of receptors exist, which are differentially stabilized by different ligands, has come the exciting realization that particular ligands or drugs can preferentially stimulate some signaling pathways above others. This phenomenon, variably referred to as biased agonism or functional selectivity, has revolutionized current GPCR research and in particular development of drugs for what is already the most abundant class of receptor drug targets. In this volume editors Zijian Li and Kunhong Xiao have pulled together chapters from a distinguished group of authors all working at the cutting edge of this field to present the first volume devoted entirely to this subject.

I've been privileged to work in the field of GPCR research and to observe its evolution and maturation over the past more than 50 years. This has given me a special perspective on these exciting developments, all of which are expertly reviewed in this timely and important volume which highlights the transformative importance of these new concepts and approaches. I offer here a few very brief historical comments.

By the late 1990s it was already clear that GPCRs activated cell signaling pathways through multiple G proteins and that these actions were desensitized or terminated through the concerted action of receptor phosphorylation by G protein–coupled receptor kinases and subsequent binding of beta-arrestins which block further G protein interaction (Lefkowitz 1998). There were also early studies that suggested that some GPCRs can activate multiple G proteins and that some ligands preferentially promoted signaling through one or the another of these G proteins (Gurwitz et al. 1994). This represented the very first evidence for functional selectivity at GPCRs. Then, beginning about 2000, my lab discovered that the beta-arrestins, which as noted we had discovered as desensitizing molecules, were also able to serve as signal transducers in their own right to effectors such as the non-receptor tyrosine kinase Src, and the map kinases JNK3 and ERK ½ (Pierce and Lefkowitz 2001). It then emerged that there were analogues of the octapeptide hormone angiotensin which were capable of promoting beta-arrestin-mediated internalization of their receptors without activating G proteins (Holloway et al. 2002). This stimulated my group to see if such ligands, e.g. SII-angiotensin, were also capable of selectively stimulating signaling to ERK ½ through beta-arrestin rather than G proteins. This turned out to be the case and represented the first evidence of beta-arrestin biased agonism (Wei et al. 2003). Subsequently many examples of both G protein biased and beta-arrestin biased agonism were discovered at numerous GPCRs. These discoveries have significant clinical and therapeutic implications. To the extent that desirable therapeutic effects might be mediated through either G proteins or beta-arrestins and undesirable side effects through the other class of transducer, then such biased ligands will provide greater selectivity and fewer side effects.

Much has also been learned about the detailed mechanistic and structural basis for biased agonism. For example, as it became clear that beta-arrestins perform multiple functions such as desensitization, endocytosis and signaling to many different effectors, the question naturally arose as to how beta-arrestins "know what to do" after interacting with the GRK phosphorylated receptor. Some years ago, we discovered that for several GPCRS, GRK2 phosphorylation of the receptor inhibits bound beta-arrestin's ability to activate ERK whereas GRK5 phosphorylation supports ERK activation (Kim et al. 2005; Ren et al. 2005). It was already known that these two GRKs phosphorylate distinct sites on the receptors. This led us, some 20 years ago, to propose the so-called barcode hypothesis. We wrote as follows: "It can be speculated that beta-arrestins bound to receptors phosphorylated on distinctive patterns of sites adopt specific conformations capable of activating different signaling effectors. The location of these phosphorylation sites may constitute a barcode that instructs the bound beta Arrestin as to its intended function" (Kim et al. 2005). In the years since, much biochemical and biophysical evidence has supported this idea but the specific barcodes are still being worked out.

As to the biophysical and structural basis for biased agonism much has also been learned through techniques such as cryo-electron microscopy, NMR, DEER spectroscopy and other approaches. All of these techniques support the idea that distinct conformational ensembles stabilized by different types of biased ligands represents one important mechanism for achieving bias. However, differences in the stoichiometry or post-translational modifications of transducers or effectors or even organelle specific factors can also mediate or modulate bias.

Another exciting development has been the discovery of biased *allosteric* modulators which further expands the range of molecular tools and therapeutic opportunities to exploit GPCR bias. Currently, less than a handful of GPCR drugs act allosterically as opposed to orthosterically. But the recent explosion of discovery of allosteric binding sites on GPCRs has opened the door to exploiting bias in new ways and the first such molecules have already been described.

All of these exciting topics are explored in detail in this timely volume which will be of interest not only to experts in the field but to anyone wishing to gain an understanding of the rapid progress made in just the last few years.

Duke Health Distinguished Professor of Medicine, Robert J. Lefkowitz
Investigator, Howard Hughes Medical Institute,
Duke University School of Medicine
Durham, NC, USA

References

Gurwitz D, Haring R, Heldman E, Fraser CM, Manor D, Fisher A (1994) Discrete activation of transduction pathways associated with acetylcholine m1 receptor by several muscarinic ligands. Eur J Pharmacol 267(1):21–31. https://doi.org/10.1016/0922-4106(94)90220. PMID: 8206127

Holloway AC, Qian H, Pipolo L, Ziogas J, Miura S, Karnik S, Southwell BR, Lew MJ, Thomas WG (2002) Side-chain substitutions within angiotensin II reveal different requirements for signaling, internalization, and phosphorylation of type 1A angiotensin receptors. Mol Pharmacol 61(4): 768–777. https://doi.org/10.1124/mol.61.4.768. PMID: 11901215

Kim J, Ahn S, Ren XR, Whalen EJ, Reiter E, Wei H, Lefkowitz RJ (2005) Functional antagonism of different G protein-coupled receptor kinases for beta-arrestin-mediated angiotensin II receptor signaling. Proc Natl Acad Sci U S A 102(5):1442–1447. https://doi.org/10.1073/pnas.0409532102. PMID: 15671181

Lefkowitz RJ (1998) G protein-coupled receptors. III. New roles for receptor kinases and beta-arrestins in receptor signaling and desensitization. J Biol Chem 273(30):18677–18680. https://doi.org/10.1074/jbc.273.30.18677. PMID: 9668034

Pierce KL, Lefkowitz RJ (2001) Classical and new roles of beta-arrestins in the regulation of G-protein-coupled receptors. Nat Rev Neurosci 2(10):727–733. https://doi.org/10.1038/35094577. PMID: 11584310

Ren XR, Reiter E, Ahn S, Kim J, Chen W, Lefkowitz RJ (2005) Different G protein-coupled receptor kinases govern G protein and beta-arrestin-mediated signaling of V2 vasopressin receptor. Proc Natl Acad Sci U S A 102(5):1448–1453. https://doi.org/10.1073/pnas.0409534102. PMID: 15671180

Wei H, Ahn S, Shenoy SK, Karnik SS, Hunyady L, Luttrell LM, Lefkowitz RJ (2003) Independent beta-arrestin 2 and G protein-mediated pathways for angiotensin II activation of extracellular signal-regulated kinases 1 and 2. Proc Natl Acad Sci U S A 100(19):10782–10787. https://doi.org/10.1073/pnas.1834556100. PMID: 12949261

Preface

G protein–coupled receptors (GPCRs) are the most prominent class of drug target, playing an essential role in both human physiology and pathophysiology. They have profoundly shaped the history of drug discovery. Traditionally, GPCR signaling was viewed as a linear cascade—from receptor activation, to heterotrimeric G proteins, and ultimately to downstream effectors. Thanks to the groundbreaking work of Dr. Bob Lefkowitz's group at Duke University alongside contributions from many others over the past three decades, this linear model has evolved into a more complex one in which GPCRs can signal through parallel pathways via both receptor-G protein and receptor-β-arrestin interactions. β-arrestins, once thought to function solely as desensitizers or terminators of G protein–mediated GPCR signaling, are now recognized as key mediators of a G protein–independent signaling network.

This discovery of parallel G protein– and β-arrestin–mediated signaling opened the door to functional selectivity, also known as biased agonism, in which a ligand can preferentially activate one signaling network over another. Such selectivity holds tremendous potential for precise pharmacological modulation, enhancing therapeutic effects while minimizing adverse effects. Most currently approved GPCR-targeting drugs activate both G protein- and β-arrestin–mediated signaling pathways, with the combined effects of these pathways contributing to both therapeutic actions and side effects, either in an intertwined manner or through separate mechanisms. Biased agonism provides a powerful new strategy for dissecting the signaling pathways responsible for therapeutic benefits versus adverse effects. Biased ligands can induce specific conformational changes in the receptor, preferentially engaging either G protein– or β-arrestin–mediated signaling. By selectively activating pathways linked to therapeutic effects while avoiding or minimizing activation of those associated with side effects, these ligands can enhance drug safety and efficacy. By doing so, they can enhance desired outcomes while reducing unwanted effects. The approval of Oliceridine, a μ-opioid receptor agonist with biased signaling properties, exemplifies the translational potential of this concept and provides a roadmap for the development of additional GPCR biased ligands for safer and more effective therapeutics.

In recent years, research has greatly advanced our understanding of GPCR biased signaling and ligands, encompassing molecular pharmacology, signaling mechanisms, structural features and dynamics, and the discovery of biased allosteric modulators. These developments have expanded the range of tools available to probe GPCR function and have opened new avenues for therapeutic innovation.

This volume provides a comprehensive overview of the latest advancements in GPCR biased signaling and ligand pharmacology. The handbook is thoughtfully structured into four key sections, Fundamentals of GPCR Biased Signaling, The Structural Basis of GPCR Biased Signaling and Ligands, Drug Discovery and Development of Biased Ligands, and Therapeutic Applications of GPCR Biased Signaling. Through this multi-disciplinary framework, we systematically present all critical aspects of GPCR bias theory, from fundamental mechanisms to clinical translation. A particular focus is given to representative GPCR systems where biased signaling has been most extensively studied and successfully applied, including β-adrenergic receptors and μ-opioid receptors. We are honored to present contributions from 15 renowned scientists and their teams, and we would like to extend our special thanks to Dr. Bob Lefkowitz for writing the foreword to this book.

This collective work aims to serve as an authoritative reference and inspiration for researchers across multiple disciplines. We hope that readers will find this volume provides them with up-to-date knowledge on GPCR biased signaling, as well as valuable insights into future directions for drug discovery and therapeutic innovation in this rapidly evolving field.

Beijing, China — Zijian Li
Pittsburgh, PA, USA — Kunhong Xiao

Contents

Part I

Fundamentals of GPCR Biased Signaling

GPCR Phospho-Barcodes and Biased Signaling

Qingtao He, Jinpeng Sun, and Shenming Huang

Contents

Q. He
Advanced Medical Research Institute, Cheeloo College of Medicine, Shandong University, Jinan, Shandong, China

J. Sun
Advanced Medical Research Institute, Cheeloo College of Medicine, Shandong University, Jinan, Shandong, China

Department of Physiology and Pathophysiology, School of Basic Medical Sciences, State Key Laboratory of Vascular Homeostasis and Remodeling, Beijing Key Laboratory of Cardiovascular Receptors Research, Peking University, Beijing, China

S. Huang (✉)
Advanced Medical Research Institute, Cheeloo College of Medicine, Shandong University, Jinan, Shandong, China

State Key Laboratory of Bioactive Molecules and Druggability Assessment, Guangdong Basic Research Center of Excellence for Natural Bioactive Molecules and Discovery of Innovative Drugs, Jinan University, Guangzhou, China
e-mail: huangshenming@jnu.edu.cn

© The Author(s), under exclusive license to Springer Nature Switzerland AG 2025
Z. Li, K. Xiao (eds.), *Pharmacology of GPCRs Biased Signaling and Agonists*,
Handbook of Experimental Pharmacology 290, https://doi.org/10.1007/164_2025_761

Abstract

G protein-coupled receptors (GPCRs), the largest family of membrane receptors in humans, primarily regulate diverse physiological and pathological processes through G protein- and arrestin-mediated signaling pathways, making them important drug targets. Notably, arrestins not only mediate GPCR desensitization and internalization but also regulate G protein-independent signal transduction. However, the mechanisms underlying arrestin-mediated biased signaling remain incompletely understood, posing significant challenges for developing targeted GPCR drugs with signaling bias. To address this knowledge gap, researchers have conducted systematic investigations and proposed innovative models, including the flute model, the polyproline sorting dock model, and the time order effects of GPCR phospho-barcodes to elucidate the dynamic processes driving biased signaling in arrestin activations. These key findings not only refine the theoretical framework of GPCR phosphorylation in biased signaling but also provide a solid foundation for developing biased drugs targeting the GPCR-arrestin pathway, offering new opportunities for precision therapeutics in diverse diseases.

Keywords

Arrestin · Biased signaling · GPCR · Phospho-barcode

1 GPCR Phosphorylation and Arrestin Signaling

GPCRs can convert extracellular stimuli into intracellular signals by the activation of G proteins and arrestin signaling. Whereas G proteins regulate the levels of intracellular second messengers to exert their effects, arrestins recruit different downstream proteins by binding to the receptor, leading to desensitization, endocytosis, or the activation of arrestin-dependent signaling pathways (Kenakin 2013; Whalen et al. 2011). The engagement between GPCRs and arrestin necessitates the receptor's phosphorylation, which plays a central role in regulating the diversity of transmembrane signaling mediated by the receptors-arrestin pathway. The phosphorylation process of GPCRs is primarily catalyzed by G protein-coupled receptor kinases (GRKs), which induce phosphorylation of the C-terminal or the third intracellular loop of GPCRs, leading to a series of phospho-barcode patterns (Gurevich and Gurevich 2006). These patterns not only determine the characteristics of GPCR directly binding to arrestin but also influence the downstream signaling pathways through indirect effects of arrestin. The arrestins critically regulate GPCR functions by mediating receptor desensitization and internalization (Peterson and Luttrell 2017) and by redirecting signaling to G protein-independent pathways via interactions with numerous downstream effector molecules, such as MAPK and c-Raf (Chavkin et al. 2014; Coffa et al. 2011). It is noteworthy that different phospho-barcodes of GPCRs can induce arrestin to form different conformational states, which affect the binding ability of arrestin to GPCRs and downstream signaling molecules, thereby regulating the efficiency and specificity of signaling transduction (Yang et al. 2015, 2017). Therefore, the phosphorylated GPCRs-arrestin signaling pathway plays key roles in integrating and coordinating the diverse downstream signaling pathways of GPCRs.

Developing biased ligands that target the arrestin signaling of GPCRs has witnessed a significant surge in research over the past few years. Currently, the drug targets the arrestin signaling pathway of the opioid receptor, Oliceridine, which has been approved for use in pain relief with reducing the side effects of vomiting and respiratory suppression. Moreover, arrestin-biased ligands targeting AT1R and M3R have demonstrated great potential in the treatment of hypertension and asthma (Jara et al. 2023; Liu et al. 2017; Tompkins et al. 2022). Therefore, a thorough investigation into the mechanisms regulating the phospho-barcode patterns of GPCRs not only contributes to a comprehensive understanding of the underlying mechanisms of the diverse signaling transduction of GPCRs but also holds great significance for the development of biased drugs targeting the arrestin signaling pathways of GPCRs for developing novel therapeutic strategies.

1.1 The "Flute Model" Theory of GPCR Phosphorylation

The phospho-barcode patterns of GPCRs are closely related to their functional diversity. In the past decade, scientists have made significant progress in exploring the mechanisms of GPCR phosphorylation and functional regulation by proposing the "flute model" theory of GPCR. The flute model for the phospho-barcoding mechanism of arrestin signaling suggests that at least ten phosphate-binding sites located in the N-terminal region of arrestin function as sensors of the phospho-message in the receptor C-tail or the intracellular loops. Just as fingers pressing different holes on a flute can produce different notes, different phosphorylation combinations can generate different functions of arrestin. By using ^{19}F-NMR to study the complexes of receptors' C-terminal peptides with different phospho-barcodes and β-arrestin-1, scientists found that a phospho-barcode of 1-4-6-7 induced by GRK2 directs clathrin recruitment and the endocytic function of arrestin, whereas a phospho-barcode of 1–5 induced by the GRK6 directs SRC recruitment and signaling, promoting cell migration and other physiological functions. Additionally, researchers observed at least three unique activated states of β-arrestin-1 in ^{19}F-NMR spectrum, whereas clathrin could only recognize one of these structural states. In the cell, specific mutations in critical amino acids at the binding sites for phosphorylated residues selectively cause the disappearance of several different functions of β-arrestin-1 downstream of the receptor, proving that the phosphorylation patterns that select specific conformations and functions of β-arrestin-1 are universal in some GPCR family members. Therefore, there are theoretically more than 1,000 phospho-barcode patterns (2^10–1 = 1,023) that produce many arrestin conformations, dictating numerous downstream effector interactions, which in turn reveals the intrinsic mechanisms of the diverse signaling transduction of GPCRs

(Yang et al. 2015). With the development of GPCR structural biology, numerous phosphorylated receptors-arrestins complexes have been solved (Cao et al. 2022; Huang et al. 2020; Lee et al. 2020; Shukla et al. 2013; Staus et al. 2020). These structural insights collectively demonstrate that the phospho-barcodes of GPCRs serve as a pivotal element in unraveling the mechanisms of GPCR recruitment and functional regulation to arrestins.

The barcode hypothesis emerged from the observation that GPCRs are differently phosphorylated at multiple sites, which are associated with different cellular contexts and functions. It offers a theoretical framework for understanding how a single receptor can engage in multiple distinct functions through arrestin. The flute model gives us a detailed and powerful complement to the barcode hypothesis to help explore mechanism of GPCR phosphorylation. The model elucidates the manner in which the phosphorylated barcode present on the ligand-bound GPCR is accurately identified by the arrestin N-terminal phosphate-binding concave, subsequently transforming into functionally selective arrestin conformations linked to distinct signaling pathways. In line with the barcode hypothesis, a biased ligand targeting a GPCR influences particular phosphorylation profiles and may solely activate a specific subset of signaling pathways. This is in contrast to a balanced ligand, which indiscriminately triggers both G protein-mediated and phosphorylation/arrestin-regulated physiological responses (Yang et al. 2015, 2017). Therefore, the barcode hypothesis holds considerable promise for developing therapeutic compounds that selectively promote advantageous pathways while avoiding those that lead to detrimental effects. The introduced flute model offers a deeper understanding of this biased agonism through the lens of arrestin conformational signaling and should benefit the development of innovative drugs based on GPCR phospho-barcodes.

1.2 The Polyproline Sorting Dock Model of GPCR Phosphorylation

Most GPCRs can transmit diverse signaling by interacting with more than 300 downstream proteins containing SH3 domains (SH3-domain-containing proteins, SH3-CPs). How the GPCRs encoded by the human genome selectively couple to these SH3-CPs to trigger specific signaling pathways is an important component of the diversity in GPCR phosphorylation-mediated signaling. To address this scientific challenge, researchers have conducted in-depth studies using unnatural amino acid incorporation techniques combined with ^{19}F-NMR, fluorescence spectroscopy, and cellular approaches to study the mechanisms underlying arrestin-mediated GPCR signaling to SH3-CPs. The research found that different phospho-barcodes in the tail of GPCRs can regulate the conformational state of the three polyproline regions in β-arrestin-1 through allosteric regulation. This conformational change further determines the selection and recruitment of different SH3-CPs, forming signaling complexes with specific functions to finely regulate cellular signaling processes. The results revealed that the three polyproline regions in β-arrestin-1 serve as key docking sites for GPCRs to connect with downstream SH3-domain proteins and found that the phospho-GPCR active arrestin conformation increases the activation of downstream kinases containing SH3 domains by disrupting its autoinhibitory structural skeletons. Based on this discovery, researchers proposed a new "arrestin polyproline sorting dock model" to elucidate such a novel mechanism of GPCR signaling through allosteric regulation. The model revealed the pivotal role of allosteric regulation in GPCR signaling, providing a new perspective for understanding the fine regulation mechanism between GPCRs and downstream signaling proteins on at least two levels. The first level lies in the distinct, functionally interrelated conformational states of arrestin, guided by the phosphorylated GPCR barcodes. The selective coupling between receptor-phosphosite binding and the precise conformational states of the three polyproline regions within β-arrestin-1 determines the selectivity and intrinsic efficacy of downstream SH3-CP recruitment. At the second level, it has elucidated that arrestins can modulate downstream kinase signaling via an allosteric mechanism in addition to acting as the scaffolding downstream effectors to receptor-arrestin complexes. Upon the attachment of an agonist-bound phosphorylated GPCR, the polyproline regions of β-arrestin-1 adopt an active conformational state, which then interacts with SH3 domains and disrupts the compact regulatory domains of SH3-CPs such as SRC, thereby significantly increasing kinase activity. The identified allosteric regulation of downstream signaling effectors by active arrestin suggests a more general and necessary mechanism underlying GPCR-regulated signaling than previously recognized. These results will elicit future interest in determining the specificity and working mechanisms of arrestin-mediated GPCR functions and might lay as a theoretical foundation for the future development of drug targets targeting GPCR signaling pathways (Yang et al. 2018).

1.3 Functional Impacts on Arrestins from Single Phosphorylation Site

A single phosphorylation site of the receptor can also regulate the diverse signaling pathways by regulating the conformational changes of arrestin. The results from FRET assay based on genetic code expansion in arrestin showed that the contribution of a single phosphorylation site of the GPCR to the affinity of the receptor-arrestin complex is different, indicating that the effect of a single different phosphorylation site on arrestin is inconsistent (Huang et al. 2019). Furthermore, the structural complexes of arrestin bound with the V2R C-tails in different phospho-barcodes directly clarified the distinct interaction modes formed by different phosphorylated tails and arrestin. Comparing the structures of inactive arrestin with those activated by different phosphorylated C-tails, it was found that these active arrestins led to significant changes in the hydrophilic exposure area of the functional regions of arrestin. Additionally, compared with the structure of arrestin activated by the V2R C-tail with full phosphorylation, the active arrestin structure lacking phosphate interaction at sites -1, -3, -4, -6-7 formed different structural conformations in several functional related structural regions (He et al. 2021).

Moreover, DeSiPher technology showed that a single deletion in the phosphorylation site of GPCR can induce a specific dynamic conformational change in the interface between arrestin and MEK and c-Raf-1 (He et al. 2021; Liu et al. 2020). Further, FlAsH-BRET was used to detect the differences in the phosphorylation patterns caused by mutations in the C-terminal phosphorylation sites of the V2R, which found that these different phosphorylation patterns could affect the recruitment ability of arrestin to MEK and c-Raf-1 (He et al. 2021). These results indicated that the individual phospho-binding of specific arrestin sites contributed to the affinity and could induce conformational changes at remote positions of arrestin and that these changes are connected well with their selective functions.

During the study of the functional regulation of arrestin by the single phosphate, an interesting discovery was made: the identification of a new phosphate-binding site on arrestin, V3′4′, which reveals a novel phosphorylation code for the arrestin on the flute model and participates in the interaction between phosphorylated GPCRs and arrestin. This discovery suggests that the binding of phosphorylation sites follows an order of priority, with the binding of certain sites potentially affecting the ability of others to bind, and there may be as-yet-undiscovered new phosphorylation code binding sites on arrestin. The individual arrestin phospho-binding pockets could be interdependent, and crosstalk between different phospho-binding pockets could be a general mechanism for signaling downstream of arrestin. The phospho-binding pattern could not be simply derived from the primary sequence, and this pattern, in addition to the strength of the phospho-arrestin interactions, is the main mechanism determining the specific conformations and selective functions of arrestin. This phenomenon is so-called as the time order effect in the phospho-barcodes of GPCRs, which is an important expansion of the flute model and the component of the GPCR phosphorylation-mediated arrestin signaling function diversity.

2 Conclusion

The agonist-dependent phosphorylation of GPCRs serves as a crucial regulator in orchestrating the signal transduction processes mediated by arrestins. This intricate phosphorylation pattern acts as a molecular switch, determining the specific conformations and functional outcomes of arrestin activation, thereby dictating the course of GPCR-arrestin-biased signaling pathways. Over the past two decades, significant advancements in research techniques and methodologies have facilitated the discovery of the flute model, the polyproline sorting dock model, and the time order effect in the phospho-barcodes of GPCRs, which has provided a clearer understanding of how GPCR phosphorylation encodes and modulates the functional diversity of arrestins. These findings elucidated the complex interplay between GPCR phosphorylation and arrestin binding, revealing that the specific phosphorylation sites and their stoichiometry on GPCRs can influence the affinity, specificity, and downstream signaling outcomes of arrestin activation, offering valuable insights for the development of targeted and selective therapeutic agents.

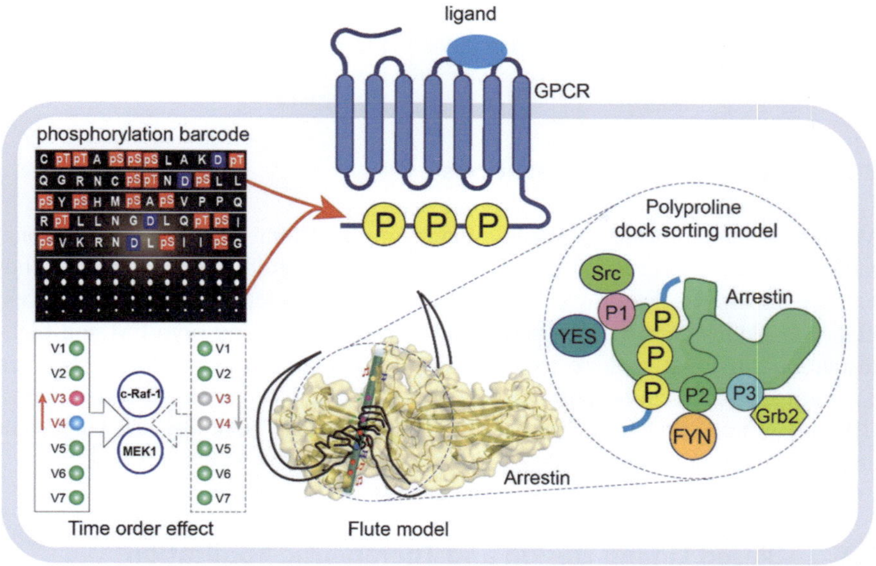

The flute model, polyproline docking sorting theory, and time order effect mechanism of GPCR phosphorylation. Yellow P: Phosphate group; Pink P1: Polyproline P1 region; Green P2: Polyproline P2 region; Cyan P3: Polyproline P3 region

3 Outlook

The field has made significant strides in understanding GPCR phosphorylation and arrestin-mediated biased signaling, driven by innovative theoretical frameworks and experimental techniques. The proposed flute model has expanded the "barcode hypothesis" by detailing how phosphorylated residues in GPCRs act as a molecular code to direct arrestin conformational changes and functional selectivity. The discovery of the polyproline sorting dock model further elucidates how phosphorylation regulates arrestin interaction with SH3-domain proteins, revealing critical allosteric mechanisms that fine-tune downstream signaling. Several critical gaps and opportunities remain in understanding GPCR phospho-barcodes and biased signaling.

3.1 Temporal Dynamics of Arrestin Activation

The time order effect of phosphorylation sites suggests a sequential activation mechanism. Investigating the kinetics of phosphorylation cascades and how they influence arrestin functional state transitions and conformational dynamics will require time-resolved techniques, such as ultrafast spectroscopy or single-molecule tracking. Understanding how upstream kinases (e.g., GRK2, GRK6) differentially regulate phosphorylation dynamics in physiological contexts could uncover context-specific signaling pathways.

3.2 Technological Innovations

Moving forward, advancing research integrating structural biology, computational modeling, and chemical biology will be essential to fully decode the phospho-barcode repertoire. Key areas of focus include (I) structural biology advances: higher-resolution imaging of arrestin-GPCR complexes using cryo-EM and high-resolution structural biology techniques, (II) computational modeling: AI-driven simulations to predict phospho-barcode-arrestin docking and allosteric modulations, (III) single-molecule studies: probing the conformational flexibility and kinetics of arrestin activation in living cells.

3.3 Biased Ligand Design and Therapeutic Application

The insights from biased agonism imply significant potential for developing arrestin-biased drugs to selectively modulate GPCR signaling cascades. For example, leveraging the polyproline sorting dock model, compounds targeting SH3-domain protein recruitment pathways could be designed to treat diseases such as cancer or metabolic disorders. Expanding biased ligand research to include novel receptor families (e.g., orphan GPCRs) and noncanonical arrestin functions (e.g., scaffolding for MAPK cascades) could provide novel therapeutic opportunities. These efforts may reveal new mechanisms for regulating GPCR signaling and unlock innovative strategies for precision medicine.

Acknowledgments This work was supported by NSFC grants 81773704, 82425105, 82304601, 32200990 and the Science and Technology Projects in Guangzhou (grant numbers 202102070001)..

Conflicts of Interest The authors have no conflicts of interest.

References

Cao C, Barros-Alvarez X, Zhang S, Kim K, Damgen MA, Panova O, Suomivuori CM, Fay JF, Zhong X, Krumm BE et al (2022) Signaling snapshots of a serotonin receptor activated by the prototypical psychedelic LSD. Neuron 110:3154–3167 e3157. https://doi.org/10.1016/j.neuron.2022.08.006

Chavkin C, Schattauer SS, Levin JR (2014) Arrestin-mediated activation of p38 MAPK: molecular mechanisms and behavioral consequences. Handb Exp Pharmacol 219:281–292. https://doi.org/10.1007/978-3-642-41199-1_14

Coffa S, Breitman M, Spiller BW, Gurevich VV (2011) A single mutation in arrestin-2 prevents ERK1/2 activation by reducing c-Raf1 binding. Biochemistry 50:6951–6958. https://doi.org/10.1021/bi200745k

Gurevich VV, Gurevich EV (2006) The structural basis of arrestin-mediated regulation of G-protein-coupled receptors. Pharmacol Ther 110:465–502. https://doi.org/10.1016/j.pharmthera.2005.09.008

He QT, Xiao P, Huang SM, Jia YL, Zhu ZL, Lin JY, Yang F, Tao XN, Zhao RJ, Gao FY et al (2021) Structural studies of phosphorylation-dependent interactions between the V2R receptor and arrestin-2. Nat Commun 12:2396. https://doi.org/10.1038/s41467-021-22731-x

Huang SM, Yang F, Cai BY, He QT, Liu Q, Qu CX, Han MJ, Kong W, Jia YL, Li F et al (2019) Genetically encoded fluorescent amino acid for monitoring protein interactions through FRET. Anal Chem 91:14936–14942. https://doi.org/10.1021/acs.analchem.9b03305

Huang W, Masureel M, Qu Q, Janetzko J, Inoue A, Kato HE, Robertson MJ, Nguyen KC, Glenn JS, Skiniotis G et al (2020) Structure of the neurotensin receptor 1 in complex with beta-arrestin 1. Nature 579:303–308. https://doi.org/10.1038/s41586-020-1953-1

Jara ZP, Harford TJ, Singh KD, Desnoyer R, Kumar A, Srinivasan D, Karnik SS (2023) Distinct mechanisms of beta-arrestin-biased agonist and blocker of AT1R in preventing aortic aneurysm and associated mortality. Hypertension 80:385–402. https://doi.org/10.1161/HYPERTENSIONAHA.122.19232

Kenakin T (2013) New concepts in pharmacological efficacy at 7TM receptors: IUPHAR review 2. Br J Pharmacol 168:554–575. https://doi.org/10.1111/j.1476-5381.2012.02223.x

Lee Y, Warne T, Nehme R, Pandey S, Dwivedi-Agnihotri H, Chaturvedi M, Edwards PC, Garcia-Nafria J, Leslie AGW, Shukla AK et al (2020) Molecular basis of beta-arrestin coupling to formoterol-bound beta(1)-adrenoceptor. Nature 583:862–866. https://doi.org/10.1038/s41586-020-2419-1

Liu CH, Gong Z, Liang ZL, Liu ZX, Yang F, Sun YJ, Ma ML, Wang YJ, Ji CR, Wang YH et al (2017) Arrestin-biased AT1R agonism induces acute catecholamine secretion through TRPC3 coupling. Nat Commun 8:14335. https://doi.org/10.1038/ncomms14335

Liu Q, He QT, Lyu X, Yang F, Zhu ZL, Xiao P, Yang Z, Zhang F, Yang ZY, Wang XY et al (2020) DeSiphering receptor core-induced and ligand-dependent conformational changes in arrestin via genetic encoded trimethylsilyl (1)H-NMR probe. Nat Commun 11:4857. https://doi.org/10.1038/s41467-020-18433-5

Peterson YK, Luttrell LM (2017) The diverse roles of Arrestin scaffolds in G protein-coupled receptor signaling. Pharmacol Rev 69:256–297. https://doi.org/10.1124/pr.116.013367

Shukla AK, Manglik A, Kruse AC, Xiao K, Reis RI, Tseng WC, Staus DP, Hilger D, Uysal S, Huang LY et al (2013) Structure of active beta-arrestin-1 bound to a G-protein-coupled receptor phosphopeptide. Nature 497:137–141. https://doi.org/10.1038/nature12120

Staus DP, Hu H, Robertson MJ, Kleinhenz ALW, Wingler LM, Capel WD, Latorraca NR, Lefkowitz RJ, Skiniotis G (2020) Structure of the M2 muscarinic receptor-beta-arrestin complex in a lipid nanodisc. Nature 579:297–302. https://doi.org/10.1038/s41586-020-1954-0

Tompkins E, Mimic B, Cuevas-Mora K, Schorsch H, Shah SD, Deshpande DA, Benovic JL, Penn RB, Pera T (2022) PD 102807 induces M3 mAChR-dependent GRK-/Arrestin-biased signaling in airway smooth muscle cells. Am J Respir Cell Mol Biol 67:550–561. https://doi.org/10.1165/rcmb.2021-0320OC

Whalen EJ, Rajagopal S, Lefkowitz RJ (2011) Therapeutic potential of beta-arrestin- and G protein-biased agonists. Trends Mol Med 17:126–139. https://doi.org/10.1016/j.molmed.2010.11.004

Yang F, Yu X, Liu C, Qu CX, Gong Z, Liu HD, Li FH, Wang HM, He DF, Yi F et al (2015) Phospho-selective mechanisms of arrestin conformations and functions revealed by unnatural amino acid incorporation and (19)F-NMR. Nat Commun 6:8202. https://doi.org/10.1038/ncomms9202

Yang Z, Yang F, Zhang D, Liu Z, Lin A, Liu C, Xiao P, Yu X, Sun JP (2017) Phosphorylation of G protein-coupled receptors: from the barcode hypothesis to the flute model. Mol Pharmacol 92:201–210. https://doi.org/10.1124/mol.116.107839

Yang F, Xiao P, Qu CX, Liu Q, Wang LY, Liu ZX, He QT, Liu C, Xu JY, Li RR et al (2018) Allosteric mechanisms underlie GPCR signaling to SH3-domain proteins through arrestin. Nat Chem Biol 14:876–886. https://doi.org/10.1038/s41589-018-0115-3

GPCR Heterodimers: Implications for Biased Signaling

Li Lin, Yizhong Li, Shenglan Zhang, Cangsong Shen, Jiyong Meng, and Jianfeng Liu

Contents

Authors Li Lin, Yizhong Li and Shenglan Zhang have equally contributed to this chapter.

L. Lin · Y. Li
Cellular Signaling laboratory, International Research Center for Sensory Biology and Technology of MOST, Key Laboratory of Molecular Biophysics of MOE, School of Life Science and Technology, Huazhong University of Science and Technology, Wuhan, China

S. Zhang
Bioland Laboratory (Guangzhou Regenerative Medicine and Health Guangdong Laboratory), Guangzhou, China

C. Shen · J. Liu (✉)
Cellular Signaling laboratory, International Research Center for Sensory Biology and Technology of MOST, Key Laboratory of Molecular Biophysics of MOE, School of Life Science and Technology, Huazhong University of Science and Technology, Wuhan, China

Bioland Laboratory (Guangzhou Regenerative Medicine and Health Guangdong Laboratory), Guangzhou, China
e-mail: jfliu@mail.hust.edu.cn

J. Meng
Institut de Génomique Fonctionnelle, Univ. Montpellier, CNRS, INSERM, Montpellier, France

© The Author(s), under exclusive license to Springer Nature Switzerland AG 2025
Z. Li, K. Xiao (eds.), *Pharmacology of GPCRs Biased Signaling and Agonists*,
Handbook of Experimental Pharmacology 290, https://doi.org/10.1007/164_2025_762

Abstract

G protein-coupled receptors (GPCRs) are key mediators of cellular signaling, participating in various physiological and pathological processes. Emerging evidence reveals that GPCRs can form functional heterodimers, wherein two distinct receptor subtypes interact mutually to generate unique signaling complexes. GPCR heterodimers play a crucial role in modulating cellular responses and are involved in biased signaling, a phenomenon where receptor activation preferentially triggers specific intracellular pathways (e.g., G protein vs. β-arrestin pathways). In this review, we will explore the molecular mechanisms underlying GPCR heterodimerization and the modulation of biased signaling in heterodimers. We first discuss the assembly and activation mechanisms based on heterodimerization in Class C GPCRs. Furthermore, we explore the impact of receptor dimerization on downstream biased signaling and the physiological relevance of these heterodimers. Next, we also summarize three criteria and essential technologies for identifying potential heterodimers. Lastly, we address the challenges and future directions in the study of GPCR heterodimers, particularly for drug discovery, highlighting their potential in designing novel therapeutics with enhanced specificity and reduced side effects.

Keywords

Biased signaling · G protein · G protein-coupled receptor · Heterodimer · β-arrestin

1 Di-/Oligomerization of G Protein-Coupled Receptors (GPCRs) and Biased Signaling

G protein-coupled receptors (GPCRs) are widely distributed throughout the human body. Approximately 3% of the human genome, encompassing about 800 genes, encodes GPCRs (Hauser et al. 2017; Zhang et al. 2006). They represent the largest family of membrane proteins and are involved in nearly all physiological and pathological responses in humans (Fredriksson et al. 2003; Rosenbaum et al. 2020). Multiple types of GPCRs can be expressed in each cell, and specific cell types may exhibit distinct GPCR expression patterns during development and physiological processes (Pin et al. 2019). Of the 800 GPCRs, 370 are non-sensory receptors predominantly expressed in the brain (Azam et al. 2020; Huang et al. 2017). These receptors play vital roles in regulating mood, appetite, pain, vision, immune responses, cognition, and synaptic transmission (Huang et al. 2017; Miyagi et al. 2020). GPCR dysfunction is directly or indirectly implicated in metabolic diseases, brain disorders, cardiovascular diseases, cancers, and other pathological conditions (Hauser et al. 2018; Schoneberg and Liebscher 2021). This makes

GPCRs the primary targets for disease therapy, with approximately one-third of all marketed drugs targeting these receptors (Alhosaini et al. 2021).

GPCRs share a common structure comprising seven transmembrane (7TM) helices, three intracellular loops (ICLs), three extracellular loops (ECLs), an extracellular N-terminus (NTD), and an intracellular C-terminus (Bockaert and Pin 1999). The canonical model of GPCR function involves ligand binding, receptor activation, and coupling to intracellular signaling molecules, primarily G proteins or β-arrestins, which are key regulators of GPCR downstream signaling (Heyder et al. 2021; Weis and Kobilka 2018). Over the past few decades, an intriguing phenomenon known as *biased signaling* has been observed in the pharmacological research of Class A GPCRs (Spengler et al. 1993; Wei et al. 2003). Upon external stimulation, these receptors preferentially trigger specific signaling pathways, such as G protein signaling ($G\alpha_i$, $G\alpha_s$, $G\alpha_q$, $G\alpha_{12/13}$) versus β-arrestin mediated signaling (Spengler et al. 1993; Wei et al. 2003). To date, several factors have been recognized to contribute to the phenomenon of *biased signaling* in GPCRs, including system bias (Fig. 1a), ligand bias (Fig. 1b), and receptor bias (Fig. 1c), highlighting the complexity and flexibility of GPCR signal transduction (Wisler et al. 2014).

GPCRs were traditionally regarded as monomeric functional units responsible for transducing external stimuli (Zhang et al. 2024). However, accumulating research have challenged the monomeric view of GPCR function, showing that many GPCRs can form stable dimeric and oligomeric functional complexes (Borroto-Escuela and Fuxe 2019b; Kniazeff et al. 2011; Moller et al. 2018). The dimerization and oligomerization of GPCRs also play a critical role in biased signaling, contributing to receptor-dependent bias (Borah et al. 2024; Ferre et al. 2014) (Fig. 1c). For example, in our recent study using the platelet-activating factor receptor (PAFR) as a model, we found that PAFR oligomers formed under low expression conditions preferentially enhance G protein activity while significantly reducing β-arrestin recruitment and agonist-induced internalization. Interestingly, β-arrestin engagement impairs the specific conformation of PAFR oligomers conversely (Liu et al. 2022). This oligomerization-induced receptor bias further underscores the profound complexity of GPCR signaling regulation.

Similarly, the effects of heterodimerization on the signaling of GPCR complexes have drawn considerable attention (Armando et al. 2014; Mores et al. 2019). The functional heterodimer comprising two distinct GPCR subtypes not only alter receptor pharmacology but also exhibit unique signaling properties that are distinct from those of homodimers or monomers. Notably, heterodimeric receptor complexes can engage in *biased signaling*. Thus, the concept of *biased signaling* is crucial for understanding how receptor heterodimeric complexes selectively activate or inhibit specific signaling cascades, offering new opportunities for designing targeted therapeutics with improved efficacy and fewer side effects (Smith et al. 2018). To elucidate these mechanisms, it is essential to identify heterodimers and investigate how they activate specific signaling pathways. The dynamic interactions between receptors and their ligands, as well as the formation of receptor complexes, determine how signals are transduced within cells, ultimately influencing cellular responses. This information not only enhances our understanding of basic biological

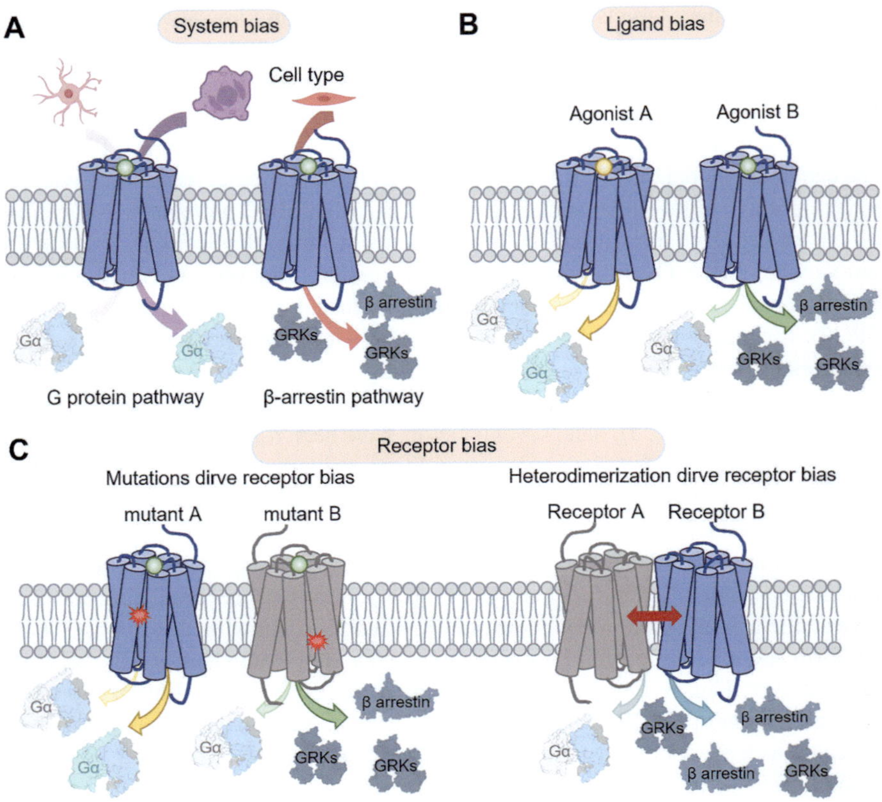

Fig. 1 Cartoons illustrating the various biased activation mechanism. (**a**) The activation mechanism in system bias. The endogenous ligand induces biased G protein pathway or β-arrestin signaling in different types of cells. (**b**) The activation mechanism in ligand bias. Different ligands targeting the same receptor will elicit different G protein pathway or β-arrestin signaling. (**c**) The activation mechanism in receptor bias driven by single point mutation (left) and heterodimerization (right). Different mutant receptors will elicit different G protein pathway or β-arrestin signaling. The mutations are shown in red pore (left). The heterodimerization between two different receptors was indicated by red arrow. The ligand was shown in green or yellow balls. Different G protein pathway was indicated in gray and light blue Gα protein, and the GRK-β-arrestin signaling was shown in sky blue. Receptor A and B was shown in gray and light blue respectively

functions but also provides valuable insights for therapeutic interventions targeting receptor-mediated signaling pathways.

In this chapter, we will focus on the molecular mechanisms underlying GPCR heterodimerization and the modulation of biased signaling in heterodimers. We first describe the formation and activation mechanisms in Class C GPCR heterodimers and compare them with dimerization mechanism of GPCRs from other classes. We also explored in detail how GPCR heterodimerization induces downstream biased signaling, such as G protein signaling and β-arrestin signaling, and examined the physiological relevance of these heterodimers through specific examples. Next, we summarize three criteria and essential technologies for identifying potential heterodimers. Lastly, we address the challenges and future directions in the study of GPCR heterodimers, particularly for drug discovery, highlighting their potential in designing novel therapeutics with enhanced specificity and reduced side effects.

2 Class C GPCR Heterodimer

The concept of GPCR homo- and heterodimerization was first proposed in studies of the β_2 adrenergic receptor in the 1980s (Borroto-Escuela and Fuxe 2019b; Fraser and Venter 1982). Since then, accumulating biochemical and physiological evidence has shown that GPCRs can form homo- or heterodimers, and even higher-order oligomeric complexes (Albizu et al. 2010; Ferre et al. 2014). Based on amino acid sequence and functional similarity, GPCRs can be classified into four groups: Class A GPCRs (rhodopsin-like receptors), Class B (adhesion-like receptors), Class C (glutamate-like receptors), and Class F (frizzled and smooth receptors). The most well-studied and well-established GPCR homo- and heterodimers belong to Class C, including neurotransmitter γ-aminobutyric acid ($GABA_B$) receptor, metabotropic glutamate (mGlu) receptor, calcium-sensing (CaS) receptor, sweet and umami taste receptor (T1Rs), and some orphan receptors such as GPR156 and GPR158 (Pin et al. 2007). Among them, the metabotropic $GABA_B$ receptor is an obligate heterodimer, composed of two subunits, $GABA_{B1}$ and $GABA_{B2}$, which play a critical role in inhibitory neurotransmission in the central nervous system (Kaupmann et al. 1998). $GABA_{B1}$ interacts with $GABA_{B2}$ between the coil-coil motifs in both subunits, masking the ER retention signal to help heterodimeric $GABA_B$ receptor trafficking to the cell surface (Fig. 2a). Both subunits are required for a functional receptor: $GABA_{B1}$ is responsible for ligand binding, while $GABA_{B2}$ is essential for $G_{i/o}$-protein activation, resulting in asymmetric signal transduction (Pin and Bettler 2016). In addition to activating $G_{i/o}$ protein, our previous results also show $GABA_B$ receptor is capable of activating G_{13} protein to mediate neuroprotection, even with slower kinetics and lower potency than $G_{i/o}$ coupling (Wang et al. 2021a). Additionally, although β-arrestin recruitment is not involved, $GABA_B$ receptor has also been reported to undergo constitutive internalization through β-arrestin-independent mechanisms (Hannan et al. 2011). These diverse signaling pathways downstream of the $GABA_B$ receptor strongly imply that this receptor can be preferentially activated by small molecules or other interacting proteins. Nevertheless, it requires further in-depth research into the structural basis of $GABA_B$ receptor activation mechanisms, such as the high-resolution cryo-electron microscopy (cryo-EM) structures of the $GABA_B$-G_{13} complex.

The mGlu receptors exist as eight distinct homodimers, stabilized by a cysteine-disulfide bond, to regulate excitatory neurotransmission (Fig. 2b). These receptors are classified into three groups based on sequence homology and pharmacological profiles: Group I (mGlu1, mGlu5), Group II (mGlu2, mGlu3), and Group III (mGlu4, mGlu6–8) (Niswender and Conn 2010). Upon activation, both subunits

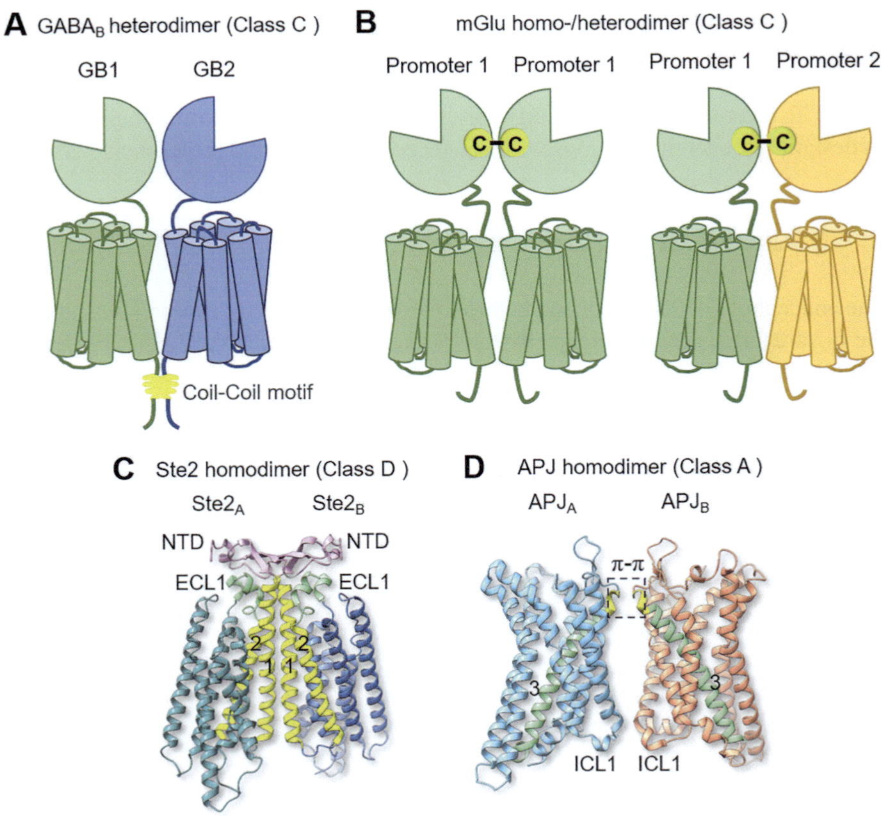

Fig. 2 The structural basis underlying the formation of homodimers and heterodimers in different GPCR families. (**a**) Class C $GABA_B$ heterodimer forms a mandatory heterodimer through the coil-coil domain (yellow) of the C-tail. GB1 and GB2 subunits are shown in green and blue. (**b**) Class C mGlu receptors form obligatory homodimers (left) or heterodimers (right) through disulfide bonds formed by cysteine residues on the VFTs of the two protomers. Protomers 1 and 2 are shown in green and orange. (**c**) Class D GPCR Ste2 forms homodimers through NTD (plum), TM1 and TM2 (yellow), and ECL1 (pale green) (PDB: 7QB9). (D) Class A GPCR APJ forms homodimers through π-π interaction (yellow) at the head of TM3 (pale green) (PDB: 7W0L). NTD, N-terminal domain

of the mGlu homodimer can couple to G proteins, but only one subunit activates the G protein at a time, demonstrating an asymmetric activation mechanism similar to that of the $GABA_B$ receptor (Pin and Bettler 2016). Meanwhile, mGlu receptors have also been reported to form 16 potential heterodimers through various subunit combinations, assembled in a manner similar to that of homodimers (Doumazane et al. 2011; Lee et al. 2020) (Fig. 2b). Although pharmacological studies have provided indirect evidence of their existence (Liu et al. 2023), determining their specific composition in native tissues remains challenging. Recently, we developed a Fluorescence Resonance Energy Transfer (FRET) assay using conformation-specific nanobodies targeting mGlu2 and mGlu4 subunits, which revealed the existence of mGlu2-4 heterodimers alongside mGlu2 and mGlu4 homodimers in various brain regions (Meng et al. 2022). Our findings showed that mGlu2-4 heterodimers are predominantly distributed outside the cerebellum compared to mGlu4 homodimers (Meng et al. 2022). Functional analyses further revealed distinct activation mechanisms in mGlu heterodimers. The mGlu1-5 heterodimer exhibits a symmetric activation mechanism, activating G proteins through both protomers to a similar extent (Werthmann et al. 2021). Negative allosteric modulators (NAMs) targeting either protomer in heterodimeric mGlu1-5 receptors partially inhibit signaling, indicating that full receptor activity requires both active 7TM domains. In contrast, the mGlu2-4 heterodimer demonstrates an asymmetric activation mechanism, where G protein activation occurs primarily through mGlu4 but not mGlu2. Positive allosteric modulators (PAMs) targeting mGlu2 or NAMs inhibiting mGlu4 can shift G protein coupling to mGlu2 (Liu et al. 2017). Similarly, the mGlu2-7 heterodimer exhibits an asymmetric activation mechanism through the mGlu7 subunit, where PAMs targeting mGlu2 can shift G protein coupling to mGlu2, whereas NAMs of mGlu7 fail to elicit same effect (Du et al. 2021).

Recent advancements in cryo-EM structures have provided valuable insights into the activation mechanisms and structural basis of GPCR heterodimerization (Figs. 3 and 4). The full-length structures of the $GABA_B$ receptors in both active and inactive states reveal that agonist binding to the $GABA_{B1}$ VFT induces its closure, bringing the stalk domain into close proximity, which then leads to the reorientation of the two 7TMs and the formation of an active TM6-TM6 interface, enabling the $GABA_{B2}$ subunit to bind and activate the G protein (Papasergi-Scott et al. 2020; Park et al. 2020; Shaye et al. 2020; Shen et al. 2021). Sequential conformational changes during the activation process are also observed in the structures of mGlu2-3 and mGlu2-4 heterodimers (Huang et al. 2024; Wang et al. 2023). Interestingly, the mGlu3 and mGlu4 protomers predominantly control the activation of the mGlu2-3 and mGlu2-4 heterodimers respectively. Furthermore, a similar Gi protein-binding pocket, composed of TM3, TM4, TM5, and the three ICLs of either $GABA_{B2}$ or the mGlu subunit, was observed without the outward movement of TM6, which is typically seen in other GPCR classes (Huang et al. 2024; Shen et al. 2021; Wang et al. 2023)(Fig. 4b). These findings suggest that the heterodimeric $GABA_B$, mGlu2-3, and mGlu2-4 receptors may share a common G protein activation mode, further confirming the asymmetric activation mechanism. Moreover, structural studies of heterodimers have revealed that their 7TMs adopt unique conformational states during activation. In the inactive "Roo" state, $GABA_B$ (Shen et al. 2021) and mGlu2-7 (Du et al. 2021) heterodimer show TM3-TM5 and TM5-TM5 interfaces, respectively. Recent studies suggest that mGlu2-3 and mGlu2-4 heterodimers may adopt two possible 7TM interaction interfaces, including TM3-TM4 and TM5-TM5, in the presence of an antagonist (Fig. 3). In contrast, in the active "Acc" state, $GABA_B$ receptor shows a TM6-TM6 interface, which is considered a hallmark of Class C GPCR activation. Of interest, mGlu2-3 and mGlu2-4 heterodimer exhibit an asymmetric TM6-TM6,7 interface, in contrast to the interfaces seen in $GABA_B$ and mGlu homodimers (Huang et al. 2024; Shen et al. 2021; Wang et al. 2023) (Fig. 4a).

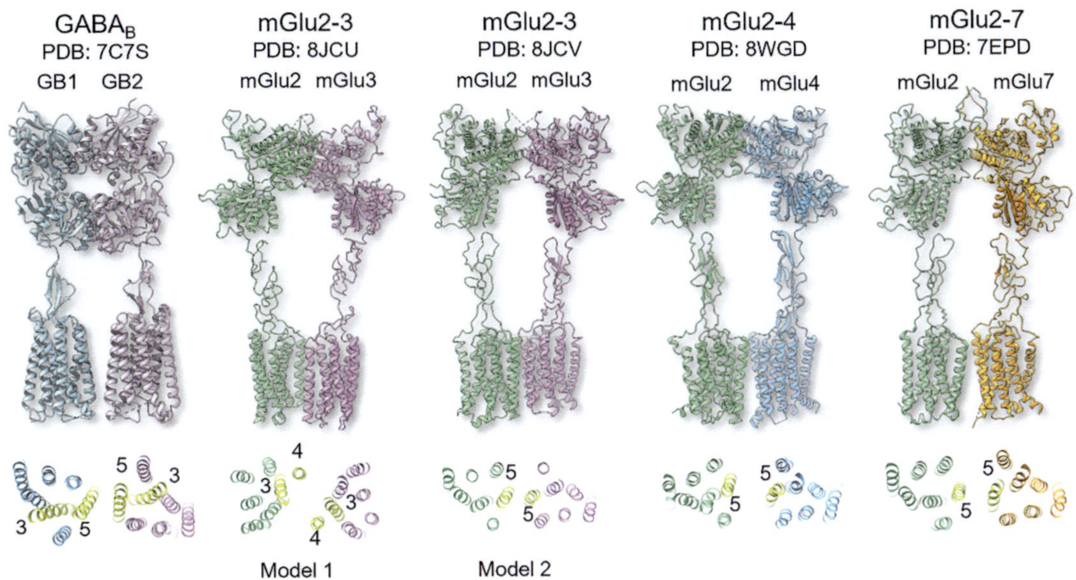

Fig. 3 Structures of GABA$_B$ and mGlu heterodimers in inactive state. Structures of the inactive conformation of GABA$_B$, mGlu2–3 (model 1 and 2), mGlu2–4, and mGlu2–7 receptors (PDB: 7C7S, 8JCU, 8JCV, 8WGD, and 7EPD) are shown in side view; interface of the TMDs of the inactive GABA$_B$, mGlu2–3 (model 1 and 2), mGlu2–4, and mGlu2–7 receptors (PDB: 7C7S, 8JCU, 8JCV, 8WGD, and 7EPD) are shown in top view. TMD helices at the interfaces are shown in yellow

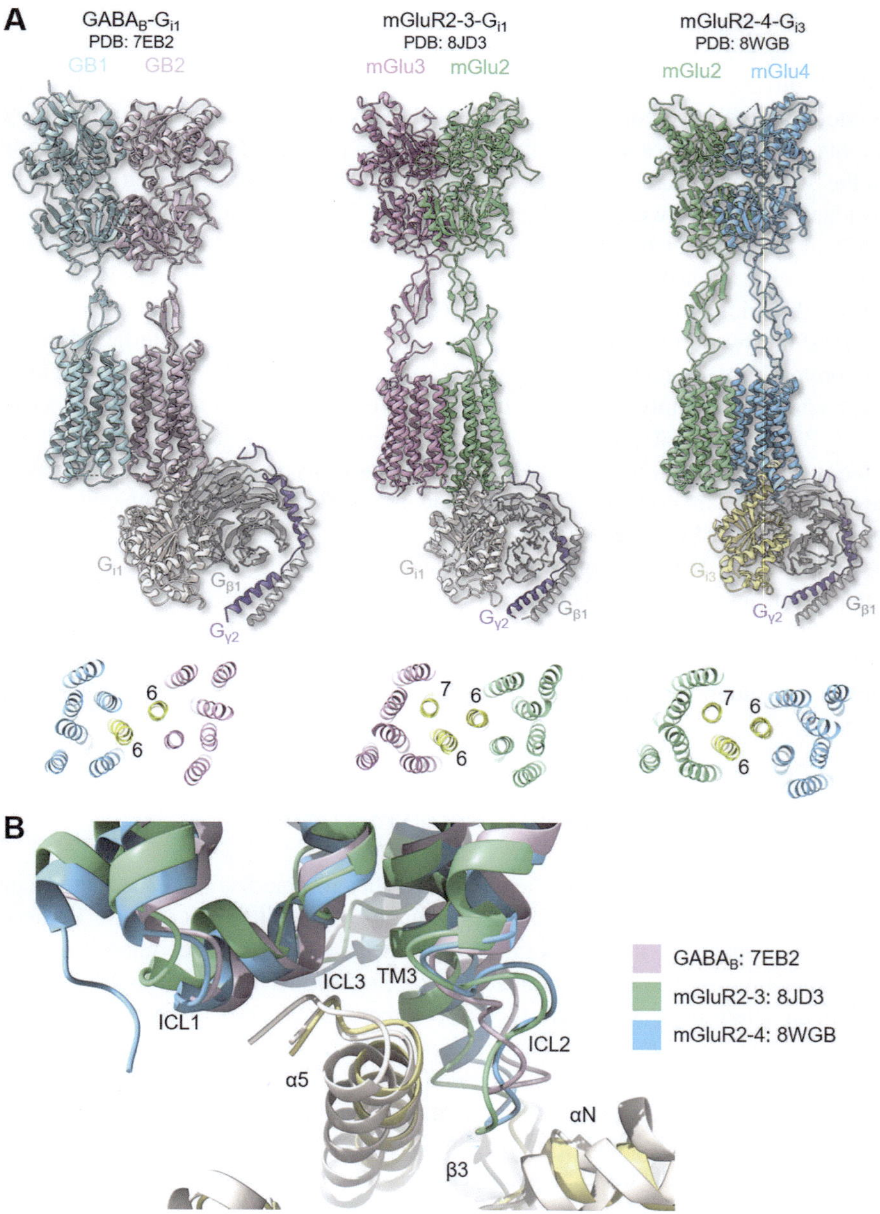

Fig. 4 Structures of $GABA_B$ and mGlu heterodimers in active state. (**a**) Structure of the active conformation of $GABA_B$, mGlu2–3, and mGlu2–4 receptors in complex with Gi (PDB: 7 EB2, 8JD3, and 8WGB) are shown in side view; interface of the TMDs of the active $GABA_B$, mGlu2–3, and mGluR2–4 receptors (PDB: 7 EB2, 8JD3, and 8WGB) are shown in top view. (**b**) Structural alignment of the G protein binding site of the structures shown in (**a**). TMD helices at the interfaces are shown in yellow

On the other hand, structural biology studies of dimerization in other GPCR families have also provided novel information into the assembly and activation of GPCR dimers. For instance, in the structure of class D fungal GPCR Ste2 homodimer with two copies of G proteins, the dimer interface is mainly formed by twenty-one specific residues within the N-terminal, TM1, TM2, and ECL1 regions of the Ste2 subunit across all the determined structures (Fig. 2c). An additional seven residues, located between the C-terminal end of TM7 and the cytoplasmic end of TM1 in the adjacent protomer, participate in contact formation only in the active conformation (Velazhahan et al. 2021; Velazhahan et al. 2022). Whereas in the fully active dimeric human apelin receptor (APJ) complexed with heterotrimeric G protein, the two protomers are arranged symmetrically with the interface formed by protein-protein interactions primarily at the tip of TM3 and ICL1. These interactions are mainly driven by limited hydrophobic and π-π interactions (Yue et al. 2022) (Fig. 2d). Moreover, pharmacological studies have shown that the monomeric APJ exhibits enhanced constitutive activity in G_i signaling and higher ligand efficacy in both the G protein and β-arrestin pathways compared to the homodimeric APJ (Yue et al. 2022).

Collectively, these findings may provide valuable insights into the allosteric interactions and activation mechanisms of potential GPCR heterodimers, extending beyond the Class C family. This could significantly advance our understanding of GPCR signaling, offering new perspectives on how receptor heterodimerization influences functional diversity and cellular responses across various biological systems.

3 Biased Signaling by Heterodimerization

Apart from obligate Class C heterodimers, heterodimerization can also occur between two different receptors from the same or different GPCR classes. In these cases, the concept of a "heterodimer" is defined as a complex composed of two functional units with specific pharmacological fingerprints distinct from those of the individual protomers. These are typically named as "receptor A-receptor B"; for example, the heterodimer formed by dopamine D1 and D2 receptors is written as the "D1-D2 receptor" (Pin et al. 2007). Heterodimeric GPCRs exhibit unique biochemical fingerprints, including distinct trafficking, ligand binding, and signaling profiles compared to their individual protomers. Several reviews have described the profiles of heterodimer-specific trafficking, recycling, and ligand binding in detail (Dale et al. 2022; Gomes et al. 2016). The allosteric interactions between protomers in heterodimers are thought to be the most likely mechanism behind these unique signaling properties. In this review, we focus on how heterodimerization drives biased signaling pathways, such as G protein coupling, β-arrestin recruitment, and internalization pathway (Table 1).

Table 1 Summary of the implication of biased signaling by heterodimerization in pathological level

Heterodimer	Biased signaling by heterodimerization	Clinical relevance	Heterodimer-targeting ligands	References
mGlu2-5-HT$_{2A}$	**G protein:** Heterodimerization enhances glutamate-elicited G_i signaling and reduces G_q signaling; **Internalization**: 5-HT$_{2A}$ agonist induces internalization of mGlu2	**Schizophrenia**	**MDL100907 – JNJ-42491293**[a]	Fribourg et al. (), Gonzalez-Maeso et al. (2008), Moreno et al. (2016), Poulie et al. (2020), Shah and Gonzalez-Maeso (2019) and Toneatti et al. (2020)
mGlu1-A1	**G protein:** Activation of A1 potentiates mGlu1-mediated G_q signaling, while activation of mGlu1 suppresses A1-mediated G_i responses	**Schizophrenia**	**ND**	Leon-Navarro et al. (2019)
mGlu5-A$_{2A}$	**G protein:** The activation of mGlu5 requires activation of A_{2A} by endogenous adenosine and vice versa; Activation of mGlu5 enhances A_{2A} mediated G_s-cAMP pathway	**PD** **Schizophrenia** **Addiction** **Autism**	**ND**	Bogenpohl et al. (2012), Borroto-Escuela et al. (2018a), Ferre et al. (2002), Nishi et al. (2003), Rodrigues et al. (2005), Sun et al. (2021) and Temido-Ferreira et al. (2020)
mGlu5-μ OR	**Internalization:** mGlu5 antagonist decreases μOR agonist-mediated internalization of μOR	**Chronic pain** **Addiction**	**MMG22**[a]	Gabra et al. (2008), Peterson et al. (2017) and Schroder et al. (2009)
mGlu5-D1	**G protein**: mGlu5-D1 couples to G_q protein and generates an atypical D1 receptor-dependent Ca^{2+} response	**PD**	**ND**	Sebastianutto et al. (2020)
D1-D2	**G protein:** D1-D2 transduces signals through Gq, while monomeric D1 and D2 transduce signals through G_s and $G_{i/o}$ respectively	**Schizophrenia** **PD** **Depression** **Addiction** **Autism**	SKF83959[b]	DelaCuesta-Barrutia et al. (2020), Hasbi et al. (2020), Lee et al. (2004), Misganaw (2021) and Rashid et al. (2007)
D1-D3	**G protein**: D3 enhances the D1 dependent AC signaling **β-arrestin:** Heterodimerization leads to the recruitment of β-arrestin-1 and activation of MAPK	**Addiction** **Schizophrenia** **PD** **L-DOPA-induced dyskinesia (LID)**	ND	Caniceiro et al. (2022), Fiorentini et al. (2010), Guitart et al. (2019), Lanza et al. (2018) and Misganaw (2021)

(continued)

Table 1 (continued)

Heterodimer	Biased signaling by heterodimerization	Clinical relevance	Heterodimer-targeting ligands	References
D2-D3	**G protein:** D3 modulates the anti-Parkinson properties of agents acting on D2 through negative allosteric crosstalk	**Schizophrenia** **PD** **Autism** **ADHD**	ND	Caniceiro et al. (2022), DelaCuesta-Barrutia et al. (2020), Maggio and Millan (2010) and Maggio et al. (2015)
D2-A_{2A}	**G protein:** Activation of A_{2A} leads to PLC signaling; **β-arrestin:** Activation of D2 leads to β-arrestin2-dependent internalization	**PD** **Schizophrenia** **Addiction**	Compound 26[a]; XCC-PPHT[a]	Borroto-Escuela et al. (2011), Borroto-Escuela et al. (2018b), Ferre et al. (2018), Misganaw (2021), Pulido et al. (2022) and Soriano et al. (2009)
A1-P2Y1	**G protein:** P2Y1 stimulation impairs the potency of A1 coupling to G_i while A1 enhances P2Y1 coupling to G_q signaling	**Brain damage; Neurodegenerative diseases**	ND	Hashimoto et al. (2001), Nakata et al. (2005), Tonazzini et al. (2007), Yoshioka et al. (2002) and Yoshioka et al. (2001)
A1-D1	**G protein:** Adenosine inhibits D1R-mediated accumulation of cAMP in heterodimer	**PD** **Schizophrenia** **Addiction** **Spinal cord injury**	Compound 1 (naphthylxanthine derivative)—SKF38393[a]	Ferre et al. (1997), Gines et al. (2000), Misganaw (2021), Rivera-Oliver et al. (2019), Shen et al. (2013), Toda et al. (2003) and Torvinen et al. (2002)
A_{2A}-CB1	**G protein:** A_{2A} activation allows CB1 to couple effective G_i protein	**PD** **Cannabinoid use disorder (CUD)**	ND	Carriba et al. (2007), Cerri et al. (2014), Chiodi et al. (2016), Ferre et al. (2023a) and Kofalvi et al. (2020)
AT1-SCT	**G protein:** Interaction leads to a diminished cAMP response to SCT stimulation and alter intracellular Ca^{2+} signaling to regulate aldosterone production	**Water intake**	ND	Bai et al. (2019), Lee et al. (2014), Lee et al. (2010) and Ng and Chow (2015)
MT1-GPR50	**G protein and β-arrestin:** GPR50 inhibits MT1's G_q coupling and β-arrestin1 binding	**Bipolar affective disorder** **Major depressive disorder**	ND	Clement et al. (2018), Jockers et al. (2008), Levoye et al. (2006a, b), and Tse and Wong (2021)

GHS_{1a}-D2	**G protein:** GHS_{1a} alters $G_{i/o}$ signaling of D2 to $G_{\beta\gamma}$ mediated PLC-IP3	**Eating disorders (anorexia or obesity)**	ND	Kern et al. (2012), Misganaw (2021), Schellekens et al. (2013) and Vucetic and Reyes (2010)
D2–$5HT_{2A}$	**G protein:** D2 increases the efficacy of DOI to activate the $G_{q/11}$ signaling pathway of 5-HT_{2A} and reduces Gi/o signaling of itself	**Schizophrenia** **Autism**	ND	Borroto-Escuela et al. (2010), DelaCuesta-Barrutia et al. (2020), Lukasiewicz et al. (2010), Misganaw (2021) and Werkman et al. (2006)
D2–$5HT_{1A}$	**G protein:** Cotreatment of clozapine and 8-OH-DPAT leads to $G_{q/11}$-dependent activation of $ERK_{1/2}$	**Schizophrenia**	scFvD2–5-HT_{1A} [a] (antibody)	Kowalik et al. (2022), Lukasiewicz et al. (2016), Szlachta et al. (2018) and Werkman et al. (2006)
D2-CB1	**G protein:** Coactivation of D2-CB1 induces G_s signaling while D2 or CB1 alone couples to $G_{i/o}$ protein **Internalization:** Internalization of D2-CB1 requires the coactivation of both two receptor	**Schizophrenia** **Autism** **PD** **Addiction**	SR141617A-PPHT[a]	Bagher et al. (2016), Bagher et al. (2020), Bonaventura et al. (2014), DelaCuesta-Barrutia et al. (2020), Grant et al. (2019), Jarrahian et al. (2004), Kearn et al. (2005), Martin et al. (2008), Misganaw (2021) and Pickel et al. (2006)
D1-H3	**G protein:** Both D1 and H3 induce $G\alpha_{i/o}$ signaling, MAPK pathway, and $ERK_{1/2}$ phosphorylation by heterodimerization, while D1 alone couples to G_s protein and H3 alone is unable to mediate MAPK pathway	**ADHD** **Schizophrenia** **Cocaine addiction**	ND	Ferrada et al. (2009), Kononoff Vanhanen et al. (2016), Misganaw (2021), Moreno et al. (2011) and Moreno et al. (2014b)
D2-TA1	**G protein:** The D2 antagonist haloperidol enhances Gs signaling of TA1	**Schizophrenia** **Anxiety**	ND	Bradaia et al. (2009), de la Mora et al. (2016), Espinoza et al. (2011) and Lindemann et al. (2008)
D2-SST5	**G protein:** D2 agonist promotes the G protein coupling downstream of SST5, while simultaneous agonist treatments results in G_i signaling	**Pituitary tumor** **Depression**	BIM-23A760[b] BIM-23A387[b]	Faron-Gorecka et al. (2013), Jaquet et al. (2005), Rocheville et al. (2000) and Szafran-Pilch et al. (2017)

(continued)

Table 1 (continued)

Heterodimer	Biased signaling by heterodimerization	Clinical relevance	Heterodimer-targeting ligands	References
D2-NTS1	**G protein:** D2 reduces NTS1-mediated Ca^{2+} response that can be abolished by D_2 antagonists The bivalent ligand 3b,c induces a distinct Gs-cAMP pathway of D_2-NTS1 **Internalization and β-arrestin:** The bivalent ligand containing NT (8–13) promotes NTS1 to recruit β-arrestin-2 at the D_2-NTS1coexpressing cells	**PD** **Schizophrenia**	CS148[a]; Eticlopride-NT(8–13)[a]; 2-methoxyphenylpiperazine-NT(8–13)[a]; Aminoindane -NT(8–13)[a]	Ferraro et al. (2008), Hubner et al. (2016), Koschatzky et al. (2011), Plach et al. (2019) and Tanganelli et al. (2012)
D2-OT	**G protein:** Heterodimerization reduces $G_{i/o}$-PKA pathway of D2 and enhances the CREB, MAPK, and G_q-PLC signaling of OT	**Anxiety** **Autism** **Fear**	ND	de la Mora et al. (2016), DelaCuesta-Barrutia et al. (2020) and Romero-Fernandez et al. (2013)
D2-D5	**G protein:** D2-D5 induces Gq signaling, while D2 and D5 are coupled to Gi/o and Gs respectively	**Depression**	ND	Centonze et al. (2003), O'Dowd et al. (2013) and So et al. (2009)
D2-AT1	**G protein:** Heterodimerization doesn't affect G_i signaling of D2 receptors but attenuate the G_q coupling of AT1	**Hypertension**	ND	Martinez-Pinilla et al. (2015)
δOR-μOR	**G protein:** Heterodimerization switches from $G_{i/o}$ to either G_z or G_q signaling **Internalization and β-arrestin:** δOR-μOR couples to β-arrestin2 to co-internalization	**Pain regulation**	D24M[a]; CYM51010[b]; MDAN21[a]	Bardoni et al. (2014), Erbs et al. (2015), Gomes et al. (2013), Gupta et al. (2010), Kabli et al. (2014), Olson et al. (2018), Portoghese et al. (2017), Wang et al. (2010)
δOR-κOR	**Internalization and β-arrestin:** Heterodimerization downregulates the δOR internalization	**Pain regulation**	6′-GNTI[b] KDAN-18[a] KDN-21[a]	Ansonoff et al. (2010), Chakrabarti et al. (2010), Daniels et al. (2005), Waldhoer et al. (2005) and Xie et al. (2005)

δOR-SNSR4	**G protein:** δOR-SNSR4 elicits Gq signaling and attenuates G_i signaling	**Pain regulation**	BAM22[a]	Breit et al. (2006)
μOR-GRPR	**G protein:** Morphine cross-activates GRPR-G_q signaling through μOR_{1D} **Internalization:** The morphine triggers internalization of both GRPR and μOR_{1D}, whereas GRP specifically triggers GRPR internalization	**Analgesia** **Itch**	ND	Benecke et al. (2013), Liu et al. (2011) and Wang et al. (2021b)
μOR-NK1	**Internalization and β-arrestin:** Protomer-selective agonists induce β-arrestin2 recruitment and enhance the internalization of μOR-NK1	**Pain regulation**	Fentanyl-L732138[a] TY027[b] AA3266[a] AA3052[a]	Aicher et al. (2000), Giri et al. (2015), Kowalczyk et al. (2016), Largent-Milnes et al. (2013), Matalinska et al. (2020), Pfeiffer et al. (2003), Vardanyan et al. (2011) and Yamamoto et al. (2007)
δOR-CB1	**G protein:** δOR reduces the Gi activity of CB1 **Internalization and β-arrestin:** Heterodimerization increases PLC-dependent β-arrestin2 recruitment and CB1 desensitization	**Pain regulation**	ND	Bushlin et al. (2012), Gomes et al. (2016), Gupta et al. (2024), Pol et al. (2006), Rios et al. (2006), Rozenfeld et al. (2012) and Shapira et al. (1998)
A_{2A}-A1	**G protein:** Under high concentrations of adenosine, A_{2A} receptor-induced Gs activation blocks A1-mediated G_i function	**Drug tolerance** **PD**	ND	Borroto-Escuela and Fuxe (2019a), Ciruela et al. (2006) and Ferre et al. (2023b)
$5HT_{2C}$-MT2	**G protein:** $5HT_{2C}$-MT2 enhances the 5-HT-mediated G_q-PLC signaling and induces melatonin-dependent transactivation of the $5\text{-}HT_{2C}$	**Depression** **Anxiety**	ND	Gerbier et al. (2021), Kamal et al. (2015) and Racagni et al. (2011)
β_1A-β_2A	**G protein**: The β_1A greatly suppresses agonist-independent G_i activity of coexisting β_2A **β-arrestin:** Heterodimerization inhibits agonist-induced β_2A internalization and $ERK_{1/2}$-MAPK pathway	**Cardiac contractility**	ND	Lavoie et al. (2002), Mercier et al. (2002) and Zhu et al. (2005)

(continued)

Table 1 (continued)

Heterodimer	Biased signaling by heterodimerization	Clinical relevance	Heterodimer-targeting ligands	References
β_2A-AT1	**G protein**: β_2A blockers interferes with AT_1-G_q coupling, while AT_1 antagonists interferes with β_2A-G_s coupling **β-arrestin:** Heterodimerization enhances β-arrestin coupling of β_2A	**Heart failure (HF)**	ND	Barki-Harrington et al. (2003), Toth et al. (2017) and Toth et al. (2012)
β_2A-EP1	**G protein**: EP1 activation prevents the β_{2A} from coupling to G_s	**Asthma**	ND	McGraw et al. (2006)
β_2A-B2	**G protein**: B2 agonist bradykinin induces transactivation of Gs-coupled pathways of B2 in presence of β_2A	**Thrombus** **Acute coronary syndrome**	ND	Aspelin et al. (2014), Haack et al. (2010)
α_{2C}A-AT1	**G protein:** Costimulation with Ang II and NEA results in G_s-cAMP-PKA signaling	**Cardiovascular diseases** **Hypertension** **HF**	ND	Bellot et al. (2015), Berg (2013) and Talaia et al. (2006)
$\alpha_{1A/B}$A-CXCR4	**G protein:** CXCR4 activation enhances α_{1B}A-induced G_q signaling **β-arrestin:** Activation of α_{1B}A leads to recruitment of β-arrestin2 to CXCR4	**Blood pressure** **Vasoreactivity** **Cancer metastases** **Autoimmune pathologies**	ND	Bach 4th et al. (2014), Gao et al. (2018a, b), Gao and Majetschak (2023) and Tripathi et al. (2015)
ETA-ETB	**G protein:** Heterodimerization precedes a sustained Gq-dependent intracellular Ca^{2+} response, while ETA and ETB regulate transient intracellular and extracellular Ca^{2+} response	**Chronic heart failure (CHF)**	ND	Evans and Walker (2008a, b), Gregan et al. (2004) and Kapsokalyvas et al. (2014)
AT1-CB1	**G protein:** Heterodimerization enables AT1 couple to G_i signaling to activate the ERK pathway rather than G_q signaling	**PD** **Anti-fibrotic** **Hypertension**	ND	Haspula and Clark (2017), Labandeira-Garcia et al. (2024) and Rozenfeld et al. (2011)

AT2-CB1	**G protein:** Heterodimerization enhances G_i-signaling **β-Arrestin:** Heterodimerization increases recruitment of β-arrestin upon co-activation	**PD**	ND	Rivas-Santisteban et al. (2023)
AT2-B2	**G protein and β-arrestin:** With bradykinin treated, Heterodimerization between AT2 and B2 enables the former to recruit G_q, G-protein kinase 2 and β-arrestin2; and enable the latter to couple to G_z	**Hypertension**	ND	Abadir et al. (2006), Gironacci et al. (2004), Johnstone et al. (2022) and Koid et al. (2014)
PAR1-PAR2	**G protein**: The thrombin-cleaved PAR1 transactivates PAR2-dependent $G\alpha_i$/Rac signaling rather than PAR1-mediated G_q and $G_{12/13}$ signaling **β-Arrestin and internalization:** PAR1-PAR2 elicits β-arrestins recruitment and constitutive co-internalization by thrombin stimulation	**Inflammatory diseases** **Sepsis** **Thrombosis**	ND	Kaneider et al. (2007), Lin et al. (2013), Lin and Trejo (2013), McEachron et al. (2010), O'Brien et al. (2000) and Sevigny et al. (2011)
PAR3-PAR4	**G protein**: PAR3 downregulates PAR4-mediated G_q-Ca^{2+} response and PKC activation	**Thrombosis**	ND	Arachiche et al. (2013), Bah et al. (2007) and Nakanishi-Matsui et al. (2000)
PAR1-PAR3	**G protein:** PAR3 enhances the activity of PAR1 to couple to G_{13}	**Vascular inflammation**	ND	Lin et al. (2013), Madhusudhan et al. (2012) and McLaughlin et al. (2007)
CXCR4-CXCR7	**G protein**: CXCR7 impairs CXCR4-promoted G_i activation and Ca^{2+} responses **β-arrestin**: Heterodimerization results in constitutive recruitment of β-arrestin2	**Colorectal cancer**	ND	Decaillot et al. (2011), Khare et al. (2021), Levoye et al. (2009), Puchert and Engele (2014), Sierro et al. (2007) and Wang et al. (2011)
ChemR23-CCR7	**G protein**: CCR7 reduces G_i signaling of ChemR23	**Atherosclerosis**	ND	de Poorter et al. (2013), van der Vorst et al. (2019)
ChemR23-CXCR4	**G protein**: CCR4 reduces G_i signaling of ChemR23	**Inflammatory and metabolic disorders**	ND	de Poorter et al. (2013), Sozzani et al. (2010)

(continued)

Table 1 (continued)

Heterodimer	Biased signaling by heterodimerization	Clinical relevance	Heterodimer-targeting ligands	References
AT1-CCR2	**G protein:** Activated AT1 inhibits the CCR2-G_i coupling **β-arrestin:** Heterodimerization enhances β-arrestin2 recruitment upon co-stimulation	**Chronic kidney disease** **Anti-inflammatory** **Hypertensive conditions**	ND	Ayoub et al. (2015), Dai et al. (2007)
μOR-CCR5	**G protein:** CCR5 agonist reduces μOR -mediated G-protein activation and vice versa **Internalization:** μOR internalization is induced by μOR agonists rather than CCR5 agonists and vice versa	**Chronic pain** **HIV infection** **AIDS** **Inflammatory arthritis pain**	Naltrexone-Maraviroc[a] MCC22[a] VZMC001[a]; VZMC013[a]	Akgun et al. (2015), Arnatt et al. (2016), Cataldo et al. (2019), Dutta et al. (2018), El-Hage et al. (2013), Huang et al. (2021), Kim et al. (2018), Suzuki et al. (2002), Szabo et al. (2002), Yuan et al. (2013) and Yuan et al. (2012)
CCR2-CCR5	**G protein:** CCR2–CCR5 recruits specifically $G_{q/11}$	**HIV infection** **PDAC** **Pulmonary arterial hypertension (PAH)**	ND	Abid et al. (2019), Fantuzzi et al. (2019), Mellado et al. (2001), Vazquez-Salat et al. (2007) and Wang et al. (2022)
CCR2-CXCR4	**G protein:** The activation of CCR2 or CXCR4 inhibits G protein signaling of the other protomer	**HIV infection** **Inflammatory**	ND	Armando et al. (2014), Rodriguez-Frade et al. (2004), See et al. (2011), Sohy et al. (2007) and Sohy et al. (2009)
CCR5-CXCR4	**G protein:** CCR5-CXCR4 couples to $G_{q/11}$ and elicit Ca^{2+}response	**HIV infection** **Autoimmune diseases**	ND	Di Marino et al. (2023), Hammad et al. (2010), Martinez-Munoz et al. (2014), Mellado et al. (2001), Molon et al. (2005) and Salanga et al. (2009)
GPR55-CB2	**G protein:** Activation of GPR55 inhibits CB2-G_i signaling	**Cancer** **Multiple sclerosis (MS)** **PD** **Inflammatory**	ND	Balenga et al. (2014), Martinez-Pinilla et al. (2016), Martinez-Pinilla et al. (2020), Menendez-Perez et al. (2024) and Moreno et al. (2014a)

MT1-MT2	**G protein:** MT1-MT2 induces G_q-dependent PLC/PKC pathway	**Sleep disorders** **Depression** **Photoreceptor function**	ND	Ayoub et al. (2004), Baba et al. (2013) and Tse and Wong (2021)
μOR-GPR139	**G protein:** GPR139 reduces the G_o signaling of μOR **β-arrestin:** GPR139 promotes μOR to recruit β-arrestin2	**Pain regulation**	ND	Wang et al. (2019), Zhang et al. (2020)
μOR-V1B	**β-arrestin:** Arginine-vasopressin (AVP) enhances morphine-induced AC superactivation of μOR-V1B via β-arrestin 2 and ERK pathways	**Pain regulation** **Morphine tolerance**	ND	Koshimizu et al. (2018), Zhang et al. (2020)
μOR-CCKB	**G protein:** Heterodimerization reduces inhibition of G_i signaling by agonist-activated μOR	**Pain regulation**	ND	Yang et al. (2018), Zhang et al. (2020)
$5HT_{1A}$-$5HT_{2A}$	**G protein:** 5-HT_{2A} allosterically inhibits 5-HT_{1A} to bind G_i protein	**Depression**	ND	Amargos-Bosch et al. (2004), Barnes et al. (2021), Butini et al. (2010), Miskiewicz et al. (2018), Mitroshina et al. (2023) and Szlachta et al. (2018)
$5HT_{2A}$-$5HT_{2B}$	**G protein:** 5-HT_{2B} makes 5-HT_{2A} capable of binding 5-HT but unable to activate G_q signaling	**Addiction** **Depression**	ND	Anastasio et al. (2015), Barnes et al. (2021), Carr et al. (2002), Mitroshina et al. (2023) and Moutkine et al. (2017)
$5HT_{2A}$-$5HT_{2C}$	**G protein:** 5-HT_{2C} makes 5-HT_{2A} capable of binding 5-HT but unable to activate G_q signaling	**Anxiety** **Depression** **Addiction**	ND	Anastasio et al. (2015), Barnes et al. (2021), Chen et al. (2023b), Felsing et al. (2018), Mitroshina et al. (2023), Moutkine et al. (2017), Muller and Homberg (2015), Pin et al. (2007) and Price et al. (2019)
$5HT_{1A}$-$5HT_7$	**G protein:** Heterodimerization downregulates 5-HT_{1A} to activate Gi, while leaving 5-HT_7-mediated signaling unaffected **β-arrestin:** Heterodimerization induces co-internalization of 5-HT_{1A} and 5-HT_7 upon serotonin treatment	**Depression** **Anxiety** **Schizophrenia** **Addiction**	ND	Barnes et al. (2021), Barnes and Sharp (1999), Li et al. (2018), Mitroshina et al. (2023), Naumenko et al. (2014) and Renner et al. (2012)

(continued)

Table 1 (continued)

Heterodimer	Biased signaling by heterodimerization	Clinical relevance	Heterodimer-targeting ligands	References
$5HT_{2A}$-OT	**G protein:** Heterodimerization attenuates G_q-dependent signaling of both receptors, which cannot be recovered by their antagonists **Internalization:** The OT increases the basal internalization of the $5\text{-}HT_{2A}$	**Anxiety** **Depression** **Autism** **Cognition**	ND	Chruscicka et al. (2019), DelaCuesta-Barrutia et al. (2020), Mottolese et al. (2014) and Yoshida et al. (2009)
$5HT_{2C}$-OT	**G protein:** $5\text{-}HT_{2C}$ reduces OT-mediated G_q signaling **Internalization:** Heterodimerization increases the basal internalization of $5\text{-}HT_{2C}$ and OT significantly	**Anxiety** **Depression** **Autism**	ND	Chruscicka et al. (2021), Mottolese et al. (2014) and Yoshida et al. (2009)
AT1-AT2	**G protein:** AT2 inhibits AT1 $G_{i/o}$ and $G_{q/11}$ signaling **β-arrestin:** AT2 may cross-inhibit AT1 internalization	**PD**	ND	AbdAlla et al. (2001), Ferrao et al. (2012), Gironacci and Bruna-Haupt (2024) and Rivas-Santisteban et al. (2020)

PD Parkinson's disease, *ADHD* Attention deficit and hyperactive disorder, *AIDS* Acquired immune deficiency syndrome, *PDAC* Pancreatic ductal *adenocarcinoma MAPK* Mitogen-activated protein kinase, *PLC* Phospholipase C, *cAMP* Cyclic adenosine monophosphate, *IP3* Inositol triphosphate, *ERK* Extracellular signal-regulated kinases, *CREB* cAMP response element binding protein, *PKA* Protein kinase A, *D1* Dopamine D1 receptor, *D2* Dopamine D2 receptor, *D3* Dopamine D3 receptor, *D5* Dopamine D5 receptor, A_{2A} Adenosine receptor A2a, *A1* Adenosine receptor A1, *P2Y1* P2Y purinoceptor 1, *CB1* Cannabinoid receptor 1, *CB2* Cannabinoid receptor 2, *AT1* Type-1 angiotensin II receptor, *AT2* Type-2 angiotensin II receptor, *SCT* Secretin receptor, *MT1* Melatonin receptor type 1A, *MT2* Melatonin receptor type 1B, *GPR50* G protein-coupled receptor 50, $GHSR_{1a}$ Growth hormone secretagogue receptor 1a, $5\text{-}HT_{1A}$ 5-hydroxytryptamine receptor 1A, $5\text{-}HT_{2A}$ 5-hydroxytryptamine receptor 2A, $5\text{-}HT_{2B}$ 5-hydroxytryptamine receptor 2B, $5\text{-}HT_{2C}$ 5-hydroxytryptamine receptor 2C, $5\text{-}HT_7$ 5-hydroxytryptamine receptor 7, *H3* Histamine H3 receptor, *TA1* Trace amine-associated receptor 1, *SST5* Somatostatin receptor type 5, *NTS1* Neurotensin receptor type 1, *OT* Oxytocin receptor, *δOR* Delta-type opioid receptor, *μOR* Mu-type opioid receptor, *κOR* Kappa-type opioid receptor, *SNSR4* Sensory neuron-specific receptor 4, *GRPR* Gastrin-releasing peptide *receptor NK1* Substance-P receptor, $\beta_1 A$ Beta-1 adrenergic receptor, $\beta_2 A$ Beta-2 adrenergic receptor, *EP1* Prostaglandin E2 receptor EP1 subtype, *B2* B2 bradykinin receptor, $\alpha_{1A}A$ Alpha-1A adrenergic receptor, $\alpha_{1B}A$ Alpha-1A adrenergic receptor, $\alpha_{2C}A$ Alpha-2C adrenergic receptor, *CXCR4* C-X-C chemokine receptor type 4, *CXCR7* Atypical chemokine receptor 3, *ETA* Endothelin-1 receptor, *ETB* Endothelin receptor type B, *PAR1* Proteinase-activated receptor 1, *PAR2* Proteinase-activated receptor 2, *PAR3* Proteinase-activated receptor 3, *PAR4* Proteinase-activated receptor 4, *ChemR23* Chemerin-like receptor 1, *CCR2* C-C chemokine receptor type 2, *CCR5* C-C chemokine receptor type 5, *CCR7* C-C chemokine receptor type 7, *GPR55* G-protein coupled receptor 55, *GPR139* Probable G-protein coupled receptor 139, *V1B* Vasopressin V1b receptor, *CCKB* Gastrin/cholecystokinin type B receptor, *mGlu1* Metabotropic glutamate receptor 1, *mGlu2* Metabotropic glutamate receptor 2, *mGlu5* Metabotropic glutamate receptor 5

[a]Bivalent ligand

[b]Heterodimer-selective ligand

4 G Protein Signaling

Heterodimerization of GPCRs enables the coupling of various G proteins ($G\alpha_i$, $G\alpha_s$, $G\alpha_q$, $G\alpha_{12/13}$) and their associated effector pathways. For example, the dopamine receptors D1 and D2 activate G_s and $G_{i/o}$ proteins, respectively. However, the well-known D1-D2 heterodimer exhibits unique G_q signaling, enhancing intracellular Ca^{2+} levels and promoting the expression of brain-derived neurotrophic factor (BDNF) in response to co-stimulation of both receptors. This effect can be blocked by antagonists of either receptor (Hasbi et al. 2009). A similar switch from $G_{i/o}$ to G_q signaling has been observed in the D2-5-HT_{1A} heterodimer, leading to the activation of $ERK_{1/2}$. In the case of the D2-CB1 heterodimer, co-activation of both receptors shifts G protein signaling from $G_{i/o}$ to G_s, resulting in biased signaling despite both protomers being $G_{i/o}$-dependent. An atypical G_s-cAMP signaling pathway has also been identified in the AT1-α_{2c}AR heterodimer, which modulates norepinephrine secretion upon co-treatment with both agonists (Bellot et al. 2015). Additionally, melatonin induces MT1-MT2 heterodimer-specific phospholipase C and protein kinase C (PLC/PKC) pathway (Baba et al. 2013) and transactivates 5-HT_{2C}-dependent PLC-G_q signaling downstream of the MT2-5-HT_{2C} heterodimer (Kamal et al. 2015).

Heterodimeric receptors also play a crucial role in modulating downstream G protein signaling pathways. In the D2-A_{2A} heterodimer, agonists for either the D2 or A_{2A} receptor reduce the activated signaling induced by the agonist of the other protomer (Borroto-Escuela et al. 2011). In δOR-μOR heterodimer, the activation of one protomer-dependent signaling is enhanced in the presence of an agonist for the other protomer. Interestingly, this heterodimer couples to G_z protein, while homomeric δOR and μOR couple to $G_{i/o}$ proteins. Moreover, in the presence of the μOR agonist DAMGO, the intracellular PLC-Ca^{2+} pathway is activated in heterodimer-expressing GH3 cells, instead of $G_{i/o}$ signaling (Baba et al. 2013). In the δOR-SNSR4 heterodimer, selective agonists for δOR and SNSR4 activate $G_{i/o}$ and G_q signaling, respectively. The bivalent agonist BAM22, which targets both receptors, preferentially favors the SNSR4-induced G_q signaling over δOR-induced $G_{i/o}$ signaling. This phenomenon is also observed when combining selective ligands for δOR and SNSR4. Additionally, BAM22-mediated G_q signaling is inhibited by the δOR antagonist naltrexone, indicating a transinhibition mechanism through δOR within the complex (Breit et al. 2006). During the heterodimerization of the μOR isoform μOR_{1D} and the gastrin-releasing peptide receptor (GRPR), the PLC-Ca^{2+} signaling is observed upon activation by morphine or GRP. Notably, μOR_{1D}-dependent calcium responses are only detected in co-expressed μOR_{1D}-GRP cells. Furthermore, the use of GRPR or μOR_{1D} antagonists effectively blocks the calcium response induced by morphine or GRP, respectively (Liu et al. 2011). In the heterodimerization of chemokine receptors CXCR4 and CXCR7, co-expression of CXCR7 triggers a Ca^{2+} response and disrupts the interaction between CXCR4 and G_i protein (Levoye et al. 2009).

5 β-Arrestin and Internalization Pathway

Heterodimerization of GPCRs can result in selective β-arrestin pathways as well. For example, the δOR-μOR heterodimer constitutively regulates the β-arrestin2-dependent $ERK_{1/2}$ pathway, which can be disrupted by co-treatment with a μOR agonist and a δOR antagonist (Rozenfeld and Devi 2007). Neither individual δOR nor μOR protomers can internalize independently of the other in the heterodimer. Selective agonists such as DAMGO, deltorphin II, and methadone enhance β-arrestin recruitment and induce heterodimer-specific internalization. Among these, methadone also promotes the degradation of the δOR-μOR heterodimer (Chen et al. 2022; Guitart et al. 2014). Another example is the proteinase-activated receptor (PAR) heterodimer, PAR1-PAR2. Thrombin cleaves the N-terminal of PAR1, which functions as an agonist for both PAR1 and PAR2. PAR1 undergoes thrombin-stimulated internalization, while PAR2 does not. Additionally, activation of PAR1 fails to sustain β-arrestin association, whereas activation of PAR2 recruits β-arrestin2, inducing substantial internalization into endocytic vesicles (Lin and Trejo 2013). The formation of the PAR1-PAR2 heterodimer displays constitutive internalization driven by PAR1 monomer trafficking. During thrombin stimulation, PAR1-PAR2 heterodimers recruit β-arrestin2 and co-internalize into endosomes, contributing to β-arrestin2-mediated $ERK_{1/2}$ activation in the cytoplasm (Lin and Trejo 2013).

On the other hand, allosteric interactions between the two protomers within a heterodimer can shift signaling from G protein-dependent pathways to β-arrestin-dependent signaling. For instance, in the D1-D3 heterodimer, coactivation of D1 and D3 downregulates adenylyl cyclase signaling, leading to β-arrestin1 recruitment, which in turn switches G protein-dependent MAPK signaling to a G protein-independent pathway. This effect is blocked by either D1 or D3 antagonists (Guitart et al. 2014). The $μOR_{1D}$-GRPR heterodimer exhibits unique internalization properties, that is, agonist morphine induces internalization of both $μOR_{1D}$ and GRPR in cells co-expressing these receptors, whereas agonist GRP does not induce $μOR_{1D}$ internalization in the same context (Liu et al. 2011). Similarly, the interaction of the D2-A_{2A} heterodimer results in a switch from $G_{i/o}$ signaling to a β-arrestin-dependent internalization process in the presence of a D2 agonist (Ferre et al. 2018). The AT1-AT2 heterodimer also modulates β-arrestin recruitment and receptor trafficking dynamics. Under normal physiological conditions, agonists bind to AT1 on the plasma membrane, triggering receptor activation. Upon activation, AT1 recruits β-arrestin2, forming a stable complex and further endocytoses into vesicles (Porrello et al. 2011; Rivas-Santisteban et al. 2020). In contrast to AT1 monomers, the AT1-AT2 heterodimer, despite being able to interact with β-arrestin2 post-activation, exhibits a reduced propensity for internalization following ligand activation. This suggests a potential cross-inhibitory mechanism, where the formation of the heterodimer may attenuate the internalization process of AT1, highlighting the complex interplay between these receptors in regulating cellular signaling (Porrello et al. 2011).

6 Heterodimers Are the Potential Therapy Target

6.1 mGlu2-5-HT_{2A} Heterodimer in Schizophrenia

The metabotropic glutamate type 2 (mGlu2) and serotonin type 2A (5-HT_{2A}) receptors are critical therapeutic targets for schizophrenia. Using co-immunoprecipitation (Co-IP), BRET, and FRET technologies, the mGlu2-5-HT_{2A} heterodimer was first identified in primary cortical neurons, transfected HEK293 cells, and tissue samples from mouse and human brains (Gonzalez-Maeso et al. 2008). Additionally, the 5-HT_{2A} receptor modulates the localization and trafficking of the mGlu2 receptor through heteromerization in HEK293 cells. Co-expression of 5-HT_{2A} favors the intracellular localization of mGlu2 in the frontal cortex of mice. Interestingly, the 5-HT_{2A} inverse agonist clozapine downregulated the levels of mGlu2 by disrupting the formation of the mGlu2-5-HT_{2A} heterodimer (Toneatti et al. 2020). The transmembrane regions TM4/5 of mGlu2 and TM4 of 5-HT_{2A} are required for the physical interaction between the two receptors (Gonzalez-Maeso et al. 2008; Moreno et al. 2016; Shah et al. 2020). Competitive binding studies revealed that the affinities of 5-HT_{2A} agonists, such as DOI, DOM, and DOB, were enhanced by the mGlu2 agonist LY379268, while the affinities of mGlu2 agonists, including LY379268, DCG-IV, and L-CCG-I, decreased in the presence of the 5-HT_{2A} agonist DOI (Gonzalez-Maeso et al. 2008). Furthermore, the mGlu2 receptor modulates the hallucinogenic $G_{i/o}$ signaling of the 5-HT_{2A} receptor within the complex, and mGlu2 activation suppresses $G_{i/o}$ signaling and associated behaviors induced by hallucinogenic drugs. Thus, the mGlu2-5-HT_{2A} complex is considered a potential target for hallucinogenic drug development (Gonzalez-Maeso et al. 2008).

The mGlu2-5-HT_{2A} heterodimer further establishes an optimal $G_{i/o}$-G_q signaling balance in response to the endogenous ligand glutamate and serotonin. The mGlu2 antagonist LY341495 and hallucinogenic 5-HT_{2A} agonists such as DOI decrease $G_{i/o}$ signaling and enhance G_q signaling, respectively. In contrast, the mGlu2 agonist LY379268 and the 5-HT_{2A} inverse agonist clozapine restore the $G_{i/o}$-G_q signaling balance (Fribourg et al. 2011). The development of bivalent ligands targeting the mGlu2-5-HT_{2A} heterodimer, based on the 5-HT_{2A} antagonist MDL-100907 and the mGlu2 ago-PAM JNJ-42491293, further confirms this functional crosstalk (Poulie et al. 2020). Finally, the mGlu2 agonist LY379268 induces G_q signaling via the 5-HT_{2A} receptor, which requires $G_{i/o}$ protein recruitment from at least one mGlu2 protomer. This LY379268-dependent G_q activation is diminished in the frontal cortex of 5-HT_{2A}-knockout mice and in the brains of schizophrenic patients (Moreno et al. 2016).

6.2 mGlu5-D1 Heterodimer in Parkinson's Disease (PD)

The metabotropic glutamate type 5 (mGlu5) and dopamine type 1 (D1) receptors modulate the glutamatergic and dopaminergic systems in striatal neurons, which are essential for controlling action selection and behavioral plasticity. These cortico-basal ganglia circuits are important therapeutic targets in Parkinson's disease (PD), particularly for addressing L-DOPA-induced dyskinesia (LID) (Bagetta et al. 2010; Surmeier et al. 2014).

The mGlu5-D1 heterodimer was first identified in overexpressed HEK293 cells, primary neurons, and rodent models of PD using BRET and bimolecular fluorescence complementation (BiFC) experiments (Sebastianutto et al. 2020). The mGlu5 and D1 receptors couple to G_q and Gs proteins, respectively, while the mGlu5-D1 heterodimer is coupled to Gq proteins. This heterocomplex synergistically activates phospholipase C (PLC) signaling and triggers intracellular Ca^{2+} release in response to glutamate or dopamine (Sebastianutto et al. 2020). Notably, the mGlu5-D1 heterodimer generates an atypical D1 receptor-dependent intracellular Ca^{2+} response. The number of mGlu5-D1 complexes is significantly increased in the DOPA-denervated striatum. The mGlu5 and D1-dependent PLC pathway is also associated with the activation of $ERK_{1/2}$ in striatal neurons, which contributes to dyskinetic behaviors in animal models treated with L-DOPA, SKF38393, or quinpirole (Sebastianutto et al. 2020). Collectively, the physical and functional crosstalk within the mGlu5-D1 heteromer enhances intracellular G_q-PLC signaling in dopamine-denervated striatal neurons, suggesting its potential as a therapeutic target in PD (Sebastianutto et al. 2020).

6.3 5-HT_{1A}-OX1 Heterodimer in Depression

Depression is a common and heterogeneous disorder. A substantial body of evidence highlights the roles of the 5-hydroxytryptamine 1A (5-HT_{1A}) receptor and orexin receptor 1 (OX1) in the pathophysiology of depression and anxiety. Using techniques such as dual immunofluorescence staining, in situ PLA, Co-IP, BRET, and FRET techniques, the co-localization and interaction between 5-HT_{1A} and OX1 were demonstrated in transfected HEK293 cells, as well as in the hippocampus and medial prefrontal cortex (mPFC) of rodent models (Zhang et al. 2022).

The 5-HT_{1A} receptor couples to Gi/o proteins, which inhibit adenylate cyclase activity (Maroteaux et al. 2019), while the OX1 receptor primarily signals through G_q coupling, triggering intracellular Ca^{2+} response release via PKC-dependent or -independent pathways (Wang et al. 2018). Interestingly, the 5-HT_{1A}-OX1 heterodimer induces a novel G protein-dependent signaling pathway, activating G_s- and $G_{12/13}$-dependent downstream signal transduction, without affecting β-arrestin recruitment to the complex (Zhang et al. 2022). In the hippocampus of rats, the number of endogenous 5-HT_{1A}-OX1 heterodimers was significantly higher in a depression model compared to the control group. Treatment with three transmembrane peptides derived from the 5-HT_{1A} TM4, TM5, and OX1 TM5 regions reduced the number of 5-HT_{1A}-OX1 heterodimers and alleviated depression-related symptoms (Zhang et al. 2022). In summary, the 5-HT_{1A}-OX1 heterodimer plays a crucial role in the pathophysiology of depression, and small molecule peptides targeting this heterodimer could represent a novel approach for developing antidepressant therapies.

7 Identification of Potential Heterodimer

Given the significant pharmacological characteristics exhibited by heterodimers in physiological and pathological processes, how can we determine whether two receptors are capable of directly forming a heterodimer? Alternatively, how can we ascertain whether these unique pharmacological properties arise from allosteric interactions between the receptors or from cross-talk within their downstream signaling pathways?

So far, three main criteria have been widely used to demonstrate heterodimer formation in both transfected in vitro and in vivo systems (Pin et al. 2007). First, the physical association or interaction between the two protomers should be observed in transfected cells and native tissues. Colocalization, co-immunoprecipitation, and proximity-based assays are commonly used to assess this criterion (Fig. 5a, b, d). For instance, in situ hybridization and antibody-based immunohistochemistry can detect the presence of receptors in the same cell or cellular compartment. Proximity ligation assays (PLA) and bimolecular fluorescence or luminescence complementation (BiFC/BiLC), including those using genetically modified animals expressing fluorescent proteins, also provide evidence for heterodimer formation. Recently, FRET has become one of the most popular and powerful techniques, as it can indicate the close proximity (within 10 nm) between protomers in real time within living cells. Moreover, Time-Resolved FRET (TR-FRET), based on antibodies or ligands, can specifically detect heterodimers in native tissues (Fig. 5e, f). To better determine the interaction regions between protomers, fluorescent tag-based Cys-Cys crosslinking experiments combined with nuclear magnetic resonance (NMR) spectroscopy and cryo-electron microscopy (cryo-EM) can provide convincing evidence (Fig. 5c).

Second, the heterodimer should exhibit specific functional properties in native tissues, beyond simple co-expression. Unlike their respective monomers, heterodimers show unique biochemical properties, which result in positive or negative crosstalk in ligand binding, G protein signaling, internalization, recycling, or other pharmacological fingerprints. These novel properties are observed in normal animals but not in deficient animals that lack one of the protomers, making heterodimers promising therapeutic targets. Notably, the identification of ligands that specifically target heterodimers will directly fulfill this criterion. The Heterodimer Identification Technology (HIT) is widely used to investigate these heterodimer-specific pharmacological properties in a mixture of monomers, dimers, and other complexes (Fig. 6a). In this system, one GPCR is tagged with one part of a proximity-based reporter system and another one is untagged. The untagged GPCR-interacting ligand, G protein or β-arrestin, is then tagged with a complementary part of the same fluorescent reporter system. Activation of one protomer or the heterodimer results in modulation of ligand-induced signal (Ayoub and Pfleger 2010). Additionally, bioluminescence resonance energy transfer (BRET) (Stoddart et al. 2015) (Fig. 6b), bimolecular complementation of donor-based BRET (CODA-RET) (Wouters et al. 2019) (Fig. 6c), TR-FRET (Hounsou et al. 2015) (Fig. 6d), and Nanoluc-based BRET ligand-binding assays (Jaeger et al. 2014; Stoddart et al. 2015)

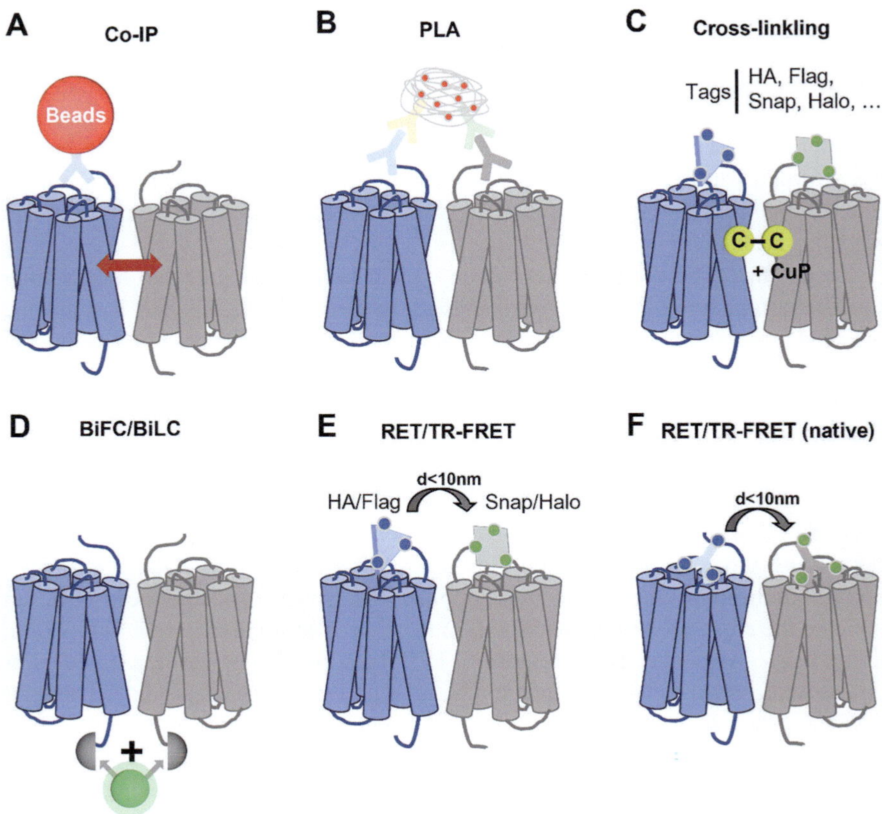

Fig. 5 Technologies to identify heterodimers. Antibodies targeting epitope-tagged or native GPCRs specifically label receptor populations to allow detection of physical interaction by coimmunoprecipitation (Co-IP) (**a**) or close proximity using in situ proximity ligation of DNA-conjugated secondary antibodies (**b**) and crosslinking experiments based on a disulfide bond between two receptors with tags or antibodies (**c**). (**d**) Fusion of fragments of luminescent or fluorescent proteins to the C-terminal tail of GPCRs allows detection of close proximity by bimolecular fluorescent (BiFC) or luminescence (BiLC) complementation. (**e**) Time-resolved FRET between fluorescent tags or tag antibodies allows detection of heterodimeric receptor. (**f**) Time-resolved FRET based on antibodies or nanobodies targeting at receptor complexes in native tissue. Two different receptors are shown in gray and light blue respectively

(Fig. 6e) are also employed to study the ligand-dependent biased signaling and allosteric interactions based on the heterodimer specific configuration.

Finally, the destruction of heterodimers should result in the loss of their specific functions. The absence of either protomer should significantly reduce the functional response by interrupting heterodimer formation. The existence and function of GPCR heterodimers in vivo can be further confirmed using RNA interference (RNAi) technology or in transgenic animals with mutational protomers that block heterodimer formation, as well as receptor protomer knockout animals. Interestingly,

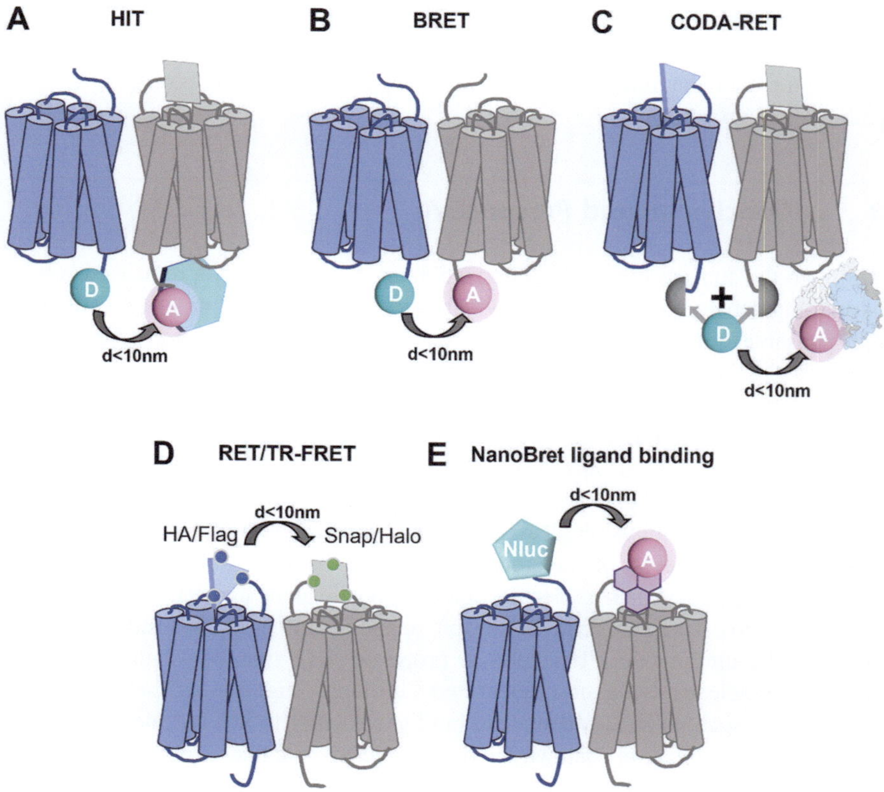

Fig. 6 Technologies to study heterodimer-specific pharmacology. (**a**) Heterodimer identification technology (HIT). (**b**) Fusion of luminescent or fluorescent donor and acceptor proteins to the C-terminal tail of GPCRs allows detection of close proximity by RET. (**c**) CODA-RET detects the interaction of GPCR dimers with intracellular signaling partners using the combination of bimolecular fluorescent complementation. (**d**) Time-resolved FRET between fluorescent tags or tag antibodies allows detection of heterodimeric receptor. (**e**) BRET between NanoLuc-tagged receptor and fluorescent ligands targeting at another receptor to measure ligand-binding affinities of GPCR heterodimer. Two different receptors are shown in gray and light blue respectively

the development of transmembrane peptides that can disrupt the interaction interface between receptor protomers provides another way to explore heterodimers in native tissues. For instance, pepducin peptides, derived from the GPCR intracellular loop, have been shown to induce striking neointimal hyperplasia in wild-type mice but not in either PAR1- or PAR2-knockout mice, by affecting the PAR1-PAR2 heterodimer formation (Sevigny et al. 2011).

To identify and validate a GPCR heterodimer, at least two of the three criteria outlined above, based on NC-IUPHAR guidelines, must be met (Pin et al. 2007). However, due to the lack of appropriate experimental tools, characterizing the existence and pharmacological properties of heterodimers in heterogeneous and native systems remains a challenge. By combining these technologies, it will be possible to define the biochemical fingerprint of emerging native GPCR heterodimers in the future, highlighting their crucial roles in physiological and pathological processes.

8 Conclusion and Perspective

Although the concept of GPCR dimerization and oligomerization remains a subject of ongoing debate, there is growing evidence that dimeric or oligomeric GPCRs play indispensable roles in both physiological and pathological processes. GPCR heterodimers have attracted significant attention as promising therapeutic targets due to their ability to reduce treatment-related side effects and generate distinct signaling profiles. Through heterodimerization, GPCRs can exhibit unique signaling behaviors, such as biased activation of G protein- or β-arrestin-dependent pathways, which are not observed in individual protomers. To better elucidate the role of GPCR heterodimers under physiological and pathological conditions, it is essential to investigate the effects of heterodimer-selective agents, including membrane-permeable peptides, small molecule ligands, and bivalent ligands, in in vitro and in vivo systems. The membrane-permeable peptides can disrupt heterodimer formation, thereby altering their biochemical properties and signaling pathways, while heterodimer-selective ligands identified through high-throughput screening technologies such as HIT systems can bind specifically to heterodimeric receptors and modulate signaling pathways in a targeted manner. Composed of two pharmacophores linked by a flexible linker, bivalent ligands simultaneously bind to both protomers within a heterodimer. They offer a promising strategy to selectively target heterodimers in native tissues while minimizing off-target effects. Importantly, the development of bivalent ligands is often more accessible due to the existing knowledge of functional properties of known drugs. Overall, these agents represent powerful tools for selectively targeting GPCR heterodimers, enabling novel therapeutic strategies for both research and clinical applications.

Despite these advancements, significant challenges remain in understanding the physical and functional interplay within GPCR heterodimers. A major limitation is the lack of high-resolution cryo-EM structures, which are critical for clarifying the structural basis of allosteric modulation and signaling integration. Recent progress in elucidating the overall structures of Class C GPCR heterodimers, as well as the homodimers of Class A APJ and Class D Ste2, has provided valuable insights. Briefly, $GABA_B$ receptors form heterodimers through coil-coil interactions at the C-terminal regions of their subunits, while mGlu receptors form heterodimers via disulfide bonds between two VFTs. The formation of Class D Ste2 dimers involve extensive polar interactions, whereas APJ dimers are stabilized through π-π interactions, involving only five residues from each protomer. The distinct assembly mechanisms of homodimers and heterodimers across different GPCR families highlight the complexity of allosteric interactions within heterodimers, as well as their structural and functional diversity. Furthermore, the structure of the class A GPCR sphingophospholipid S1P1 receptor complex with transmembrane protein CD19 demonstrated how CD19 allosterically activates the receptor (Cao et al. 2022). Similar structural allosteric effects have been observed in class B GPCR complexes with receptor activity-modifying proteins (RAMPs), such as the glucagon and calcitonin/amylin receptors (Chen et al. 2023a; Krishna Kumar et al. 2023). These findings mark an important step forward in understanding the molecular and structural mechanisms of GPCR heterodimerization. Although recent molecular dynamics studies have revealed the dynamic behaviors of GPCR heterodimers (Di Marino et al. 2023), further advancements are needed to develop more efficient and effective technologies to investigate the dynamic conformational changes and unique functional fingerprints of heterodimers in vivo. Our nanobody-based FRET experiments offer a novel approach to clarify the subunit composition of GPCR heterodimers in native environments, providing a foundation for future studies.

To address existing challenges, comprehensive biochemical, pharmacological, and structural studies are required. Advancing experimental techniques to investigate heterodimer-specific signaling dynamics will be crucial for identifying functional signatures of GPCR heterodimers. Such progress will pave the way for the development of innovative drugs that precisely target GPCR heterodimers to regulate signaling pathways with high specificity and efficacy. In conclusion, the traditional understanding of GPCR biased signaling must be revisited and updated to include heterodimerization-induced biased signaling mechanisms. Sustained research in this area holds great significance and promises to significantly expand our knowledge of GPCR signal transduction, ultimately driving the development of novel therapeutic strategies to target GPCR heterodimers.

Acknowledgments This work was supported by grants from National Key R&D Program of China (grant number 2022YFE0116600 and 2021ZD0203302 to J.L.), the National Natural Science Foundation of China (NSFC) (grant number 32330049, 82320108021, and 32421003 to J.L and grant number 32300598 to C.S.), the Major Project of Guangzhou National Laboratory (grant No. GZNL2023A03007 to J.L.), and the Key Technologies R&D Program of Guangdong Province (grant no. 2010A080813001 to J.L.). This work was partially supported by the Interdisciplinary Research Program of HUST (grant number 5003170102 to J.L) and the Postdoctoral Innovative Talent Support Program (grant number BX20220122 to C.S.).

Disclosures No conflicts of interest, financial or otherwise, are declared by the authors.

Author Contributions J.L. conceived and supervised the whole review; L.L., Y.L., and S.Z. drafted the manuscript; L.L., Y.L, S.Z., C.S., and J.M. prepared figures; L.L. and J.L. edited and revised the manuscript; L.L., Y.L., S.Z., and J.L. approved the final version of the manuscript.

References

Abadir PM, Periasamy A, Carey RM, Siragy HM (2006) Angiotensin II type 2 receptor-bradykinin B2 receptor functional heterodimerization. Hypertension 48:316–322. https://doi.org/10.1161/01.HYP.0000228997.88162.a8

AbdAlla S, Lother H, Abdel-tawab AM, Quitterer U (2001) The angiotensin II AT2 receptor is an AT1 receptor antagonist. J Biol Chem 276:39721–39726. https://doi.org/10.1074/jbc.M105253200

Abid S, Marcos E, Parpaleix A, Amsellem V, Breau M, Houssaini A, Vienney N, Lefevre M, Derumeaux G, Evans S, Hubeau C, Delcroix M, Quarck R, Adnot S, Lipskaia L (2019) CCR2/CCR5-mediated macrophage-smooth muscle cell crosstalk in pulmonary hypertension. Eur Respir J 54. https://doi.org/10.1183/13993003.02308-2018

Aicher SA, Sharma S, Cheng PY, Liu-Chen LY, Pickel VM (2000) Dual ultrastructural localization of mu-opiate receptors and substance p in the dorsal horn. Synapse 36:12–20. https://doi.org/10.1002/(SICI)1098-2396(200004)36:1<12::AID-SYN2>3.0.CO;2-E

Akgun E, Javed MI, Lunzer MM, Powers MD, Sham YY, Watanabe Y, Portoghese PS (2015) Inhibition of inflammatory and neuropathic pain by targeting a mu opioid receptor/chemokine Receptor5 Heteromer (MOR-CCR5). J Med Chem 58:8647–8657. https://doi.org/10.1021/acs.jmedchem.5b01245

Albizu L, Cottet M, Kralikova M, Stoev S, Seyer R, Brabet I, Roux T, Bazin H, Bourrier E, Lamarque L, Breton C, Rives ML, Newman A, Javitch J, Trinquet E, Manning M, Pin JP, Mouillac B, Durroux T (2010) Time-resolved FRET between GPCR ligands reveals oligomers in native tissues. Nat Chem Biol 6:587–594. https://doi.org/10.1038/nchembio.396

Alhosaini K, Azhar A, Alonazi A, Al-Zoghaibi F (2021) GPCRs: the most promiscuous druggable receptor of the mankind. Saudi Pharm J 29:539–551. https://doi.org/10.1016/j.jsps.2021.04.015

Amargos-Bosch M, Bortolozzi A, Puig MV, Serrats J, Adell A, Celada P, Toth M, Mengod G, Artigas F (2004) Co-expression and in vivo interaction of serotonin1A and serotonin2A receptors in pyramidal neurons of prefrontal cortex. Cereb Cortex 14:281–299. https://doi.org/10.1093/cercor/bhg128

Anastasio NC, Stutz SJ, Fink LH, Swinford-Jackson SE, Sears RM, DiLeone RJ, Rice KC, Moeller FG, Cunningham KA (2015) Serotonin (5-HT) 5-HT2A receptor (5-HT2AR):5-HT2CR imbalance in medial prefrontal cortex associates with motor impulsivity. ACS Chem Neurosci 6:1248–1258. https://doi.org/10.1021/acschemneuro.5b00094

Ansonoff MA, Portoghese PS, Pintar JE (2010) Consequences of opioid receptor mutation on actions of univalent and bivalent kappa and delta ligands. Psychopharmacology 210:161–168. https://doi.org/10.1007/s00213-010-1826-7

Arachiche A, de la Fuente M, Nieman MT (2013) Calcium mobilization and protein kinase C activation downstream of protease activated receptor 4 (PAR4) is negatively regulated by PAR3 in mouse platelets. PLoS One 8:e55740. https://doi.org/10.1371/journal.pone.0055740

Armando S, Quoyer J, Lukashova V, Maiga A, Percherancier Y, Heveker N, Pin JP, Prezeau L, Bouvier M (2014) The chemokine CXC4 and CC2 receptors form homo- and heterooligomers that can engage their signaling G-protein effectors and betaarrestin. FASEB J 28:4509–4523. https://doi.org/10.1096/fj.13-242446

Arnatt CK, Falls BA, Yuan Y, Raborg TJ, Masvekar RR, El-Hage N, Selley DE, Nicola AV, Knapp PE, Hauser KF, Zhang Y (2016) Exploration of bivalent ligands targeting putative mu opioid receptor and chemokine receptor CCR5 dimerization. Bioorg Med Chem 24:5969–5987. https://doi.org/10.1016/j.bmc.2016.09.059

Aspelin T, Eriksen M, Ilebekk A, Cataliotti A, Carlson CR, Lyberg T (2014) Beta-blockade abolishes the augmented cardiac tPA release induced by transactivation of heterodimerised bradykinin receptor-2 and beta2-adrenergic receptor in vivo. Thromb Haemost 112:951–959. https://doi.org/10.1160/TH14-01-0059

Ayoub MA, Pfleger KD (2010) Recent advances in bioluminescence resonance energy transfer technologies to study GPCR heteromerization. Curr Opin Pharmacol 10:44–52. https://doi.org/10.1016/j.coph.2009.09.012

Ayoub MA, Levoye A, Delagrange P, Jockers R (2004) Preferential formation of MT1/MT2 melatonin receptor heterodimers with distinct ligand interaction properties compared with MT2 homodimers. Mol Pharmacol 66:312–321. https://doi.org/10.1124/mol.104.000398

Ayoub MA, Zhang Y, Kelly RS, See HB, Johnstone EK, McCall EA, Williams JH, Kelly DJ, Pfleger KD (2015) Functional interaction between angiotensin II receptor type 1 and chemokine (C-C motif) receptor 2 with implications for chronic kidney disease. PLoS One 10:e0119803. https://doi.org/10.1371/journal.pone.0119803

Azam S, Haque ME, Jakaria M, Jo SH, Kim IS, Choi DK (2020) G-protein-coupled receptors in CNS: a potential therapeutic target for intervention in neurodegenerative disorders and associated cognitive deficits. Cells 9. https://doi.org/10.3390/cells9020506

Baba K, Benleulmi-Chaachoua A, Journe AS, Kamal M, Guillaume JL, Dussaud S, Gbahou F, Yettou K, Liu C, Contreras-Alcantara S, Jockers R, Tosini G (2013) Heteromeric MT1/MT2 melatonin receptors modulate photoreceptor function. Sci Signal 6:ra89. https://doi.org/10.1126/scisignal.2004302

Bach HH 4th, Wong YM, Tripathi A, Nevins AM, Gamelli RL, Volkman BF, Byron KL, Majetschak M (2014) Chemokine (C-X-C motif) receptor 4 and atypical chemokine receptor 3 regulate vascular alpha(1)-adrenergic receptor function. Mol Med 20:435–447. https://doi.org/10.2119/molmed.2014.00101

Bagetta V, Ghiglieri V, Sgobio C, Calabresi P, Picconi B (2010) Synaptic dysfunction in Parkinson's disease. Biochem Soc Trans 38:493–497. https://doi.org/10.1042/BST0380493

Bagher AM, Laprairie RB, Kelly ME, Denovan-Wright EM (2016) Antagonism of dopamine receptor 2 Long affects cannabinoid receptor 1 signaling in a cell culture model of striatal medium spiny projection neurons. Mol Pharmacol 89:652–666. https://doi.org/10.1124/mol.116.103465

Bagher AM, Young AP, Laprairie RB, Toguri JT, Kelly MEM, Denovan-Wright EM (2020) Heteromer formation between cannabinoid type 1 and dopamine type 2 receptors is altered by combination cannabinoid and antipsychotic treatments. J Neurosci Res 98:2496–2509. https://doi.org/10.1002/jnr.24716

Bah A, Chen Z, Bush-Pelc LA, Mathews FS, Di Cera E (2007) Crystal structures of murine thrombin in complex with the extracellular fragments of murine protease-activated receptors PAR3 and PAR4. Proc Natl Acad Sci USA 104:11603–11608. https://doi.org/10.1073/pnas.0704409104

Bai J, Duraisamy K, Mak SOK, Allam A, Ajarem J, Li Z, Chow BKC (2019) Role of SCTR/AT1aR heteromer in mediating ANGII-induced aldosterone secretion. PLoS One 14:e0222005. https://doi.org/10.1371/journal.pone.0222005

Balenga NA, Martinez-Pinilla E, Kargl J, Schroder R, Peinhaupt M, Platzer W, Balint Z, Zamarbide M, Dopeso-Reyes IG, Ricobaraza A, Perez-Ortiz JM, Kostenis E, Waldhoer M, Heinemann A, Franco R (2014) Heteromerization of GPR55 and cannabinoid CB2 receptors modulates signalling. Br J Pharmacol 171:5387–5406. https://doi.org/10.1111/bph.12850

Bardoni R, Tawfik VL, Wang D, Francois A, Solorzano C, Shuster SA, Choudhury P, Betelli C, Cassidy C, Smith K, de Nooij JC, Mennicken F, O'Donnell D, Kieffer BL, Woodbury CJ, Basbaum AI, MacDermott AB, Scherrer G (2014) Delta opioid receptors presynaptically regulate cutaneous mechanosensory neuron input to the spinal cord dorsal horn. Neuron 81:1312–1327. https://doi.org/10.1016/j.neuron.2014.01.044

Barki-Harrington L, Luttrell LM, Rockman HA (2003) Dual inhibition of beta-adrenergic and angiotensin II receptors by a single antagonist: a functional role for receptor-receptor interaction in vivo. Circulation 108:1611–1618. https://doi.org/10.1161/01.CIR.0000092166.30360.78

Barnes NM, Sharp T (1999) A review of central 5-HT receptors and their function. Neuropharmacology 38:1083–1152. https://doi.org/10.1016/s0028-3908(99)00010-6

Barnes NM, Ahern GP, Becamel C, Bockaert J, Camilleri M, Chaumont-Dubel S, Claeysen S, Cunningham KA, Fone KC, Gershon M, Di Giovanni G, Goodfellow NM, Halberstadt AL, Hartley RM, Hassaine G, Herrick-Davis K, Hovius R, Lacivita E, Lambe EK, Leopoldo M, Levy FO, Lummis SCR, Marin P, Maroteaux L, McCreary AC, Nelson DL, Neumaier JF, Newman-Tancredi A, Nury H, Roberts A, Roth BL, Roumier A, Sanger GJ, Teitler M, Sharp T, Villalon CM, Vogel H, Watts SW, Hoyer D (2021) International Union of Basic and Clinical

Pharmacology. CX. Classification of receptors for 5-hydroxytryptamine; pharmacology and function. Pharmacol Rev 73:310–520. https://doi.org/10.1124/pr.118.015552

Bellot M, Galandrin S, Boularan C, Matthies HJ, Despas F, Denis C, Javitch J, Mazeres S, Sanni SJ, Pons V, Seguelas MH, Hansen JL, Pathak A, Galli A, Senard JM, Gales C (2015) Dual agonist occupancy of AT1-R-alpha2C-AR heterodimers results in atypical Gs-PKA signaling. Nat Chem Biol 11:271–279. https://doi.org/10.1038/nchembio.1766

Benecke H, Lotts T, Stander S (2013) Investigational drugs for pruritus. Expert Opin Investig Drugs 22:1167–1179. https://doi.org/10.1517/13543784.2013.813932

Berg T (2013) Angiotensin AT1 – alpha2C-adrenoceptor interaction disturbs alpha2A-auto-inhibition of catecholamine release in hypertensive rats. Front Neurol 4:70. https://doi.org/10.3389/fneur.2013.00070

Bockaert J, Pin JP (1999) Molecular tinkering of G protein-coupled receptors: an evolutionary success. EMBO J 18:1723–1729. https://doi.org/10.1093/emboj/18.7.1723

Bogenpohl JW, Ritter SL, Hall RA, Smith Y (2012) Adenosine A2A receptor in the monkey basal ganglia: ultrastructural localization and colocalization with the metabotropic glutamate receptor 5 in the striatum. J Comp Neurol 520:570–589. https://doi.org/10.1002/cne.22751

Bonaventura J, Rico AJ, Moreno E, Sierra S, Sanchez M, Luquin N, Farre D, Muller CE, Martinez-Pinilla E, Cortes A, Mallol J, Armentero MT, Pinna A, Canela EI, Lluis C, McCormick PJ, Lanciego JL, Casado V, Franco R (2014) L-DOPA-treatment in primates disrupts the expression of A(2A) adenosine-CB(1) cannabinoid-D(2) dopamine receptor heteromers in the caudate nucleus. Neuropharmacology 79:90–100. https://doi.org/10.1016/j.neuropharm.2013.10.036

Borah MP, Trakroo D, Soni N, Kumari P, Baidya M (2024) Exploring bias in GPCR signaling and its implication in drug development: a one-sided affair. Biochemistry. https://doi.org/10.1021/acs.biochem.4c00676

Borroto-Escuela DO, Fuxe K (2019a) Adenosine heteroreceptor complexes in the basal ganglia are implicated in Parkinson's disease and its treatment. J Neural Transm (Vienna) 126:455–471. https://doi.org/10.1007/s00702-019-01969-2

Borroto-Escuela DO, Fuxe K (2019b) Oligomeric receptor complexes and their allosteric receptor-receptor interactions in the plasma membrane represent a new biological principle for integration of signals in the CNS. Front Mol Neurosci 12. https://doi.org/10.3389/fnmol.2019.00230

Borroto-Escuela DO, Romero-Fernandez W, Tarakanov AO, Marcellino D, Ciruela F, Agnati LF, Fuxe K (2010) Dopamine D2 and 5-hydroxytryptamine 5-HT((2)a) receptors assemble into functionally interacting heteromers. Biochem Biophys Res Commun 401:605–610. https://doi.org/10.1016/j.bbrc.2010.09.110

Borroto-Escuela DO, Romero-Fernandez W, Tarakanov AO, Ciruela F, Agnati LF, Fuxe K (2011) On the existence of a possible A2A-D2-beta-Arrestin2 complex: A2A agonist modulation of D2 agonist-induced beta-arrestin2 recruitment. J Mol Biol 406:687–699. https://doi.org/10.1016/j.jmb.2011.01.022

Borroto-Escuela DO, Hinz S, Navarro G, Franco R, Muller CE, Fuxe K (2018a) Understanding the role of adenosine A2AR Heteroreceptor complexes in neurodegeneration and neuroinflammation. Front Neurosci 12:43. https://doi.org/10.3389/fnins.2018.00043

Borroto-Escuela DO, Wydra K, Filip M, Fuxe K (2018b) A2AR-D2R Heteroreceptor complexes in cocaine reward and addiction. Trends Pharmacol Sci 39:1008–1020. https://doi.org/10.1016/j.tips.2018.10.007

Bradaia A, Trube G, Stalder H, Norcross RD, Ozmen L, Wettstein JG, Pinard A, Buchy D, Gassmann M, Hoener MC, Bettler B (2009) The selective antagonist EPPTB reveals TAAR1-mediated regulatory mechanisms in dopaminergic neurons of the mesolimbic system. Proc Natl Acad Sci USA 106:20081–20086. https://doi.org/10.1073/pnas.0906522106

Breit A, Gagnidze K, Devi LA, Lagace M, Bouvier M (2006) Simultaneous activation of the delta opioid receptor (deltaOR)/sensory neuron-specific receptor-4 (SNSR-4) hetero-oligomer by the mixed bivalent agonist bovine adrenal medulla peptide 22 activates SNSR-4 but inhibits deltaOR signaling. Mol Pharmacol 70:686–696. https://doi.org/10.1124/mol.106.022897

Bushlin I, Gupta A, Stockton SD Jr, Miller LK, Devi LA (2012) Dimerization with cannabinoid receptors allosterically modulates delta opioid receptor activity during neuropathic pain. PLoS One 7:e49789. https://doi.org/10.1371/journal.pone.0049789

Butini S, Campiani G, Franceschini S, Trotta F, Kumar V, Guarino E, Borrelli G, Fiorini I, Novellino E, Fattorusso C, Persico M, Orteca N, Sandager-Nielsen K, Jacobsen TA, Madsen K, Scheel-Kruger J, Gemma S (2010) Discovery of bishomo(hetero)arylpiperazines as novel multifunctional ligands targeting dopamine D(3) and serotonin 5-HT(1A) and 5-HT (2A) receptors. J Med Chem 53:4803–4807. https://doi.org/10.1021/jm100294b

Caniceiro AB, Bueschbell B, Schiedel AC, Moreira IS (2022) Class A and C GPCR dimers in neurodegenerative diseases. Curr Neuropharmacol 20:2081–2141. https://doi.org/10.2174/1570159X20666220327221830

Cao J, Belousoff MJ, Liang YL, Johnson RM, Josephs TM, Fletcher MM, Christopoulos A, Hay DL, Danev R, Wootten D, Sexton PM (2022) A structural basis for amylin receptor phenotype. Science 375:eabm9609. https://doi.org/10.1126/science.abm9609

Carr DB, Cooper DC, Ulrich SL, Spruston N, Surmeier DJ (2002) Serotonin receptor activation inhibits sodium current and dendritic excitability in prefrontal cortex via a protein kinase C-dependent mechanism. J Neurosci 22:6846–6855

Carriba P, Ortiz O, Patkar K, Justinova Z, Stroik J, Themann A, Muller C, Woods AS, Hope BT, Ciruela F, Casado V, Canela EI, Lluis C, Goldberg SR, Moratalla R, Franco R, Ferre S (2007) Striatal adenosine A2A and cannabinoid CB1 receptors form functional heteromeric complexes that mediate the motor effects of cannabinoids. Neuropsychopharmacology 32:2249–2259. https://doi.org/10.1038/sj.npp.1301375

Cataldo G, Erb SJ, Lunzer MM, Luong N, Akgun E, Portoghese PS, Olson JK, Simone DA (2019) The bivalent ligand MCC22 potently attenuates hyperalgesia in a mouse model of cisplatin-evoked neuropathic pain without tolerance or reward. Neuropharmacology 158:107598. https://doi.org/10.1016/j.neuropharm.2019.04.004

Centonze D, Grande C, Usiello A, Gubellini P, Erbs E, Martin AB, Pisani A, Tognazzi N, Bernardi G, Moratalla R, Borrelli E, Calabresi P (2003) Receptor subtypes involved in the presynaptic and postsynaptic actions of dopamine on striatal interneurons. J Neurosci 23:6245–6254. https://doi.org/10.1523/JNEUROSCI.23-15-06245.2003

Cerri S, Levandis G, Ambrosi G, Montepeloso E, Antoninetti GF, Franco R, Lanciego JL, Baqi Y, Muller CE, Pinna A, Blandini F, Armentero MT (2014) Neuroprotective potential of adenosine A2A and cannabinoid CB1 receptor antagonists in an animal model of Parkinson disease. J Neuropathol Exp Neurol 73:414–424. https://doi.org/10.1097/NEN.0000000000000064

Chakrabarti S, Liu NJ, Gintzler AR (2010) Formation of mu−/kappa-opioid receptor heterodimer is sex-dependent and mediates female-specific opioid analgesia. Proc Natl Acad Sci USA 107: 20115–20119. https://doi.org/10.1073/pnas.1009923107

Chen X, Yuan Y, Chen Y, Yu J, Wang J, Chen J, Guo Y, Pu X (2022) Biased activation mechanism induced by GPCR Heterodimerization: observations from muOR/deltaOR dimers. J Chem Inf Model 62:5581–5600. https://doi.org/10.1021/acs.jcim.2c00962

Chen H, Qin Y, Chou M, Cyster JG, Li X (2023a) Transmembrane protein CD69 acts as an S1PR1 agonist. elife 12. https://doi.org/10.7554/eLife.88204

Chen J, Garcia EJ, Merritt CR, Zamora JC, Bolinger AA, Pazdrak K, Stafford SJ, Mifflin RC, Wold EA, Wild CT, Chen H, Anastasio NC, Cunningham KA, Zhou J (2023b) Discovery of novel Oleamide analogues as brain-penetrant positive allosteric serotonin 5-HT(2C) receptor and dual 5-HT(2C)/5-HT(2A) receptor modulators. J Med Chem 66:9992–10009. https://doi.org/10.1021/acs.jmedchem.3c00908

Chiodi V, Ferrante A, Ferraro L, Potenza RL, Armida M, Beggiato S, Pezzola A, Bader M, Fuxe K, Popoli P, Domenici MR (2016) Striatal adenosine-cannabinoid receptor interactions in rats over-expressing adenosine A2A receptors. J Neurochem 136:907–917. https://doi.org/10.1111/jnc.13421

Chruscicka B, Wallace Fitzsimons SE, Borroto-Escuela DO, Druelle C, Stamou P, Nally K, Dinan TG, Cryan JF, Fuxe K, Schellekens H (2019) Attenuation of oxytocin and serotonin 2A receptor signaling through novel Heteroreceptor formation. ACS Chem Neurosci 10:3225–3240. https://doi.org/10.1021/acschemneuro.8b00665

Chruscicka B, Cowan CSM, Wallace Fitzsimons SE, Borroto-Escuela DO, Druelle CM, Stamou P, Bergmann CA, Dinan TG, Slattery DA, Fuxe K, Cryan JF, Schellekens H (2021) Molecular, biochemical and behavioural evidence for a novel oxytocin receptor and serotonin 2C receptor heterocomplex. Neuropharmacology 183:108394. https://doi.org/10.1016/j.neuropharm.2020.108394

Ciruela F, Casado V, Rodrigues RJ, Lujan R, Burgueno J, Canals M, Borycz J, Rebola N, Goldberg SR, Mallol J, Cortes A, Canela EI, Lopez-Gimenez JF, Milligan G, Lluis C, Cunha RA, Ferre S, Franco R (2006) Presynaptic control of striatal glutamatergic neurotransmission by adenosine A1-A2A receptor heteromers. J Neurosci 26:2080–2087. https://doi.org/10.1523/JNEUROSCI.3574-05.2006

Clement N, Renault N, Guillaume JL, Cecon E, Journe AS, Laurent X, Tadagaki K, Coge F, Gohier A, Delagrange P, Chavatte P, Jockers R (2018) Importance of the second extracellular loop for melatonin MT(1) receptor function and absence of melatonin binding in GPR50. Br J Pharmacol 175:3281–3297. https://doi.org/10.1111/bph.14029

Dai Q, Xu M, Yao M, Sun B (2007) Angiotensin AT1 receptor antagonists exert anti-inflammatory effects in spontaneously hypertensive rats. Br J Pharmacol 152:1042–1048. https://doi.org/10.1038/sj.bjp.0707454

Dale NC, Johnstone EKM, Pfleger KDG (2022) GPCR heteromers: an overview of their classification, function and physiological relevance. Front Endocrinol (Lausanne) 13:931573. https://doi.org/10.3389/fendo.2022.931573

Daniels DJ, Kulkarni A, Xie Z, Bhushan RG, Portoghese PS (2005) A bivalent ligand (KDAN-18) containing delta-antagonist and kappa-agonist pharmacophores bridges delta2 and kappa1 opioid receptor phenotypes. J Med Chem 48:1713–1716. https://doi.org/10.1021/jm034234f

de la Mora MP, Perez-Carrera D, Crespo-Ramirez M, Tarakanov A, Fuxe K, Borroto-Escuela DO (2016) Signaling in dopamine D2 receptor-oxytocin receptor heterocomplexes and its relevance for the anxiolytic effects of dopamine and oxytocin interactions in the amygdala of the rat. Biochim Biophys Acta 1862:2075–2085. https://doi.org/10.1016/j.bbadis.2016.07.004

de Poorter C, Baertsoen K, Lannoy V, Parmentier M, Springael JY (2013) Consequences of ChemR23 heteromerization with the chemokine receptors CXCR4 and CCR7. PLoS One 8:e58075. https://doi.org/10.1371/journal.pone.0058075

Decaillot FM, Kazmi MA, Lin Y, Ray-Saha S, Sakmar TP, Sachdev P (2011) CXCR7/CXCR4 heterodimer constitutively recruits beta-arrestin to enhance cell migration. J Biol Chem 286:32188–32197. https://doi.org/10.1074/jbc.M111.277038

DelaCuesta-Barrutia J, Penagarikano O, Erdozain AM (2020) G protein-coupled receptor heteromers as putative pharmacotherapeutic targets in autism. Front Cell Neurosci 14:588662. https://doi.org/10.3389/fncel.2020.588662

Di Marino D, Conflitti P, Motta S, Limongelli V (2023) Structural basis of dimerization of chemokine receptors CCR5 and CXCR4. Nat Commun 14:6439. https://doi.org/10.1038/s41467-023-42082-z

Doumazane E, Scholler P, Zwier JM, Trinquet E, Rondard P, Pin JP (2011) A new approach to analyze cell surface protein complexes reveals specific heterodimeric metabotropic glutamate receptors. FASEB J 25:66–77. https://doi.org/10.1096/fj.10-163147

Du J, Wang D, Fan H, Xu C, Tai L, Lin S, Han S, Tan Q, Wang X, Xu T, Zhang H, Chu X, Yi C, Liu P, Wang X, Zhou Y, Pin JP, Rondard P, Liu H, Liu J, Sun F, Wu B, Zhao Q (2021) Structures of human mGlu2 and mGlu7 homo- and heterodimers. Nature 594:589–593. https://doi.org/10.1038/s41586-021-03641-w

Dutta R, Lunzer MM, Auger JL, Akgun E, Portoghese PS, Binstadt BA (2018) A bivalent compound targeting CCR5 and the mu opioid receptor treats inflammatory arthritis pain in mice without inducing pharmacologic tolerance. Arthritis Res Ther 20:154. https://doi.org/10.1186/s13075-018-1661-5

El-Hage N, Dever SM, Podhaizer EM, Arnatt CK, Zhang Y, Hauser KF (2013) A novel bivalent HIV-1 entry inhibitor reveals fundamental differences in CCR5-mu-opioid receptor interactions between human astroglia and microglia. AIDS 27:2181–2190. https://doi.org/10.1097/QAD.0b013e3283639804

Erbs E, Faget L, Scherrer G, Matifas A, Filliol D, Vonesch JL, Koch M, Kessler P, Hentsch D, Birling MC, Koutsourakis M, Vasseur L, Veinante P, Kieffer BL, Massotte D (2015) A mu-delta opioid receptor brain atlas reveals neuronal co-occurrence in subcortical networks. Brain Struct Funct 220:677–702. https://doi.org/10.1007/s00429-014-0717-9

Espinoza S, Salahpour A, Masri B, Sotnikova TD, Messa M, Barak LS, Caron MG, Gainetdinov RR (2011) Functional interaction between trace amine-associated receptor 1 and dopamine D2 receptor. Mol Pharmacol 80:416–425. https://doi.org/10.1124/mol.111.073304

Evans NJ, Walker JW (2008a) Endothelin receptor dimers evaluated by FRET, ligand binding, and calcium mobilization. Biophys J 95:483–492. https://doi.org/10.1529/biophysj.107.119206

Evans NJ, Walker JW (2008b) Sustained Ca2+ signaling and delayed internalization associated with endothelin receptor heterodimers linked through a PDZ finger. Can J Physiol Pharmacol 86:526–535. https://doi.org/10.1139/Y08-050

Fantuzzi L, Tagliamonte M, Gauzzi MC, Lopalco L (2019) Dual CCR5/CCR2 targeting: opportunities for the cure of complex disorders. Cell Mol Life Sci 76:4869–4886. https://doi.org/10.1007/s00018-019-03255-6

Faron-Gorecka A, Kusmider M, Solich J, Kolasa M, Szafran K, Zurawek D, Pabian P, Dziedzicka-Wasylewska M (2013) Involvement of prolactin and somatostatin in depression and the mechanism of action of antidepressant drugs. Pharmacol Rep 65:1640–1646. https://doi.org/10.1016/s1734-1140(13)71525-1

Felsing DE, Anastasio NC, Miszkiel JM, Gilbertson SR, Allen JA, Cunningham KA (2018) Biophysical validation of serotonin 5-HT2A and 5-HT2C receptor interaction. PLoS One 13: e0203137. https://doi.org/10.1371/journal.pone.0203137

Ferrada C, Moreno E, Casado V, Bongers G, Cortes A, Mallol J, Canela EI, Leurs R, Ferre S, Lluis C, Franco R (2009) Marked changes in signal transduction upon heteromerization of dopamine D1 and histamine H3 receptors. Br J Pharmacol 157:64–75. https://doi.org/10.1111/j.1476-5381.2009.00152.x

Ferrao FM, Lara LS, Axelband F, Dias J, Carmona AK, Reis RI, Costa-Neto CM, Vieyra A, Lowe J (2012) Exposure of luminal membranes of LLC-PK1 cells to ANG II induces dimerization of AT1/AT2 receptors to activate SERCA and to promote Ca2+ mobilization. Am J Physiol Renal Physiol 302:F875–F883. https://doi.org/10.1152/ajprenal.00381.2011

Ferraro L, Tomasini MC, Mazza R, Fuxe K, Fournier J, Tanganelli S, Antonelli T (2008) Neurotensin receptors as modulators of glutamatergic transmission. Brain Res Rev 58:365–373. https://doi.org/10.1016/j.brainresrev.2007.11.001

Ferre S, Fredholm BB, Morelli M, Popoli P, Fuxe K (1997) Adenosine-dopamine receptor-receptor interactions as an integrative mechanism in the basal ganglia. Trends Neurosci 20:482–487. https://doi.org/10.1016/s0166-2236(97)01096-5

Ferre S, Karcz-Kubicha M, Hope BT, Popoli P, Burgueno J, Gutierrez MA, Casado V, Fuxe K, Goldberg SR, Lluis C, Franco R, Ciruela F (2002) Synergistic interaction between adenosine A2A and glutamate mGlu5 receptors: implications for striatal neuronal function. Proc Natl Acad Sci USA 99:11940–11945. https://doi.org/10.1073/pnas.172393799

Ferre S, Casado V, Devi LA, Filizola M, Jockers R, Lohse MJ, Milligan G, Pin JP, Guitart X (2014) G protein-coupled receptor oligomerization revisited: functional and pharmacological perspectives. Pharmacol Rev 66:413–434. https://doi.org/10.1124/pr.113.008052

Ferre S, Bonaventura J, Zhu W, Hatcher-Solis C, Taura J, Quiroz C, Cai NS, Moreno E, Casado-Anguera V, Kravitz AV, Thompson KR, Tomasi DG, Navarro G, Cordomi A, Pardo L, Lluis C, Dessauer CW, Volkow ND, Casado V, Ciruela F, Logothetis DE, Zwilling D (2018) Essential control of the function of the Striatopallidal neuron by pre-coupled complexes of adenosine a (2A)-dopamine D(2) receptor Heterotetramers and adenylyl cyclase. Front Pharmacol 9:243. https://doi.org/10.3389/fphar.2018.00243

Ferre S, Kofalvi A, Ciruela F, Justinova Z, Pistis M (2023a) Targeting corticostriatal transmission for the treatment of cannabinoid use disorder. Trends Pharmacol Sci 44:495–506. https://doi.org/10.1016/j.tips.2023.05.003

Ferre S, Sarasola LI, Quiroz C, Ciruela F (2023b) Presynaptic adenosine receptor heteromers as key modulators of glutamatergic and dopaminergic neurotransmission in the striatum. Neuropharmacology 223:109329. https://doi.org/10.1016/j.neuropharm.2022.109329

Fiorentini C, Busi C, Spano P, Missale C (2010) Dimerization of dopamine D1 and D3 receptors in the regulation of striatal function. Curr Opin Pharmacol 10:87–92. https://doi.org/10.1016/j.coph.2009.09.008

Fraser CM, Venter JC (1982) The size of the mammalian lung beta 2-adrenergic receptor as determined by target size analysis and immunoaffinity chromatography. Biochem Biophys Res Commun 109:21–29. https://doi.org/10.1016/0006-291x(82)91560-1

Fredriksson R, Lagerstrom MC, Lundin LG, Schioth HB (2003) The G-protein-coupled receptors in the human genome form five main families. Phylogenetic analysis, paralogon groups, and fingerprints. Mol Pharmacol 63:1256–1272. https://doi.org/10.1124/mol.63.6.1256

Fribourg M, Moreno JL, Holloway T, Provasi D, Baki L, Mahajan R, Park G, Adney SK, Hatcher C, Eltit JM, Ruta JD, Albizu L, Li Z, Umali A, Shim J, Fabiato A, MacKerell AD Jr, Brezina V, Sealfon SC, Filizola M, Gonzalez-Maeso J, Logothetis DE (2011) Decoding the signaling of a GPCR heteromeric complex reveals a unifying mechanism of action of antipsychotic drugs. Cell 147:1011–1023. https://doi.org/10.1016/j.cell.2011.09.055

Gabra BH, Smith FL, Navarro HA, Carroll FI, Dewey WL (2008) mGluR5 antagonists that block calcium mobilization in vitro also reverse (S)-3,5-DHPG-induced hyperalgesia and morphine antinociceptive tolerance in vivo. Brain Res 1187:58–66. https://doi.org/10.1016/j.brainres.2007.10.007

Gao X, Majetschak M (2023) G protein activation via chemokine (C-X-C motif) receptor 4 and alpha(1b) -adrenoceptor is ligand and heteromer-dependent. FEBS Lett 597:2017–2027. https://doi.org/10.1002/1873-3468.14692

Gao X, Abdelkarim H, Albee LJ, Volkman BF, Gaponenko V, Majetschak M (2018a) Partial agonist activity of alpha1-adrenergic receptor antagonists for chemokine (C-X-C motif) receptor 4 and atypical chemokine receptor 3. PLoS One 13:e0204041. https://doi.org/10.1371/journal.pone.0204041

Gao X, Albee LJ, Volkman BF, Gaponenko V, Majetschak M (2018b) Asymmetrical ligand-induced cross-regulation of chemokine (C-X-C motif) receptor 4 by alpha(1)-adrenergic receptors at the heteromeric receptor complex. Sci Rep 8:2730. https://doi.org/10.1038/s41598-018-21096-4

Gerbier R, Ndiaye-Lobry D, Martinez de Morentin PB, Cecon E, Heisler LK, Delagrange P, Gbahou F, Jockers R (2021) Pharmacological evidence for transactivation within melatonin MT(2) and serotonin 5-HT(2C) receptor heteromers in mouse brain. FASEB J 35:e21161. https://doi.org/10.1096/fj.202000305R

Gines S, Hillion J, Torvinen M, Le Crom S, Casado V, Canela EI, Rondin S, Lew JY, Watson S, Zoli M, Agnati LF, Verniera P, Lluis C, Ferre S, Fuxe K, Franco R (2000) Dopamine D1 and adenosine A1 receptors form functionally interacting heteromeric complexes. Proc Natl Acad Sci USA 97:8606–8611. https://doi.org/10.1073/pnas.150241097

Giri AK, Apostol CR, Wang Y, Forte BL, Largent-Milnes TM, Davis P, Rankin D, Molnar G, Olson KM, Porreca F, Vanderah TW, Hruby VJ (2015) Discovery of novel multifunctional ligands with mu/delta opioid agonist/Neurokinin-1 (NK1) antagonist activities for the treatment of pain. J Med Chem 58:8573–8583. https://doi.org/10.1021/acs.jmedchem.5b01170

Gironacci MM, Bruna-Haupt E (2024) Unraveling the crosstalk between renin-angiotensin system receptors. Acta Physiol (Oxf) 240:e14134. https://doi.org/10.1111/apha.14134

Gironacci MM, Valera MS, Yujnovsky I, Pena C (2004) Angiotensin-(1-7) inhibitory mechanism of norepinephrine release in hypertensive rats. Hypertension 44:783–787. https://doi.org/10.1161/01.HYP.0000143850.73831.9d

Gomes I, Fujita W, Gupta A, Saldanha SA, Negri A, Pinello CE, Eberhart C, Roberts E, Filizola M, Hodder P, Devi LA (2013) Identification of a mu-delta opioid receptor heteromer-biased agonist with antinociceptive activity. Proc Natl Acad Sci USA 110:12072–12077. https://doi.org/10.1073/pnas.1222044110

Gomes I, Ayoub MA, Fujita W, Jaeger WC, Pfleger KD, Devi LA (2016) G protein-coupled receptor Heteromers. Annu Rev Pharmacol Toxicol 56:403–425. https://doi.org/10.1146/annurev-pharmtox-011613-135952

Gonzalez-Maeso J, Ang RL, Yuen T, Chan P, Weisstaub NV, Lopez-Gimenez JF, Zhou M, Okawa Y, Callado LF, Milligan G, Gingrich JA, Filizola M, Meana JJ, Sealfon SC (2008) Identification of a serotonin/glutamate receptor complex implicated in psychosis. Nature 452:93–97. https://doi.org/10.1038/nature06612

Grant PS, Kahlcke N, Govindpani K, Hunter M, MacDonald C, Brimble MA, Glass M, Furkert DP (2019) Divalent cannabinoid-1 receptor ligands: a linker attachment point survey of SR141716A for development of high-affinity CB1R molecular probes. Bioorg Med Chem Lett 29:126644. https://doi.org/10.1016/j.bmcl.2019.126644

Gregan B, Jurgensen J, Papsdorf G, Furkert J, Schaefer M, Beyermann M, Rosenthal W, Oksche A (2004) Ligand-dependent differences in the internalization of endothelin A and endothelin B receptor heterodimers. J Biol Chem 279:27679–27687. https://doi.org/10.1074/jbc.M403601200

Guitart X, Navarro G, Moreno E, Yano H, Cai NS, Sanchez-Soto M, Kumar-Barodia S, Naidu YT, Mallol J, Cortes A, Lluis C, Canela EI, Casado V, McCormick PJ, Ferre S (2014) Functional selectivity of allosteric interactions within G protein-coupled receptor oligomers: the dopamine D1-D3 receptor heterotetramer. Mol Pharmacol 86:417–429. https://doi.org/10.1124/mol.114.093096

Guitart X, Moreno E, Rea W, Sanchez-Soto M, Cai NS, Quiroz C, Kumar V, Bourque L, Cortes A, Canela EI, Bishop C, Newman AH, Casado V, Ferre S (2019) Biased G protein-independent signaling of dopamine D(1)-D(3) receptor Heteromers in the nucleus Accumbens. Mol Neurobiol 56:6756–6769. https://doi.org/10.1007/s12035-019-1564-8

Gupta A, Mulder J, Gomes I, Rozenfeld R, Bushlin I, Ong E, Lim M, Maillet E, Junek M, Cahill CM, Harkany T, Devi LA (2010) Increased abundance of opioid receptor heteromers after chronic morphine administration. Sci Signal 3:ra54. https://doi.org/10.1126/scisignal.2000807

Gupta A, Gomes I, Osman A, Fujita W, Devi LA (2024) Regulation of cannabinoid and opioid receptor levels by endogenous and pharmacological chaperones. J Pharmacol Exp Ther 391:279–288. https://doi.org/10.1124/jpet.124.002187

Haack KK, Tougas MR, Jones KT, El-Dahr SS, Radhakrishna H, McCarty NA (2010) A novel bioassay for detecting GPCR heterodimerization: transactivation of beta 2 adrenergic receptor by bradykinin receptor. J Biomol Screen 15:251–260. https://doi.org/10.1177/1087057109360254

Hammad MM, Kuang YQ, Yan R, Allen H, Dupre DJ (2010) Na+/H+ exchanger regulatory factor-1 is involved in chemokine receptor homodimer CCR5 internalization and signal transduction but does not affect CXCR4 homodimer or CXCR4-CCR5 heterodimer. J Biol Chem 285:34653–34664. https://doi.org/10.1074/jbc.M110.106591

Hannan S, Wilkins ME, Dehghani-Tafti E, Thomas P, Baddeley SM, Smart TG (2011) Gamma-aminobutyric acid type B (GABA(B)) receptor internalization is regulated by the R2 subunit. J Biol Chem 286:24324–24335. https://doi.org/10.1074/jbc.M110.220814

Hasbi A, Fan T, Alijaniaram M, Nguyen T, Perreault ML, O'Dowd BF, George SR (2009) Calcium signaling cascade links dopamine D1-D2 receptor heteromer to striatal BDNF production and neuronal growth. Proc Natl Acad Sci USA 106:21377–21382. https://doi.org/10.1073/pnas.0903676106

Hasbi A, Sivasubramanian M, Milenkovic M, Komarek K, Madras BK, George SR (2020) Dopamine D1-D2 receptor heteromer expression in key brain regions of rat and higher species: upregulation in rat striatum after cocaine administration. Neurobiol Dis 143:105017. https://doi.org/10.1016/j.nbd.2020.105017

Hashimoto Y, Niikura T, Tajima H, Yasukawa T, Sudo H, Ito Y, Kita Y, Kawasumi M, Kouyama K, Doyu M, Sobue G, Koide T, Tsuji S, Lang J, Kurokawa K, Nishimoto I (2001) A rescue factor abolishing neuronal cell death by a wide spectrum of familial Alzheimer's disease genes and Abeta. Proc Natl Acad Sci USA 98:6336–6341. https://doi.org/10.1073/pnas.101133498

Haspula D, Clark MA (2017) MAPK activation patterns of AT1R and CB1R in SHR versus Wistar astrocytes: evidence of CB1R hypofunction and crosstalk between AT1R and CB1R. Cell Signal 40:81–90. https://doi.org/10.1016/j.cellsig.2017.09.002

Hauser AS, Attwood MM, Rask-Andersen M, Schioth HB, Gloriam DE (2017) Trends in GPCR drug discovery: new agents, targets and indications. Nat Rev Drug Discov 16:829–842. https://doi.org/10.1038/nrd.2017.178

Hauser AS, Chavali S, Masuho I, Jahn LJ, Martemyanov KA, Gloriam DE, Babu MM (2018) Pharmacogenomics of GPCR drug targets. Cell 172:41-+. https://doi.org/10.1016/j.cell.2017.11.033

Heyder NA, Kleinau G, Speck D, Schmidt A, Paisdzior S, Szczepek M, Bauer B, Koch A, Gallandi M, Kwiatkowski D, Burger J, Mielke T, Beck-Sickinger AG, Hildebrand PW, Spahn CMT, Hilger D, Schacherl M, Biebermann H, Hilal T, Kuhnen P, Kobilka BK, Scheerer P (2021) Structures of active melanocortin-4 receptor-Gs-protein complexes with NDP-alpha-MSH and setmelanotide. Cell Res 31:1176–1189. https://doi.org/10.1038/s41422-021-00569-8

Hounsou C, Margathe JF, Oueslati N, Belhocine A, Dupuis E, Thomas C, Mann A, Ilien B, Rognan D, Trinquet E, Hibert M, Pin JP, Bonnet D, Durroux T (2015) Time-resolved FRET binding assay to investigate hetero-oligomer binding properties: proof of concept with dopamine D1/D3 heterodimer. ACS Chem Biol 10:466–474. https://doi.org/10.1021/cb5007568

Huang Y, Todd N, Thathiah A (2017) The role of GPCRs in neurodegenerative diseases: avenues for therapeutic intervention. Curr Opin Pharmacol 32:96–110. https://doi.org/10.1016/j.coph.2017.02.001

Huang B, Wang H, Zheng Y, Li M, Kang G, Barreto-de-Souza V, Nassehi N, Knapp PE, Selley DE, Hauser KF, Zhang Y (2021) Structure-based design and development of chemical probes targeting putative MOR-CCR5 heterodimers to inhibit opioid exacerbated HIV-1 infectivity. J Med Chem 64:7702–7723. https://doi.org/10.1021/acs.jmedchem.1c00408

Huang W, Jin N, Guo J, Shen C, Xu C, Xi K, Bonhomme L, Quast RB, Shen DD, Qin J, Liu YR, Song Y, Gao Y, Margeat E, Rondard P, Pin JP, Zhang Y, Liu J (2024) Structural basis of orientated asymmetry in a mGlu heterodimer. Nat Commun 15:10345. https://doi.org/10.1038/s41467-024-54744-7

Hubner H, Schellhorn T, Gienger M, Schaab C, Kaindl J, Leeb L, Clark T, Moller D, Gmeiner P (2016) Structure-guided development of heterodimer-selective GPCR ligands. Nat Commun 7:12298. https://doi.org/10.1038/ncomms12298

Jaeger WC, Armstrong SP, Hill SJ, Pfleger KD (2014) Biophysical detection of diversity and bias in GPCR function. Front Endocrinol (Lausanne) 5:26. https://doi.org/10.3389/fendo.2014.00026

Jaquet P, Gunz G, Saveanu A, Barlier A, Dufour H, Taylor J, Dong J, Kim S, Moreau JP, Culler MD (2005) BIM-23A760, a chimeric molecule directed towards somatostatin and dopamine receptors, vs universal somatostatin receptors ligands in GH-secreting pituitary adenomas partial responders to octreotide. J Endocrinol Investig 28:21–27

Jarrahian A, Watts VJ, Barker EL (2004) D2 dopamine receptors modulate Galpha-subunit coupling of the CB1 cannabinoid receptor. J Pharmacol Exp Ther 308:880–886. https://doi.org/10.1124/jpet.103.057620

Jockers R, Maurice P, Boutin JA, Delagrange P (2008) Melatonin receptors, heterodimerization, signal transduction and binding sites: what's new? Br J Pharmacol 154:1182–1195. https://doi.org/10.1038/bjp.2008.184

Johnstone EKM, Ayoub MA, Hertzman RJ, See HB, Abhayawardana RS, Seeber RM, Pfleger KDG (2022) Novel pharmacology following Heteromerization of the angiotensin II type 2 receptor and the bradykinin type 2 receptor. Front Endocrinol (Lausanne) 13:848816. https://doi.org/10.3389/fendo.2022.848816

Kabli N, Fan T, O'Dowd BF, George SR (2014) mu-delta opioid receptor heteromer-specific signaling in the striatum and hippocampus. Biochem Biophys Res Commun 450:906–911. https://doi.org/10.1016/j.bbrc.2014.06.099

Kamal M, Gbahou F, Guillaume JL, Daulat AM, Benleulmi-Chaachoua A, Luka M, Chen P, Kalbasi Anaraki D, Baroncini M, Mannoury la Cour C, Millan MJ, Prevot V, Delagrange P, Jockers R (2015) Convergence of melatonin and serotonin (5-HT) signaling at MT2/5-HT2C receptor heteromers. J Biol Chem 290:11537–11546. https://doi.org/10.1074/jbc.M114.559542

Kaneider NC, Leger AJ, Agarwal A, Nguyen N, Perides G, Derian C, Covic L, Kuliopulos A (2007) 'Role reversal' for the receptor PAR1 in sepsis-induced vascular damage. Nat Immunol 8:1303–1312. https://doi.org/10.1038/ni1525

Kapsokalyvas D, Schiffers PM, Maij N, Suylen DP, Hackeng TM, van Zandvoort MA, De Mey JG (2014) Imaging evidence for endothelin ETA/ETB receptor heterodimers in isolated rat mesenteric resistance arteries. Life Sci 111:36–41. https://doi.org/10.1016/j.lfs.2014.07.007

Kaupmann K, Malitschek B, Schuler V, Heid J, Froest W, Beck P, Mosbacher J, Bischoff S, Kulik A, Shigemoto R, Karschin A, Bettler B (1998) GABA(B)-receptor subtypes assemble into functional heteromeric complexes. Nature 396:683–687. https://doi.org/10.1038/25360

Kearn CS, Blake-Palmer K, Daniel E, Mackie K, Glass M (2005) Concurrent stimulation of cannabinoid CB1 and dopamine D2 receptors enhances heterodimer formation: a mechanism for receptor cross-talk? Mol Pharmacol 67:1697–1704. https://doi.org/10.1124/mol.104.006882

Kern A, Albarran-Zeckler R, Walsh HE, Smith RG (2012) Apo-ghrelin receptor forms heteromers with DRD2 in hypothalamic neurons and is essential for anorexigenic effects of DRD2 agonism. Neuron 73:317–332. https://doi.org/10.1016/j.neuron.2011.10.038

Khare T, Bissonnette M, Khare S (2021) CXCL12-CXCR4/CXCR7 Axis in colorectal cancer: therapeutic target in preclinical and clinical studies. Int J Mol Sci 22. https://doi.org/10.3390/ijms22147371

Kim S, Hahn YK, Podhaizer EM, McLane VD, Zou S, Hauser KF, Knapp PE (2018) A central role for glial CCR5 in directing the neuropathological interactions of HIV-1 Tat and opiates. J Neuroinflammation 15:285. https://doi.org/10.1186/s12974-018-1320-4

Kniazeff J, Prezeau L, Rondard P, Pin JP, Goudet C (2011) Dimers and beyond: the functional puzzles of class C GPCRs. Pharmacol Ther 130:9–25. https://doi.org/10.1016/j.pharmthera.2011.01.006

Kofalvi A, Moreno E, Cordomi A, Cai NS, Fernandez-Duenas V, Ferreira SG, Guixa-Gonzalez R, Sanchez-Soto M, Yano H, Casado-Anguera V, Cunha RA, Sebastiao AM, Ciruela F, Pardo L, Casado V, Ferre S (2020) Control of glutamate release by complexes of adenosine and cannabinoid receptors. BMC Biol 18:9. https://doi.org/10.1186/s12915-020-0739-0

Koid SS, Ziogas J, Campbell DJ (2014) Aliskiren reduces myocardial ischemia-reperfusion injury by a bradykinin B2 receptor- and angiotensin AT2 receptor-mediated mechanism. Hypertension 63:768–773. https://doi.org/10.1161/HYPERTENSIONAHA.113.02902

Kononoff Vanhanen J, Nuutinen S, Tuominen M, Panula P (2016) Histamine H3 receptor regulates sensorimotor gating and dopaminergic signaling in the striatum. J Pharmacol Exp Ther 357:264–272. https://doi.org/10.1124/jpet.115.230771

Koschatzky S, Tschammer N, Gmeiner P (2011) Cross-receptor interactions between dopamine D2L and neurotensin NTS1 receptors modulate binding affinities of dopaminergics. ACS Chem Neurosci 2:308–316. https://doi.org/10.1021/cn200020y

Koshimizu TA, Honda K, Nagaoka-Uozumi S, Ichimura A, Kimura I, Nakaya M, Sakai N, Shibata K, Ushijima K, Fujimura A, Hirasawa A, Kurose H, Tsujimoto G, Tanoue A, Takano Y (2018) Complex formation between the vasopressin 1b receptor, beta-arrestin-2, and the mu-opioid receptor underlies morphine tolerance. Nat Neurosci 21:820–833. https://doi.org/10.1038/s41593-018-0144-y

Kowalczyk A, Kleczkowska P, Rekawek M, Kulik K, Lesniak A, Erdei A, Borics A, Martin C, Pawlik K, Lipkowski AW, Benyhe S, Makulska-Nowak H, Ballet S, Bujalska-Zadrozny M (2016) Biological evaluation and molecular docking studies of AA3052, a compound containing a mu-selective opioid peptide agonist DALDA and d-Phe-Phe-d-Phe-Leu-Leu-

NH2, a substance P analogue. Eur J Pharm Sci 93:11–20. https://doi.org/10.1016/j.ejps.2016.07.009
Kowalik A, Majerek M, Mrowiec K, Solich J, Faron-Gorecka A, Woznicka O, Dziedzicka-Wasylewska M, Lukasiewicz S (2022) Dopamine D(2) and serotonin 5-HT(1A) dimeric receptor-binding monomeric antibody scFv as a potential ligand for carrying drugs targeting selected areas of the brain. Biomolecules 12:749. https://doi.org/10.3390/biom12060749
Krishna Kumar K, O'Brien ES, Habrian CH, Latorraca NR, Wang H, Tuneew I, Montabana E, Marqusee S, Hilger D, Isacoff EY, Mathiesen JM, Kobilka BK (2023) Negative allosteric modulation of the glucagon receptor by RAMP2. Cell 186:1465–1477 e18. https://doi.org/10.1016/j.cell.2023.02.028
Labandeira-Garcia JL, Labandeira CM, Guerra MJ, Rodriguez-Perez AI (2024) The role of the brain renin-angiotensin system in Parkinson s disease. Transl Neurodegener 13:22. https://doi.org/10.1186/s40035-024-00410-3
Lanza K, Meadows SM, Chambers NE, Nuss E, Deak MM, Ferre S, Bishop C (2018) Behavioral and cellular dopamine D(1) and D(3) receptor-mediated synergy: implications for L-DOPA-induced dyskinesia. Neuropharmacology 138:304–314. https://doi.org/10.1016/j.neuropharm.2018.06.024
Largent-Milnes TM, Brookshire SW, Skinner DP Jr, Hanlon KE, Giuvelis D, Yamamoto T, Davis P, Campos CR, Nair P, Deekonda S, Bilsky EJ, Porreca F, Hruby VJ, Vanderah TW (2013) Building a better analgesic: multifunctional compounds that address injury-induced pathology to enhance analgesic efficacy while eliminating unwanted side effects. J Pharmacol Exp Ther 347:7–19. https://doi.org/10.1124/jpet.113.205245
Lavoie C, Mercier JF, Salahpour A, Umapathy D, Breit A, Villeneuve LR, Zhu WZ, Xiao RP, Lakatta EG, Bouvier M, Hebert TE (2002) Beta 1/beta 2-adrenergic receptor heterodimerization regulates beta 2-adrenergic receptor internalization and ERK signaling efficacy. J Biol Chem 277:35402–35410. https://doi.org/10.1074/jbc.M204163200
Lee SP, So CH, Rashid AJ, Varghese G, Cheng R, Lanca AJ, O'Dowd BF, George SR (2004) Dopamine D1 and D2 receptor Co-activation generates a novel phospholipase C-mediated calcium signal. J Biol Chem 279:35671–35678. https://doi.org/10.1074/jbc.M401923200
Lee VH, Lee LT, Chu JY, Lam IP, Siu FK, Vaudry H, Chow BK (2010) An indispensable role of secretin in mediating the osmoregulatory functions of angiotensin II. FASEB J 24:5024–5032. https://doi.org/10.1096/fj.10-165399
Lee LT, Ng SY, Chu JY, Sekar R, Harikumar KG, Miller LJ, Chow BK (2014) Transmembrane peptides as unique tools to demonstrate the in vivo action of a cross-class GPCR heterocomplex. FASEB J 28:2632–2644. https://doi.org/10.1096/fj.13-246868
Lee J, Munguba H, Gutzeit VA, Singh DR, Kristt M, Dittman JS, Levitz J (2020) Defining the homo- and Heterodimerization propensities of metabotropic glutamate receptors. Cell Rep 31: 107891. https://doi.org/10.1016/j.celrep.2020.107891
Leon-Navarro DA, Albasanz JL, Martin M (2019) Functional cross-talk between adenosine and metabotropic glutamate receptors. Curr Neuropharmacol 17:422–437. https://doi.org/10.2174/1570159X16666180416093717
Levoye A, Dam J, Ayoub MA, Guillaume JL, Couturier C, Delagrange P, Jockers R (2006a) The orphan GPR50 receptor specifically inhibits MT1 melatonin receptor function through heterodimerization. EMBO J 25:3012–3023. https://doi.org/10.1038/sj.emboj.7601193
Levoye A, Dam J, Ayoub MA, Guillaume JL, Jockers R (2006b) Do orphan G-protein-coupled receptors have ligand-independent functions? New insights from receptor heterodimers. EMBO Rep 7:1094–1098. https://doi.org/10.1038/sj.embor.7400838
Levoye A, Balabanian K, Baleux F, Bachelerie F, Lagane B (2009) CXCR7 heterodimerizes with CXCR4 and regulates CXCL12-mediated G protein signaling. Blood 113:6085–6093. https://doi.org/10.1182/blood-2008-12-196618
Li YH, Xiang K, Xu X, Zhao X, Li Y, Zheng L, Wang J (2018) Co-activation of both 5-HT(1A) and 5-HT(7) receptors induced attenuation of glutamatergic synaptic transmission in the rat visual cortex. Neurosci Lett 686:122–126. https://doi.org/10.1016/j.neulet.2018.09.013

Lin H, Trejo J (2013) Transactivation of the PAR1-PAR2 heterodimer by thrombin elicits beta-arrestin-mediated endosomal signaling. J Biol Chem 288:11203–11215. https://doi.org/10.1074/jbc.M112.439950

Lin H, Liu AP, Smith TH, Trejo J (2013) Cofactoring and dimerization of proteinase-activated receptors. Pharmacol Rev 65:1198–1213. https://doi.org/10.1124/pr.111.004747

Lindemann L, Meyer CA, Jeanneau K, Bradaia A, Ozmen L, Bluethmann H, Bettler B, Wettstein JG, Borroni E, Moreau JL, Hoener MC (2008) Trace amine-associated receptor 1 modulates dopaminergic activity. J Pharmacol Exp Ther 324:948–956. https://doi.org/10.1124/jpet.107.132647

Liu XY, Liu ZC, Sun YG, Ross M, Kim S, Tsai FF, Li QF, Jeffry J, Kim JY, Loh HH, Chen ZF (2011) Unidirectional cross-activation of GRPR by MOR1D uncouples itch and analgesia induced by opioids. Cell 147:447–458. https://doi.org/10.1016/j.cell.2011.08.043

Liu J, Zhang Z, Moreno-Delgado D, Dalton JA, Rovira X, Trapero A, Goudet C, Llebaria A, Giraldo J, Yuan Q, Rondard P, Huang S, Liu J, Pin JP (2017) Allosteric control of an asymmetric transduction in a G protein-coupled receptor heterodimer. elife 6. https://doi.org/10.7554/eLife.26985

Liu J, Tang H, Xu C, Zhou S, Zhu X, Li Y, Prezeau L, Xu T, Pin JP, Rondard P, Ji W, Liu J (2022) Biased signaling due to oligomerization of the G protein-coupled platelet-activating factor receptor. Nat Commun 13:6365. https://doi.org/10.1038/s41467-022-34056-4

Liu L, Lin L, Shen C, Rondard P, Pin JP, Xu C, Liu J (2023) Asymmetric activation of dimeric GABA(B) and metabotropic glutamate receptors. Am J Physiol Cell Physiol 325:C79–C89. https://doi.org/10.1152/ajpcell.00150.2022

Lukasiewicz S, Polit A, Kedracka-Krok S, Wedzony K, Mackowiak M, Dziedzicka-Wasylewska M (2010) Hetero-dimerization of serotonin 5-HT(2A) and dopamine D(2) receptors. Biochim Biophys Acta 1803:1347–1358. https://doi.org/10.1016/j.bbamcr.2010.08.010

Lukasiewicz S, Blasiak E, Szafran-Pilch K, Dziedzicka-Wasylewska M (2016) Dopamine D2 and serotonin 5-HT1A receptor interaction in the context of the effects of antipsychotics – in vitro studies. J Neurochem 137:549–560. https://doi.org/10.1111/jnc.13582

Madhusudhan T, Wang H, Straub BK, Grone E, Zhou Q, Shahzad K, Muller-Krebs S, Schwenger V, Gerlitz B, Grinnell BW, Griffin JH, Reiser J, Grone HJ, Esmon CT, Nawroth PP, Isermann B (2012) Cytoprotective signaling by activated protein C requires protease-activated receptor-3 in podocytes. Blood 119:874–883. https://doi.org/10.1182/blood-2011-07-365973

Maggio R, Millan MJ (2010) Dopamine D2-D3 receptor heteromers: pharmacological properties and therapeutic significance. Curr Opin Pharmacol 10:100–107. https://doi.org/10.1016/j.coph.2009.10.001

Maggio R, Scarselli M, Capannolo M, Millan MJ (2015) Novel dimensions of D3 receptor function: focus on heterodimerisation, transactivation and allosteric modulation. Eur Neuropsychopharmacol 25:1470–1479. https://doi.org/10.1016/j.euroneuro.2014.09.016

Maroteaux L, Bechade C, Roumier A (2019) Dimers of serotonin receptors: impact on ligand affinity and signaling. Biochimie 161:23–33. https://doi.org/10.1016/j.biochi.2019.01.009

Martin AB, Fernandez-Espejo E, Ferrer B, Gorriti MA, Bilbao A, Navarro M, Rodriguez de Fonseca F, Moratalla R (2008) Expression and function of CB1 receptor in the rat striatum: localization and effects on D1 and D2 dopamine receptor-mediated motor behaviors. Neuropsychopharmacology 33:1667–1679. https://doi.org/10.1038/sj.npp.1301558

Martinez-Munoz L, Barroso R, Dyrhaug SY, Navarro G, Lucas P, Soriano SF, Vega B, Costas C, Munoz-Fernandez MA, Santiago C, Rodriguez Frade JM, Franco R, Mellado M (2014) CCR5/CD4/CXCR4 oligomerization prevents HIV-1 gp120IIIB binding to the cell surface. Proc Natl Acad Sci USA 111:E1960–E1969. https://doi.org/10.1073/pnas.1322887111

Martinez-Pinilla E, Rodriguez-Perez AI, Navarro G, Aguinaga D, Moreno E, Lanciego JL, Labandeira-Garcia JL, Franco R (2015) Dopamine D2 and angiotensin II type 1 receptors form functional heteromers in rat striatum. Biochem Pharmacol 96:131–142. https://doi.org/10.1016/j.bcp.2015.05.006

Martinez-Pinilla E, Rabal O, Reyes-Resina I, Zamarbide M, Navarro G, Sanchez-Arias JA, de Miguel I, Lanciego JL, Oyarzabal J, Franco R (2016) Two affinity sites of the cannabinoid subtype 2 receptor identified by a novel homogeneous binding assay. J Pharmacol Exp Ther 358:580–587. https://doi.org/10.1124/jpet.116.234948

Martinez-Pinilla E, Rico AJ, Rivas-Santisteban R, Lillo J, Roda E, Navarro G, Lanciego JL, Franco R (2020) Expression of GPR55 and either cannabinoid CB(1) or CB(2) heteroreceptor complexes in the caudate, putamen, and accumbens nuclei of control, parkinsonian, and dyskinetic non-human primates. Brain Struct Funct 225:2153–2164. https://doi.org/10.1007/s00429-020-02116-4

Matalinska J, Lipinski PFJ, Kosson P, Kosinska K, Misicka A (2020) In vivo, in vitro and in silico studies of the hybrid compound AA3266, an opioid agonist/NK1R antagonist with selective cytotoxicity. Int J Mol Sci 21. https://doi.org/10.3390/ijms21207738

McEachron TA, Pawlinski R, Richards KL, Church FC, Mackman N (2010) Protease-activated receptors mediate crosstalk between coagulation and fibrinolysis. Blood 116:5037–5044. https://doi.org/10.1182/blood-2010-06-293126

McGraw DW, Mihlbachler KA, Schwarb MR, Rahman FF, Small KM, Almoosa KF, Liggett SB (2006) Airway smooth muscle prostaglandin-EP1 receptors directly modulate beta2-adrenergic receptors within a unique heterodimeric complex. J Clin Invest 116:1400–1409. https://doi.org/10.1172/JCI25840

McLaughlin JN, Patterson MM, Malik AB (2007) Protease-activated receptor-3 (PAR3) regulates PAR1 signaling by receptor dimerization. Proc Natl Acad Sci USA 104:5662–5667. https://doi.org/10.1073/pnas.0700763104

Mellado M, Rodriguez-Frade JM, Vila-Coro AJ, Fernandez S, Martin de Ana A, Jones DR, Toran JL, Martinez AC (2001) Chemokine receptor homo- or heterodimerization activates distinct signaling pathways. EMBO J 20:2497–2507. https://doi.org/10.1093/emboj/20.10.2497

Menendez-Perez C, Rivas-Santisteban R, Del Valle E, Tolivia J, Navarro A, Franco R, Martinez-Pinilla E (2024) Heteromers formed by GPR55 and either cannabinoid CB(1) or CB(2) receptors are upregulated in the prefrontal cortex of multiple sclerosis patients. Int J Mol Sci 25. https://doi.org/10.3390/ijms25084176

Meng J, Xu C, Lafon P-A, Roux S, Mathieu M, Zhou R, Scholler P, Blanc E, Becker JAJ, Le Merrer J, González-Maeso J, Chames P, Liu J, Pin J-P, Rondard P (2022) Nanobody-based sensors reveal a high proportion of mGlu heterodimers in the brain. Nat Chem Biol 18. https://doi.org/10.1038/s41589-022-01050-2

Mercier JF, Salahpour A, Angers S, Breit A, Bouvier M (2002) Quantitative assessment of beta 1- and beta 2-adrenergic receptor homo- and heterodimerization by bioluminescence resonance energy transfer. J Biol Chem 277:44925–44931. https://doi.org/10.1074/jbc.M205767200

Misganaw D (2021) Heteromerization of dopaminergic receptors in the brain: pharmacological implications. Pharmacol Res 170:105600. https://doi.org/10.1016/j.phrs.2021.105600

Miskiewicz A, Kowalczyk P, Oraibi SM, Cybulska K, Misiewicz A (2018) Bird feathers as potential sources of pathogenic microorganisms: a new look at old diseases. Antonie Van Leeuwenhoek 111:1493–1507. https://doi.org/10.1007/s10482-018-1048-2

Mitroshina EV, Marasanova EA, Vedunova MV (2023) Functional dimerization of serotonin receptors: role in health and depressive disorders. Int J Mol Sci 24. https://doi.org/10.3390/ijms242216416

Miyagi H, Asada H, Suzuki M, Takahashi Y, Yasunaga M, Suno C, Iwata S, Saito JI (2020) The discovery of a new antibody for BRIL-fused GPCR structure determination. Sci Rep 10:11669. https://doi.org/10.1038/s41598-020-68355-x

Moller TC, Hottin J, Clerte C, Zwier JM, Durroux T, Rondard P, Prezeau L, Royer CA, Pin JP, Margeat E, Kniazeff J (2018) Oligomerization of a G protein-coupled receptor in neurons controlled by its structural dynamics. Sci Rep 8:10414. https://doi.org/10.1038/s41598-018-28682-6

Molon B, Gri G, Bettella M, Gomez-Mouton C, Lanzavecchia A, Martinez AC, Manes S, Viola A (2005) T cell costimulation by chemokine receptors. Nat Immunol 6:465–471. https://doi.org/10.1038/ni1191

Moreno E, Hoffmann H, Gonzalez-Sepulveda M, Navarro G, Casado V, Cortes A, Mallol J, Vignes M, McCormick PJ, Canela EI, Lluis C, Moratalla R, Ferre S, Ortiz J, Franco R (2011) Dopamine D1-histamine H3 receptor heteromers provide a selective link to MAPK signaling in GABAergic neurons of the direct striatal pathway. J Biol Chem 286:5846–5854. https://doi.org/10.1074/jbc.M110.161489

Moreno E, Andradas C, Medrano M, Caffarel MM, Perez-Gomez E, Blasco-Benito S, Gomez-Canas M, Pazos MR, Irving AJ, Lluis C, Canela EI, Fernandez-Ruiz J, Guzman M, McCormick PJ, Sanchez C (2014a) Targeting CB2-GPR55 receptor heteromers modulates cancer cell signaling. J Biol Chem 289:21960–21972. https://doi.org/10.1074/jbc.M114.561761

Moreno E, Moreno-Delgado D, Navarro G, Hoffmann HM, Fuentes S, Rosell-Vilar S, Gasperini P, Rodriguez-Ruiz M, Medrano M, Mallol J, Cortes A, Casado V, Lluis C, Ferre S, Ortiz J, Canela E, McCormick PJ (2014b) Cocaine disrupts histamine H3 receptor modulation of dopamine D1 receptor signaling: sigma1-D1-H3 receptor complexes as key targets for reducing cocaine's effects. J Neurosci 34:3545–3558. https://doi.org/10.1523/JNEUROSCI.4147-13.2014

Moreno JL, Miranda-Azpiazu P, Garcia-Bea A, Younkin J, Cui M, Kozlenkov A, Ben-Ezra A, Voloudakis G, Fakira AK, Baki L, Ge Y, Georgakopoulos A, Moron JA, Milligan G, Lopez-Gimenez JF, Robakis NK, Logothetis DE, Meana JJ, Gonzalez-Maeso J (2016) Allosteric signaling through an mGlu2 and 5-HT2A heteromeric receptor complex and its potential contribution to schizophrenia. Sci Signal 9:ra5. https://doi.org/10.1126/scisignal.aab0467

Mores KL, Cassell RJ, van Rijn RM (2019) Arrestin recruitment and signaling by G protein-coupled receptor heteromers. Neuropharmacology 152:15–21. https://doi.org/10.1016/j.neuropharm.2018.11.010

Mottolese R, Redoute J, Costes N, Le Bars D, Sirigu A (2014) Switching brain serotonin with oxytocin. Proc Natl Acad Sci USA 111:8637–8642. https://doi.org/10.1073/pnas.1319810111

Moutkine I, Quentin E, Guiard BP, Maroteaux L, Doly S (2017) Heterodimers of serotonin receptor subtypes 2 are driven by 5-HT2C protomers. J Biol Chem 292:6352–6368. https://doi.org/10.1074/jbc.M117.779041

Muller CP, Homberg JR (2015) The role of serotonin in drug use and addiction. Behav Brain Res 277:146–192. https://doi.org/10.1016/j.bbr.2014.04.007

Nakanishi-Matsui M, Zheng YW, Sulciner DJ, Weiss EJ, Ludeman MJ, Coughlin SR (2000) PAR3 is a cofactor for PAR4 activation by thrombin. Nature 404:609–613. https://doi.org/10.1038/35007085

Nakata H, Yoshioka K, Kamiya T, Tsuga H, Oyanagi K (2005) Functions of heteromeric association between adenosine and P2Y receptors. J Mol Neurosci 26:233–238. https://doi.org/10.1385/JMN:26:2-3:233

Naumenko VS, Popova NK, Lacivita E, Leopoldo M, Ponimaskin EG (2014) Interplay between serotonin 5-HT1A and 5-HT7 receptors in depressive disorders. CNS Neurosci Ther 20:582–590. https://doi.org/10.1111/cns.12247

Ng HK, Chow BK (2015) Oligomerization of family B GPCRs: exploration in inter-family oligomer formation. Front Endocrinol (Lausanne) 6:10. https://doi.org/10.3389/fendo.2015.00010

Nishi A, Liu F, Matsuyama S, Hamada M, Higashi H, Nairn AC, Greengard P (2003) Metabotropic mGlu5 receptors regulate adenosine A2A receptor signaling. Proc Natl Acad Sci USA 100:1322–1327. https://doi.org/10.1073/pnas.0237126100

Niswender CM, Conn PJ (2010) Metabotropic glutamate receptors: physiology, pharmacology, and disease. Annu Rev Pharmacol Toxicol 50:295–322. https://doi.org/10.1146/annurev.pharmtox.011008.145533

O'Brien PJ, Prevost N, Molino M, Hollinger MK, Woolkalis MJ, Woulfe DS, Brass LF (2000) Thrombin responses in human endothelial cells. Contributions from receptors other than PAR1 include the transactivation of PAR2 by thrombin-cleaved PAR1. J Biol Chem 275:13502–13509. https://doi.org/10.1074/jbc.275.18.13502

O'Dowd BF, Nguyen T, Ji X, George SR (2013) D5 dopamine receptor carboxyl tail involved in D5-D2 heteromer formation. Biochem Biophys Res Commun 431:586–589. https://doi.org/10.1016/j.bbrc.2012.12.139

Olson KM, Keresztes A, Tashiro JK, Daconta LV, Hruby VJ, Streicher JM (2018) Synthesis and evaluation of a novel bivalent selective antagonist for the Mu-Delta opioid receptor heterodimer that reduces morphine withdrawal in mice. J Med Chem 61:6075–6086. https://doi.org/10.1021/acs.jmedchem.8b00403

Papasergi-Scott MM, Robertson MJ, Seven AB, Panova O, Mathiesen JM, Skiniotis G (2020) Structures of metabotropic GABAB receptor. Nature 584:310–314. https://doi.org/10.1038/s41586-020-2469-4

Park J, Fu Z, Frangaj A, Liu J, Mosyak L, Shen T, Slavkovich VN, Ray KM, Taura J, Cao B, Geng Y, Zuo H, Kou Y, Grassucci R, Chen S, Liu Z, Lin X, Williams JP, Rice WJ, Eng ET, Huang RK, Soni RK, Kloss B, Yu Z, Javitch JA, Hendrickson WA, Slesinger PA, Quick M, Graziano J, Yu H, Fiehn O, Clarke OB, Frank J, Fan QR (2020) Structure of human GABAB receptor in an inactive state. Nature 584:304–309. https://doi.org/10.1038/s41586-020-2452-0

Peterson CD, Kitto KF, Akgun E, Lunzer MM, Riedl MS, Vulchanova L, Wilcox GL, Portoghese PS, Fairbanks CA (2017) Bivalent ligand that activates mu opioid receptor and antagonizes mGluR5 receptor reduces neuropathic pain in mice. Pain 158:2431–2441. https://doi.org/10.1097/j.pain.0000000000001050

Pfeiffer M, Kirscht S, Stumm R, Koch T, Wu D, Laugsch M, Schroder H, Hollt V, Schulz S (2003) Heterodimerization of substance P and mu-opioid receptors regulates receptor trafficking and resensitization. J Biol Chem 278:51630–51637. https://doi.org/10.1074/jbc.M307095200

Pickel VM, Chan J, Kearn CS, Mackie K (2006) Targeting dopamine D2 and cannabinoid-1 (CB1) receptors in rat nucleus accumbens. J Comp Neurol 495:299–313. https://doi.org/10.1002/cne.20881

Pin JP, Bettler B (2016) Organization and functions of mGlu and GABAB receptor complexes. Nature 540:60–68. https://doi.org/10.1038/nature20566

Pin JP, Neubig R, Bouvier M, Devi L, Filizola M, Javitch JA, Lohse MJ, Milligan G, Palczewski K, Parmentier M, Spedding M (2007) International Union of Basic and Clinical Pharmacology. LXVII. Recommendations for the recognition and nomenclature of G protein-coupled receptor heteromultimers. Pharmacol Rev 59:5–13. https://doi.org/10.1124/pr.59.1.5

Pin JP, Kniazeff J, Prezeau L, Liu JF, Rondard P (2019) GPCR interaction as a possible way for allosteric control between receptors. Mol Cell Endocrinol 486:89–95. https://doi.org/10.1016/j.mce.2019.02.019

Plach M, Schafer T, Borroto-Escuela DO, Weikert D, Gmeiner P, Fuxe K, Friedland K (2019) Differential allosteric modulation within dopamine D(2)R – neurotensin NTS1R and D(2)R – serotonin 5-HT(2A)R receptor complexes gives bias to intracellular calcium signalling. Sci Rep 9:16312. https://doi.org/10.1038/s41598-019-52540-8

Pol O, Murtra P, Caracuel L, Valverde O, Puig MM, Maldonado R (2006) Expression of opioid receptors and c-fos in CB1 knockout mice exposed to neuropathic pain. Neuropharmacology 50:123–132. https://doi.org/10.1016/j.neuropharm.2005.11.002

Porrello ER, Pfleger KD, Seeber RM, Qian H, Oro C, Abogadie F, Delbridge LM, Thomas WG (2011) Heteromerization of angiotensin receptors changes trafficking and arrestin recruitment profiles. Cell Signal 23:1767–1776. https://doi.org/10.1016/j.cellsig.2011.06.011

Portoghese PS, Akgun E, Lunzer MM (2017) Heteromer induction: an approach to unique pharmacology? ACS Chem Neurosci 8:426–428. https://doi.org/10.1021/acschemneuro.7b00002

Poulie CBM, Liu N, Jensen AA, Bunch L (2020) Design, synthesis, and pharmacological characterization of Heterobivalent ligands for the putative 5-HT2A/mGlu2 receptor complex. J Med Chem 63:9928–9949. https://doi.org/10.1021/acs.jmedchem.0c01058

Price AE, Sholler DJ, Stutz SJ, Anastasio NC, Cunningham KA (2019) Endogenous serotonin 5-HT (2A) and 5-HT(2C) receptors associate in the medial prefrontal cortex. ACS Chem Neurosci 10: 3241–3248. https://doi.org/10.1021/acschemneuro.8b00669

Puchert M, Engele J (2014) The peculiarities of the SDF-1/CXCL12 system: in some cells, CXCR4 and CXCR7 sing solos, in others, they sing duets. Cell Tissue Res 355:239–253. https://doi.org/10.1007/s00441-013-1747-y

Pulido D, Casado-Anguera V, Gomez-Autet M, Llopart N, Moreno E, Casajuana-Martin N, Ferre S, Pardo L, Casado V, Royo M (2022) Heterobivalent ligand for the adenosine A(2A)-dopamine D (2) receptor Heteromer. J Med Chem 65:616–632. https://doi.org/10.1021/acs.jmedchem.1c01763

Racagni G, Riva MA, Molteni R, Musazzi L, Calabrese F, Popoli M, Tardito D (2011) Mode of action of agomelatine: synergy between melatonergic and 5-HT2C receptors. World J Biol Psychiatry 12:574–587. https://doi.org/10.3109/15622975.2011.595823

Rashid AJ, So CH, Kong MM, Furtak T, El-Ghundi M, Cheng R, O'Dowd BF, George SR (2007) D1-D2 dopamine receptor heterooligomers with unique pharmacology are coupled to rapid activation of Gq/11 in the striatum. Proc Natl Acad Sci USA 104:654–659. https://doi.org/10.1073/pnas.0604049104

Renner U, Zeug A, Woehler A, Niebert M, Dityatev A, Dityateva G, Gorinski N, Guseva D, Abdel-Galil D, Frohlich M, Doring F, Wischmeyer E, Richter DW, Neher E, Ponimaskin EG (2012) Heterodimerization of serotonin receptors 5-HT1A and 5-HT7 differentially regulates receptor signalling and trafficking. J Cell Sci 125:2486–2499. https://doi.org/10.1242/jcs.101337

Rios C, Gomes I, Devi LA (2006) mu opioid and CB1 cannabinoid receptor interactions: reciprocal inhibition of receptor signaling and neuritogenesis. Br J Pharmacol 148:387–395. https://doi.org/10.1038/sj.bjp.0706757

Rivas-Santisteban R, Rodriguez-Perez AI, Munoz A, Reyes-Resina I, Labandeira-Garcia JL, Navarro G, Franco R (2020) Angiotensin AT(1) and AT(2) receptor heteromer expression in the hemilesioned rat model of Parkinson's disease that increases with levodopa-induced dyskinesia. J Neuroinflammation 17:243. https://doi.org/10.1186/s12974-020-01908-z

Rivas-Santisteban R, Lillo J, Raich I, Munoz A, Lillo A, Rodriguez-Perez AI, Labandeira-Garcia JL, Navarro G, Franco R (2023) The cannabinoid CB(1) receptor interacts with the angiotensin AT(2) receptor. Overexpression of AT(2)-CB(1) receptor heteromers in the striatum of 6-hydroxydopamine hemilesioned rats. Exp Neurol 362:114319. https://doi.org/10.1016/j.expneurol.2023.114319

Rivera-Oliver M, Moreno E, Alvarez-Bagnarol Y, Ayala-Santiago C, Cruz-Reyes N, Molina-Castro GC, Clemens S, Canela EI, Ferre S, Casado V, Diaz-Rios M (2019) Adenosine A(1)-Dopamine D(1) receptor Heteromers control the excitability of the spinal Motoneuron. Mol Neurobiol 56: 797–811. https://doi.org/10.1007/s12035-018-1120-y

Rocheville M, Lange DC, Kumar U, Patel SC, Patel RC, Patel YC (2000) Receptors for dopamine and somatostatin: formation of hetero-oligomers with enhanced functional activity. Science 288:154–157. https://doi.org/10.1126/science.288.5463.154

Rodrigues RJ, Alfaro TM, Rebola N, Oliveira CR, Cunha RA (2005) Co-localization and functional interaction between adenosine A(2A) and metabotropic group 5 receptors in glutamatergic nerve terminals of the rat striatum. J Neurochem 92:433–441. https://doi.org/10.1111/j.1471-4159.2004.02887.x

Rodriguez-Frade JM, del Real G, Serrano A, Hernanz-Falcon P, Soriano SF, Vila-Coro AJ, de Ana AM, Lucas P, Prieto I, Martinez AC, Mellado M (2004) Blocking HIV-1 infection via CCR5 and CXCR4 receptors by acting in trans on the CCR2 chemokine receptor. EMBO J 23:66–76. https://doi.org/10.1038/sj.emboj.7600020

Romero-Fernandez W, Borroto-Escuela DO, Agnati LF, Fuxe K (2013) Evidence for the existence of dopamine D2-oxytocin receptor heteromers in the ventral and dorsal striatum with facilitatory receptor-receptor interactions. Mol Psychiatry 18:849–850. https://doi.org/10.1038/mp.2012.103

Rosenbaum MI, Clemmensen LS, Bredt DS, Bettler B, Stromgaard K (2020) Targeting receptor complexes: a new dimension in drug discovery. Nat Rev Drug Discov 19:884–901. https://doi.org/10.1038/s41573-020-0086-4

Rozenfeld R, Devi LA (2007) Receptor heterodimerization leads to a switch in signaling: beta-arrestin2-mediated ERK activation by mu-delta opioid receptor heterodimers. FASEB J 21: 2455–2465. https://doi.org/10.1096/fj.06-7793com

Rozenfeld R, Gupta A, Gagnidze K, Lim MP, Gomes I, Lee-Ramos D, Nieto N, Devi LA (2011) AT1R-CB(1)R heteromerization reveals a new mechanism for the pathogenic properties of angiotensin II. EMBO J 30:2350–2363. https://doi.org/10.1038/emboj.2011.139

Rozenfeld R, Bushlin I, Gomes I, Tzavaras N, Gupta A, Neves S, Battini L, Gusella GL, Lachmann A, Ma'ayan A, Blitzer RD, Devi LA (2012) Receptor heteromerization expands the repertoire of cannabinoid signaling in rodent neurons. PLoS One 7:e29239. https://doi.org/10.1371/journal.pone.0029239

Salanga CL, O'Hayre M, Handel T (2009) Modulation of chemokine receptor activity through dimerization and crosstalk. Cell Mol Life Sci 66:1370–1386. https://doi.org/10.1007/s00018-008-8666-1

Schellekens H, Dinan TG, Cryan JF (2013) Taking two to tango: a role for ghrelin receptor heterodimerization in stress and reward. Front Neurosci 7:148. https://doi.org/10.3389/fnins.2013.00148

Schoneberg T, Liebscher I (2021) Mutations in G protein-coupled receptors: mechanisms, pathophysiology and potential therapeutic approaches. Pharmacol Rev 73:89–119. https://doi.org/10.1124/pharmrev.120.000011

Schroder H, Wu DF, Seifert A, Rankovic M, Schulz S, Hollt V, Koch T (2009) Allosteric modulation of metabotropic glutamate receptor 5 affects phosphorylation, internalization, and desensitization of the micro-opioid receptor. Neuropharmacology 56:768–778. https://doi.org/10.1016/j.neuropharm.2008.12.010

Sebastianutto I, Goyet E, Andreoli L, Font-Ingles J, Moreno-Delgado D, Bouquier N, Jahannault-Talignani C, Moutin E, Di Menna L, Maslava N, Pin JP, Fagni L, Nicoletti F, Ango F, Cenci MA, Perroy J (2020) D1-mGlu5 heteromers mediate noncanonical dopamine signaling in Parkinson's disease. J Clin Invest 130:1168–1184. https://doi.org/10.1172/JCI126361

See HB, Seeber RM, Kocan M, Eidne KA, Pfleger KD (2011) Application of G protein-coupled receptor-heteromer identification technology to monitor beta-arrestin recruitment to G protein-coupled receptor heteromers. Assay Drug Dev Technol 9:21–30. https://doi.org/10.1089/adt.2010.0336

Sevigny LM, Austin KM, Zhang P, Kasuda S, Koukos G, Sharifi S, Covic L, Kuliopulos A (2011) Protease-activated receptor-2 modulates protease-activated receptor-1-driven neointimal hyperplasia. Arterioscler Thromb Vasc Biol 31:e100–e106. https://doi.org/10.1161/ATVBAHA.111.238261

Shah UH, Gonzalez-Maeso J (2019) Serotonin and glutamate interactions in preclinical schizophrenia models. ACS Chem Neurosci 10:3068–3077. https://doi.org/10.1021/acschemneuro.9b00044

Shah UH, Toneatti R, Gaitonde SA, Shin JM, Gonzalez-Maeso J (2020) Site-specific incorporation of genetically encoded photo-crosslinkers locates the Heteromeric Interface of a GPCR complex in living cells. Cell Chem Biol 27(1308–1317):e4. https://doi.org/10.1016/j.chembiol.2020.07.006

Shapira M, Gafni M, Sarne Y (1998) Independence of, and interactions between, cannabinoid and opioid signal transduction pathways in N18TG2 cells. Brain Res 806:26–35. https://doi.org/10.1016/s0006-8993(98)00697-0

Shaye H, Ishchenko A, Lam JH, Han GW, Xue L, Rondard P, Pin JP, Katritch V, Gati C, Cherezov V (2020) Structural basis of the activation of a metabotropic GABA receptor. Nature 584:298–303. https://doi.org/10.1038/s41586-020-2408-4

Shen J, Zhang L, Song WL, Meng T, Wang X, Chen L, Feng LY, Xu YC, Shen JK (2013) Design, synthesis and biological evaluation of bivalent ligands against A(1)-D(1) receptor heteromers. Acta Pharmacol Sin 34:441–452. https://doi.org/10.1038/aps.2012.151

Shen C, Mao C, Xu C, Jin N, Zhang H, Shen DD, Shen Q, Wang X, Hou T, Chen Z, Rondard P, Pin JP, Zhang Y, Liu J (2021) Structural basis of GABAB receptor-Gi protein coupling. Nature 594: 594–598. https://doi.org/10.1038/s41586-021-03507-1

Sierro F, Biben C, Martinez-Munoz L, Mellado M, Ransohoff RM, Li M, Woehl B, Leung H, Groom J, Batten M, Harvey RP, Martinez AC, Mackay CR, Mackay F (2007) Disrupted cardiac development but normal hematopoiesis in mice deficient in the second CXCL12/SDF-1 receptor, CXCR7. Proc Natl Acad Sci USA 104:14759–14764. https://doi.org/10.1073/pnas.0702229104

Smith JS, Lefkowitz RJ, Rajagopal S (2018) Biased signalling: from simple switches to allosteric microprocessors. Nat Rev Drug Discov 17:243–260. https://doi.org/10.1038/nrd.2017.229

So CH, Verma V, Alijaniaram M, Cheng R, Rashid AJ, O'Dowd BF, George SR (2009) Calcium signaling by dopamine D5 receptor and D5-D2 receptor hetero-oligomers occurs by a mechanism distinct from that for dopamine D1-D2 receptor hetero-oligomers. Mol Pharmacol 75:843–854. https://doi.org/10.1124/mol.108.051805

Sohy D, Parmentier M, Springael JY (2007) Allosteric transinhibition by specific antagonists in CCR2/CXCR4 heterodimers. J Biol Chem 282:30062–30069. https://doi.org/10.1074/jbc.M705302200

Sohy D, Yano H, de Nadai P, Urizar E, Guillabert A, Javitch JA, Parmentier M, Springael JY (2009) Hetero-oligomerization of CCR2, CCR5, and CXCR4 and the protean effects of "selective" antagonists. J Biol Chem 284:31270–31279. https://doi.org/10.1074/jbc.M109.054809

Soriano A, Ventura R, Molero A, Hoen R, Casado V, Cortes A, Fanelli F, Albericio F, Lluis C, Franco R, Royo M (2009) Adenosine A2A receptor-antagonist/dopamine D2 receptor-agonist bivalent ligands as pharmacological tools to detect A2A-D2 receptor heteromers. J Med Chem 52:5590–5602. https://doi.org/10.1021/jm900298c

Sozzani S, Vermi W, Del Prete A, Facchetti F (2010) Trafficking properties of plasmacytoid dendritic cells in health and disease. Trends Immunol 31:270–277. https://doi.org/10.1016/j.it.2010.05.004

Spengler D, Waeber C, Pantaloni C, Holsboer F, Bockaert J, Seeburg PH, Journot L (1993) Differential signal transduction by five splice variants of the PACAP receptor. Nature 365: 170–175. https://doi.org/10.1038/365170a0

Stoddart LA, Johnstone EKM, Wheal AJ, Goulding J, Robers MB, Machleidt T, Wood KV, Hill SJ, Pfleger KDG (2015) Application of BRET to monitor ligand binding to GPCRs. Nat Methods 12:661–663. https://doi.org/10.1038/nmeth.3398

Sun L, Li X, Guan H, Chen S, Fan X, Zhou C, Yang H, Xiao W (2021) A novel role of A(2A)R in the maintenance of intestinal barrier function of enteric glia from hypoxia-induced injury by combining with mGluR5. Front Pharmacol 12:633403. https://doi.org/10.3389/fphar.2021.633403

Surmeier DJ, Graves SM, Shen W (2014) Dopaminergic modulation of striatal networks in health and Parkinson's disease. Curr Opin Neurobiol 29:109–117. https://doi.org/10.1016/j.conb.2014.07.008

Suzuki S, Chuang LF, Yau P, Doi RH, Chuang RY (2002) Interactions of opioid and chemokine receptors: oligomerization of mu, kappa, and delta with CCR5 on immune cells. Exp Cell Res 280:192-200. https://doi.org/10.1006/excr.2002.5638

Szabo I, Chen XH, Xin L, Adler MW, Howard OM, Oppenheim JJ, Rogers TJ (2002) Heterologous desensitization of opioid receptors by chemokines inhibits chemotaxis and enhances the perception of pain. Proc Natl Acad Sci USA 99:10276–10281. https://doi.org/10.1073/pnas.102327699

Szafran-Pilch K, Faron-Gorecka A, Kolasa M, Zurawek D, Szlachta M, Solich J, Kusmider M, Dziedzicka-Wasylewska M (2017) Antidepressants promote formation of heterocomplexes of dopamine D2 and somatostatin subtype 5 receptors in the mouse striatum. Brain Res Bull 135: 92–97. https://doi.org/10.1016/j.brainresbull.2017.10.003

Szlachta M, Kusmider M, Pabian P, Solich J, Kolasa M, Zurawek D, Dziedzicka-Wasylewska M, Faron-Gorecka A (2018) Repeated clozapine increases the level of serotonin 5-HT1AR Heterodimerization with 5-HT2A or dopamine D2 receptors in the mouse cortex. Front Mol Neurosci 11:40. https://doi.org/10.3389/fnmol.2018.00040

Talaia C, Queiroz G, Pinheiro H, Moura D, Goncalves J (2006) Involvement of G-protein betagamma subunits on the influence of inhibitory alpha2-autoreceptors on the angiotensin AT1-receptor modulation of noradrenaline release in the rat vas deferens. Neurochem Int 49: 698–707. https://doi.org/10.1016/j.neuint.2006.07.002

Tanganelli S, Antonelli T, Tomasini MC, Beggiato S, Fuxe K, Ferraro L (2012) Relevance of dopamine D(2)/neurotensin NTS1 and NMDA/neurotensin NTS1 receptor interaction in psychiatric and neurodegenerative disorders. Curr Med Chem 19:304–316. https://doi.org/10.2174/092986712803414268

Temido-Ferreira M, Ferreira DG, Batalha VL, Marques-Morgado I, Coelho JE, Pereira P, Gomes R, Pinto A, Carvalho S, Canas PM, Cuvelier L, Buee-Scherrer V, Faivre E, Baqi Y, Muller CE, Pimentel J, Schiffmann SN, Buee L, Bader M, Outeiro TF, Blum D, Cunha RA, Marie H, Pousinha PA, Lopes LV (2020) Age-related shift in LTD is dependent on neuronal adenosine A (2A) receptors interplay with mGluR5 and NMDA receptors. Mol Psychiatry 25:1876–1900. https://doi.org/10.1038/s41380-018-0110-9

Toda S, Alguacil LF, Kalivas PW (2003) Repeated cocaine administration changes the function and subcellular distribution of adenosine A1 receptor in the rat nucleus accumbens. J Neurochem 87: 1478–1484. https://doi.org/10.1046/j.1471-4159.2003.02121.x

Tonazzini I, Trincavelli ML, Storm-Mathisen J, Martini C, Bergersen LH (2007) Co-localization and functional cross-talk between A1 and P2Y1 purine receptors in rat hippocampus. Eur J Neurosci 26:890–902. https://doi.org/10.1111/j.1460-9568.2007.05697.x

Toneatti R, Shin JM, Shah UH, Mayer CR, Saunders JM, Fribourg M, Arsenovic PT, Janssen WG, Sealfon SC, Lopez-Gimenez JF, Benson DL, Conway DE, Gonzalez-Maeso J (2020) Interclass GPCR heteromerization affects localization and trafficking. Sci Signal 13. https://doi.org/10.1126/scisignal.aaw3122

Torvinen M, Gines S, Hillion J, Latini S, Canals M, Ciruela F, Bordoni F, Staines W, Pedata F, Agnati LF, Lluis C, Franco R, Ferre S, Fuxe K (2002) Interactions among adenosine deaminase, adenosine A(1) receptors and dopamine D(1) receptors in stably cotransfected fibroblast cells and neurons. Neuroscience 113:709–719. https://doi.org/10.1016/s0306-4522(02)00058-1

Toth DJ, Toth JT, Gulyas G, Balla A, Balla T, Hunyady L, Varnai P (2012) Acute depletion of plasma membrane phosphatidylinositol 4,5-bisphosphate impairs specific steps in endocytosis of the G-protein-coupled receptor. J Cell Sci 125:2185–2197. https://doi.org/10.1242/jcs.097279

Toth AD, Gyombolai P, Szalai B, Varnai P, Turu G, Hunyady L (2017) Angiotensin type 1A receptor regulates beta-arrestin binding of the beta(2)-adrenergic receptor via heterodimerization. Mol Cell Endocrinol 442:113–124. https://doi.org/10.1016/j.mce.2016.11.027

Tripathi A, Vana PG, Chavan TS, Brueggemann LI, Byron KL, Tarasova NI, Volkman BF, Gaponenko V, Majetschak M (2015) Heteromerization of chemokine (C-X-C motif) receptor 4 with alpha1A/B-adrenergic receptors controls alpha1-adrenergic receptor function. Proc Natl Acad Sci USA 112:E1659–E1668. https://doi.org/10.1073/pnas.1417564112

Tse LH, Wong YH (2021) Modeling the heterodimer interfaces of melatonin receptors. Front Cell Neurosci 15:725296. https://doi.org/10.3389/fncel.2021.725296

van der Vorst EPC, Mandl M, Muller M, Neideck C, Jansen Y, Hristov M, Gencer S, Peters LJF, Meiler S, Feld M, Geiselhoringer AL, de Jong RJ, Ohnmacht C, Noels H, Soehnlein O, Drechsler M, Weber C, Doring Y (2019) Hematopoietic ChemR23 (Chemerin receptor 23) fuels atherosclerosis by sustaining an M1 macrophage-phenotype and guidance of plasmacytoid

dendritic cells to murine lesions-brief report. Arterioscler Thromb Vasc Biol 39:685–693. https://doi.org/10.1161/ATVBAHA.119.312386
Vardanyan R, Kumirov VK, Nichol GS, Davis P, Liktor-Busa E, Rankin D, Varga E, Vanderah T, Porreca F, Lai J, Hruby VJ (2011) Synthesis and biological evaluation of new opioid agonist and neurokinin-1 antagonist bivalent ligands. Bioorg Med Chem 19:6135–6142. https://doi.org/10.1016/j.bmc.2011.08.027
Vazquez-Salat N, Yuhki N, Beck T, O'Brien SJ, Murphy WJ (2007) Gene conversion between mammalian CCR2 and CCR5 chemokine receptor genes: a potential mechanism for receptor dimerization. Genomics 90:213–224. https://doi.org/10.1016/j.ygeno.2007.04.009
Velazhahan V, Ma N, Pandy-Szekeres G, Kooistra AJ, Lee Y, Gloriam DE, Vaidehi N, Tate CG (2021) Structure of the class D GPCR Ste2 dimer coupled to two G proteins. Nature 589:148–153. https://doi.org/10.1038/s41586-020-2994-1
Velazhahan V, Ma N, Vaidehi N, Tate CG (2022) Activation mechanism of the class D fungal GPCR dimer Ste2. Nature 603:743–748. https://doi.org/10.1038/s41586-022-04498-3
Vucetic Z, Reyes TM (2010) Central dopaminergic circuitry controlling food intake and reward: implications for the regulation of obesity. Wiley Interdiscip Rev Syst Biol Med 2:577–593. https://doi.org/10.1002/wsbm.77
Waldhoer M, Fong J, Jones RM, Lunzer MM, Sharma SK, Kostenis E, Portoghese PS, Whistler JL (2005) A heterodimer-selective agonist shows in vivo relevance of G protein-coupled receptor dimers. Proc Natl Acad Sci USA 102:9050–9055. https://doi.org/10.1073/pnas.0501112102
Wang HB, Zhao B, Zhong YQ, Li KC, Li ZY, Wang Q, Lu YJ, Zhang ZN, He SQ, Zheng HC, Wu SX, Hokfelt TG, Bao L, Zhang X (2010) Coexpression of delta- and mu-opioid receptors in nociceptive sensory neurons. Proc Natl Acad Sci USA 107:13117–13122. https://doi.org/10.1073/pnas.1008382107
Wang Y, Li G, Stanco A, Long JE, Crawford D, Potter GB, Pleasure SJ, Behrens T, Rubenstein JL (2011) CXCR4 and CXCR7 have distinct functions in regulating interneuron migration. Neuron 69:61–76. https://doi.org/10.1016/j.neuron.2010.12.005
Wang C, Wang Q, Ji B, Pan Y, Xu C, Cheng B, Bai B, Chen J (2018) The orexin/receptor system: molecular mechanism and therapeutic potential for neurological diseases. Front Mol Neurosci 11:220. https://doi.org/10.3389/fnmol.2018.00220
Wang D, Stoveken HM, Zucca S, Dao M, Orlandi C, Song C, Masuho I, Johnston C, Opperman KJ, Giles AC, Gill MS, Lundquist EA, Grill B, Martemyanov KA (2019) Genetic behavioral screen identifies an orphan anti-opioid system. Science 365:1267–1273. https://doi.org/10.1126/science.aau2078
Wang Y, Gai S, Zhang W, Huang X, Ma S, Huo Y, Wu Y, Tu H, Pin JP, Rondard P, Xu C, Liu J (2021a) The GABAB receptor mediates neuroprotection by coupling to G13. Sci Signal 14: eaaz4112. https://doi.org/10.1126/scisignal.aaz4112
Wang Z, Jiang C, Yao H, Chen O, Rahman S, Gu Y, Zhao J, Huh Y, Ji RR (2021b) Central opioid receptors mediate morphine-induced itch and chronic itch via disinhibition. Brain 144:665–681. https://doi.org/10.1093/brain/awaa430
Wang J, Saung MT, Li K, Fu J, Fujiwara K, Niu N, Muth S, Wang J, Xu Y, Rozich N, Zlomke H, Chen S, Espinoza B, Henderson M, Funes V, Herbst B, Ding D, Twyman-Saint Victor C, Zhao Q, Narang A, He J, Zheng L (2022) CCR2/CCR5 inhibitor permits the radiation-induced effector T cell infiltration in pancreatic adenocarcinoma. J Exp Med 219. https://doi.org/10.1084/jem.20211631
Wang X, Wang M, Xu T, Feng Y, Shao Q, Han S, Chu X, Xu Y, Lin S, Zhao Q, Wu B (2023) Structural insights into dimerization and activation of the mGlu2-mGlu3 and mGlu2-mGlu4 heterodimers. Cell Res 33:762–774. https://doi.org/10.1038/s41422-023-00830-2
Wei H, Ahn S, Shenoy SK, Karnik SS, Hunyady L, Luttrell LM, Lefkowitz RJ (2003) Independent beta-arrestin 2 and G protein-mediated pathways for angiotensin II activation of extracellular signal-regulated kinases 1 and 2. Proc Natl Acad Sci USA 100:10782–10787. https://doi.org/10.1073/pnas.1834556100

Weis WI, Kobilka BK (2018) The molecular basis of G protein-coupled receptor activation. Annu Rev Biochem 87:897–919. https://doi.org/10.1146/annurev-biochem-060614-033910

Werkman TR, Glennon JC, Wadman WJ, McCreary AC (2006) Dopamine receptor pharmacology: interactions with serotonin receptors and significance for the aetiology and treatment of schizophrenia. CNS Neurol Disord Drug Targets 5:3–23. https://doi.org/10.2174/187152706784111614

Werthmann RC, Tzouros M, Lamerz J, Augustin A, Fritzius T, Trovo L, Stawarski M, Raveh A, Diener C, Fischer C, Gassmann M, Lindemann L, Bettler B (2021) Symmetric signal transduction and negative allosteric modulation of heterodimeric mGlu1/5 receptors. Neuropharmacology 190:108426. https://doi.org/10.1016/j.neuropharm.2020.108426

Wisler JW, Xiao K, Thomsen AR, Lefkowitz RJ (2014) Recent developments in biased agonism. Curr Opin Cell Biol 27:18–24. https://doi.org/10.1016/j.ceb.2013.10.008

Wouters E, Vasudevan L, Crans RAJ, Saini DK, Stove CP (2019) Luminescence- and fluorescence-based complementation assays to screen for GPCR oligomerization: current state of the art. Int J Mol Sci 20. https://doi.org/10.3390/ijms20122958

Xie Z, Bhushan RG, Daniels DJ, Portoghese PS (2005) Interaction of bivalent ligand KDN21 with heterodimeric delta-kappa opioid receptors in human embryonic kidney 293 cells. Mol Pharmacol 68:1079–1086. https://doi.org/10.1124/mol.105.012070

Yamamoto T, Nair P, Davis P, Ma SW, Navratilova E, Moye S, Tumati S, Lai J, Vanderah TW, Yamamura HI, Porreca F, Hruby VJ (2007) Design, synthesis, and biological evaluation of novel bifunctional C-terminal-modified peptides for delta/mu opioid receptor agonists and neurokinin-1 receptor antagonists. J Med Chem 50:2779–2786. https://doi.org/10.1021/jm061369n

Yang Y, Li Q, He QH, Han JS, Su L, Wan Y (2018) Heteromerization of mu-opioid receptor and cholecystokinin B receptor through the third transmembrane domain of the mu-opioid receptor contributes to the anti-opioid effects of cholecystokinin octapeptide. Exp Mol Med 50:1–16. https://doi.org/10.1038/s12276-018-0090-5

Yoshida M, Takayanagi Y, Inoue K, Kimura T, Young LJ, Onaka T, Nishimori K (2009) Evidence that oxytocin exerts anxiolytic effects via oxytocin receptor expressed in serotonergic neurons in mice. J Neurosci 29:2259–2271. https://doi.org/10.1523/JNEUROSCI.5593-08.2009

Yoshioka K, Saitoh O, Nakata H (2001) Heteromeric association creates a P2Y-like adenosine receptor. Proc Natl Acad Sci USA 98:7617–7622. https://doi.org/10.1073/pnas.121587098

Yoshioka K, Hosoda R, Kuroda Y, Nakata H (2002) Hetero-oligomerization of adenosine A1 receptors with P2Y1 receptors in rat brains. FEBS Lett 531:299–303. https://doi.org/10.1016/s0014-5793(02)03540-8

Yuan Y, Arnatt CK, Li G, Haney KM, Ding D, Jacob JC, Selley DE, Zhang Y (2012) Design and synthesis of a bivalent ligand to explore the putative heterodimerization of the mu opioid receptor and the chemokine receptor CCR5. Org Biomol Chem 10:2633–2646. https://doi.org/10.1039/c2ob06801j

Yuan Y, Arnatt CK, El-Hage N, Dever SM, Jacob JC, Selley DE, Hauser KF, Zhang Y (2013) A bivalent ligand targeting the putative mu opioid receptor and chemokine receptor CCR5 heterodimers: binding affinity versus functional activities. Medchemcomm 4:847–851. https://doi.org/10.1039/C3MD00080J

Yue Y, Liu L, Wu LJ, Wu Y, Wang L, Li F, Liu J, Han GW, Chen B, Lin X, Brouillette RL, Breault E, Longpre JM, Shi S, Lei H, Sarret P, Stevens RC, Hanson MA, Xu F (2022) Structural insight into apelin receptor-G protein stoichiometry. Nat Struct Mol Biol 29:688–697. https://doi.org/10.1038/s41594-022-00797-5

Zhang Y, Devries ME, Skolnick J (2006) Structure modeling of all identified G protein-coupled receptors in the human genome. PLoS Comput Biol 2:e13. https://doi.org/10.1371/journal.pcbi.0020013

Zhang L, Zhang JT, Hang L, Liu T (2020) Mu opioid receptor heterodimers emerge as novel therapeutic targets: recent Progress and future perspective. Front Pharmacol 11:1078. https://doi.org/10.3389/fphar.2020.01078

Zhang R, Li D, Mao H, Wei X, Xu M, Zhang S, Jiang Y, Wang C, Xin Q, Chen X, Li G, Ji B, Yan M, Cai X, Dong B, Randeva HS, Liu C, Chen J (2022) Disruption of 5-hydroxytryptamine 1A receptor and orexin receptor 1 heterodimer formation affects novel G protein-dependent signaling pathways and has antidepressant effects in vivo. Transl Psychiatry 12:122. https://doi.org/10.1038/s41398-022-01886-1

Zhang M, Chen T, Lu X, Lan X, Chen Z, Lu S (2024) G protein-coupled receptors (GPCRs): advances in structures, mechanisms, and drug discovery. Signal Transduct Target Ther 9:88. https://doi.org/10.1038/s41392-024-01803-6

Zhu WZ, Chakir K, Zhang S, Yang D, Lavoie C, Bouvier M, Hebert TE, Lakatta EG, Cheng H, Xiao RP (2005) Heterodimerization of beta1- and beta2-adrenergic receptor subtypes optimizes beta-adrenergic modulation of cardiac contractility. Circ Res 97:244–251. https://doi.org/10.1161/01.RES.0000176764.38934.86

Structure-Encoded Location Biased Signaling in a Class B GPCR: Focus on the PTH Type 1 Receptor

Karina A. Peña and Jean-Pierre Vilardaga

Contents

Abstract

Research conducted over the last 15 years indicates that cAMP is generated not just from the plasma membrane but also from intracellular compartments, particularly in endosomes, where receptors are redistributed during the endocytosis process. This review centers on the parathyroid hormone type 1 receptor (PTH_1R) as a model for a peptide hormone GPCRs that generates cAMP from various

K. A. Peña
Department of Pharmacology and Chemical Biology, University of Pittsburgh School of Medicine, Pittsburgh, PA, USA

J.-P. Vilardaga (✉)
Department of Pharmacology and Chemical Biology, University of Pittsburgh School of Medicine, Pittsburgh, PA, USA

U.S. Department of Veterans Affairs, Pittsburgh Healthcare System, Pittsburgh, PA, USA
e-mail: jpv@pitt.edu; Jean-Pierre.Vilardaga@va.gov

© The Author(s), under exclusive license to Springer Nature Switzerland AG 2025

Z. Li, K. Xiao (eds.), *Pharmacology of GPCRs Biased Signaling and Agonists*, Handbook of Experimental Pharmacology 290, https://doi.org/10.1007/164_2025_763

locations with distinct duration and pharmacological effectiveness. We discuss how structural dynamics simulations aid in designing ligands that induce cAMP location bias, ultimately answering how the spatiotemporal generation of cAMP affects pharmacological responses mediated by the PTH_1R.

Keywords

Biased ligand · Endosomal signaling · G protein-coupled receptor · Location bias signaling · Parathyroid hormone · Structural dynamics

Abbreviations

ANM	anisotropic network model
ASRT	actin-SNX27-retromer-tubule
GAGs	glycosaminoglycans
GPCR	G protein-coupled receptor
GRK	G protein-coupled receptor kinase
LA-PTH	long-acting PTH
PIP_2	$PtdIns(4,5)P_2$
PIP_3	$PtdIns(3,4,5)P_3$
$PI3K_\beta$	phosphoinositide-3 kinase β
PTH	parathyroid hormone
PTHrP	PTH-related protein
PTH_1R	parathyroid hormone type 1 receptor
TM	transmembrane helix
SNX	sortin nexin
VPS	vacuolar protein sorting
βarr	β-arrestin

1 Overview of PTH_1R's Function in Human Physiology and Pathology

The parathyroid hormone (PTH) type 1 receptor (PTH_1R) is a class B G protein-coupled receptor (GPCR) that plays a crucial role in regulating skeletal development, bone remodeling, and calcium and phosphate homeostasis in the body (Cheloha et al. 2015) and is expressed and active through the cardiovascular system (Towler 2024). It serves as the cognate cell surface receptor for the native agonists parathyroid hormone (PTH) and PTH-related protein (PTHrP). The parathyroid glands secrete PTH as an 84-amino-acid peptide, which is the primary regulator of serum calcium (Ca^{2+}) and phosphate (PO_4^{3-}) ions balance by acting on bone and kidney cells. In hypocalcemia, PTH secretion is stimulated when serum Ca^{2+} levels drop below the homeostatic point (1.2 ± 0.1 mM) to increase Ca^{2+} levels by promoting bone remodeling and Ca^{2+} reabsorption in the kidneys (Horwitz et al. 2005; Drueke 1995). Activation of PTH_1R by PTH in osteoblasts and osteocytes stimulates bone matrix reabsorption releasing Ca^{2+} into systemic circulation (Silva et al. 2011; Boyce et al. 2012; O'Brien et al. 2013; Saini et al. 2013). In the kidneys, PTH has a twofold mineral ion regulatory effect. In distal tubule cells, PTH increases the reabsorption of Ca^{2+} by regulating the expression and activation of Ca^{2+} transport proteins. Meanwhile, in proximal tubule cells, it decreases the expression of the plasma membrane sodium-dependent phosphate transporter, resulting in reduced inorganic phosphate absorption (van Abel et al. 2005; de Groot et al. 2009; Biber et al. 2009; Picard et al. 2010; Nagai et al. 2011). Furthermore, PTH regulates the circulating levels of active vitamin D_3 (VitD) by inducing the expression of the rate-limiting enzyme 25-hydroxyvitamin D 1α-hydroxylase in proximal tubule cells of the kidney. In turn, VitD promotes the absorption of Ca^{2+} from the small intestine (Ogawa et al. 2022).

Unlike PTH, PTHrP acts primarily as a paracrine hormone, synthesized by different tissues and secreted as a 139-, 141-, or 171-amino-acid protein. However, PTHrP can exert similar effects on bone and kidneys as PTH. This comparable action is not surprising due to the similarities in the amino acid sequence between PTH and PTHrP, particularly at the N-terminal region, which is crucial for PTH_1R activation (Goltzman 2018; Suva et al. 1987; Nissenson et al. 1988; McCauley and Martin 2012). Once identified as the cause of hypercalcemia in cancer patients, PTHrP is now understood to play a significant role in the normal growth and development of various tissues, including bone, mammary glands, and teeth (McCauley and Martin 2012; Karaplis et al. 1994; Wysolmerski and Stewart 1998; Philbrick et al. 1998; Philbrick et al. 1996). While both ligands naturally exist as full-length proteins, synthetic or recombinant N-terminal fragments of PTH (PTH_{1-34} or teriparatide, brand name Forteo) and PTHrP ($PTHrP_{1-36}$) have been experimentally shown to retain full activity and are commonly used in research (Goltzman 2018; Nissenson et al. 1988; Dean et al. 2008; White et al. 2019; Potts Jr et al. 1971).

Dysfunction of PTH_1R signaling leads to several diseases, which have been extensively discussed elsewhere (Cheloha et al. 2015). For instance, Blomstrand chondrodysplasia, which results in fetal mortality, is caused by homozygous mutations in PTH_1R that lead to receptor inactivation (Jobert et al. 1998; Hoogendam et al. 2007). Various single mutations in PTH_1R, which cause constitutive activation of the receptor, induce Jansen metaphyseal chondrodysplasia, a rare disease characterized by short-limbed dwarfism and hypercalcemia. These mutations are located in the transmembrane (TM) helices of the receptor, either in TM2 (H223R), TM6 (T410P), or TM7 (I458R) (Schipani et al. 1995, 1996, 1999). Additionally, mutations in the coding sequence of PTH also cause diseases. In patients with idiopathic hypoparathyroidism, a single Arg-to-Cys mutation in

PTH's residue 25 (PTH^{R25C}) affects cAMP signaling and Ca^{2+} homeostasis (Pena 2022; Lee et al. 2015). Abnormal hormone levels are also associated with diseases characterized by PTH_1R dysfunction. Humoral hypercalcemia of malignancy present in about 25% of cancer patients is caused by the oversecretion of PTHrP by tumor cells, resulting in overactive PTH_1R signaling and subsequent elevation of serum Ca^{2+} (Feldenzer and Sarno 2018). Hyper- and under-secretion of PTH by the parathyroid glands causes hyper- and hypoparathyroidism, respectively. Hyperparathyroidism is typically treated by surgical removal of the parathyroid glands (Giovanella et al. 2021), though this may result in complications such as hypocalcemia. To mitigate this, pharmacological intervention often involves using calcimimetics, a group of positive allosteric modulators of the calcium-sensing receptor (CaSR), a class C GPCR that negatively regulates PTH secretion by the parathyroid glands (Wuthrich et al. 2007). On the other hand, hypoparathyroidism can be managed by oral calcium supplements, active VitD, and daily subcutaneous injections of recombinant human PTH (Rubin 2020); Furthermore, other metabolic diseases can affect bone homeostasis and PTH_1R function. For instance, diabetes mellitus induces bone fragility syndrome, characterized by increased osteocyte apoptosis and altered expression of the PTH_1R-regulated gene *SOST*, which inhibits bone formation (Marino and Bellido 2024).

In humans, pharmacological administration of synthetic PTH_1R ligands can modulate bone and Ca^{2+} homeostasis. Continuous infusion of $PTH_{1–34}$ promotes net bone catabolism in young adults (Horwitz et al. 2005; Canalis et al. 2007), while its daily subcutaneous injection induces net bone anabolism and is an FDA-approved treatment for severe cases of osteoporosis (Cohen et al. 2020; Ono et al. 2021; Neer et al. 2001). A synthetic analog of $PTHrP_{1–34}$, (abaloparatide or ABL, brand name Tymlos) is used to treat osteoporosis in postmenopausal women. Studies have reported that ABL can be more effective at inducing bone formation than $PTH_{1–34}$, lessening hypercalcemic effects (Leder et al. 2015; Sleeman and Clements 2019; Miller et al. 2019; Arlt et al. 2020). Osteoporosis treatment by PTH analogs is, however, limited to 18 months due to the risk of osteosarcoma and hypercalcemia. More recently, ABL has been shown to reduce the effects of epididymitis and orchitis in human and mouse males by lessening inflammatory responses via Gq and β-arrestin-1 (βarr1) signaling (Wang et al. 2021). The long-acting PTH (LA-PTH), which is a modified $PTH_{1–15}/PTHrP_{16–34}$ chimera, is in phase 3 to evaluate its efficacy to normalize the serum Ca^{2+} level for the treatment of hyperparathyroidism (Rejnmark 2024; Clarke et al. 2024).

The molecular mechanisms controlling the different effects of PTH_1R in calcemic response in humans are yet to be fully understood. One possible explanation comes from studies using recombinant PTH_1R in cultured cells, which show that $PTH_{1–34}$ and ABL stabilize different PTH_1R conformations (White et al. 2019; Hattersley et al. 2016). This ligand-dependent PTH_1R conformation selectivity likely results in distinct ligand residence times at the receptor, which may affect the spatiotemporal components of PTH_1R signaling. The mechanisms underlying this emerging paradigm are discussed in the following paragraphs.

2 Moving Toward a Paradigm Shift in GPCR Signaling

2.1 PTH_1R Signals via cAMP from Endosomes

In the classical model of GPCR signaling, cAMP is produced at the plasma membrane. In this model, ligand binding stabilizes an active conformation of the receptor, which couples to and activates the stimulatory Gs protein for transmembrane adenylate cyclases. G protein activation involves the release of GDP from the Gα subunit, followed by the binding of GTP and the dissociation or conformational rearrangement of the Gα subunit from the Gβγ heterodimer. The free Gα-GTP and Gβγ subunits independently regulate proteins involved in second messenger production, such as cAMP (Oldham and Hamm 2006). Signaling is terminated when GPCR kinases (GRKs) phosphorylate the receptor, leading to the recruitment of β-arrestins, which initiate the internalization of the ligand-bound receptor-βarr complex into endosomes. In this classical model, receptor desensitization occurs within minutes (2–5 min) after ligand binding. Recruitment of β-arrestins and receptor internalization into endosomes lead to the termination of cAMP signaling. From early endosomes, GPCRs are typically trafficked through the endocytic pathway for lysosomal degradation or recycled back to the cell surface. However, this model fails to explain the sustained cAMP signaling observed for some GPCRs. Notably, PTH_1R does not colocalize with late endosomal markers, and β-arrestins recruitment in response to PTH_{1-84}, PTH_{1-34}, or LA-PTH does not terminate cAMP production. Instead, β-arrestin2 promotes cAMP from early endosomes (Ferrandon et al. 2009; Feinstein et al. 2011). Therefore, alternative termination mechanisms regulate PTH_1R signaling.

PTH_1R primarily signals through Gs and Gq/11 in response to PTH or PTHrP binding. Activation of Gs leads to the production of cAMP by adenylyl cyclases and further activation of protein kinase A (PKA) (Juppner et al. 1991; Abou-Samra et al. 1992), while Gq/11 activates phospholipase Cβ (PLCβ), which catalyzes the production of diacylglycerol (DAG) and inositol (1,4,5)-triphosphate (IP_3) from phosphatidylinositol 4,5-bisphosphate (PIP_2) located in the plasma membrane. IP_3 diffuses through the cytosol and activates IP3 receptors in the endoplasmic reticulum (ER) membrane, releasing stored Ca^{2+} into the cytosol. This, in turn, promotes protein kinase C (PKC) translocation to the plasma membrane and its activation by DAG. Although less studied, PTH_1R also couples to $G_{12/13}$ proteins (Singh et al. 2005a; b) and inhibitory Gi proteins (Avet et al. 2022).

When PTH_{1-34} is infused into humans, it increases blood Ca^{2+}, vitamin D, urinary phosphate ion, and bone resorption. However, $PTHrP_{1-36}$ infusion does not similarly increase these physiological parameters (Horwitz et al. 2005), despite PTH and $PTHrP_{1-36}$ sharing similar pharmacological properties at equilibrium, such as binding affinity and potency (EC_{50}) for stimulating Gs and Gq signaling pathways (Vilardaga et al. 2023; Fraher et al. 1992). This discrepancy prompted spatiotemporal investigations of PTH_1R signaling in living cells in real time to understand better how PTH and $PTHrP_{1-36}$ differentiate themselves. Advances in microscopy techniques coupled with the development and use of biosensors revealed that the interaction between $PTHrP_{1-36}$ and PTH_1R is reversible (Dean et al. 2008; Ferrandon et al. 2009) and leads to transient cAMP, while PTH has an extended residence time ($1/t_{off}$, where t_{off} is the dissociation time constant) in the receptor that permits sustained cAMP production after receptor internalization into endosmes (Ferrandon et al. 2009). Initially, this prolonged cAMP response challenged the traditional model of GPCR desensitization, which involves rapid termination of G protein-dependent signaling after receptor phosphorylation by GRKs and recruitment of β-arrestins, leading to G protein uncoupling and ligand-bound GPCR internalization. However, the findings show that blocking PTH_1R internalization prevents the prolonged cAMP response in cells expressing either the recombinant or the native receptor (Ferrandon et al. 2009; Jean-Alphonse et al. 2017). Additional studies show that PTH causes sustained cAMP signaling from early endosomes following the internalization of a PTH_1R–Gβγ − β-arrestin complex (Wehbi et al. 2013).

This ternary complex reassembles in the endosome with diffusing Gαs to induce a second and sustained pool of cAMP. Additionally, blocking receptor internalization by expressing the dominant-negative form of dynamin (Dyn^{K44A}) eliminates the sustained phase of cAMP production in response to PTH_{1-34} in cells expressing the recombinant or native receptor (Ferrandon et al. 2009), providing further evidence for cAMP generation from endosomes in PTH_1R signaling (Fig. 1a, b).

The ability of PTH_1R ligands to induce endosomal cAMP signaling can be partly attributed to their varying potency in stabilizing two specific high-affinity receptor conformations, named R_0 and R_G, in reference to prior studies conducted with another class B GPCR, the CRF receptor (Hoare et al. 2003, 2004). The R_G conformation is the classical G protein-dependent high-affinity receptor conformation. In contrast, the R_0 conformation is not dependent on G protein coupling but can display high-affinity ligand binding. The R_0 and R_G conformations are differentiated using membrane-based radioligand competition binding assays at equilibrium (Dean et al. 2006, 2008; Hoare et al. 1999). The R_0 conformation is assessed using ^{125}I-PTH_{1-34} as a radioligand in the presence of GTPγS, a non-hydrolyzable GTP analog that prevents receptor and G protein coupling. The R_G conformation is assessed using ^{125}I-M-PTH_{1-15} (a modified $PTH_{1\text{-}15}$ where M is Ala/Aib_1, Aib_3, Gln_{10}, Har_{11}, Ala_{12}, Trp_{14}, Arg_{19}), and in the presence of a dominant negative $G\alpha_S$ mutant that binds the receptor irreversibly (Ferrandon et al. 2009; Berlot 2002). Analysis of competition binding experiments in which PTH_1R agonists displace the radioligand revealed that the selectivity to R_0 correlates with the efficacy of a ligand to induce endosomal cAMP signaling. As shown in Fig. 1, the enhanced selectivity of LA-PTH and PTH for the R_0 conformation, compared to $PTHrP_{1-36}$ (Fig. 1c, d), is accompanied by a significantly prolonged endosomal cAMP production (Fig. 1e).

Another mechanism by which PTH_1R ligands sustain cAMP is advanced from cryo-EM structures of the LAPTH-PTH_1R-Gs complex, which show three distinct conformations of LA-PTH (Fig. 2a, b) (Zhao et al. 2019). In these active receptor conformations, the interactions between ligand's residue E4 and receptor's residues $R233^{2.60b}$ in TM2 (superscript refers to Wootten's class B GPCR nomenclature) and $Y195^{1.47b}$ in TM1 induce the formation of a polar interaction network with

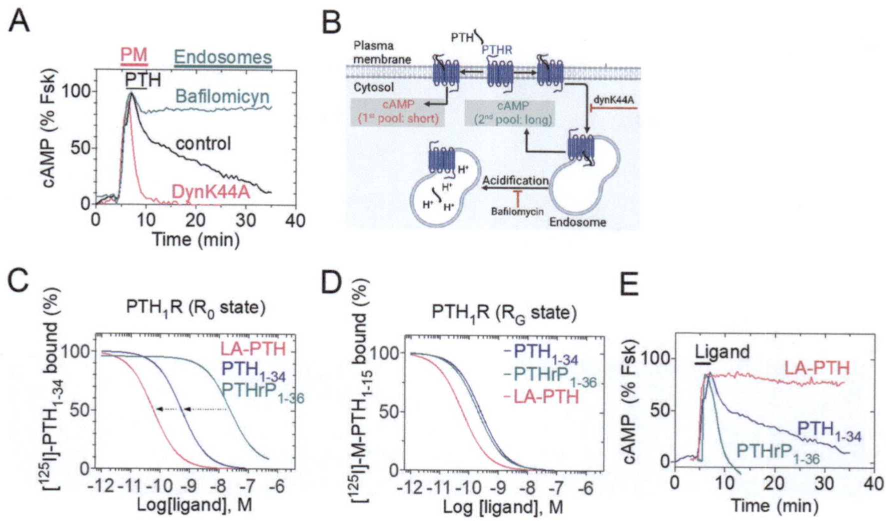

Fig. 1 PTH_1R signaling and ligand binding properties. (**a**) Time courses of cAMP in response to PTH for control cells (*black*) and when either internalization is inhibited by the dynamin mutant DynK44A (*pink*), or endosomal acidification is blocked by bafilomycin (*green*). (**b**) Modes of cAMP production in PTH_1R signaling. (**c, d**) Binding to the R_0 (**c**) and R_G (**d**) conformations of PTH_1R determined by competition isotherms using plasma membrane extracts from HEK293 cells. (**e**) Time courses of cAMP in response to PTH_1R agonists

$H420^{6.52b}$ and $Y421^{6.53b}$ in TM6. These interactions stabilize a sharp kink with the conserved class B GPCR PxxG motif at the center of TM6 ($P415^{6.47b}$xx $G418^{6.50b}$) as illustrated in a close-up view with interacting residues in stick format (Fig. 2c). In two of the Gs-coupled PTH_1R conformations, LA-PTH forms an α-helix that connects the extracellular domain (ECD) of the receptor's N-terminal to the transmembrane domain. In the third conformation, the peptide ligand's C-terminal residues 18–34 are detached from the ECD (Fig. 2b). This suggests that the C-terminal residue of the ligand may experience multiple association and dissociation cycles while the ligand's N-domain (residues 1–17) remains anchored to the TM domain of the receptor, facilitating extended periods of G protein coupling and activation even when the receptor is located in endosomes.

2.2 Mechanisms Terminating Endosomal cAMP Signaling

One mechanism involved in the termination of endosomal PTH_1R signaling via cAMP is the sorting of PTH_1R from early endosomes to the trans-Golgi via the retromer complex. Involved in the recycling of numerous transmembrane proteins, the retromer complex consists of two endosomal-bound sorting nexins (SNX1 and SNX2) and a soluble heterodimer formed by three vacuolar protein sorting (VPS) subunits: VPS26, VPS29, and VPS35 (Collins 2008). In endosomes, PTH_1R is

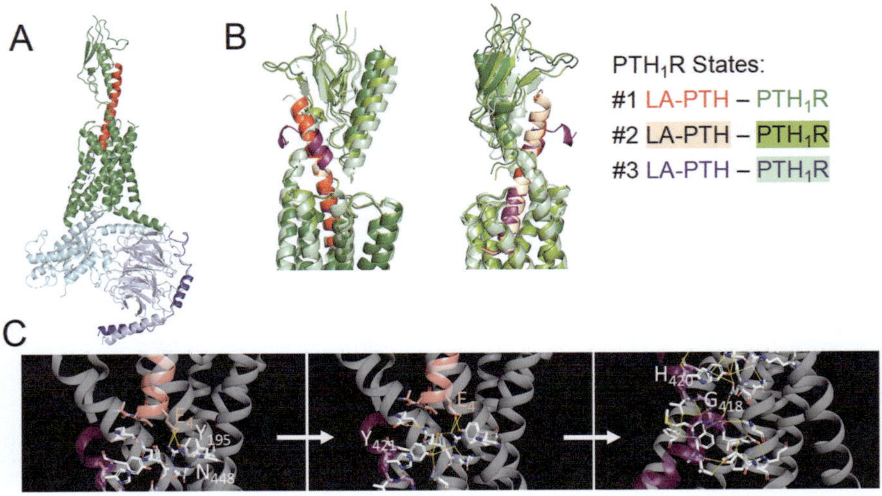

Fig. 2 Gs-coupled PTH_1R structures. (**a**) Overall cryo-EM structure of the LAPTH-PTH_1R-Gs complex in one of the conformations with PTH_1R in green, LAPTH in red, $G\alpha_s$ in gray, $G\beta\gamma$ in purple. (**b**) Three distinct conformational states of the LAPTH–PTH_1R-Gs complex. The oscillation of the N-terminal domain of PTH_1R ($PTHR^{ECD}$) is evident, while the TMD core shows a higher degree of stability. Notably, state #3 captures the partial dissociation of LAPTH's C-domain from $PTHR^{ECD}$. (**c**) A close-up and sequential view proposes establishing key activating polar interactions between LAPTH and PTH_1R

associated with the retromer complex after dissociating from PTH, βarr, and Gβγ, resulting in the termination of endosomal cAMP production (Feinstein et al. 2011). This process is directly regulated by the retromer complex, as overexpression of VPS subunits reduces the duration of endosomal cAMP production. Conversely, knockdown of VPS subunits via siRNA prolongs cAMP production in response to PTH (Feinstein et al. 2011).

Additionally, the retromer is a component of the actin-SNX27-retromer-tubule (ASRT) complex, which is involved in the sorting of proteins from endosomes to the plasma membrane. A PDZ (post-synaptic density protein 95/disc-large/zona occludens-1 protein) domain in SNX27 serves as a cargo selector for the retromer complex and is responsible for its interaction with the PDZ ligand, ETMV, located at the end of the PTH_1R's C-terminus (McGarvey et al. 2016; Chan et al. 2016). The SNX27-PTH_1R interaction and the ASRT complex are determinants for receptor recycling to the plasma membrane, as depletion of either SNX27 or VPS35 or actin depolymerization decreases the rate of PTH_1R recycling (McGarvey et al. 2016). This mechanism depends on a negative feedback loop in which PTH-induced PKA activation leads to endosomal v-ATPase phosphorylation and subsequent acidification of the endosomal lumen (Gidon et al. 2014). Lowering the endosomal pH results in the dissociation of the ternary PTH_1R-βarr-Gβγ complex, allowing inactive PTH_1R to associate with the retromer (Feinstein et al. 2011; Gidon et al. 2014).

Conversely, blocking endosomal acidification with bafilomycin A1 (v-ATPase inhibitor) maintains the PTH_1R's active signaling state in endosomes (Fig. 1a, b).

2.3 Mechanisms Regulating Endosomal cAMP Signaling

2.3.1 Gq Protein and β-Arrestin as Inducer of Endosomal cAMP Signaling

Upon activation of PTH_1R by PTH, both the Gs/cAMP/PKA and Gq/PLC/Ca^{2+} signaling pathways are activated. While the role of Gs in PTH_1R endosomal signaling is well established (Ferrandon et al. 2009), only recently has the crucial role of Gq/11 been discovered in initiating endosomal cAMP production. This discovery stemmed from the observation that Gs-biased PTH analogs, which do not activate Gq/11, also show impaired β-arrestin recruitment to PTH_1R and, consequently, cannot trigger prolonged cAMP responses (Liu et al. 2018, 2019) The absence or selective inhibition of Gq/11 activation consistently reduces sustained cAMP production in response to PTH1–34 in various recombinant and native cell types (White et al. 2020), thus suggesting that Gq/11 activation is required for inducing sustained endosomal cAMP signaling.

Although Gβγ subunits can mediate β-arrestin recruitment by translocating GRK2/3 to the plasma membrane (Gurevich and Gurevich 2019), the lack of Gq/11 expression does not affect PTH_1R phosphorylation status, indicating that Gq/11-driven β-arrestin recruitment is independent of PTH_1R phosphorylation (White et al. 2020). The mechanism underlying β-arrestin recruitment to the PTH_1R involves the activation of phosphoinositide-3 kinase β (PI3Kβ) by Gq/11-released Gβγ subunits, which catalyzes the formation of PtdIns(3,4,5)P_3 (PIP_3) from PtdIns(4,5)P_2 (PIP_2). Thus, Gq/11 regulates endosomal cAMP production by promoting PIP_3 synthesis through Gβγ-dependent PI3Kβ activation, facilitating β-arrestin recruitment to PTH_1R and internalization of the PTH_1R-βarr-Gβγ complex into endosomes (White et al. 2020). For class A GPCRs, PIP_2 is thought to be the primary plasma membrane phosphatidylinositol driving β-arrestin recruitment and activation (Janetzko et al. 2022). However, β-arrestin recruitment to PTH_1R is mediated by PIP_3 generated by Gq/11 activation. Recent findings show that PIP_3 directly binds to β-arrestin2 in response to PTH_{1-34}, inducing a conformational change that enables its interaction with PTH-bound PTH_1R within clathrin-coated regions of the plasma membrane (Pacheco et al. 2024). The ternary signaling complex is subsequently internalized into endosomes to prolong cAMP production (Fig. 3).

2.3.2 Allosteric Regulation of PTH_1R Signaling

GPCRs are allosterically modulated by ions such as Na^+, Mg^{2+}, Ca^{2+}, and Mn^{2+} (Katritch et al. 2014; Urwyler 2011; Rodriguez et al. 1992; Mazzoni et al. 1993). Extracellular Ca^{2+} acts as a positive allosteric modulator of PTH_1R by increasing the residence time of PTH_{1-34} or ABL binding the active receptor conformation. Ca^{2+} allostery prolongs PTH_1R activation and increases cAMP production from

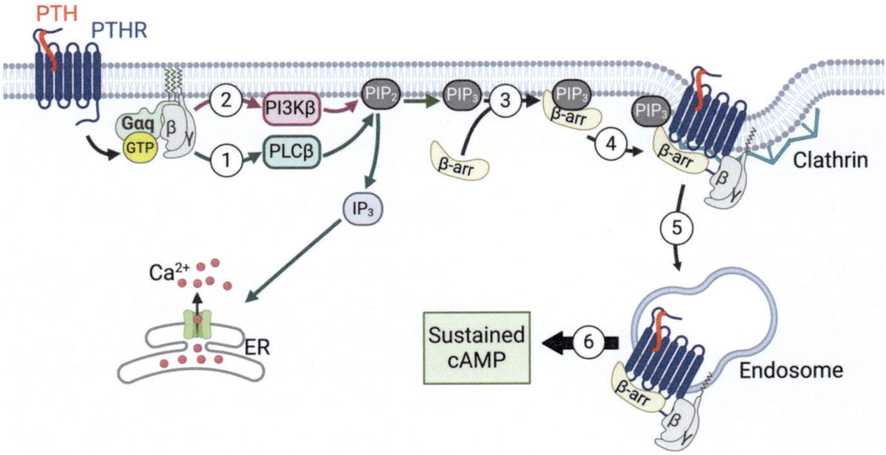

Fig. 3 Regulation of endosomal cAMP signaling by Gq/11. Activation of heterotrimeric Gs (not depicted) and Gq/11 proteins occurs upon PTH binding to PTH_1R. Gs activation leads to transient cAMP generation from the plasma membrane, while Gq/11 activation results in PLCβ activation, leading to IP_3 generation and consequent release of Ca^{2+} from the ER (step 1). Gβγ subunits derived from Gq/11 activate PI3Kβ, resulting in increased production of PIP_3 from PIP_2 (step 2). PIP_3 binds to βarr at the plasma membrane, leading to the assembly of the signaling complex (PTH-PTH_1R-β arr-Gβγ) in clathrin-coated pits (step 4), followed by its internalization into endosomes (step 5). The internalized signaling complex generates sustained cAMP from endosomes (step 6). Generated with BioRender.com. (Adapted from Pena et al. Mol Cell Endocrinol (2024) 1:581:112107)

endosomes (White et al. 2019). This modulation is likely physiologically relevant, as the mutant PTH^{R25C} associated with idiopathic hyperparathyroidism is unaffected by extracellular Ca^{2+} and fails to induce endosomal cAMP production upon PTH_1R binding (Lee et al. 2015).

Residue R25 in PTH can form ionic interactions with negatively charged residues in extracellular loop 1 (ECL1) of the receptor, facilitating allosteric modulation by extracellular Ca^{2+} (Li et al. 2021). Thus, Ca^{2+} may stabilize ligand-PTH_1R interaction, promoting sustained cAMP production. While cell-based assays show that increasing Ca^{2+} concentrations (0.1 to 10 mM) lower the ligand concentration required to activate PTH_1R (White et al. 2019), bone cells in the body can be exposed to significantly higher Ca^{2+} levels due to bone resorption, resulting in a Ca^{2+}-rich microenvironment where concentrations may reach as high as 40 mM (Silver et al. 1988). Therefore, Ca^{2+} can allosterically promote PTH_1R signaling in bone cells exposed to circulating picomolar PTH levels.

PTH_1R can also be allosterically modulated by nucleotides. Extracellular ATP and CMP enhance PTH-induced cAMP production, β-arrestin recruitment, and activation of cAMP response element-binding protein (CREB) (Kim et al. 2018). This enhancement occurs independently of activating the purine P_2X_7 receptor or ATP hydrolysis (Kim et al. 2018). Although the precise mechanism underlying nucleotide modulation remains unclear, the presence of a sugar-phosphate is sufficient to potentiate PTH activity. Studies suggest that ribose-5-phosphate (R5P) acts as a positive allosteric modulator of PTH_1R (Kim et al. 2019). Differentiated osteoblasts release ATP in response to PTH stimulation (Wang et al. 2013), potentially establishing an autocrine feedback loop where released ATP modulates PTH-PTH_1R signaling in bone cells. Therefore, nucleotide allostery of PTH_1R is a potential regulator of bone homeostasis.

More recently, studies have shown that PTH_1R can be modulated by receptor-activity modifying proteins (RAMPs), single-transmembrane helix proteins that regulate the signaling properties of several GPCRs (Nemec et al. 2022). RAMP2 interacts with PTH_1R under co-expression conditions in HEK293 cells, inducing a pre-activated receptor state that allows faster activation upon ligand binding (Nemec et al. 2022). RAMP2 enhances G-protein signaling and β-arrestin recruitment to PTH_1R in a ligand-dependent manner, with more pronounced effects observed for PTH_{1-34} than $PTHrP_{1-36}$. Although further studies are needed to verify RAMP2's role under native conditions, RAMP2-knockout mice exhibit placental dysfunction and impaired PTH_1R regulation (Kadmiel et al. 2017).

3 Structure-Encoded Allosteric Modulation of PTH_1R Signaling

The design of biased PTH peptides has been facilitated after the functional determinants in PTH were identified through the in silico analysis of dynamics and flexibility of the PTH-bound PTH_1R using the Anisotropic Network Model (ANM) (Clark et al. 2020). The ANM uses the cryo-EM structure of the PTH_1R (PDB: 6NBF) to depict each receptor's residue as a single node, with the α-carbon (Cα) atom at the center. The nodes located within a distance of <15 Å are interconnected with springs to illustrate residue interactions influenced by the six normal vibrational modes (asymmetric and symmetric bond stretching, wagging, twisting, scissoring, and rocking). Unlike isotropic models, ANM considers direction-dependent (anisotropic) motions and is thus ideally suited to capture allosteric conformational changes in the receptor and, thus, its molecular mechanisms of action. The ANM analysis showed that the opening and closing of the receptor's third intracellular region (ICL3) are allosterically coupled to structural changes at residues interacting with PTH residues 1–14. Given that PTH residues 1–4 are crucial for the ON-and-OFF activation switch of the receptor (Zhao et al. 2019) and residues 15-34 are determinant for the binding affinity of PTH to the reecptor, PTH's residues 5–14 are predictably a signal-selectivity epitope involved in the selectivity of PTH_1R signaling via G proteins and β-arrestin. This prediction was verified and allowed the development of a location-biased PTH analog, PTH^{7d} (Leu 7 is epimerized, see Fig. 4a), which stabilizes the outward receptor's TM6 kink better than PTH by enhancing the polar network of the PTH residue E4 (Fig. 4b). These changes result in improved coupling of PTH_1R to Gs but a lack of coupling to βarr, favoring sustained cAMP signaling at the plasma membrane over endosomes. Remarkably, while PTH^{7d} induces cAMP responses comparable in magnitude and duration to those

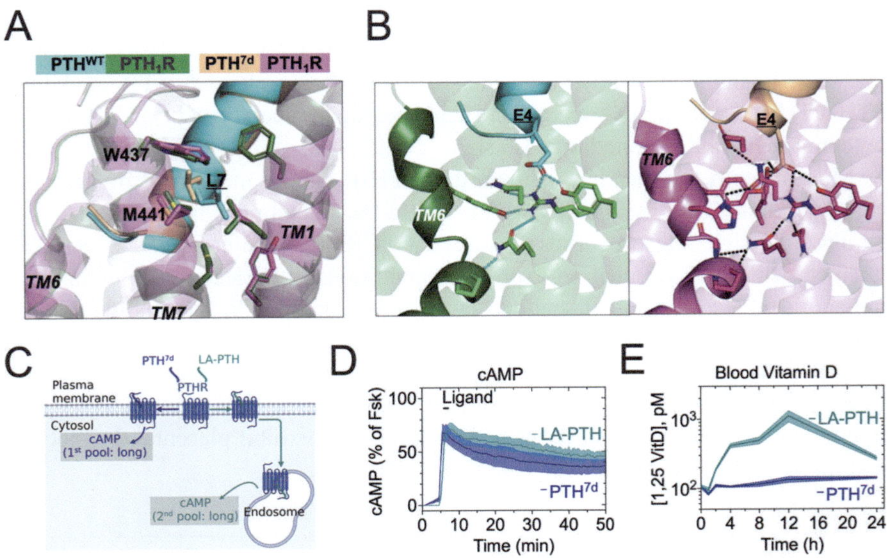

Fig. 4 Location-biased structural and pharmacological properties of PTH^{7d}. (**a**) Structural models of PTH_1R bound to PTH^{7L} (PTH^{wt}, *cyan*) and its epimer PTH^{7d} (*wheat*) with PTH_1R in *dark green* when bound to PTH^{7L}, and *violet* when bound to PTH^{7d}. (**b**) Comparison of the interaction network of the ligand E4 residue when the receptor is bound to PTH^{WT} (left panel) or PTH^{7d} (right panel) and receptor residues, (**c, d**) LA-PTH and PTH^{7d} are biased PTH agonists that elicit comparable, sustained cAMP production from different cellular locations: the plasma membrane vs endosomal. (**e**) When administered to mice, only LA-PTH significantly boosts vitamin D levels

triggered by LA-PTH, its signaling is limited to the plasma membrane, whereas LA-PTH drives endosomal cAMP production (White et al. 2021) (Fig. 4c, d).

ANM analysis of PTH_1R dynamics identified another PTH residue, H9, which mutated into Ala generates a location-biased PTH analog (PTH^{H9A}) that signals transiently from the plasma membrane and is unable to recruit βarr and induce endosomal cAMP signaling (Clark et al. 2020). A combination of NMR and computational approaches revealed that interactions between His9 and PTH_1R are critical for correctly inserting the PTH peptide within the PTH_1R's TMD (Fig. 5), and inducing a conformational change in the receptor's ICL3 that permits interactions with β-arrestin's finger loop (Clark et al. 2020).

4 Location-Biased cAMP Signaling

The concept of location-biased cAMP signaling involves the spatially confined production and regulation of cAMP from distinct subcellular membrane compartments, such as endosomes, Golgi, and the endoplasmic reticulum (ER). Research on PTH_1R was crucial in revealing this concept by showing that once activated by PTH, the receptor internalizes and continues to induce cAMP

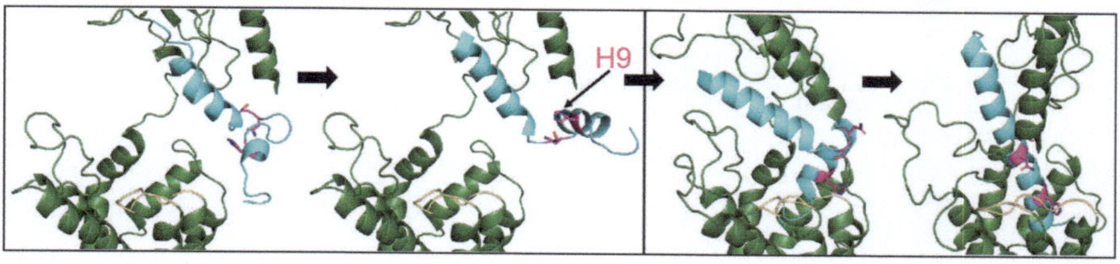

Fig. 5 Binding mechanism. PTH$_1$R is dark green, with ECL2 in light orange, and PTH is cyan, with residues His9, Asn16, and Ser17 displayed as magenta sticks. In the fast initial steps, binding the PTH's C-terminal part to PTHR^{ECD} (Step 1) rigidifies the C-terminal helix and residues 6–15 within the N-terminal part of PTH (Step 2). These conformational changes may expand the small N-terminal helix from residues 6–9 to 6–15. In the slow following steps, the N-terminal part of PTH is inserted into PTH$_1$R's TMD (Step 3). Interactions between the N-terminal portion of PTH and PTH$_1$R's TMD and ECL2 residues promote the formation of a continuous PTH helix (Step 4)

production from early endosomes. This results in sustained signaling with distinct cellular and pharmacological outcomes when compared to cAMP generated from the plasma membrane production. Following this discovery, additional GPCRs demonstrated endosomal cAMP signaling, indicating that location-biased cAMP generation is a mechanism many other receptors share to regulate cell functions (Table 1).

4.1 Pharmacological Relevance

Pharmacological functions mediated by PTH$_1$R depend on the location of cAMP signaling (endosomes *vs.* plasma membrane) (Fig. 4c–e). Supporting this, studies in mice show that LAPTH stimulates significantly greater bone formation and serum vitamin D elevation than PTH^{7d}, although both LA-PTH and PTH^{7d} induce a similar duration of cAMP production in cells (Fig. 4c–e). LAPTH or PTH-mediated cAMP in renal proximal epithelial tubular cells induces the expression of the 1-α-hydroxylase, the rate-limiting enzyme in the formation of the active vitamin D (White et al. 2021). However, PTH^{7d} fails to elevate 1-α hydroxylase expression in polarized MDCK cells, suggesting that vitamin D production requires endosomal cAMP production by PTH$_1$R (White et al. 2021). The concept of location-biased GPCR signaling has gained considerable interest over the past 15 years. Since the discovery of endosomal cAMP production by PTH$_1$R, several class A and class B GPCRs have been identified to exhibit similar endosomal signaling capabilities (Table 1). A key focus has been understanding the physiological impact of endosomal cAMP production. Recent studies indicate that cAMP produced from

Table 1 Examples of GPCRs that engage endosomal signaling via heterotrimeric Gs protein and cAMP

Ligand type	GPCR		Class	Discovery year	Pharmacological function	Human disease relevance
Peptide	PTH* type 1 receptor	PTH_1R	B	Ferrandon et al. (2009)	Ca^{2+} homeostasis (White et al. 2021)	HPT[a] (Lee et al. 2015)
Peptide	TSH* receptor	TSHR	A	Calebiro et al. (2009)	Gene transcription (Godbole et al. 2017)	ND
Non-peptide	Dopamine receptor D_1	D_1R	A	Kotowski et al. (2011)	ND	ND
Peptide	Vasopressin type 2 receptor	V_2R	A	(Feinstein et al. 2013)	H_2O homeostasis (Feinstein et al. 2013)	ND
Peptide	Glucagon-like peptide 1 receptor	GLP_1R	B	Kuna et al. (2013)	Sugar homeostasis (Kuna et al. 2013)	ND
Peptide	PACAP* type 1 receptor	PAC_1R	B	May and Parsons (2017)	Neuronal excitability (May and Parsons 2017; Merriam et al. 2013)	ND
Non-peptide	β_2-adrenergic receptor	β_2AR	A	Irannejad et al. (2013)	ND	ND
Peptide	Calcitonin receptor	CTR	B	Andreassen et al. (2014)	ND	ND
Peptide	Luteinizing hormone receptor	LHR	A	Lyga et al. (2016)	Oogenesis process (Lyga et al. 2016)	ND
Peptide	Calcitonin-like receptor	CLR	B	Yarwood et al. (2017)	Nociception (Yarwood et al. 2017)	ND

*Abbreviations. *HPT* hypoparathyroidism, *PACAP* Pituitary adenylate cyclase-activating polypeptide, *PTH* parathyroid hormone, *TSH* Thyroid-stimulating hormone endosomes elicits more robust transcriptional responses than cAMP generated at the plasma membrane (Tsvetanova et al. 2021; Peng et al. 2021; Willette et al. 2024). This difference may stem from endosomes being physically closer to the nucleus, enabling cAMP to rapidly activate PKA, which phosphorylates the cAMP-response element-binding protein (CREB) in the nucleus, driving gene transcription. Indeed, blocking endocytosis using Dyn^{K44A} expression or clathrin knockdown reduces nuclear PKA catalytic subunit accumulation and suppresses CREB phosphorylation (Tsvetanova et al. 2021; Peng et al. 2021). Additionally, the spatial origin of cAMP signaling affects global phosphoproteomic profiles (Tsvetanova et al. 2021). This may be attributed to endosomal receptors colliding with PKA clusters, emphasizing the importance of the spatiotemporal regulation of cAMP production in transcriptional control (Peng et al. 2021). These findings underscore the critical role of endosomal signaling in fine-tuning cellular responses through precise spatial and temporal cAMP dynamics. However, additional studies are needed to fully understand the importance of localized cAMP signaling in native cell systems of physiological relevance. For instance, the aforementioned studies (Tsvetanova et al. 2021; Peng et al. 2021; Willette et al. 2024) were conducted in non-native cells (HEK cells) using isoproterenol, a synthetic ligand for the β2-adrenergic receptor (β2-AR). It remains unclear whether β2-AR can engage cAMP generation from endosomes in response to its native ligand, adrenaline. Therefore, future studies using native ligands are crucial to unveil the physiological effects of spatiotemporal regulation of cAMP signaling.

4.2 The Role of the Extracellular Matrix

Glycosaminoglycans (GAGs) are intriguing extracellular matrix molecules that influence the location-biased signaling of PTH_1R via the native PTHrP. Its N-terminal fragment, $PTHrP_{1–36}$, has been utilized in basic and preclinical studies as a proxy for the native PTHrP and is notable for inducing transient cAMP production from the plasma membrane (Ferrandon et al. 2009; Pena et al. 2022). However, the signaling mechanism of native PTHrP through PTH_1R was not fully understood until recently. Unlike $PTHrP_{1–36}$, the native 141-amino acid PTHrP, $PTHrP_{1–141}$, triggers sustained cAMP production at the plasma membrane, akin to the response elicited by the location-biased PTH analog PTH^{7d} (Pena et al. 2022). Cell-based studies reveal that blocking receptor internalization does not impact the cAMP production induced by $PTHrP_{1–141}$, indicating that the native hormone does not depend on internalized PTH_1R for sustained cAMP production. Furthermore, a cell-impermeable antagonist, [D-W_{12}, Y_{34})-$PTH_{7–34}$, which inhibits PTH_1R signaling at the plasma membrane, reduces cAMP levels to baseline after stimulation with $PTHrP_{1–141}$, thus supporting that the native PTHrP is a location-biased agonist (Pena et al. 2022) .

Heparin/heparan sulfate, a type of GAG, is a linear polysaccharide characterized by diverse sulfation patterns and charge densities, which makes it an essential component of the extracellular matrix (Bu and Jin 2021). Due to their proximity to the plasma membrane, GAGs can modulate signal transduction by binding to, stabilizing, and activating various extracellular protein ligands (Bu and Jin 2021). Prior studies have shown that heparin binds with PTH without affecting its bioactivity in cAMP accumulation assays (Kamerzell et al. 2007), though these experiments do not differentiate between plasma membrane and endosomal signaling. Secretin, another class B GPCR peptide agonist, has also been identified as a heparan sulfate-binding ligand (Quittot et al. 2017). The addition of soluble heparin, which acts as a decoy to block potential $PTHrP_{1-141}$-GAG interactions, significantly reduces the magnitude and duration of cAMP production in response to $PTHrP_{1-141}$ but does not affect responses to $PTHrP_{1-36}$ or PTH_{1-34}. These findings suggest that GAGs play distinct roles in modulating PTH_1R ligand signaling, possibly by binding to native $PTHrP_{1-141}$ and anchoring it near the receptor to sustain signaling (Pena et al. 2022) (Fig. 6). Despite this emerging evidence, the precise role of GAGs in GPCR signaling remains incompletely understood. Future research could provide valuable insights into how GAGs regulate PTH_1R signaling and reveal novel pharmacological targets for therapeutic intervention.

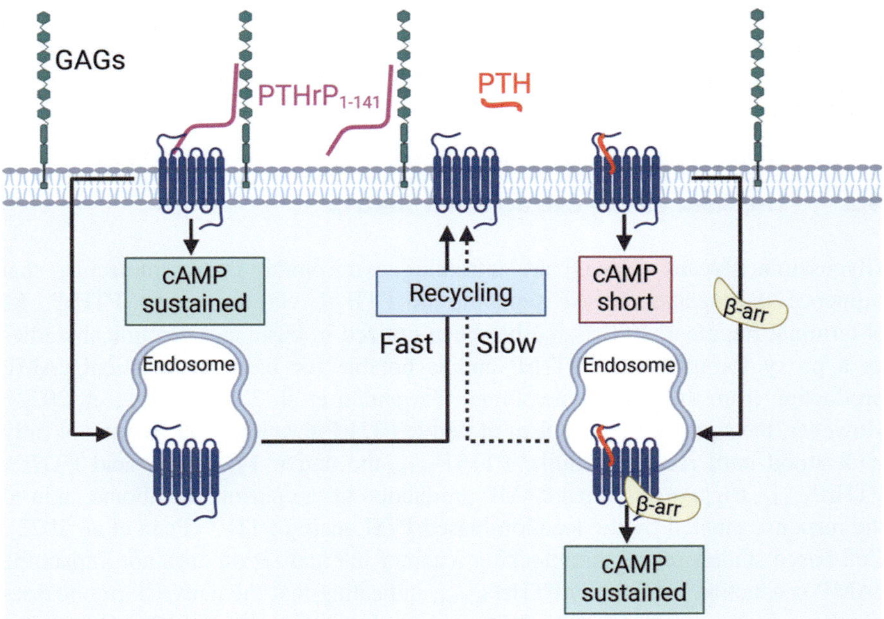

Fig. 6 Proposed model for the role of GAGs in spatial bias for the native $PTHrP_{1-141}$. Cell surface-anchored glycosaminoglycans (GAGs) bind to $PTHrP_{1-141}$, favoring sustained cAMP signaling from the plasma membrane. Though PTH_1R is internalized into endosomes upon $PTHrP_{1-141}$ binding, $PTHrP_{1-141}$ remains bound to GAGs at the cell surface. This allows for fast receptor recycling and reactivation by the anchored ligand. In contrast, PTH_{1-34} is internalized into endosomes with the receptor and β-arr, resulting in sustained cAMP production from the endosomes. Generated with BioRender.com (Adapted from Pena et al. Mol Cell Endocrinol (2024) 1:581:112107)

5 Conclusions

Over the years, PTH_1R has emerged as a model for how GPCRs can signal through cAMP from endosomes. Since endosomal cAMP regulates key physiological and pharmacological processes mediated by PTH_1R, such as vitamin D synthesis and serum Ca^{2+} homeostasis, endosomal G protein signaling by other GPCRs is likely to have pharmacological and biological significance for human health. Gaining a deeper understanding of the mechanisms and rate-limiting biochemical processes that regulate endosomal GPCR signaling is essential for developing therapies.

Acknowledgments The redaction of this chapter was supported by the National Institute of Diabetes and Digestive and Kidney Diseases (NIDKK), the National Institute of Dental and Craniofacial Research (NIDCR) of the US National Institutes of Health (NIH) under Award Numbers R01DK116780 (to J.-P.V.), and R21DE032478 (to J.-P.V.), and by the U.S. Department of Veterans Affairs (VA) under grant I01BX006371 (to J.-P.V). The content is solely the responsibility of the authors and does not necessarily represent the official views of the NIH or the VA. We thank Lisa J. Clark for the preparation of Fig. 4.

References

Abou-Samra AB et al (1992) Expression cloning of a common receptor for parathyroid hormone and parathyroid hormone-related peptide from rat osteoblast-like cells: a single receptor stimulates intracellular accumulation of both cAMP and inositol trisphosphates and increases intracellular free calcium. Proc Natl Acad Sci USA 89(7):2732–2736

Andreassen KV et al (2014) Prolonged calcitonin receptor signaling by salmon, but not human calcitonin, reveals ligand bias. PLoS One 9(3):e92042

Arlt H et al (2020) Effects of abaloparatide and teriparatide on bone resorption and bone formation in female mice. Bone Rep 13:100291

Avet C et al (2022) Effector membrane translocation biosensors reveal G protein and betaarrestin coupling profiles of 100 therapeutically relevant GPCRs. elife 11:e74101

Berlot CH (2002) A highly effective dominant negative alpha s construct containing mutations that affect distinct functions inhibits multiple Gs-coupled receptor signaling pathways. J Biol Chem 277(23):21080–21085

Biber J et al (2009) Regulation of phosphate transport in proximal tubules. Pflugers Arch 458(1): 39–52

Boyce BF et al (2012) The osteoclast, bone remodelling and treatment of metabolic bone disease. Eur J Clin Investig 42(12):1332–1341

Bu C, Jin L (2021) NMR characterization of the interactions between Glycosaminoglycans and proteins. Front Mol Biosci 8:646808

Calebiro D et al (2009) Persistent cAMP-signals triggered by internalized G-protein-coupled receptors. PLoS Biol 7(8):e1000172

Canalis E, Giustina A, Bilezikian JP (2007) Mechanisms of anabolic therapies for osteoporosis. N Engl J Med 357(9):905–916

Chan AS et al (2016) Sorting nexin 27 couples PTHR trafficking to retromer for signal regulation in osteoblasts during bone growth. Mol Biol Cell 27(8):1367–1382

Cheloha RW et al (2015) PTH receptor-1 signalling-mechanistic insights and therapeutic prospects. Nat Rev Endocrinol 11(12):712–724

Clark LJ et al (2020) Allosteric interactions in the parathyroid hormone GPCR-arrestin complex formation. Nat Chem Biol 16(10):1096–1104

Clarke BL et al (2024) Efficacy and safety of TransCon PTH in adults with hypoparathyroidism: 52-week results from the phase 3 PaTHway trial. J Clin Endocrinol Metab. https://doi.org/10.1210/clinem/dgae693
Cohen A et al (2020) Effect of Teriparatide on bone remodeling and density in premenopausal idiopathic osteoporosis: a phase II trial. J Clin Endocrinol Metab 105(10):e3540–e3556
Collins BM (2008) The structure and function of the retromer protein complex. Traffic 9(11): 1811–1822
de Groot T et al (2009) Parathyroid hormone activates TRPV5 via PKA-dependent phosphorylation. J Am Soc Nephrol 20(8):1693–1704
Dean T et al (2006) Mechanisms of ligand binding to the PTH/PTHrp receptor: selectivity of a modified PTH(1-15) Radioligand for G{alpha}S-coupled receptor conformations. Mol Endocrinol 20:931–942
Dean T et al (2008) Altered selectivity of parathyroid hormone (PTH) and PTH-related protein (PTHrP) for distinct conformations of the PTH/PTHrP receptor. Mol Endocrinol 22(1):156–166
Drueke TB (1995) The pathogenesis of parathyroid gland hyperplasia in chronic renal failure. Kidney Int 48(1):259–272
Feinstein TN et al (2011) Retromer terminates the generation of cAMP by internalized PTH receptors. Nat Chem Biol 7(5):278–284
Feinstein TN et al (2013) Noncanonical control of vasopressin receptor type 2 signaling by retromer and arrestin. J Biol Chem 288(39):27849–27860
Feldenzer KL, Sarno J (2018) Hypercalcemia of malignancy. J Adv Pract Oncol 9(5):496–504
Ferrandon S et al (2009) Sustained cyclic AMP production by parathyroid hormone receptor endocytosis. Nat Chem Biol 5(10):734–742
Fraher LJ et al (1992) A comparison of the in vivo biochemical responses to exogenous parathyroid hormone-(1-34) [PTH-(1-34)] and PTH-related peptide-(1-34) in man. J Clin Endocrinol Metab 75(2):417–423
Gidon A et al (2014) Endosomal GPCR signaling turned off by negative feedback actions of PKA and v-ATPase. Nat Chem Biol 10(9):707–709
Giovanella L et al (2021) Will (18)F-fluorocholine PET/CT replace other methods of preoperative parathyroid imaging? Endocrine 71(2):285–297
Godbole A et al (2017) Internalized TSH receptors en route to the TGN induce local G(s)-protein signaling and gene transcription. Nat Commun 8(1):443
Goltzman D (2018) Physiology of parathyroid hormone. Endocrinol Metab Clin N Am 47(4): 743–758
Gurevich VV, Gurevich EV (2019) GPCR signaling regulation: the role of GRKs and Arrestins. Front Pharmacol 10:125
Hattersley G et al (2016) Binding selectivity of Abaloparatide for PTH-Type-1-receptor conformations and effects on downstream signaling. Endocrinology 157(1):141–149
Hoare SR, de Vries G, Usdin TB (1999) Measurement of agonist and antagonist ligand-binding parameters at the human parathyroid hormone type 1 receptor: evaluation of receptor states and modulation by guanine nucleotide. J Pharmacol Exp Ther 289(3):1323–1333
Hoare SR et al (2003) Conformational states of the corticotropin releasing factor 1 (CRF1) receptor: detection, and pharmacological evaluation by peptide ligands. Peptides 24(12):1881–1897
Hoare SR et al (2004) Ligand affinity for amino-terminal and juxtamembrane domains of the corticotropin releasing factor type I receptor: regulation by G-protein and nonpeptide antagonists. Biochemistry 43(13):3996–4011
Hoogendam J et al (2007) Novel mutations in the parathyroid hormone (PTH)/PTH-related peptide receptor type 1 causing Blomstrand osteochondrodysplasia types I and II. J Clin Endocrinol Metab 92(3):1088–1095
Horwitz MJ et al (2005) Continuous PTH and PTHrP infusion causes suppression of bone formation and discordant effects on 1,25(OH)2 vitamin D. J Bone Miner Res 20(10):1792–1803
Irannejad R et al (2013) Conformational biosensors reveal GPCR signalling from endosomes. Nature 495(7442):534–538

Janetzko J et al (2022) Membrane phosphoinositides regulate GPCR-beta-arrestin complex assembly and dynamics. Cell 185(24):4560–4573 e19

Jean-Alphonse FG et al (2017) beta(2)-adrenergic receptor control of endosomal PTH receptor signaling via Gbetagamma. Nat Chem Biol 13(3):259–261

Jobert AS et al (1998) Absence of functional receptors for parathyroid hormone and parathyroid hormone-related peptide in Blomstrand chondrodysplasia. J Clin Invest 102(1):34–40

Juppner H et al (1991) A G protein-linked receptor for parathyroid hormone and parathyroid hormone-related peptide. Science 254(5034):1024–1026

Kadmiel M et al (2017) Loss of receptor activity-modifying protein 2 in mice causes placental dysfunction and alters PTH1R regulation. PLoS One 12(7):e0181597

Kamerzell TJ et al (2007) Parathyroid hormone is a heparin/polyanion binding protein: binding energetics and structure modification. Protein Sci 16(6):1193–1203

Karaplis AC et al (1994) Lethal skeletal dysplasia from targeted disruption of the parathyroid hormone-related peptide gene. Genes Dev 8(3):277–289

Katritch V et al (2014) Allosteric sodium in class A GPCR signaling. Trends Biochem Sci 39(5): 233–244

Kim BH et al (2018) Extracellular nucleotides enhance agonist potency at the parathyroid hormone 1 receptor. Cell Signal 46:103–112

Kim BH et al (2019) Toward defining the pharmacophore for positive allosteric modulation of PTH1 receptor signaling by extracellular nucleotides. ACS Pharmacol Transl Sci 2(3):155–167

Kotowski SJ et al (2011) Endocytosis promotes rapid dopaminergic signaling. Neuron 71(2): 278–290

Kuna RS et al (2013) Glucagon-like peptide-1 receptor-mediated endosomal cAMP generation promotes glucose-stimulated insulin secretion in pancreatic beta-cells. Am J Physiol Endocrinol Metab 305(2):E161–E170

Leder BZ et al (2015) Effects of abaloparatide, a human parathyroid hormone-related peptide analog, on bone mineral density in postmenopausal women with osteoporosis. J Clin Endocrinol Metab 100(2):697–706

Lee S et al (2015) A homozygous [Cys25]PTH(1-84) mutation that impairs PTH/PTHrP receptor activation defines a novel form of hypoparathyroidism. J Bone Miner Res 30(10):1803–1813

Li M, Li M, Guo J (2021) Molecular mechanism of Ca(2+) in the allosteric regulation of human parathyroid hormone receptor-1. J Chem Inf Model. https://doi.org/10.1021/acs.jcim.1c00471

Liu S et al (2018) Receptor selectivity from minimal backbone modification of a polypeptide agonist. Proc Natl Acad Sci USA 115(49):12383–12388

Liu S et al (2019) Use of backbone modification to enlarge the spatiotemporal diversity of parathyroid hormone Receptor-1 signaling via biased Agonism. J Am Chem Soc 141(37): 14486–14490

Lyga S et al (2016) Persistent cAMP signaling by internalized LH receptors in ovarian follicles. Endocrinology 157(4):1613–1621

Marino S, Bellido T (2024) PTH receptor signalling, osteocytes and bone disease induced by diabetes mellitus. Nat Rev Endocrinol 20(11):661–672

May V, Parsons RL (2017) G protein-coupled receptor endosomal signaling and regulation of neuronal excitability and stress responses: signaling options and lessons from the PAC1 receptor. J Cell Physiol 232(4):698–706

Mazzoni MR, Martini C, Lucacchini A (1993) Regulation of agonist binding to A2A adenosine receptors: effects of guanine nucleotides (GDP[S] and GTP[S]) and Mg2+ ion. Biochim Biophys Acta 1220(1):76–84

McCauley LK, Martin TJ (2012) Twenty-five years of PTHrP progress: from cancer hormone to multifunctional cytokine. J Bone Miner Res 27(6):1231–1239

McGarvey JC et al (2016) Actin-sorting nexin 27 (SNX27)-Retromer complex mediates rapid parathyroid hormone receptor recycling. J Biol Chem 291(21):10986–11002

Merriam LA et al (2013) Pituitary adenylate cyclase 1 receptor internalization and endosomal signaling mediate the pituitary adenylate cyclase activating polypeptide-induced increase in guinea pig cardiac neuron excitability. J Neurosci 33(10):4614–4622
Miller PD et al (2019) Bone mineral density response rates are greater in patients treated with abaloparatide compared with those treated with placebo or teriparatide: results from the ACTIVE phase 3 trial. Bone 120:137–140
Nagai S et al (2011) Acute down-regulation of sodium-dependent phosphate transporter NPT2a involves predominantly the cAMP/PKA pathway as revealed by signaling-selective parathyroid hormone analogs. J Biol Chem 286(2):1618–1626
Neer RM et al (2001) Effect of parathyroid hormone (1-34) on fractures and bone mineral density in postmenopausal women with osteoporosis. N Engl J Med 344(19):1434–1441
Nemec K et al (2022) Functional modulation of PTH1R activation and signaling by RAMP2. Proc Natl Acad Sci USA 119(32):e2122037119
Nissenson RA, Diep D, Strewler GJ (1988) Synthetic peptides comprising the amino-terminal sequence of a parathyroid hormone-like protein from human malignancies. Binding to parathyroid hormone receptors and activation of adenylate cyclase in bone cells and kidney. J Biol Chem 263(26):12866–12871
O'Brien CA, Nakashima T, Takayanagi H (2013) Osteocyte control of osteoclastogenesis. Bone 54(2):258–263
Ogawa M et al (2022) Hypercalcemia associated with the ectopic expression of 25-hydroxyvitamin D3-1alpha-hydroxylase in diffuse large B-cell lymphoma. Intern Med 61(16):2489–2495
Oldham WM, Hamm HE (2006) Structural basis of function in heterotrimeric G proteins. Q Rev Biophys 39(2):117–166
Ono K et al (2021) Evaluations of daily teriparatide using finite-element analysis over 12 months in rheumatoid arthritis patients. J Bone Miner Metab 39(2):270–277
Pacheco J et al (2024) Fast-diffusing receptor collisions with slow-diffusing peptide ligand assemble the ternary parathyroid hormone-GPCR-arrestin complex. Nat Commun 15(1):10499
Pena KA (2022) Endosomal parathyroid hormone receptor signaling. Am J Physiol Cell Physiol 323(3):C783–C790
Pena KA et al (2022) Biased GPCR signaling by the native parathyroid hormone-related protein 1 to 141 relative to its N-terminal fragment 1 to 36. J Biol Chem 298(9):102332
Peng GE et al (2021) Spatial decoding of endosomal cAMP signals by a metastable cytoplasmic PKA network. Nat Chem Biol 17(5):558–566
Philbrick WM et al (1996) Defining the roles of parathyroid hormone-related protein in normal physiology. Physiol Rev 76(1):127–173
Philbrick WM et al (1998) Parathyroid hormone-related protein is required for tooth eruption. Proc Natl Acad Sci USA 95(20):11846–11851
Picard N et al (2010) Acute parathyroid hormone differentially regulates renal brush border membrane phosphate cotransporters. Pflugers Arch 460(3):677–687
Potts JT Jr et al (1971) Synthesis of a biologically active N-terminal tetratriacontapeptide of parathyroid hormone. Proc Natl Acad Sci USA 68(1):63–67
Quittot N et al (2017) Identification of a conformational heparin-recognition motif on the peptide hormone secretin: key role for cell surface binding. Biochem J 474(13):2249–2260
Rejnmark L (2024) Treatment of hypoparathyroidism by re-establishing the effects of parathyroid hormone. Endocrinol Metab (Seoul) 39(2):262–266
Rodriguez FD, Bardaji E, Traynor JR (1992) Differential effects of Mg2+ and other divalent cations on the binding of tritiated opioid ligands. J Neurochem 59(2):467–472
Rubin MR (2020) Recent advances in understanding and managing hypoparathyroidism. F1000Res 9:F1000
Saini V et al (2013) Parathyroid hormone (PTH)/PTH-related peptide type 1 receptor (PPR) signaling in osteocytes regulates anabolic and catabolic skeletal responses to PTH. J Biol Chem 288(28):20122–20134

Schipani E, Kruse K, Juppner H (1995) A constitutively active mutant PTH-PTHrP receptor in Jansen-type metaphyseal chondrodysplasia. Science 268(5207):98–100
Schipani E et al (1996) Constitutively activated receptors for parathyroid hormone and parathyroid hormone-related peptide in Jansen's metaphyseal chondrodysplasia. N Engl J Med 335(10): 708–714
Schipani E et al (1999) A novel parathyroid hormone (PTH)/PTH-related peptide receptor mutation in Jansen's metaphyseal chondrodysplasia. J Clin Endocrinol Metab 84(9):3052–3057
Silva BC et al (2011) Catabolic and anabolic actions of parathyroid hormone on the skeleton. J Endocrinol Investig 34(10):801–810
Silver IA, Murrills RJ, Etherington DJ (1988) Microelectrode studies on the acid microenvironment beneath adherent macrophages and osteoclasts. Exp Cell Res 175(2):266–276
Singh AT et al (2005a) G alpha12/G alpha13 subunits of heterotrimeric G proteins mediate parathyroid hormone activation of phospholipase D in UMR-106 osteoblastic cells. Endocrinology 146(5):2171–2175
Singh AT, Frohman MA, Stern PH (2005b) Parathyroid hormone stimulates phosphatidylethanolamine hydrolysis by phospholipase D in osteoblastic cells. Lipids 40(11):1135–1140
Sleeman A, Clements JN (2019) Abaloparatide: a new pharmacological option for osteoporosis. Am J Health Syst Pharm 76(3):130–135
Suva LJ et al (1987) A parathyroid hormone-related protein implicated in malignant hypercalcemia: cloning and expression. Science 237(4817):893–896
Towler DA (2024) Parathyroid hormone-PTH1R signaling in cardiovascular disease and homeostasis. Trends Endocrinol Metab. https://doi.org/10.1016/j.tem.2024.02.005
Tsvetanova NG et al (2021) Endosomal cAMP production broadly impacts the cellular phosphoproteome. J Biol Chem 297(1):100907
Urwyler S (2011) Allosteric modulation of family C G-protein-coupled receptors: from molecular insights to therapeutic perspectives. Pharmacol Rev 63(1):59–126
van Abel M et al (2005) Coordinated control of renal Ca(2+) transport proteins by parathyroid hormone. Kidney Int 68(4):1708–1721
Vilardaga JP et al (2023) Molecular mechanisms of PTH/PTHrP class B GPCR signaling and pharmacological implications. Endocr Rev 44(3):474–491
Wang B et al (2013) NHERF1 regulation of PTH-dependent bimodal Pi transport in osteoblasts. Bone 52(1):268–277
Wang MW et al (2021) Activation of PTH1R alleviates epididymitis and orchitis through Gq and beta-arrestin-1 pathways. Proc Natl Acad Sci USA 118(45):e2107363118
Wehbi VL et al (2013) Noncanonical GPCR signaling arising from a PTH receptor-arrestin-Gbetagamma complex. Proc Natl Acad Sci USA 110(4):1530–1535
White AD et al (2019) Ca(2+) allostery in PTH-receptor signaling. Proc Natl Acad Sci USA 116(8): 3294–3299
White AD et al (2020) Gq/11-dependent regulation of endosomal cAMP generation by parathyroid hormone class B GPCR. Proc Natl Acad Sci USA 117(13):7455–7460
White AD et al (2021) Spatial bias in cAMP generation determines biological responses to PTH type 1 receptor activation. Sci Signal 14(703):eabc5944
Willette BKA et al (2024) Endosome positioning coordinates spatially selective GPCR signaling. Nat Chem Biol 20(2):151–161
Wuthrich RP, Martin D, Bilezikian JP (2007) The role of calcimimetics in the treatment of hyperparathyroidism. Eur J Clin Investig 37(12):915–922
Wysolmerski JJ, Stewart AF (1998) The physiology of parathyroid hormone-related protein: an emerging role as a developmental factor. Annu Rev Physiol 60:431–460
Yarwood RE et al (2017) Endosomal signaling of the receptor for calcitonin gene-related peptide mediates pain transmission. Proc Natl Acad Sci USA 114(46):12309–12314
Zhao LH et al (2019) Structure and dynamics of the active human parathyroid hormone receptor-1. Science 364(6436):148–153

Mechanisms of Location Bias in G Protein-Coupled Receptors

Uyen Pham, Anand Chundi, and Sudarshan Rajagopal

Contents

Abstract

GPCRs are known for their versatile signaling roles at the plasma membrane; however, recent studies have revealed that these receptors also function within various intracellular compartments, such as endosomes, the Golgi apparatus, and

U. Pham
Department of Biochemistry, Duke University School of Medicine, Durham, NC, USA

A. Chundi · S. Rajagopal (✉)
Department of Medicine, Duke University Medical Center, Durham, NC, USA
e-mail: sudarshan.rajagopal@duke.edu

© The Author(s), under exclusive license to Springer Nature Switzerland AG 2025
Z. Li, K. Xiao (eds.), *Pharmacology of GPCRs Biased Signaling and Agonists*,
Handbook of Experimental Pharmacology 290, https://doi.org/10.1007/164_2025_764

the endoplasmic reticulum. This spatially distinct signaling, termed location bias, allows GPCRs to initiate unique signaling cascades and influence cellular processes—including cAMP production, calcium mobilization, and protein phosphorylation—in a compartment-specific manner. By mapping the impact of GPCR signaling from these subcellular locations, this chapter emphasizes the mechanisms underlying signaling from intracellular receptor pools in diversifying receptor functionality. Such mechanistic insights into location-biased signaling open up novel therapeutic strategies aimed at targeting GPCRs within specific organelles, promising new levels of precision in therapeutic modulation and potential improvements in treatment efficacy and specificity.

Keywords

Endocytosis · G protein-coupled receptor · Location bias · Nanodomains · Subcellular locations · Trafficking

1 Introduction

G protein-coupled receptors (GPCRs) are a vast and versatile family of membrane proteins that play a pivotal role in transmitting signals from the external environment to the interior of cells. With over 800 distinct receptors encoded in the human genome, these receptors respond to a wide array of extracellular stimuli, including hormones, neurotransmitters, and sensory signals like light and odors, and are essential for regulating numerous physiological processes such as metabolism, immune responses, and neuronal activity (Lagerstrom and Schioth 2008). Upon binding to their specific ligands in the extracellular space, GPCRs undergo conformational changes and activate intracellular signaling pathways through their interaction with G proteins, β-arrestins, and GPCR kinases (GRKs), ultimately leading to diverse cellular responses like gene expression, metabolic regulation, and immune activation (Wootten et al. 2018). Due to their broad influence on human physiology and their involvement in numerous conditions, including cardiovascular diseases, cancer, neurodegenerative disorders, and metabolic syndromes, GPCRs are the target of a significant portion of modern pharmaceuticals, making them a critical focus in drug discovery and therapeutic development (Lagerstrom and Schioth 2008; Zhang et al. 2024).

In the classical model of GPCR signaling transduction, GPCRs are located on the plasma membrane, where upon ligand binding, they undergo a conformational change that promotes the activation of intracellular heterotrimeric G proteins, composed of Gα, Gβ, and Gγ subunits. Once activated, the Gα subunit dissociates from the Gβγ complex, allowing both components to regulate downstream effectors such as adenylyl cyclase, phospholipase C, or ion channels. These effectors then generate second messengers like cyclic AMP (cAMP), diacylglycerol, and inositol trisphosphate, leading to a cascade of intracellular events, including changes in gene expression, cell metabolism, or motility (Pierce et al. 2002; Rosenbaum et al.

2009). After a short time, GPCR signaling is typically terminated through a process called desensitization, where proteins like G protein-coupled receptor kinases (GRKs) phosphorylate the receptor, leading to the recruitment of β-arrestins (Gurevich and Gurevich 2019). The β-arrestins uncouple the receptor from G proteins and facilitate receptor internalization through clathrin-mediated endocytosis, bringing GPCRs into the cell for either recycling or degradation (Lohse et al. 1990; Smith and Rajagopal 2016).

The discovery that GPCRs can signal from multiple intracellular sites challenges the long-held notion that these receptors operate solely from the cell surface and suggests that GPCRs are far more versatile and context-dependent than previously appreciated (Calebiro et al. 2009; Ferrandon et al. 2009; Irannejad et al. 2013; Luttrell et al. 2001). This emerging concept of "location bias" adds a nuanced dimension to this classical model by recognizing that GPCR signaling can continue – or even initiate – inside the cell from different subcellular compartments (Eiger et al. 2023; Mohammad Nezhady et al. 2020). Instead of viewing receptor internalization as merely a mechanism to shut off signaling, recent research shows that GPCRs can signal from within the cell, specifically from endosomes, the Golgi apparatus, and other intracellular compartments (Fig. 1). This chapter highlights recent progress in understanding the mechanisms that regulate intracellular GPCRs as key contributors

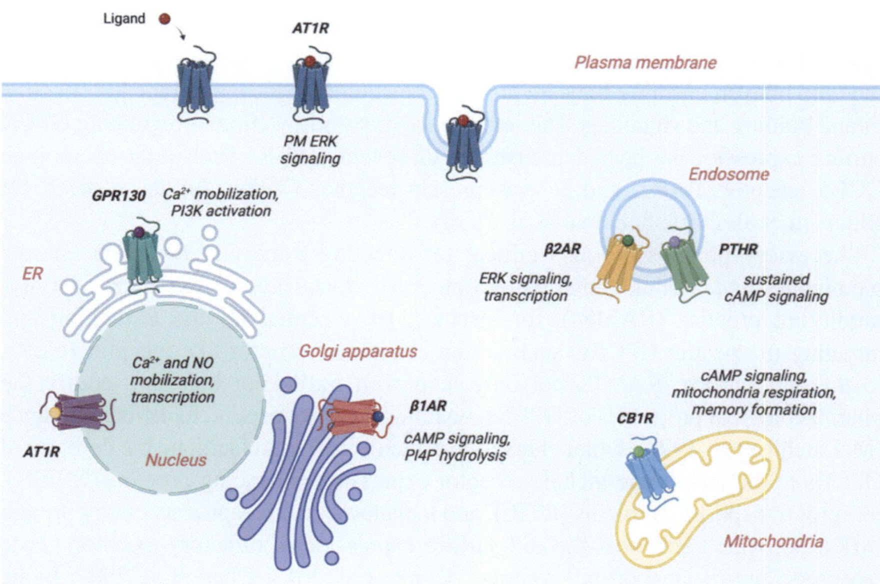

Fig. 1 Examples of location-biased GPCR signaling from different subcellular compartments. Signaling by these different receptors in different subcellular locations is regulated through different mechanisms, e.g., trafficking, pools of receptors in different locations, etc. AT1R – type 1 angiotensin II receptor. β1AR – β1 adrenergic receptor. β2AR – β2 adrenergic receptor. PTHR – parathyroid hormone receptor. CB1R –cannabinoid type 1 receptor

to signaling bias, explores unresolved challenges in the field, and discusses their potential implications for therapeutic development.

2 Cellular Expression and Signaling of GPCRs

2.1 Cell Surface Expression of GPCRs

GPCRs on the cell surface interact with extracellular ligands and activate intracellular signaling pathways. The expression of GPCRs at the plasma membrane is a highly regulated process, influenced by several factors that ensure proper receptor function and localization.

Post-translational modifications (PTMs) play a crucial role in the maturation, stability, and surface expression of GPCRs. Glycosylation, ubiquitination, phosphorylation, and palmitoylation are among the key modifications that enhance receptor folding, trafficking, and targeting to the cell surface (Patwardhan et al. 2021). Glycosylation, in particular, is essential for stabilizing GPCRs in the endoplasmic reticulum (ER) and assisting their proper folding, which is a prerequisite for trafficking to the plasma membrane. Disruption of N-glycosylation was shown to perturb the cell surface expression of certain GPCRs, such as the bradykinin B2 receptor (B2R), angiotensin type 1 receptor (AT1R), dopamine D5 receptor (D5R), and protease-activated receptor 2 (PAR2) (Compton et al. 2002; Karpa et al. 1999; Lanctot et al. 1999; Michineau et al. 2004). Palmitoylation is important for efficient transport of receptors through the biosynthetic pathway and helps anchor GPCRs to the lipid bilayer, ensuring they are properly positioned in the membrane for effective ligand binding and signaling. The importance of palmitoylation in regulating GPCR surface expression has been demonstrated for several GPCRs, such as the chemokine CCR5 receptor, PAR2, and V_2 vasopressin receptor (V2R) (Adams et al. 2011; Blanpain et al. 2001; Schulein et al. 1996).

Accessory proteins are also critical for directing some GPCRs to the plasma membrane and maintaining their functional localization. Receptor activity-modifying proteins (RAMPs), for instance, are essential for the trafficking and targeting of specific GPCRs, such as the calcitonin receptor-like receptor (CLR), to the cell surface. RAMPs not only help with trafficking but also modify the pharmacological properties of GPCRs, enabling them to respond to different ligands (McLatchie et al. 1998). Other chaperone proteins known to facilitate the delivery of GPCRs to the membrane include receptor expression enhancing proteins (REEPs), receptor transporting proteins (RTPs), and melanocortin 2 receptor accessory protein (MRAPs), which enhances the cell surface expression of olfactory receptors, taste receptors, and melanocortin 2 receptor (Bjork et al. 2013; Chan et al. 2009; Inoue et al. 2023).

GPCR expression on the plasma membrane is not uniform. Several factors, including cell type, membrane properties, and the existence of specialized membrane domains, contribute to the heterogeneity of GPCR expression. The lipid composition of the plasma membrane also affects the distribution and function of GPCRs.

Additionally, GPCRs are often localized in specific membrane microdomains, such as lipid rafts, caveolae, or clathrin-coated pits (Chini and Parenti 2004). Lipid rafts and caveolae are small, dynamic, and self-assembled microdomains enriched with cholesterol and sphingolipids that provide platforms for efficient receptor signaling. Cholesterol-rich regions have also been found to promote GPCR stability and enhance receptor-ligand interactions. Clathrin-coated pits are involved in the internalization of GPCRs following ligand binding, contributing to receptor desensitization and recycling (Wolfe and Trejo 2007).

2.2 Endosomal GPCRs

GPCR endocytosis is a process that is classically downstream of ligand binding and receptor activation, although a number of GPCRs constitutively recycle between the endosomal compartment and the plasma membrane. Upon activation, GPCRs are typically phosphorylated by G protein-coupled receptor kinases (GRKs), which promotes the recruitment of β-arrestins. β-arrestins serve dual functions: they terminate G protein signaling at the plasma membrane and facilitate receptor internalization by recruiting components of the clathrin-mediated endocytic machinery (Lefkowitz and Shenoy 2005). Once internalized, GPCRs are trafficked into early endosomes, where they are either recycled back to the plasma membrane or directed toward lysosomal degradation (Sorkin and von Zastrow 2009). Initially, the main role of internalization was thought to be desensitization, as receptor removal from the cell surface prevents excessive signaling. However, the discovery that GPCRs signal from endosomes has transformed our understanding of receptor signaling dynamics. Endosomes provide a unique microenvironment that can modulate GPCR signaling. Factors such as acidic pH, lipid composition, and the presence of specific effectors within endosomes can alter GPCR conformation and its interaction with downstream signaling molecules. This enables the initiation of different signaling pathways compared to plasma membrane signals, adding versatility to GPCR-mediated responses (Klauer et al. 2024).

Early evidence of β-arrestin-dependent endosomal signaling came from studies using dominant negative mutant of dynamin to block clathrin-dependent endocytosis, revealing that β2AR internalization is essential for full activation of extracellular signal-regulated kinase 1/2 (ERK1/2) by the β2AR agonist isoproterenol (Daaka et al. 1998). Subsequent research demonstrated that certain GPCRs such as the V2 vasopressin receptor (V2R) can remain bound to β-arrestin in endosomes, which is largely dictated by the specific phosphorylatable motifs in the receptor C-terminal tail (Oakley et al. 1999). Other research showed that GPCRs can form a multiprotein signaling complex with β-arrestins and various kinases of the mitogen-activated protein kinase (MAPK) signaling cascades in endosomes (DeFea et al. 2000; Luttrell et al. 2001; McDonald et al. 2000). This β-arrestin-driven signaling from endosomes was found to exhibit distinct temporal and spatial activation patterns from the transient G protein signaling initiated at the plasma membrane (Ahn et al. 2004).

It was later found that GPCRs can also activate G protein-dependent signaling from endosomes. Research with the metabotropic glutamate receptor 5 (mGlu5), parathyroid hormone receptor type 1 (PTHR), and the thyroid-stimulating hormone receptor (TSHR) provided the initial evidence of sustained signaling of G protein-mediated pathways, such as cAMP and intracellular calcium response, that requires internalized receptors (Calebiro et al. 2009; Ferrandon et al. 2009; Jong et al. 2005). Using nanobodies which selectively recognizes the active state of β2-adrenergic receptor (β2AR) and its cognate G protein, Gαs, it was subsequently shown that the β2AR continues to activate the cAMP pathway following internalization into endosomes with spatially distinct and sustained signals compared to those initiated at the plasma membrane (Irannejad et al. 2013).

Subsequent studies further supported the idea of "signaling endosome" with a diverse array of G proteins, such as Gαs, Gαi/o, and Gαq, and GPCRs (Eiger et al. 2022; Jensen et al. 2017; Kotowski et al. 2011; Kwon et al. 2022; Tsvetanova et al. 2021; Tsvetanova and von Zastrow 2014; Yarwood et al. 2017). For instance, CXCR3, a chemokine receptor, exhibits biased signaling depending on its localization and the type of ligand that binds to it. CXCR3 can engage different downstream pathways, either through G protein-dependent or β-arrestin-dependent mechanisms, depending on whether it is activated by its ligand CXCL9, CXCL10, or CXCL11. CXCR3 biased signaling has been implicated in immune responses, particularly in inflammatory diseases, where biased signaling from endosomes leads to sustained activation of ERK1/2 in the nucleus (Eiger et al. 2022). This prolonged signaling is critical for regulating T-cell transcription responses and inflammatory pathways (Eiger et al. 2022; Smith et al. 2018).

Besides the discreet G protein- and β-arrestin-dependent signaling pathways, it was also found that GPCRs can form complexes with both G protein and β-arrestin in endosomes, called "megaplexes." This signaling complex, in which the receptor simultaneously interacts with G protein through its core regions and with β-arrestin via the phosphorylated C-terminus, promotes sustained G protein activation and cAMP signaling from internalized compartments (Nguyen et al. 2019; Thomsen et al. 2016).

2.3 Nuclear GPCRs

Expression at the nuclear membrane has been described for over 40 receptors, such as the AT1R and the prostaglandin EP1 receptor, which regulate key signaling pathways and exhibit functional consequences distinct from their plasma membrane counterparts (Bhattacharya et al. 1998; Lu et al. 1998). These receptors not only play roles in modulating intracellular calcium and cAMP levels but also participate in phosphorylation of key signaling intermediates like ERK and protein kinase C (PKC), further emphasizing their diverse signaling outputs (Cattaneo et al. 2016; O'Malley et al. 2003; Valdehita et al. 2010; Wright et al. 2008; Wu et al. 2014). AT1R has been shown to translocate to the nucleus upon ligand stimulation, leading to downstream signaling via pathways such as PKC and NOX4-mediated reactive oxygen species (ROS) generation (Lu et al. 1998; Pendergrass et al. 2009).

Nuclear GPCRs are believed to signal through both the inner and outer nuclear membranes (Tadevosyan et al. 2012). In this model, the receptor's N-terminus is localized within the lumen of the nuclear membrane, while the C-terminus may reside in the cytoplasm or the nucleus. This orientation suggests that nuclear GPCRs may activate classical signaling pathways inside the nucleus, akin to cytoplasmic GPCR activation, but with nuclear-specific downstream effects. For instance, studies show that angiotensin II (AngII) interacts with nuclear AT1R and angiotensin type 2 receptor (AT2R) in atrial cardiac fibroblasts and renal cortex, which can stimulate NOX4-mediated ROS production, calcium and nitric oxide (NO) mobilization, contributing to cellular oxidative stress responses and influencing processes like RNA synthesis, gene transcription, cell proliferation, and collagen secretion (Gwathmey et al. 2009; Pendergrass et al. 2009; Tadevosyan et al. 2017). In cardiomyocytes, the AngII receptors have been found to promote nuclear calcium mobilization, transcriptional initiation, and nuclear factor-κB (Nf-κB) gene expression (Tadevosyan et al. 2010). Furthermore, clathrin-dependent internalization of AT1R from the plasma membrane to the nucleus is essential for expression of cyclooxygenase-2 (COX-2) in vascular smooth muscle cells, leading to cell proliferation and migration (Hu et al. 2002; Morinelli et al. 2008; Ohnaka et al. 2000).

The protease-activated receptor 2 (PAR2) translocates from the plasma membrane to the nucleus, where it interacts with the Sp1 transcription factor to promote vascular endothelial growth factor A (VEGFA) expression, leading to neovascularization (Joyal et al. 2014). Other nuclear GPCRs, such as the oxytocin receptor (OXTR), have been linked to osteoblastic transcriptional induction, which is important for bone formation (Di Benedetto et al. 2014; Kinsey et al. 2007). Endogenous α1-adrenergic receptor (α1-AR) have been found to form both homo- and hetero-oligomers when localized to the nuclear membrane in cardiomyocytes, which is required for ERK activation at the plasma membrane, an essential signaling pathway that mediates α1-AR's physiological role in normal cardiomyocyte hypertrophy and adaptive response to cardiac stress (O'Connell et al. 2003, 2006; Wright et al. 2008, 2012).

The mechanisms enabling GPCR translocation to the nucleus are not fully understood. One key method is the engagement of nuclear localization signals (NLS), sequences within the receptor that are recognized by importins, which transport GPCRs across the nuclear envelope (Lu et al. 2021). Lipid microdomains and nuclear bodies could provide environments conducive to embedding the hydrophobic regions of GPCRs within the nucleus. These domains, reported to participate in transcription and RNA transport, might harbor GPCRs through invaginations from the nuclear envelope or as part of membrane-less organelles (Cascianelli et al. 2008; Fricker et al. 1997; Zimber et al. 2004). Additionally, emerging evidence points to phase separation as a possible mechanism for nuclear GPCR organization, where hydrophobic domains of GPCRs could interact with other multivalent proteins, forming functional complexes involved in transcriptional regulation (Maccaroni et al. 2022; Pinheiro et al. 2023). This hypothesis suggests that

GPCRs may adopt different conformations or shapes based on their nuclear environment, enabling a broader range of functions compared to their traditional cylindrical structure.

2.4 Mitochondrial GPCRs

An increasing number of GPCRs can localize on the mitochondrial membranes, where they participate in intracellular signaling. Mitochondrial GPCRs regulate several vital processes, such as cellular metabolism, ROS production, and apoptosis, linking extracellular signals directly to the mitochondria. For instance, both the AT1R and AT2R have been identified in the mitochondria of various tissues and cell types where they mediate energy regulation and cellular stress responses with AT2R appearing with much greater abundance (Abadir et al. 2011; Valenzuela et al. 2016). In dopaminergic neurons, activation of mitochondrial AngII receptors results in opposite effects on respiratory activity. Activation of mitochondrial AT2R leads to NO production, which inhibits mitochondrial respiration and has antiapoptotic effects, and its expression level increases significantly upon treatment with oxidative stress inducers while decreases with aging. In contrast, AngII stimulation of AT1R induces NOX4-mediated superoxide production, which increases respiration and oxidative stress, and its mitochondrial level increases with aging and after treatment of cells with antioxidants such as N-acetyl cysteine (NAC) (Valenzuela et al. 2016). Other receptors such as the cannabinoid type 1 receptors (CB1R) have been found to localize on the mitochondrial membranes of mouse hippocampal neurons, where they demonstrate key roles in modulating cAMP production, PKA activity, mitochondrial respiration, ATP production, and memory formation (Benard et al. 2012; Hebert-Chatelain et al. 2016).

The presence of GPCRs in mitochondria opens up new avenues for drug development, especially in diseases where mitochondrial dysfunction is a key factor, such as neurodegenerative disorders, cancer, and metabolic syndromes (Zong et al. 2024). Targeting mitochondrial GPCRs could provide a novel strategy to restore mitochondrial function, regulate apoptosis, and improve energy metabolism. For instance, modulating mitochondrial AT1R activation could help reduce neuroinflammation, oxidative stress, and the degeneration of dopaminergic neurons in Parkinson's disease.

2.5 ER and Golgi GPCRs

The Golgi apparatus and endoplasmic reticulum (ER) play crucial roles in the maturation, post-translational modification, and trafficking of GPCRs. The ER is the site of GPCR synthesis and initial folding, while the Golgi processes receptors through glycosylation and sorting for delivery to their final destinations (Dong et al. 2007). However, distinguishing transiently trafficking GPCRs from functionally active resident receptors in these organelles is challenging, as these compartments are central to receptor maturation.

Nanobodies – single-domain antibodies that selectively bind to active GPCR conformations – have helped differentiate actively signaling GPCRs from those merely passing through the Golgi and ER. For example, studies using nanobodies have demonstrated that the β1AR is active not only at the plasma membrane but also in the Golgi, where it contributes significantly to the overall cellular cAMP response and activates PLCε, leading to the hydrolysis of phosphatidylinositol-4-phosphate (PI4P) (Irannejad et al. 2013; Nash et al. 2019). Furthermore, the activation of this endogenous pool of Golgi-localized β1AR is independent of its activation at the plasma membrane, and this signaling plays a physiological role, as demonstrated by research showing that blocking Golgi-localized β1AR inhibits norepinephrine-induced hypertrophic responses in cardiac myocytes, a key factor in heart disease (Nash et al. 2019). Other examples of GPCRs that localize and signal from the Golgi include the dopamine D1 receptor (D1R), which can be activated by dopamine to promote cAMP production and protein kinase A (PKA) activation in murine striatal medium spiny neurons (Puri et al. 2022). The Golgi pool of μ-opioid (MOR) and δ-opioid (DOR) receptors can initiate distinct signaling pathways and transcriptional responses compared to those at the plasma membrane (Radoux-Mergault et al. 2023; Stoeber et al. 2018).

In contrast, signaling by the parathyroid hormone receptor type 1 (PTHR) is terminated by trafficking to the Golgi via retromer, a heteropentameric complex that facilitates the retrograde transport of internalized receptors, thus halting the cAMP signal (Feinstein et al. 2011). This underscores that different GPCRs in the Golgi can either sustain signaling or act as a checkpoint for signal termination.

The ER also hosts active GPCRs that regulate key intracellular processes, particularly calcium signaling. GPR30, an estrogen receptor, is predominantly expressed in the ER and upon binding to estrogen, initiates intracellular calcium mobilization and phosphoinositide 3-kinase (PI3K) activation, triggering specific signaling pathways (Revankar et al. 2005). Another receptor of interest in the ER is metabotropic glutamate receptor 5 (mGluR5), which has been detected abundantly on the intracellular membranes of both the ER and nucleus, as well as at the plasma membrane of rat hippocampal neurons. Using caged ligands and nanobodies to control activation in specific cellular regions, researchers have shown that intracellular mGluR5 activation leads to sustained calcium release and gene expression, highlighting its role in calcium homeostasis and hippocampal synaptic plasticity (Jong et al. 2009; Purgert et al. 2014).

One intriguing aspect of GPCR localization on intracellular membranes is that for their endogenous ligands to interact with the receptor's binding site, these ligands must either be membrane-permeable or actively transported into the organelle. This is especially relevant for GPCRs located in compartments such as the ER or Golgi apparatus, where the receptor's binding pocket is embedded within the organelle's lumen, necessitating specific mechanisms for ligand access to initiate intracellular signaling. Different ligands have been found to reach intracellular receptors through various transport mechanisms. For example, mGluR5 in the ER is activated by glutamate, a non-membrane-permeable ligand which is transported intracellularly via sodium-dependent excitatory amino acid transporters and the cystine/glutamate exchanger (Purgert et al. 2014). Similarly, cell-impermeant ligands like those for β1AR and D1R in the Golgi are transported by organic cation transporters (OCTs) (Irannejad et al. 2017; Jong et al. 2009; Puri et al. 2022). On the other hand, GPR30 on the ER binds estrogen, a membrane-permeable ligand, which easily accesses its binding site within the organelle (Revankar et al. 2005).

3 Intracellular Expression of GPCR Effectors

3.1 G Proteins

Traditionally, G proteins have been viewed as plasma membrane-associated signal transducers that relay information from activated GPCRs at the cell surface to intracellular effectors. In this classical model, ligand binding to GPCRs at the cell surface leads to the activation of heterotrimeric G proteins composed of Gα, Gβ, and Gγ subunits. Upon activation, the Gα subunit dissociates from the Gβγ dimer, initiating distinct downstream signaling cascades. This plasma membrane-centric view of G protein function has been a cornerstone of cellular signaling research for decades. However, growing evidence has demonstrated that G proteins are also expressed and functional in various intracellular organelles, where they modulate localized signaling events.

Endosomes are key intracellular compartments where GPCRs continue to signal after internalization from the plasma membrane. G proteins, particularly Gαs, have been shown to localize to early and late endosomes, where they engage in sustained signaling. For instance, the β2-adrenergic receptor (β2AR) can activate Gαs in endosomes, leading to prolonged production of the second messenger cAMP and activation of downstream effectors such as extracellular signal-regulated kinase (ERK) (Kwon et al. 2022; Liccardo et al. 2022). This extended signaling from endosomes contrasts with the transient nature of G protein activation at the plasma membrane and contributes to longer-term cellular responses such as gene transcription (Kwon et al. 2022).

The Golgi apparatus is another site of intracellular G protein signaling. Gαq/11 and Gαs have been localized to the cis-Golgi, where they regulate critical processes such as protein trafficking and secretion. For instance, the KDEL receptor (KDELR) has been found to activate Gαs, Gαq/11, and Gαo at the Golgi (Cancino et al. 2014; Giannotta et al. 2012; Solis et al. 2017). While Gαs signaling in the Golgi is involved in the retrograde transport of ER-resident chaperones, Gαq/11-Src signaling promotes the intra-Golgi transport of proteins destined for the plasma membrane (Cancino et al. 2014; Giannotta et al. 2012). Gβγ subunits have also been shown to localize in the Golgi and regulate signaling pathways (Jamora et al. 1999; Klayman and Wedegaertner 2017; Masuho et al. 2021; Wei and Smrcka 2024).

G proteins have also been detected in the nucleus, where they are involved in nuclear signaling pathways that influence gene expression (Bhatnagar et al. 2013;

Dahl et al. 2018; Sato et al. 2011; Zhang et al. 2001). For instance, Gβγ has been shown to interact with chromatin and regulate transcription factor activity, and the nuclear localization of the Gβ2 subunit was crucial for modulating the activity of Myocyte enhancer factor 2A (MEF2A), a transcription factor involved in muscle differentiation. This suggests that G protein signaling can influence transcription by directly interacting with nuclear components (Bhatnagar et al. 2013).

Studies have identified the presence of Gαi in mitochondria, where it inhibits cAMP signaling and regulates the melatonin type 1 receptor (MT1R) to block stress-mediated cytochrome c release in neuronal mitochondria (Lyssand and Bajjalieh 2007; Suofu et al. 2017). Additionally, Gβ2 has been demonstrated to modulate the activity of mitofusin 1 (Mfn1) on the surface of mitochondria, affecting mitochondrial fusion (Zhang et al. 2010). Furthermore, Gα12 has been found to contain a mitochondrial targeting sequence and affect mitochondrial membrane potential and mitochondrial motility (Andreeva et al. 2008).

3.2 β-arrestins

β-arrestins are multifunctional adapter proteins that regulate GPCR signaling, desensitization and trafficking. Traditionally, β-arrestin activation was believed to primarily occur in the plasma membrane, where they bind to activated GPCRs following ligand stimulation. This interaction inhibits further G protein signaling and initiates receptor internalization, a crucial step in receptor desensitization (Ahn et al. 2003; Cahill 3rd et al. 2017; Hausdorff et al. 1990). Beyond their role at the plasma membrane, β-arrestins are also critical for receptor trafficking and signaling in intracellular compartments.

In endosomes, β-arrestins scaffold signaling complexes, enabling sustained signaling after receptor internalization. This endosomal localization of receptor complexes allows for prolonged second messenger and MAPK/ERK signaling, which has been observed in GPCRs such as the β2-adrenergic receptor (Luttrell et al. 1999; Luttrell et al. 2001; McDonald et al. 2000; Thomsen et al. 2016). Additionally, β-arrestins help regulate the fate of internalized receptors, determining whether they are recycled back to the plasma membrane or directed toward degradation (Noor et al. 2011).

While both β-arrestins 1 and 2 contain nuclear import sequences, β-arrestin 2 also contains a C-terminal leucine-rich nuclear export sequence, resulting in its expression being primarily limited to the cytoplasm while β-arrestin 1 is expressed in both the nucleus and cytoplasm (Scott et al. 2002). This nuclear localization allows β-arrestins to regulate transcription directly by binding to cofactors such as p300 and cAMP-response element-binding protein (CREB) and indirectly through interactions with E3 ubiquitin ligase Mdm2 (Ahmed et al. 2011; Beaulieu and Caron 2005).

β-arrestins in the cytoplasm act as scaffolds for various signaling complexes, including those that activate MAPK pathways such as c-Jun N-terminal kinases (JNK), p38, and ERK (Eishingdrelo et al. 2015; Tan et al. 2009; Zhan et al. 2014).

This cytoplasmic scaffolding function of β-arrestins positions them as versatile regulators of intracellular signaling beyond their classical GPCR desensitization role. β-arrestins are also present in the intermembrane space of neuronal mitochondria along with the MT1R in the outer mitochondrial membrane, where they regulate MT1R signaling and contribute to the neuroprotective effect of melatonin (Suofu et al. 2017). β-arrestins also play a crucial role in lysosomal trafficking by mediating the degradation of GPCRs through their interaction with ubiquitinated receptors. For example, β-arrestin 2 works alongside the Nedd4 E3 ubiquitin ligase to ubiquitinate receptors like mGlu7, facilitating their endocytosis and directing them toward lysosomal degradation (Lee et al. 2019). This process is essential for downregulating receptor signaling, preventing overstimulation, and maintaining cellular homeostasis.

A recent study explores how β-arrestins adopt distinct conformational states depending on their subcellular location, isoform, and ligand type, which influences AT1R-biased signaling outcomes. These location-specific conformations impact the downstream ERK signaling cascade differently, enabling ligand-specific signaling responses. For example, at the plasma membrane, catalytically active β-arrestins exhibit ligand-independent conformations and ERK activation, while for β-arrestins in complex with receptor at the cell surface and in endosomes, distinct ligand effects are observed in their conformations and ERK signaling. Furthermore, the subcellular distribution of ERK activity is greatly dependent on receptor endocytosis, as it inhibits plasma membrane ERK activation and traffics the ERK signaling complexes intracellularly to the endosomes, nucleus, cytosol. These findings underscore the spatial and functional diversity of β-arrestin's role in regulating GPCR signaling pathways, suggesting new avenues for therapeutic targeting based on receptor location and β-arrestin conformation.

3.3 GRKs

GRKs are a diverse family of kinases that regulate GPCR signaling by phosphorylating activated receptors, thus initiating processes like β-arrestin recruitment, desensitization, and receptor internalization. There are seven GRKs divided into three subfamilies based on their structural similarities: GRK1 subfamily (GRK1, GRK7), GRK2 subfamily (GRK2, GRK3), and GRK4 subfamily (GRK4, GRK5, GRK6). These kinases are found in various cellular compartments, and their subcellular localization is critical in determining their role in signaling.

The GRK1 subfamily consists of GRK1 (rhodopsin kinase) and GRK7, which are both membrane-bound via farnesylation and geranylgeranylation, respectively (Hisatomi et al. 1998; Millette et al. 2022). GRK1 is primarily found in rod photoreceptors, where it phosphorylates light-activated rhodopsin to terminate the visual signal, but it is also expressed in cones, though at lower levels than GRK7 (Osawa and Weiss 2012). GRK7 is the dominant kinase in cones, responsible for phosphorylating cone opsins, particularly under bright light conditions (Osawa and

Weiss 2012). The precise localization of these kinases in the outer segments of rods and cones ensures rapid and specific visual signal termination.

The GRK2 subfamily includes GRK2 and GRK3, which are cytoplasmic kinases that are recruited to the plasma membrane upon receptor activation via their pleckstrin homology (PH) domain's interaction with free Gβγ subunits (Touhara et al. 1994). The GRK4 subfamily is composed of GRK4, GRK5, and GRK6, with GRK5 and GRK6 constitutively localized at the plasma membrane (Jiang et al. 2007; Thiyagarajan et al. 2004). GRK5 is unique in its ability to localize to the nucleus, where it can bind directly to DNA and activate the NF-κB pathway through phosphorylation of Iκ-Bα, regulating gene expression linked to cell growth and apoptosis (Islam et al. 2013; Johnson et al. 2004; Patial et al. 2009; So et al. 2012). This nuclear role of GRK5 demonstrates the expanded, non-canonical functions of GRKs beyond GPCR desensitization.

GRKs have been demonstrated to display location bias in their activity, with activity that varies at the plasma membrane or endosomal compartments depending on the agonist used to stimulate the receptor. At CXCR3, while GRK2, GRK3, GRK5, and GRK6 are all recruited to the receptor at the plasma membrane, only GRK2, GRK3, and GRK5 are recruited to endosomes following stimulation with the endogenous chemokines, CXCL9, CXCL10, and CXCL11, and different synthetic agonists. The localization of each kinase modulates distinct aspects of CXCR3 signaling, including β-arrestin engagement, receptor internalization, and downstream ERK activation, indicating that the spatial context of GRKs significantly influences biased signaling pathways in GPCRs (Gardner et al. 2024).

3.4 RGS Proteins

Regulators of G protein signaling (RGS) proteins play an integral role in terminating GPCR signaling by enhancing the GTPase activity of Gα subunits. Recent studies have revealed their dynamic intracellular localization, including within the nucleus, plasma membrane, and other cellular compartments. These findings suggest that RGS proteins contribute to compartment-specific signaling regulation, broadening their functional roles in the cell.

Several RGS proteins, such as RGS10 and RGS14, shuttle between the cytoplasm and nucleus, modulating transcriptional and stress response pathways. RGS14 is particularly notable for its localization in chromatin-rich regions of the nucleus and juxtanuclear membranes, where it influences synaptic plasticity and learning-related processes (Branch and Hepler 2017; Burchett 2003). Nuclear RGS14 is thought to regulate gene transcription through interactions with nuclear signaling components, extending its functional scope beyond traditional GTPase-accelerating activity (Branch and Hepler 2017; Burchett 2003).

The trafficking of RGS proteins into the nucleus is tightly regulated by nuclear localization signals (NLS) and nuclear export signals (NES). This regulated shuttling enables RGS proteins to participate in nuclear processes, such as modulating the transcription of stress-related genes. For example, RGS10 has been implicated in stress response regulation, suggesting that nuclear RGS proteins may serve as critical mediators in cellular stress signaling (Burchett 2003; Huang and Fisher 2009).

RGS proteins also exhibit dynamic translocation between the plasma membrane and intracellular compartments in response to signaling events. RGS8, for example, translocates from the cytoplasm to the plasma membrane upon activation by Gα subunits. This translocation is essential for regulating GPCR signaling at the plasma membrane by enhancing GTP hydrolysis on Gα, thereby accelerating signal termination. The mechanism of RGS8 plasma membrane translocation involves direct interaction with activated Gα subunits, which induces its movement to membrane domains (Masuho et al. 2004).

The subcellular localization of RGS proteins is further regulated by post-translational modifications such as phosphorylation. For instance, melatonin signaling through PKCα alters the nuclear-cytoplasmic distribution of RGS proteins like RGS2, RGS4, and RGS10, demonstrating the impact of hormonal signals on RGS localization and function (Rimler et al. 2006). These phosphorylation events highlight how external signals, such as hormonal or metabolic cues, can control the spatial distribution of RGS proteins, influencing their activity in distinct cellular compartments.

In neural tissues, RGS proteins such as RGS7 and RGS9–2 form complexes with Gβ5 and R7BP (R7 binding protein), a scaffold protein that facilitates their movement between the plasma membrane and nucleus. R7BP plays a pivotal role in regulating the localization of these RGS-Gβ5 complexes, with reversible palmitoylation controlling their shuttling. This process is critical in modulating non-canonical signaling pathways, particularly in the brain, where these RGS complexes influence neurotransmitter signaling, neuroplasticity, and other neural processes (Hepler 2005). The interaction between R7BP and RGS proteins underscores the importance of scaffold proteins in regulating the intracellular dynamics and functional specificity of RGS proteins.

RGS proteins are dynamically localized within various intracellular compartments, including the nucleus, plasma membrane, and cytoplasm, where they regulate signaling pathways in a compartment-specific manner. Their ability to shuttle between different cellular locations allows RGS proteins to integrate multiple signaling inputs, thereby fine-tuning GPCR signaling and modulating cellular processes such as transcription, stress response, and synaptic plasticity. Understanding the spatial regulation of RGS proteins provides critical insight into their broader functional roles in both normal physiological and pathophysiological contexts.

3.5 Second Messengers

Second messengers play an integral role in the propagation and amplification of signals initiated by GPCRs. These small molecules, such as cAMP, inositol trisphosphate (IP3), diacylglycerol (DAG), calcium, and key downstream effectors like MAPKs and AKT, are produced or activated in response to extracellular signals and regulate a wide array of cellular processes. Their localization within distinct subcellular compartments allows for spatially and temporally precise control over signaling pathways. This compartmentalization ensures that second messenger activity is highly regulated and targeted, preventing inappropriate or excessive signaling that could lead to cellular dysfunction. Below, we explore the expression and role of these second messengers and effectors in various intracellular organelles.

Compartmentalized cAMP Signaling

cAMP is synthesized by adenylyl cyclases, a family of enzymes localized primarily to the plasma membrane and endosomes in response to GPCR activation. cAMP functions as a second messenger by activating protein kinase A (PKA), which subsequently phosphorylates a variety of target proteins to regulate processes such as metabolism, gene transcription, and cell growth (Sassone-Corsi 2012). Importantly, cAMP signaling is spatially compartmentalized within the cell through the action of A-kinase anchoring proteins (AKAPs), which tether PKA to specific organelles such as the mitochondria and sarcoplasmic reticulum. This ensures that cAMP signaling remains confined to localized areas, providing precise regulation of its downstream effects (Lygren et al. 2007; Means et al. 2011).

Recent studies have explored the role of receptor-associated cAMP nanodomains, referred to as RAINs, in generating highly localized and specific cAMP signals at the cell membrane. These nanodomains are formed and regulated by interactions with specific proteins that cluster around the GPCR, effectively creating a microenvironment that restricts cAMP diffusion and sustains high local concentrations near the receptor (Anton et al. 2022; Zhang et al. 2020). For example, anchoring proteins such as AKAPs help tether components of the cAMP pathway, including adenylyl cyclases and phosphodiesterases (PDEs), near the GPCR within the RAIN. AKAPs bind to both PKA and phosphodiesterases, allowing for rapid feedback regulation of cAMP levels through concurrent synthesis and degradation within the nanodomain. This precise balance ensures that RAINs can generate cAMP pulses that are both brief and spatially restricted, further enhancing the specificity of the signaling cascade. These cAMP nanodomains allow receptors such as glucagon-like peptide 1 (GLP-1) and β2-adrenergic receptors to produce highly localized cAMP responses within just a few nanometers, ensuring that the cAMP generated by one receptor does not diffuse to other areas of the cell (Anton et al. 2022). Notably, the regulatory subunit I alpha (RIα) of protein kinase A (PKA) also undergoes liquid–liquid phase separation (LLPS), which creates distinct intracellular compartments that concentrate cAMP, effectively forming specialized PKA signaling “nanodomains” within the cell. Importantly, disruptions in the LLPS process can contribute to oncogenesis, as loss of RIα phase separation from expressing RIα LLPS mutants results in increased cell proliferation and anchorage-independent growth in non-tumorigenic hepatocytic cells (Zhang et al. 2020). This compartmentalization of cAMP has profound implications for cellular signaling and normal cell growth, as it allows for the coexistence of multiple, simultaneous signals within a single cell, contributing to the fine-tuning of GPCR functions in different cellular contexts.

In addition to the plasma membrane, cAMP and its related effectors, such as PKA, adenylyl cyclase, AKAPs, and PDEs, have been identified in most intracellular organelles, including the nucleus (Brown et al. 2003; Coghlan et al. 1994; Haj Slimane et al. 2014; Pizzoni et al. 2023; Sample et al. 2012), mitochondria (Acin-Perez et al. 2009a, b; Lefkimmiatis et al. 2013; Means et al. 2011), Golgi apparatus (Godbole et al. 2017; Shanks et al. 2002), and the ER (Yamamoto et al. 1998).

Phosphoinositides at Intracellular Organelles

Inositol trisphosphate (IP3) and diacylglycerol (DAG) are second messengers produced by the cleavage of phosphatidylinositol 4,5-bisphosphate (PIP2) by phospholipase C (PLC), a process that can occur at both the plasma membrane and Golgi apparatus (Katan and Cockcroft 2020; Madukwe et al. 2018; Malik et al. 2015). IP3 diffuses through the cytoplasm to bind to its receptor on the ER, triggering the release of calcium ions from intracellular stores (Prole and Taylor 2019). This release creates localized calcium microdomains that activate calcium-dependent enzymes such as calmodulin and calcium/calmodulin-dependent kinases (CaMKs), which play crucial roles in synaptic plasticity and muscle contraction (Robison and Colbran 2013; Yang and Tsai 2022). DAG remains anchored in the plasma membrane or Golgi, where it recruits protein kinase C (PKC), driving processes such as cell proliferation and differentiation (Kolczynska et al. 2020; Litvak et al. 2005; Zhang et al. 2021). Additionally, functional PLC, PLD, and PLA isoforms as well as IP3 and DAG are present in various intracellular organelles, including the nucleus (Kumar et al. 2008; Schievella et al. 1995), Golgi apparatus (Freyberg et al. 2001; Zhang et al. 2013), mitochondria (Knox et al. 2004), and ER (Schievella et al. 1995).

MAPK and AKT Signaling Pathways

Emerging evidence have also identified the presence major components of GPCR signaling downstream cascades in intracellular compartments. The MAPK signaling pathways are central to cell proliferation, differentiation, and stress responses. The subcellular localization of MAPK pathway components – including ERK1/2, JNK, and p38 – adds a layer of regulation to these pathways (Wainstein and Seger 2016). Localization affects the duration, intensity, and outcome of the signaling cascade, with different compartments contributing unique regulatory contexts and signaling effects. The MAPK cascade generally initiates at the plasma membrane, where extracellular ligands activate the GPCRs (Plotnikov et al. 2011). Following activation, ERK1/2 translocates to the nucleus to regulate gene expression by phosphorylating nuclear transcription factors like c-Fos, Elk-1, and c-Myc, driving important processes such as cell proliferation and differentiation (Kwon et al. 2022; Turjanski et al. 2007). Similarly, activated JNK and p38 MAPKs can translocate to the nucleus, where they regulate transcription factors like ATF-2, p53, and NF-κB, influencing genes involved in stress response and cell cycle control (Turjanski et al. 2007). Certain MAPK pathway components, particularly ERK1/2, JNK, and p38, localize to mitochondria under specific conditions, such as during cellular stress (Chambers and LoGrasso 2011; Heslop et al. 2020; Rasola et al. 2010; Sarg et al. 2024). ERK1/2 activation at the Golgi can influence Golgi-related processes, such as protein trafficking and vesicular transport (Aebersold et al. 2004; Torii et al. 2004). For example, Golgi-localized ERK1c is known for its role in Golgi fragmentation during mitosis, where it participates in cell cycle-dependent signaling (Aebersold et al. 2004).

AKT is a key regulator of cell survival, metabolism, and growth and is activated by GPCR signaling at the plasma membrane via the phosphoinositide 3-kinase (PI3K) pathway (Desale et al. 2021). Importantly, AKT signaling is also compartmentalized within the Golgi, ER, mitochondria, and nucleus (Bijur and Jope 2003; Lee et al. 2008; Sasaki et al. 2003). This spatial localization of AKT ensures that its activity is finely tuned to regulate cell survival and metabolism in specific organelles.

4 Mechanisms of GPCR Trafficking

The trafficking and translocation of GPCRs is a dynamic process that regulates receptor signaling and desensitization. GPCRs undergo complex movement between the cell surface and intracellular compartments, influencing the intensity, duration, and specificity of cellular responses.

4.1 Arrestins/GRK-Mediated Trafficking

In the classical homologous desensitization pathway, GPCRs are phosphorylated by GRKs after repeated stimulation by their ligands (Krupnick and Benovic 1998). This phosphorylation promotes the association of β-arrestins, which not only terminate G protein signaling but also direct GPCRs into clathrin-mediated endocytic pathways. This β-arrestin-receptor complex then interacts with clathrin and adaptor proteins, such as AP2, facilitating the receptor's incorporation into clathrin-coated pits (Goodman Jr. et al. 1996). Once internalized, GPCRs are trafficked into endosomes where they can either be recycled back to the plasma membrane or targeted for degradation in lysosomes (Noor et al. 2011). Importantly, β-arrestins also scaffold various signaling proteins such as MAPKs, Src, and AKT, allowing internalized receptors to continue signaling within endosomes (Peterson and Luttrell 2017).

There are a few examples of a role for β-arrestins in trafficking receptors to intracellular organelles. One study demonstrated the essential role of β-arrestin in transporting the oxytocin receptor (OXTR) to the nucleus in osteoblasts. Upon oxytocin binding, β-arrestins facilitate OXTR's nuclear translocation by interacting with other transport proteins, such as Rab5 and importin-β, enabling OXTR to directly influence osteoblast differentiation by activating key genes like osterix and osteocalcin without affecting ERK phosphorylation (Di Benedetto et al. 2014).

4.2 Arrestin-Independent Trafficking

In addition to the well-characterized arrestin-dependent pathways, several GPCRs utilize arrestin-independent endocytosis mechanisms, involving distinct cellular machinery that can lead to varying signaling and trafficking outcomes. These arrestin-independent pathways allow GPCRs to maintain functional versatility in response to external stimuli, often influencing how the receptors recycle, degrade, or sustain intracellular signaling.

A notable example of arrestin-independent internalization involves caveolae-mediated endocytosis. Caveolae are small, flask-shaped invaginations in the plasma membrane, enriched in cholesterol and sphingolipids (Brown and Rose 1992; Ortegren et al. 2004). They are stabilized by structural caveolin proteins, which are essential for maintaining their integrity (Ludwig et al. 2013; Rothberg et al. 1992). Caveolae function as lipid raft domains, organizing specific proteins and receptors for selective internalization. The process begins with the clustering of caveolin-associated proteins, followed by vesicle formation, which is slower than clathrin-mediated endocytosis but allows for the compartmentalization of signaling molecules (Rejman et al. 2005). Receptors such as the glucagon-like peptide-1 receptor (GLP-1R) have been shown to internalize independently of β-arrestin (Jones et al. 2018), instead relying on both caveolin-1 and dynamin (Jones et al. 2018; Syme et al. 2006).

In some cases, clathrin-mediated endocytosis can occur independently of β-arrestins. For example, the proteinase-activated receptor 1 (PAR1) interacts directly with the adaptor protein AP-2 to facilitate internalization via clathrin-coated pits (Paing et al. 2006; Paing et al. 2002). PAR1 contains a specific YXXL motif that binds to AP-2, allowing for receptor internalization without arrestins. Other examples of β-arrestin-independent clathrin-mediated endocytosis include the chemokine receptor ACKR3, vasoactive intestinal peptide receptor 1 (VIPR1), apelin receptor (APJ), proteinase-activated receptor 4 (PAR4), and the M1 muscarinic receptor (M1R) (Blythe and von Zastrow 2024; Lee et al. 1998; Pope et al. 2016; Smith et al. 2016; Vogler et al. 1998; Zarca et al. 2021).

Fast endophilin-mediated endocytosis (FEME) is another mechanism of arrestin- and clathrin-independent internalization. Receptors such as the dopamine D3 and D4 receptors and the M4 muscarinic receptor use this pathway for rapid internalization within seconds of receptor activation (Boucrot et al. 2015; Lee et al. 1998). This mechanism is triggered almost instantly upon receptor activation, with vesicles forming within seconds after receptor stimulation (Boucrot et al. 2015). A key element in FEME is the involvement of endophilins, which are proteins containing Bin/amphiphysin/Rvs (BAR) domains (Boucrot et al. 2015). Endophilins facilitate plasma membrane curvature through their BAR domains and their ability to insert amphipathic helices into the membrane, promoting membrane invagination (Boucrot et al. 2015). The FEME pathway is dynamically primed, where endophilin-enriched domains are assembled on the plasma membrane before receptor activation (Boucrot et al. 2015). This priming involves interaction with proteins like Cdc42-interacting protein 4 (CIP4) and formin-binding protein 17 (FBP17), which helps recruit SHIP1/

2 phosphatases to increase the local concentration of phosphatidylinositol-3,4-bisphosphate (Chan Wah Hak et al. 2018). The accumulation of this phosphatidylinositol species enables the recruitment of endophilins, which then bind to receptor motifs upon ligand activation, triggering the formation of FEME vesicles. After recruitment, the scission of vesicles is mediated by dynamin to release the endocytic vesicle into the cytoplasm (Boucrot et al. 2015).

5 Applications of Location Bias in GPCR Drug Discovery

Several challenges remain in targeting GPCRs at these intracellular sites, and location-biased drugs must therefore be carefully designed to access their target receptors. One major issue is the delivery of drugs to specific intracellular compartments. Since traditional drugs are designed to target cell surface receptors, developing molecules that can penetrate cells and reach internal compartments like the Golgi, ER, or endosomes poses a significant hurdle. Many drugs, especially those that are hydrophilic, struggle to cross the plasma membrane, reducing their efficacy when targeting intracellular GPCRs. For instance, studies on nanobodies targeting the chemokine receptor US28 showed only partial inhibition of tumor cell growth, largely due to the nanobodies' inability to penetrate the membrane and reach the intracellular receptor pools (Heukers et al. 2018).

However, promising efforts to develop drugs that target specific intracellular GPCRs have begun to emerge. For example, neurokinin 1 receptor (NK1R) antagonists are being designed to target endosomal signaling that contributes to sustained nociception for the treatment of chronic pain. Lipophilic NK1R antagonists that are not charged at the acidic pH of endosomes have demonstrated enhanced localization within endosomes, leading to improved efficacy in inhibiting pain responses compared to those targeting only plasma membrane receptors (Jensen et al. 2017; Latorre et al. 2022; Mai et al. 2021). Other examples include β1AR signaling at the Golgi that can be modulated by hydrophobic ligands like metoprolol, which can passively diffuse through membranes and inhibit β1AR at both the plasma membrane and the Golgi. This results in greater reductions in cAMP and heart rate compared to other hydrophilic antagonists that cannot access intracellular pools (Irannejad et al. 2017).

In addition to small molecules, location-biased peptide drugs have also shown potential. For example, the fentanyl analog NFEPP, which preferentially activates MOR in acidified environments such as endosomes and diseased tissues, has demonstrated strong antinociceptive effects in diseased tissue without the common side effects seen in other tissues, indicating a promising approach to reduce side effects in opioid therapy (Jimenez-Vargas et al. 2022; Spahn et al. 2017).

The ability to target intracellular receptor pools can also enhance signaling duration and efficacy. Parathyroid hormone 1–34 (PTH1–34) promotes a more robust PTHR response compared to parathyroid hormone-related peptide 1–36 (PTHrP1–36), as PTH1–34 can continue signaling from endosomes, whereas PTHrP1–36 is restricted to surface-level signaling (Dean et al. 2008; Ferrandon et al. 2009). Similarly, the synthetic drug FTY720 induces prolonged sphingosine-1-phosphate receptor (S1P1) signaling by promoting its endosomal localization, which in turn enhances chemokinetic migration in endothelial cells (Mullershausen et al. 2009).

6 Conclusions

GPCRs are highly versatile in their signaling capabilities, and their localization within different cellular compartments plays a critical role in determining the specific outcomes of their signaling pathways. By dynamically translocating between the plasma membrane and intracellular organelles, such as endosomes, the Golgi apparatus, mitochondria, and the nucleus, GPCRs can initiate distinct signaling cascades that regulate diverse cellular processes. The spatial context in which a GPCR resides influences not only which downstream effectors are activated but also the intensity and duration of signaling. Thus, location-biased GPCR therapeutics represent a promising advancement in precision pharmacology, offering targeted control of GPCR activity at specific intracellular locations. By tailoring drugs to exploit the unique signaling mechanisms of GPCRs within subcellular compartments, researchers can unlock new avenues for the treatment of diseases such as heart disease, cancer, and chronic pain, where traditional surface receptor-targeted therapies fall short. Advances in nanotechnology and drug delivery systems, such as nanoparticles or conjugation to transport peptides, may help overcome the current challenges in design location-specific drugs. As the field of intracellular GPCR signaling continues to evolve, future drug discovery efforts will likely focus on improving delivery methods and developing highly selective compounds that harness the full potential of location-biased GPCR modulation.

Acknowledgment This work was supported by a National Institute of Health grant 1R01GM122798, the Mandel Foundation from Duke Cardiovascular Research Center (S.R.), and the American Heart Association Predoctoral Fellowship 23PRE1019796 (U.P.).

References

Abadir PM, Foster DB, Crow M, Cooke CA, Rucker JJ, Jain A, Smith BJ, Burks TN, Cohn RD, Fedarko NS, Carey RM, O'Rourke B, Walston JD (2011) Identification and characterization of a functional mitochondrial angiotensin system. Proc Natl Acad Sci USA 108(36):14849–14854. https://doi.org/10.1073/pnas.1101507108

Acin-Perez R, Salazar E, Brosel S, Yang H, Schon EA, Manfredi G (2009a) Modulation of mitochondrial protein phosphorylation by soluble adenylyl cyclase ameliorates cytochrome oxidase defects. EMBO Mol Med 1(8–9):392–406. https://doi.org/10.1002/emmm.200900046

Acin-Perez R, Salazar E, Kamenetsky M, Buck J, Levin LR, Manfredi G (2009b) Cyclic AMP produced inside mitochondria regulates oxidative phosphorylation. Cell Metab 9(3):265–276. https://doi.org/10.1016/j.cmet.2009.01.012

Adams MN, Christensen ME, He Y, Waterhouse NJ, Hooper JD (2011) The role of palmitoylation in signalling, cellular trafficking and plasma membrane localization of protease-activated receptor-2. PLoS One 6(11):e28018. https://doi.org/10.1371/journal.pone.0028018

Aebersold DM, Shaul YD, Yung Y, Yarom N, Yao Z, Hanoch T, Seger R (2004) Extracellular signal-regulated kinase 1c (ERK1c), a novel 42-kilodalton ERK, demonstrates unique modes of regulation, localization, and function. Mol Cell Biol 24(22):10000–10015. https://doi.org/10.1128/MCB.24.22.10000-10015.2004

Ahmed MR, Zhan X, Song X, Kook S, Gurevich VV, Gurevich EV (2011) Ubiquitin ligase parkin promotes Mdm2-arrestin interaction but inhibits arrestin ubiquitination. Biochemistry 50(18):3749–3763. https://doi.org/10.1021/bi200175q

Ahn S, Nelson CD, Garrison TR, Miller WE, Lefkowitz RJ (2003) Desensitization, internalization, and signaling functions of β-arrestins demonstrated by RNA interference. Proc Natl Acad Sci 100(4):1740–1744. https://doi.org/10.1073/pnas.262789099

Ahn S, Shenoy SK, Wei H, Lefkowitz RJ (2004) Differential kinetic and spatial patterns of beta-arrestin and G protein-mediated ERK activation by the angiotensin II receptor. J Biol Chem 279(34):35518–35525. https://doi.org/10.1074/jbc.M405878200

Andreeva AV, Kutuzov MA, Voyno-Yasenetskaya TA (2008) G alpha12 is targeted to the mitochondria and affects mitochondrial morphology and motility. FASEB J 22(8):2821–2831. https://doi.org/10.1096/fj.07-104224

Anton SE, Kayser C, Maiellaro I, Nemec K, Moller J, Koschinski A, Zaccolo M, Annibale P, Falcke M, Lohse MJ, Bock A (2022) Receptor-associated independent cAMP nanodomains mediate spatiotemporal specificity of GPCR signaling. Cell 185(7):1130–1142 e1111. https://doi.org/10.1016/j.cell.2022.02.011

Beaulieu JM, Caron MG (2005) Beta-arrestin goes nuclear. Cell 123(5):755–757. https://doi.org/10.1016/j.cell.2005.11.010

Benard G, Massa F, Puente N, Lourenco J, Bellocchio L, Soria-Gomez E, Matias I, Delamarre A, Metna-Laurent M, Cannich A, Hebert-Chatelain E, Mulle C, Ortega-Gutierrez S, Martin-Fontecha M, Klugmann M, Guggenhuber S, Lutz B, Gertsch J, Chaouloff F et al (2012) Mitochondrial CB(1) receptors regulate neuronal energy metabolism. Nat Neurosci 15(4):558–564. https://doi.org/10.1038/nn.3053

Bhatnagar A, Unal H, Jagannathan R, Kaveti S, Duan Z-H, Yong S, Vasanji A, Kinter M, Desnoyer R, Karnik SS (2013) Interaction of G-protein βγ complex with chromatin modulates GPCR-dependent gene regulation. PLoS One 8(1):e52689. https://doi.org/10.1371/journal.pone.0052689

Bhattacharya M, Peri KG, Almazan G, Ribeiro-da-Silva A, Shichi H, Durocher Y, Abramovitz M, Hou X, Varma DR, Chemtob S (1998) Nuclear localization of prostaglandin E2 receptors. Proc Natl Acad Sci USA 95(26):15792–15797. https://doi.org/10.1073/pnas.95.26.15792

Bijur GN, Jope RS (2003) Rapid accumulation of Akt in mitochondria following phosphatidylinositol 3-kinase activation. J Neurochem 87(6):1427–1435. https://doi.org/10.1046/j.1471-4159.2003.02113.x

Bjork S, Hurt CM, Ho VK, Angelotti T (2013) REEPs are membrane shaping adapter proteins that modulate specific g protein-coupled receptor trafficking by affecting ER cargo capacity. PLoS One 8(10):e76366. https://doi.org/10.1371/journal.pone.0076366

Blanpain C, Wittamer V, Vanderwinden JM, Boom A, Renneboog B, Lee B, Le Poul E, El Asmar L, Govaerts C, Vassart G, Doms RW, Parmentier M (2001) Palmitoylation of CCR5 is critical for receptor trafficking and efficient activation of intracellular signaling pathways. J Biol Chem 276(26):23795–23804. https://doi.org/10.1074/jbc.M100583200

Blythe EE, von Zastrow M (2024) beta-Arrestin-independent endosomal cAMP signaling by a polypeptide hormone GPCR. Nat Chem Biol 20(3):323–332. https://doi.org/10.1038/s41589-023-01412-4

Boucrot E, Ferreira APA, Almeida-Souza L, Debard S, Vallis Y, Howard G, Bertot L, Sauvonnet N, McMahon HT (2015) Endophilin marks and controls a clathrin-independent endocytic pathway. Nature 517(7535):460–465. https://doi.org/10.1038/nature14067

Branch MR, Hepler JR (2017) Endogenous RGS14 is a cytoplasmic-nuclear shuttling protein that localizes to juxtanuclear membranes and chromatin-rich regions of the nucleus. PLoS One 12(9):e0184497. https://doi.org/10.1371/journal.pone.0184497

Brown DA, Rose JK (1992) Sorting of GPI-anchored proteins to glycolipid-enriched membrane subdomains during transport to the apical cell surface. Cell 68(3):533–544. https://doi.org/10.1016/0092-8674(92)90189-j

Brown RL, August SL, Williams CJ, Moss SB (2003) AKAP7gamma is a nuclear RI-binding AKAP. Biochem Biophys Res Commun 306(2):394–401. https://doi.org/10.1016/s0006-291x(03)00982-3

Burchett SA (2003) In through the out door: nuclear localization of the regulators of G protein signaling. J Neurochem 87(3):551–559. https://doi.org/10.1046/j.1471-4159.2003.02047.x

Cahill TJ 3rd, Thomsen AR, Tarrasch JT, Plouffe B, Nguyen AH, Yang F, Huang LY, Kahsai AW, Bassoni DL, Gavino BJ, Lamerdin JE, Triest S, Shukla AK, Berger B, Little JT, Antar A, Blanc A, Qu CX, Chen X et al (2017) Distinct conformations of GPCR-β-arrestin complexes mediate desensitization, signaling, and endocytosis. Proc Natl Acad Sci USA 114(10): 2562–2567. https://doi.org/10.1073/pnas.1701529114

Calebiro D, Nikolaev VO, Gagliani MC, de Filippis T, Dees C, Tacchetti C, Persani L, Lohse MJ (2009) Persistent cAMP-signals triggered by internalized G-protein-coupled receptors. PLoS Biol 7(8):e1000172. https://doi.org/10.1371/journal.pbio.1000172

Cancino J, Capalbo A, Di Campli A, Giannotta M, Rizzo R, Jung JE, Di Martino R, Persico M, Heinklein P, Sallese M, Luini A (2014) Control systems of membrane transport at the interface between the endoplasmic reticulum and the Golgi. Dev Cell 30(3):280–294. https://doi.org/10.1016/j.devcel.2014.06.018

Cascianelli G, Villani M, Tosti M, Marini F, Bartoccini E, Magni MV, Albi E (2008) Lipid microdomains in cell nucleus. Mol Biol Cell 19(12):5289–5295. https://doi.org/10.1091/mbc.e08-05-0517

Cattaneo F, Parisi M, Fioretti T, Sarnataro D, Esposito G, Ammendola R (2016) Nuclear localization of formyl-peptide receptor 2 in human cancer cells. Arch Biochem Biophys 603:10–19. https://doi.org/10.1016/j.abb.2016.05.006

Chambers JW, LoGrasso PV (2011) Mitochondrial c-Jun N-terminal kinase (JNK) signaling initiates physiological changes resulting in amplification of reactive oxygen species generation. J Biol Chem 286(18):16052–16062. https://doi.org/10.1074/jbc.M111.223602

Chan Wah Hak L, Khan S, Di Meglio I, Law A-L, Lucken-Ardjomande Häsler S, Quintaneiro LM, Ferreira APA, Krause M, McMahon HT, Boucrot E (2018) FBP17 and CIP4 recruit SHIP2 and lamellipodin to prime the plasma membrane for fast endophilin-mediated endocytosis. Nat Cell Biol 20(9):1023–1031. https://doi.org/10.1038/s41556-018-0146-8

Chan LF, Webb TR, Chung TT, Meimaridou E, Cooray SN, Guasti L, Chapple JP, Egertova M, Elphick MR, Cheetham ME, Metherell LA, Clark AJ (2009) MRAP and MRAP2 are bidirectional regulators of the melanocortin receptor family. Proc Natl Acad Sci USA 106(15): 6146–6151. https://doi.org/10.1073/pnas.0809918106

Chini B, Parenti M (2004) G-protein coupled receptors in lipid rafts and caveolae: how, when and why do they go there? J Mol Endocrinol 32(2):325–338. https://doi.org/10.1677/jme.0.0320325

Coghlan VM, Langeberg LK, Fernandez A, Lamb NJ, Scott JD (1994) Cloning and characterization of AKAP 95, a nuclear protein that associates with the regulatory subunit of type II cAMP-dependent protein kinase. J Biol Chem 269(10):7658–7665. https://www.ncbi.nlm.nih.gov/pubmed/8125992

Compton SJ, Sandhu S, Wijesuriya SJ, Hollenberg MD (2002) Glycosylation of human proteinase-activated receptor-2 (hPAR2): role in cell surface expression and signalling. Biochem J 368 (Pt 2):495–505. https://doi.org/10.1042/BJ20020706

Daaka Y, Luttrell LM, Ahn S, Della Rocca GJ, Ferguson SS, Caron MG, Lefkowitz RJ (1998) Essential role for G protein-coupled receptor endocytosis in the activation of mitogen-activated protein kinase. J Biol Chem 273(2):685–688. https://doi.org/10.1074/jbc.273.2.685

Dahl EF, Wu SC, Healy CL, Harsch BA, Shearer GC, O'Connell TD (2018) Subcellular compartmentalization of proximal Galpha(q)-receptor signaling produces unique hypertrophic phenotypes in adult cardiac myocytes. J Biol Chem 293(23):8734–8749. https://doi.org/10.1074/jbc.RA118.002283

Dean T, Vilardaga JP, Potts JT Jr, Gardella TJ (2008) Altered selectivity of parathyroid hormone (PTH) and PTH-related protein (PTHrP) for distinct conformations of the PTH/PTHrP receptor. Mol Endocrinol 22(1):156–166. https://doi.org/10.1210/me.2007-0274

DeFea KA, Zalevsky J, Thoma MS, Dery O, Mullins RD, Bunnett NW (2000) beta-arrestin-dependent endocytosis of proteinase-activated receptor 2 is required for intracellular targeting of activated ERK1/2. J Cell Biol 148(6):1267–1281. https://doi.org/10.1083/jcb.148.6.1267

Desale SE, Chidambaram H, Chinnathambi S (2021) G-protein coupled receptor, PI3K and rho signaling pathways regulate the cascades of tau and amyloid-β in Alzheimer's disease. Mol Biomed 2(1):17. https://doi.org/10.1186/s43556-021-00036-1

Di Benedetto A, Sun L, Zambonin CG, Tamma R, Nico B, Calvano CD, Colaianni G, Ji Y, Mori G, Grano M, Lu P, Colucci S, Yuen T, New MI, Zallone A, Zaidi M (2014) Osteoblast regulation via ligand-activated nuclear trafficking of the oxytocin receptor. Proc Natl Acad Sci USA 111(46):16502–16507. https://doi.org/10.1073/pnas.1419349111

Dong C, Filipeanu CM, Duvernay MT, Wu G (2007) Regulation of G protein-coupled receptor export trafficking. Biochim Biophys Acta 1768(4):853–870. https://doi.org/10.1016/j.bbamem.2006.09.008

Eiger DS, Boldizsar N, Honeycutt CC, Gardner J, Kirchner S, Hicks C, Choi I, Pham U, Zheng K, Warman A, Smith JS, Zhang JY, Rajagopal S (2022) Location bias contributes to functionally selective responses of biased CXCR3 agonists. Nat Commun 13(1):5846. https://doi.org/10.1038/s41467-022-33569-2

Eiger DS, Hicks C, Gardner J, Pham U, Rajagopal S (2023) Location bias: a "Hidden variable" in GPCR pharmacology. BioEssays 45(11):e2300123. https://doi.org/10.1002/bies.202300123

Eishingdrelo H, Sun W, Li H, Wang L, Eishingdrelo A, Dai S, McKew JC, Zheng W (2015) ERK and β-arrestin interaction: a converging point of signaling pathways for multiple types of cell surface receptors. J Biomol Screen 20(3):341–349. https://doi.org/10.1177/1087057114557233

Feinstein TN, Wehbi VL, Ardura JA, Wheeler DS, Ferrandon S, Gardella TJ, Vilardaga JP (2011) Retromer terminates the generation of cAMP by internalized PTH receptors. Nat Chem Biol 7(5):278–284. https://doi.org/10.1038/nchembio.545

Ferrandon S, Feinstein TN, Castro M, Wang B, Bouley R, Potts JT, Gardella TJ, Vilardaga JP (2009) Sustained cyclic AMP production by parathyroid hormone receptor endocytosis. Nat Chem Biol 5(10):734–742. https://doi.org/10.1038/nchembio.206

Freyberg Z, Sweeney D, Siddhanta A, Bourgoin S, Frohman M, Shields D (2001) Intracellular localization of phospholipase D1 in mammalian cells. Mol Biol Cell 12(4):943–955. https://doi.org/10.1091/mbc.12.4.943

Fricker M, Hollinshead M, White N, Vaux D (1997) Interphase nuclei of many mammalian cell types contain deep, dynamic, tubular membrane-bound invaginations of the nuclear envelope. J Cell Biol 136(3):531–544. https://doi.org/10.1083/jcb.136.3.531

Gardner J, Eiger DS, Hicks C, Choi I, Pham U, Chundi A, Namjoshi O, Rajagopal S (2024) GPCR kinases differentially modulate biased signaling downstream of CXCR3 depending on their subcellular localization. Sci Signal 17(823):eadd9139. https://doi.org/10.1126/scisignal.add9139

Giannotta M, Ruggiero C, Grossi M, Cancino J, Capitani M, Pulvirenti T, Consoli GM, Geraci C, Fanelli F, Luini A, Sallese M (2012) The KDEL receptor couples to Gαq/11 to activate Src kinases and regulate transport through the Golgi. EMBO J 31(13):2869–2881. https://doi.org/10.1038/emboj.2012.134

Godbole A, Lyga S, Lohse MJ, Calebiro D (2017) Internalized TSH receptors en route to the TGN induce local G(s)-protein signaling and gene transcription. Nat Commun 8(1):443. https://doi.org/10.1038/s41467-017-00357-2

Goodman OB Jr, Krupnick JG, Santini F, Gurevich VV, Penn RB, Gagnon AW, Keen JH, Benovic JL (1996) Beta-arrestin acts as a clathrin adaptor in endocytosis of the beta2-adrenergic receptor. Nature 383(6599):447–450. https://doi.org/10.1038/383447a0

Gurevich VV, Gurevich EV (2019) GPCR signaling regulation: the role of GRKs and Arrestins. Front Pharmacol 10:125. https://doi.org/10.3389/fphar.2019.00125

Gwathmey TM, Shaltout HA, Pendergrass KD, Pirro NT, Figueroa JP, Rose JC, Diz DI, Chappell MC (2009) Nuclear angiotensin II type 2 (AT2) receptors are functionally linked to nitric oxide production. Am J Physiol Renal Physiol 296(6):F1484–F1493. https://doi.org/10.1152/ajprenal.90766.2008

Haj Slimane Z, Bedioune I, Lechene P, Varin A, Lefebvre F, Mateo P, Domergue-Dupont V, Dewenter M, Richter W, Conti M, El-Armouche A, Zhang J, Fischmeister R, Vandecasteele G (2014) Control of cytoplasmic and nuclear protein kinase A by phosphodiesterases and phosphatases in cardiac myocytes. Cardiovasc Res 102(1):97–106. https://doi.org/10.1093/cvr/cvu029

Hausdorff WP, Caron MG, Lefkowitz RJ (1990) Turning off the signal: desensitization of beta-adrenergic receptor function. FASEB J 4(11):2881–2889

Hebert-Chatelain E, Desprez T, Serrat R, Bellocchio L, Soria-Gomez E, Busquets-Garcia A, Pagano Zottola AC, Delamarre A, Cannich A, Vincent P, Varilh M, Robin LM, Terral G, Garcia-Fernandez MD, Colavita M, Mazier W, Drago F, Puente N, Reguero L et al (2016) A cannabinoid link between mitochondria and memory. Nature 539(7630):555–559. https://doi.org/10.1038/nature20127

Hepler JR (2005) R7BP: a surprising new link between G proteins, RGS proteins, and nuclear signaling in the brain. Sci STKE 2005(294):pe38. https://doi.org/10.1126/stke.2942005pe38

Heslop KA, Rovini A, Hunt EG, Fang D, Morris ME, Christie CF, Gooz MB, DeHart DN, Dang Y, Lemasters JJ, Maldonado EN (2020) JNK activation and translocation to mitochondria mediates mitochondrial dysfunction and cell death induced by VDAC opening and sorafenib in hepatocarcinoma cells. Biochem Pharmacol 171:113728. https://doi.org/10.1016/j.bcp.2019.113728

Heukers R, Fan TS, de Wit RH, van Senten JR, De Groof TWM, Bebelman MP, Lagerweij T, Vieira J, de Munnik SM, Smits-de Vries L, van Offenbeek J, Rahbar A, van Hoorick D, Soderberg-Naucler C, Wurdinger T, Leurs R, Siderius M, Vischer HF, Smit MJ (2018) The constitutive activity of the virally encoded chemokine receptor US28 accelerates glioblastoma growth. Oncogene 37(30):4110–4121. https://doi.org/10.1038/s41388-018-0255-7

Hisatomi O, Matsuda S, Satoh T, Kotaka S, Imanishi Y, Tokunaga F (1998) A novel subtype of G-protein-coupled receptor kinase, GRK7, in teleost cone photoreceptors. FEBS Lett 424(3):159–164. https://doi.org/10.1016/s0014-5793(98)00162-8

Hu ZW, Kerb R, Shi XY, Wei-Lavery T, Hoffman BB (2002) Angiotensin II increases expression of cyclooxygenase-2: implications for the function of vascular smooth muscle cells. J Pharmacol Exp Ther 303(2):563–573. https://doi.org/10.1124/jpet.102.037705

Huang J, Fisher RA (2009) Nuclear trafficking of regulator of G protein signaling proteins and their roles in the nucleus. Prog Mol Biol Transl Sci 86:115–156. https://doi.org/10.1016/s1877-1173(09)86005-5

Inoue R, Fukutani Y, Niwa T, Matsunami H, Yohda M (2023) Identification and characterization of proteins that are involved in RTP1S-dependent transport of olfactory receptors. Int J Mol Sci 24(9). https://doi.org/10.3390/ijms24097829

Irannejad R, Tomshine JC, Tomshine JR, Chevalier M, Mahoney JP, Steyaert J, Rasmussen SG, Sunahara RK, El-Samad H, Huang B, von Zastrow M (2013) Conformational biosensors reveal GPCR signalling from endosomes. Nature 495(7442):534–538. https://doi.org/10.1038/nature12000

Irannejad R, Pessino V, Mika D, Huang B, Wedegaertner PB, Conti M, von Zastrow M (2017) Functional selectivity of GPCR-directed drug action through location bias. Nat Chem Biol 13(7):799–806. https://doi.org/10.1038/nchembio.2389

Islam KN, Bae J-W, Gao E, Koch WJ (2013) Regulation of nuclear factor κB (NF-κB) in the nucleus of Cardiomyocytes by G protein-coupled receptor kinase 5 (GRK5)*. J Biol Chem 288(50):35683–35689. https://doi.org/10.1074/jbc.M113.529347

Jamora C, Yamanouye N, Van Lint J, Laudenslager J, Vandenheede JR, Faulkner DJ, Malhotra V (1999) Gbetagamma-mediated regulation of Golgi organization is through the direct activation of protein kinase D. Cell 98(1):59–68. https://doi.org/10.1016/S0092-8674(00)80606-6

Jensen DD, Lieu T, Halls ML, Veldhuis NA, Imlach WL, Mai QN, Poole DP, Quach T, Aurelio L, Conner J, Herenbrink CK, Barlow N, Simpson JS, Scanlon MJ, Graham B, McCluskey A, Robinson PJ, Escriou V, Nassini R et al (2017) Neurokinin 1 receptor signaling in endosomes mediates sustained nociception and is a viable therapeutic target for prolonged pain relief. Sci Transl Med 9(392). https://doi.org/10.1126/scitranslmed.aal3447

Jiang X, Benovic JL, Wedegaertner PB (2007) Plasma membrane and nuclear localization of G protein coupled receptor kinase 6A. Mol Biol Cell 18(8):2960–2969. https://doi.org/10.1091/mbc.e07-01-0013

Jimenez-Vargas NN, Yu Y, Jensen DD, Bok DD, Wisdom M, Latorre R, Lopez C, Jaramillo-Polanco JO, Degro C, Guzman-Rodriguez M, Tsang Q, Snow Z, Schmidt BL, Reed DE, Lomax AE, Margolis KG, Stein C, Bunnett NW, Vanner SJ (2022) Agonist that activates the micro-opioid receptor in acidified microenvironments inhibits colitis pain without side effects. Gut 71(4):695–704. https://doi.org/10.1136/gutjnl-2021-324070

Johnson LR, Scott MG, Pitcher JA (2004) G protein-coupled receptor kinase 5 contains a DNA-binding nuclear localization sequence. Mol Cell Biol 24(23):10169–10179. https://doi.org/10.1128/MCB.24.23.10169-10179.2004

Jones B, Buenaventura T, Kanda N, Chabosseau P, Owen BM, Scott R, Goldin R, Angkathunyakul N, Corrêa IR Jr, Bosco D, Johnson PR, Piemonti L, Marchetti P, Shapiro AMJ, Cochran BJ, Hanyaloglu AC, Inoue A, Tan T, Rutter GA et al (2018) Targeting GLP-1 receptor trafficking to improve agonist efficacy. Nat Commun 9(1):1602. https://doi.org/10.1038/s41467-018-03941-2

Jong YJ, Kumar V, Kingston AE, Romano C, O'Malley KL (2005) Functional metabotropic glutamate receptors on nuclei from brain and primary cultured striatal neurons. Role of transporters in delivering ligand. J Biol Chem 280(34):30469–30480. https://doi.org/10.1074/jbc.M501775200

Jong YJ, Kumar V, O'Malley KL (2009) Intracellular metabotropic glutamate receptor 5 (mGluR5) activates signaling cascades distinct from cell surface counterparts. J Biol Chem 284(51): 35827–35838. https://doi.org/10.1074/jbc.M109.046276

Joyal JS, Nim S, Zhu T, Sitaras N, Rivera JC, Shao Z, Sapieha P, Hamel D, Sanchez M, Zaniolo K, St-Louis M, Ouellette J, Montoya-Zavala M, Zabeida A, Picard E, Hardy P, Bhosle V, Varma DR, Gobeil F Jr et al (2014) Subcellular localization of coagulation factor II receptor-like 1 in neurons governs angiogenesis. Nat Med 20(10):1165–1173. https://doi.org/10.1038/nm.3669

Karpa KD, Lidow MS, Pickering MT, Levenson R, Bergson C (1999) N-linked glycosylation is required for plasma membrane localization of D5, but not D1, dopamine receptors in transfected mammalian cells. Mol Pharmacol 56(5):1071–1078. https://doi.org/10.1124/mol.56.5.1071

Katan M, Cockcroft S (2020) Phosphatidylinositol(4,5)bisphosphate: diverse functions at the plasma membrane. Essays Biochem 64(3):513–531. https://doi.org/10.1042/ebc20200041

Kinsey CG, Bussolati G, Bosco M, Kimura T, Pizzorno MC, Chernin MI, Cassoni P, Novak JF (2007) Constitutive and ligand-induced nuclear localization of oxytocin receptor. J Cell Mol Med 11(1):96–110. https://doi.org/10.1111/j.1582-4934.2007.00015.x

Klauer MJ, Willette BKA, Tsvetanova NG (2024) Functional diversification of cell signaling by GPCR localization. J Biol Chem 300(3):105668. https://doi.org/10.1016/j.jbc.2024.105668

Klayman LM, Wedegaertner PB (2017) Inducible inhibition of Gbetagamma reveals localization-dependent functions at the plasma membrane and Golgi. J Biol Chem 292(5):1773–1784. https://doi.org/10.1074/jbc.M116.750430

Knox CD, Belous AE, Pierce JM, Wakata A, Nicoud IB, Anderson CD, Pinson CW, Chari RS (2004) Novel role of phospholipase C-delta1: regulation of liver mitochondrial Ca2+ uptake.

Am J Physiol Gastrointest Liver Physiol 287(3):G533–G540. https://doi.org/10.1152/ajpgi.00050.2004

Kolczynska K, Loza-Valdes A, Hawro I, Sumara G (2020) Diacylglycerol-evoked activation of PKC and PKD isoforms in regulation of glucose and lipid metabolism: a review. Lipids Health Dis 19(1):113. https://doi.org/10.1186/s12944-020-01286-8

Kotowski SJ, Hopf FW, Seif T, Bonci A, von Zastrow M (2011) Endocytosis promotes rapid dopaminergic signaling. Neuron 71(2):278–290. https://doi.org/10.1016/j.neuron.2011.05.036

Krupnick JG, Benovic JL (1998) The role of receptor kinases and arrestins in G protein-coupled receptor regulation. Annu Rev Pharmacol Toxicol 38:289–319. https://doi.org/10.1146/annurev.pharmtox.38.1.289

Kumar V, Jong YJ, O'Malley KL (2008) Activated nuclear metabotropic glutamate receptor mGlu5 couples to nuclear Gq/11 proteins to generate inositol 1,4,5-trisphosphate-mediated nuclear Ca2+ release. J Biol Chem 283(20):14072–14083. https://doi.org/10.1074/jbc.M708551200

Kwon Y, Mehta S, Clark M, Walters G, Zhong Y, Lee HN, Sunahara RK, Zhang J (2022) Non-canonical beta-adrenergic activation of ERK at endosomes. Nature 611(7934):173–179. https://doi.org/10.1038/s41586-022-05343-3

Lagerstrom MC, Schioth HB (2008) Structural diversity of G protein-coupled receptors and significance for drug discovery. Nat Rev Drug Discov 7(4):339–357. https://doi.org/10.1038/nrd2518

Lanctot PM, Leclerc PC, Escher E, Leduc R, Guillemette G (1999) Role of N-glycosylation in the expression and functional properties of human AT1 receptor. Biochemistry 38(27):8621–8627. https://doi.org/10.1021/bi9830516

Latorre R, Ramirez-Garcia PD, Hegron A, Grace JL, Retamal JS, Shenoy P, Tran M, Aurelio L, Flynn B, Poole DP, Klein-Cloud R, Jensen DD, Davis TP, Schmidt BL, Quinn JF, Whittaker MR, Veldhuis NA, Bunnett NW (2022) Sustained endosomal release of a neurokinin-1 receptor antagonist from nanostars provides long-lasting relief of chronic pain. Biomaterials 285: 121536. https://doi.org/10.1016/j.biomaterials.2022.121536

Lee KB, Pals-Rylaarsdam R, Benovic JL, Hosey MM (1998) Arrestin-independent internalization of the m1, m3, and m4 subtypes of muscarinic cholinergic receptors. J Biol Chem 273(21): 12967–12972. https://doi.org/10.1074/jbc.273.21.12967

Lee SB, Xuan Nguyen TL, Choi JW, Lee KH, Cho SW, Liu Z, Ye K, Bae SS, Ahn JY (2008) Nuclear Akt interacts with B23/NPM and protects it from proteolytic cleavage, enhancing cell survival. Proc Natl Acad Sci USA 105(43):16584–16589. https://doi.org/10.1073/pnas.0807668105

Lee S, Park S, Lee H, Han S, Song J-M, Han D, Suh YH (2019) Nedd4 E3 ligase and beta-arrestins regulate ubiquitination, trafficking, and stability of the mGlu7 receptor. eLife 8:e44502. https://doi.org/10.7554/eLife.44502

Lefkimmiatis K, Leronni D, Hofer AM (2013) The inner and outer compartments of mitochondria are sites of distinct cAMP/PKA signaling dynamics. J Cell Biol 202(3):453–462. https://doi.org/10.1083/jcb.201303159

Lefkowitz RJ, Shenoy SK (2005) Transduction of receptor signals by beta-arrestins. Science 308(5721):512–517. https://doi.org/10.1126/science.1109237

Liccardo F, Luini A, Di Martino R (2022) Endomembrane-based signaling by GPCRs and G-proteins. Cells 11(3). https://doi.org/10.3390/cells11030528

Litvak V, Dahan N, Ramachandran S, Sabanay H, Lev S (2005) Maintenance of the diacylglycerol level in the Golgi apparatus by the Nir2 protein is critical for Golgi secretory function. Nat Cell Biol 7(3):225–234. https://doi.org/10.1038/ncb1221

Lohse MJ, Benovic JL, Codina J, Caron MG, Lefkowitz RJ (1990) beta-Arrestin: a protein that regulates beta-adrenergic receptor function. Science 248(4962):1547–1550. https://doi.org/10.1126/science.2163110

Lu D, Yang H, Shaw G, Raizada MK (1998) Angiotensin II-induced nuclear targeting of the angiotensin type 1 (AT1) receptor in brain neurons. Endocrinology 139(1):365–375. https://doi.org/10.1210/endo.139.1.5679

Lu J, Wu T, Zhang B, Liu S, Song W, Qiao J, Ruan H (2021) Types of nuclear localization signals and mechanisms of protein import into the nucleus. Cell Commun Signal 19(1):60. https://doi.org/10.1186/s12964-021-00741-y

Ludwig A, Howard G, Mendoza-Topaz C, Deerinck T, Mackey M, Sandin S, Ellisman MH, Nichols BJ (2013) Molecular composition and ultrastructure of the caveolar coat complex. PLoS Biol 11(8):e1001640. https://doi.org/10.1371/journal.pbio.1001640

Luttrell LM, Ferguson SS, Daaka Y, Miller WE, Maudsley S, Della Rocca GJ, Lin F, Kawakatsu H, Owada K, Luttrell DK, Caron MG, Lefkowitz RJ (1999) Beta-arrestin-dependent formation of beta2 adrenergic receptor-Src protein kinase complexes. Science 283(5402):655–661. https://doi.org/10.1126/science.283.5402.655

Luttrell LM, Roudabush FL, Choy EW, Miller WE, Field ME, Pierce KL, Lefkowitz RJ (2001) Activation and targeting of extracellular signal-regulated kinases by beta-arrestin scaffolds. Proc Natl Acad Sci USA 98(5):2449–2454. https://doi.org/10.1073/pnas.041604898

Lygren B, Carlson CR, Santamaria K, Lissandron V, McSorley T, Litzenberg J, Lorenz D, Wiesner B, Rosenthal W, Zaccolo M, Taskén K, Klussmann E (2007) AKAP complex regulates Ca2+ re-uptake into heart sarcoplasmic reticulum. EMBO Rep 8(11):1061–1067. https://doi.org/10.1038/sj.embor.7401081

Lyssand JS, Bajjalieh SM (2007) The heretotrimeric G protein subunit Gαi is present on mitochondria. FEBS Lett 581(30):5765–5768. https://doi.org/10.1016/j.febslet.2007.11.044

Maccaroni K, La Torre M, Burla R, Saggio I (2022) Phase separation in the nucleus and at the nuclear periphery during post-mitotic nuclear envelope reformation. Cells 11(11). https://doi.org/10.3390/cells11111749

Madukwe JC, Garland-Kuntz EE, Lyon AM, Smrcka AV (2018) G protein βγ subunits directly interact with and activate phospholipase cϵ. J Biol Chem 293(17):6387–6397. https://doi.org/10.1074/jbc.RA118.002354

Mai QN, Shenoy P, Quach T, Retamal JS, Gondin AB, Yeatman HR, Aurelio L, Conner JW, Poole DP, Canals M, Nowell CJ, Graham B, Davis TP, Briddon SJ, Hill SJ, Porter CJH, Bunnett NW, Halls ML, Veldhuis NA (2021) A lipid-anchored neurokinin 1 receptor antagonist prolongs pain relief by a three-pronged mechanism of action targeting the receptor at the plasma membrane and in endosomes. J Biol Chem 296:100345. https://doi.org/10.1016/j.jbc.2021.100345

Malik S, deRubio RG, Trembley M, Irannejad R, Wedegaertner PB, Smrcka AV (2015) G protein βγ subunits regulate cardiomyocyte hypertrophy through a perinuclear Golgi phosphatidylinositol 4-phosphate hydrolysis pathway. Mol Biol Cell 26(6):1188–1198. https://doi.org/10.1091/mbc.E14-10-1476

Masuho I, Itoh M, Itoh H, Saitoh O (2004) The mechanism of membrane-translocation of regulator of G-protein signaling (RGS) 8 induced by Galpha expression. J Neurochem 88(1):161–168. https://doi.org/10.1046/j.1471-4159.2003.02139.x

Masuho I, Skamangas NK, Muntean BS, Martemyanov KA (2021) Diversity of the Gbetagamma complexes defines spatial and temporal bias of GPCR signaling. Cell Syst 12(4):324–337 e325. https://doi.org/10.1016/j.cels.2021.02.001

McDonald PH, Chow CW, Miller WE, Laporte SA, Field ME, Lin FT, Davis RJ, Lefkowitz RJ (2000) Beta-arrestin 2: a receptor-regulated MAPK scaffold for the activation of JNK3. Science 290(5496):1574–1577. https://doi.org/10.1126/science.290.5496.1574

McLatchie LM, Fraser NJ, Main MJ, Wise A, Brown J, Thompson N, Solari R, Lee MG, Foord SM (1998) RAMPs regulate the transport and ligand specificity of the calcitonin-receptor-like receptor. Nature 393(6683):333–339. https://doi.org/10.1038/30666

Means CK, Lygren B, Langeberg LK, Jain A, Dixon RE, Vega AL, Gold MG, Petrosyan S, Taylor SS, Murphy AN, Ha T, Santana LF, Tasken K, Scott JD (2011) An entirely specific type I A-kinase anchoring protein that can sequester two molecules of protein kinase A at mitochondria. Proc Natl Acad Sci USA 108(48):E1227–E1235. https://doi.org/10.1073/pnas.1107182108

Michineau S, Muller L, Pizard A, Alhenc-Gelas F, Rajerison RM (2004) N-linked glycosylation of the human bradykinin B2 receptor is required for optimal cell-surface expression and coupling. Biol Chem 385(1):49–57. https://doi.org/10.1515/BC.2004.007

Millette M-A, Roy S, Salesse C (2022) Farnesylation and lipid unsaturation are critical for the membrane binding of the C-terminal segment of G-protein receptor kinase 1. Colloids Surf B: Biointerfaces 211:112315. https://doi.org/10.1016/j.colsurfb.2021.112315

Mohammad Nezhady MA, Rivera JC, Chemtob S (2020) Location Bias as emerging paradigm in GPCR biology and drug discovery. iScience 23(10):101643. https://doi.org/10.1016/j.isci.2020.101643

Morinelli TA, Walker LP, Ullian ME (2008) COX-2 expression stimulated by angiotensin II depends upon AT1 receptor internalization in vascular smooth muscle cells. Biochim Biophys Acta 1783(6):1048–1054. https://doi.org/10.1016/j.bbamcr.2008.01.012

Mullershausen F, Zecri F, Cetin C, Billich A, Guerini D, Seuwen K (2009) Persistent signaling induced by FTY720-phosphate is mediated by internalized S1P1 receptors. Nat Chem Biol 5(6): 428–434. https://doi.org/10.1038/nchembio.173

Nash CA, Wei W, Irannejad R, Smrcka AV (2019) Golgi localized beta1-adrenergic receptors stimulate Golgi PI4P hydrolysis by PLCepsilon to regulate cardiac hypertrophy. elife 8. https://doi.org/10.7554/eLife.48167

Nguyen AH, Thomsen ARB, Cahill TJ 3rd, Huang R, Huang LY, Marcink T, Clarke OB, Heissel S, Masoudi A, Ben-Hail D, Samaan F, Dandey VP, Tan YZ, Hong C, Mahoney JP, Triest S, Little JT, Chen X, Sunahara R et al (2019) Structure of an endosomal signaling GPCR-G protein-beta-arrestin megacomplex. Nat Struct Mol Biol 26(12):1123–1131. https://doi.org/10.1038/s41594-019-0330-y

Noor N, Patel CB, Rockman HA (2011) B-arrestin: a signaling molecule and potential therapeutic target for heart failure. J Mol Cell Cardiol 51(4):534–541. https://doi.org/10.1016/j.yjmcc.2010.11.005

O'Connell TD, Ishizaka S, Nakamura A, Swigart PM, Rodrigo MC, Simpson GL, Cotecchia S, Rokosh DG, Grossman W, Foster E, Simpson PC (2003) The alpha(1A/C)- and alpha(1B)-adrenergic receptors are required for physiological cardiac hypertrophy in the double-knockout mouse. J Clin Invest 111(11):1783–1791. https://doi.org/10.1172/JCI16100

O'Connell TD, Swigart PM, Rodrigo MC, Ishizaka S, Joho S, Turnbull L, Tecott LH, Baker AJ, Foster E, Grossman W, Simpson PC (2006) Alpha1-adrenergic receptors prevent a maladaptive cardiac response to pressure overload. J Clin Invest 116(4):1005–1015. https://doi.org/10.1172/JCI22811

O'Malley KL, Jong YJ, Gonchar Y, Burkhalter A, Romano C (2003) Activation of metabotropic glutamate receptor mGlu5 on nuclear membranes mediates intranuclear Ca2+ changes in heterologous cell types and neurons. J Biol Chem 278(30):28210–28219. https://doi.org/10.1074/jbc.M300792200

Oakley RH, Laporte SA, Holt JA, Barak LS, Caron MG (1999) Association of beta-arrestin with G protein-coupled receptors during clathrin-mediated endocytosis dictates the profile of receptor resensitization. J Biol Chem 274(45):32248–32257. https://doi.org/10.1074/jbc.274.45.32248

Ohnaka K, Numaguchi K, Yamakawa T, Inagami T (2000) Induction of cyclooxygenase-2 by angiotensin II in cultured rat vascular smooth muscle cells. Hypertension 35(1 Pt 1):68–75. https://doi.org/10.1161/01.hyp.35.1.68

Ortegren U, Karlsson M, Blazic N, Blomqvist M, Nystrom FH, Gustavsson J, Fredman P, Strålfors P (2004) Lipids and glycosphingolipids in caveolae and surrounding plasma membrane of primary rat adipocytes. Eur J Biochem 271(10):2028–2036. https://doi.org/10.1111/j.1432-1033.2004.04117.x

Osawa S, Weiss ER (2012) A tale of two kinases in rods and cones. Adv Exp Med Biol 723:821–827. https://doi.org/10.1007/978-1-4614-0631-0_105

Paing MM, Stutts AB, Kohout TA, Lefkowitz RJ, Trejo J (2002) β-arrestins regulate protease-activated receptor-1 desensitization but not internalization or Down-regulation. J Biol Chem 277(2):1292–1300. https://doi.org/10.1074/jbc.M109160200

Paing MM, Johnston CA, Siderovski DP, Trejo J (2006) Clathrin adaptor AP2 regulates thrombin receptor constitutive internalization and endothelial cell resensitization. Mol Cell Biol 26(8): 3231–3242. https://doi.org/10.1128/mcb.26.8.3231-3242.2006

Patial S, Luo J, Porter KJ, Benovic JL, Parameswaran N (2009) G-protein-coupled-receptor kinases mediate TNFα-induced NFκB signalling via direct interaction with and phosphorylation of IκBα. Biochem J 425(1):169–178. https://doi.org/10.1042/bj20090908

Patwardhan A, Cheng N, Trejo J (2021) Post-translational modifications of G protein-coupled receptors control cellular signaling dynamics in space and time. Pharmacol Rev 73(1):120–151. https://doi.org/10.1124/pharmrev.120.000082

Pendergrass KD, Gwathmey TM, Michalek RD, Grayson JM, Chappell MC (2009) The angiotensin II-AT1 receptor stimulates reactive oxygen species within the cell nucleus. Biochem Biophys Res Commun 384(2):149–154. https://doi.org/10.1016/j.bbrc.2009.04.126

Peterson YK, Luttrell LM (2017) The diverse roles of Arrestin scaffolds in G protein-coupled receptor signaling. Pharmacol Rev 69(3):256–297. https://doi.org/10.1124/pr.116.013367

Pierce KL, Premont RT, Lefkowitz RJ (2002) Seven-transmembrane receptors. Nat Rev Mol Cell Biol 3(9):639–650. https://doi.org/10.1038/nrm908

Pinheiro EDS, Preato AM, Petrucci TVB, Dos Santos LS, Glezer I (2023) Phase-separation: a possible new layer for transcriptional regulation by glucocorticoid receptor. Front Endocrinol (Lausanne) 14:1160238. https://doi.org/10.3389/fendo.2023.1160238

Pizzoni A, Zhang X, Naim N, Altschuler DL (2023) Soluble cyclase-mediated nuclear cAMP synthesis is sufficient for cell proliferation. Proc Natl Acad Sci USA 120(4):e2208749120. https://doi.org/10.1073/pnas.2208749120

Plotnikov A, Zehorai E, Procaccia S, Seger R (2011) The MAPK cascades: signaling components, nuclear roles and mechanisms of nuclear translocation. Biochim Biophys Acta 1813(9): 1619–1633. https://doi.org/10.1016/j.bbamcr.2010.12.012

Pope GR, Tilve S, McArdle CA, Lolait SJ, O'Carroll AM (2016) Agonist-induced internalization and desensitization of the apelin receptor. Mol Cell Endocrinol 437:108–119. https://doi.org/10.1016/j.mce.2016.07.040

Prole DL, Taylor CW (2019) Structure and function of IP(3) receptors. Cold Spring Harb Perspect Biol 11(4). https://doi.org/10.1101/cshperspect.a035063

Purgert CA, Izumi Y, Jong YJ, Kumar V, Zorumski CF, O'Malley KL (2014) Intracellular mGluR5 can mediate synaptic plasticity in the hippocampus. J Neurosci 34(13):4589–4598. https://doi.org/10.1523/JNEUROSCI.3451-13.2014

Puri NM, Romano GR, Lin TY, Mai QN, Irannejad R (2022) The organic cation transporter 2 regulates dopamine D1 receptor signaling at the Golgi apparatus. elife 11. https://doi.org/10.7554/eLife.75468

Radoux-Mergault A, Oberhauser L, Aureli S, Gervasio FL, Stoeber M (2023) Subcellular location defines GPCR signal transduction. Sci Adv 9(16):eadf6059. https://doi.org/10.1126/sciadv.adf6059

Rasola A, Sciacovelli M, Chiara F, Pantic B, Brusilow WS, Bernardi P (2010) Activation of mitochondrial ERK protects cancer cells from death through inhibition of the permeability transition. Proc Natl Acad Sci USA 107(2):726–731. https://doi.org/10.1073/pnas.0912742107

Rejman J, Bragonzi A, Conese M (2005) Role of clathrin- and caveolae-mediated endocytosis in gene transfer mediated by lipo- and polyplexes. Mol Ther 12(3):468–474. https://doi.org/10.1016/j.ymthe.2005.03.038

Revankar CM, Cimino DF, Sklar LA, Arterburn JB, Prossnitz ER (2005) A transmembrane intracellular estrogen receptor mediates rapid cell signaling. Science 307(5715):1625–1630. https://doi.org/10.1126/science.1106943

Rimler A, Jockers R, Lupowitz Z, Sampson SR, Zisapel N (2006) Differential effects of melatonin and its downstream effector PKCalpha on subcellular localization of RGS proteins. J Pineal Res 40(2):144–152. https://doi.org/10.1111/j.1600-079X.2005.00290.x

Robison AJ, Colbran RJ (2013) Calcium/calmodulin-dependent protein kinases. In: Lennarz WJ, Lane MD (eds) Encyclopedia of biological chemistry, 2nd edn. Academic, pp 304–309. https://doi.org/10.1016/B978-0-12-378630-2.00493-X

Rosenbaum DM, Rasmussen SG, Kobilka BK (2009) The structure and function of G-protein-coupled receptors. Nature 459(7245):356–363. https://doi.org/10.1038/nature08144

Rothberg KG, Heuser JE, Donzell WC, Ying YS, Glenney JR, Anderson RG (1992) Caveolin, a protein component of caveolae membrane coats. Cell 68(4):673–682. https://doi.org/10.1016/0092-8674(92)90143-z

Sample V, DiPilato LM, Yang JH, Ni Q, Saucerman JJ, Zhang J (2012) Regulation of nuclear PKA revealed by spatiotemporal manipulation of cyclic AMP. Nat Chem Biol 8(4):375–382. https://doi.org/10.1038/nchembio.799

Sarg NH, Zaher DM, Abu Jayab NN, Mostafa SH, Ismail HH, Omar HA (2024) The interplay of p38 MAPK signaling and mitochondrial metabolism, a dynamic target in cancer and pathological contexts. Biochem Pharmacol 225:116307. https://doi.org/10.1016/j.bcp.2024.116307

Sasaki K, Sato M, Umezawa Y (2003) Fluorescent indicators for Akt/protein kinase B and dynamics of Akt activity visualized in living cells*. J Biol Chem 278(33):30945–30951. https://doi.org/10.1074/jbc.M212167200

Sassone-Corsi P (2012) The cyclic AMP pathway. Cold Spring Harb Perspect Biol 4(12). https://doi.org/10.1101/cshperspect.a011148

Sato M, Hiraoka M, Suzuki H, Bai Y, Kurotani R, Yokoyama U, Okumura S, Cismowski MJ, Lanier SM, Ishikawa Y (2011) Identification of transcription factor E3 (TFE3) as a receptor-independent activator of Galpha16: gene regulation by nuclear Galpha subunit and its activator. J Biol Chem 286(20):17766–17776. https://doi.org/10.1074/jbc.M111.219816

Schievella AR, Regier MK, Smith WL, Lin LL (1995) Calcium-mediated translocation of cytosolic phospholipase A2 to the nuclear envelope and endoplasmic reticulum. J Biol Chem 270(51):30749–30754. https://doi.org/10.1074/jbc.270.51.30749

Schulein R, Liebenhoff U, Muller H, Birnbaumer M, Rosenthal W (1996) Properties of the human arginine vasopressin V2 receptor after site-directed mutagenesis of its putative palmitoylation site. Biochem J 313(Pt 2):611–616. https://doi.org/10.1042/bj3130611

Scott MGH, Le Rouzic E, Périanin A, Pierotti V, Enslen H, Benichou S, Marullo S, Benmerah A (2002) Differential nucleocytoplasmic shuttling of β-Arrestins: characterization of a leucine-rich nuclear export signal in β-Arrestin2*. J Biol Chem 277(40):37693–37701. https://doi.org/10.1074/jbc.M207552200

Shanks RA, Steadman BT, Schmidt PH, Goldenring JR (2002) AKAP350 at the Golgi apparatus. I. Identification of a distinct Golgi apparatus targeting motif in AKAP350. J Biol Chem 277(43):40967–40972. https://doi.org/10.1074/jbc.M203307200

Smith JS, Rajagopal S (2016) The beta-Arrestins: multifunctional regulators of G protein-coupled receptors. J Biol Chem 291(17):8969–8977. https://doi.org/10.1074/jbc.R115.713313

Smith TH, Coronel LJ, Li JG, Dores MR, Nieman MT, Trejo J (2016) Protease-activated receptor-4 signaling and trafficking is regulated by the Clathrin adaptor protein Complex-2 independent of beta-Arrestins. J Biol Chem 291(35):18453–18464. https://doi.org/10.1074/jbc.M116.729285

Smith JS, Nicholson LT, Suwanpradid J, Glenn RA, Knape NM, Alagesan P, Gundry JN, Wehrman TS, Atwater AR, Gunn MD, MacLeod AS, Rajagopal S (2018) Biased agonists of the chemokine receptor CXCR3 differentially control chemotaxis and inflammation. Sci Signal 11(555). https://doi.org/10.1126/scisignal.aaq1075

So CH, Michal AM, Mashayekhi R, Benovic JL (2012) G protein-coupled receptor kinase 5 phosphorylates nucleophosmin and regulates cell sensitivity to polo-like kinase 1 inhibition. J Biol Chem 287(21):17088–17099. https://doi.org/10.1074/jbc.M112.353854

Solis GP, Bilousov O, Koval A, Lüchtenborg AM, Lin C, Katanaev VL (2017) Golgi-resident gαo promotes protrusive membrane dynamics. Cell 170(5):939–955.e924. https://doi.org/10.1016/j.cell.2017.07.015

Sorkin A, von Zastrow M (2009) Endocytosis and signalling: intertwining molecular networks. Nat Rev Mol Cell Biol 10(9):609–622. https://doi.org/10.1038/nrm2748

Spahn V, Del Vecchio G, Labuz D, Rodriguez-Gaztelumendi A, Massaly N, Temp J, Durmaz V, Sabri P, Reidelbach M, Machelska H, Weber M, Stein C (2017) A nontoxic pain killer designed by modeling of pathological receptor conformations. Science 355(6328):966–969. https://doi.org/10.1126/science.aai8636

Stoeber M, Jullie D, Lobingier BT, Laeremans T, Steyaert J, Schiller PW, Manglik A, von Zastrow M (2018) A genetically encoded biosensor reveals location Bias of opioid drug action. Neuron 98(5):963–976 e965. https://doi.org/10.1016/j.neuron.2018.04.021

Suofu Y, Li W, Jean-Alphonse FG, Jia J, Khattar NK, Li J, Baranov SV, Leronni D, Mihalik AC, He Y, Cecon E, Wehbi VL, Kim J, Heath BE, Baranova OV, Wang X, Gable MJ, Kretz ES, Di Benedetto G et al (2017) Dual role of mitochondria in producing melatonin and driving GPCR signaling to block cytochrome c release. Proc Natl Acad Sci USA 114(38):E7997–E8006. https://doi.org/10.1073/pnas.1705768114

Syme CA, Zhang L, Bisello A (2006) Caveolin-1 regulates cellular trafficking and function of the glucagon-like Peptide 1 receptor. Mol Endocrinol 20(12):3400–3411. https://doi.org/10.1210/me.2006-0178

Tadevosyan A, Maguy A, Villeneuve LR, Babin J, Bonnefoy A, Allen BG, Nattel S (2010) Nuclear-delimited angiotensin receptor-mediated signaling regulates cardiomyocyte gene expression. J Biol Chem 285(29):22338–22349. https://doi.org/10.1074/jbc.M110.121749

Tadevosyan A, Vaniotis G, Allen BG, Hebert TE, Nattel S (2012) G protein-coupled receptor signalling in the cardiac nuclear membrane: evidence and possible roles in physiological and pathophysiological function. J Physiol 590(6):1313–1330. https://doi.org/10.1113/jphysiol.2011.222794

Tadevosyan A, Xiao J, Surinkaew S, Naud P, Merlen C, Harada M, Qi X, Chatenet D, Fournier A, Allen BG, Nattel S (2017) Intracellular angiotensin-II interacts with nuclear angiotensin receptors in cardiac fibroblasts and regulates RNA synthesis, cell proliferation, and collagen secretion. J Am Heart Assoc 6(4). https://doi.org/10.1161/JAHA.116.004965

Tan M, Walwyn WM, Evans CJ, Xie CW (2009) p38 MAPK and beta-arrestin 2 mediate functional interactions between endogenous micro-opioid and alpha2A-adrenergic receptors in neurons. J Biol Chem 284(10):6270–6281. https://doi.org/10.1074/jbc.M806742200

Thiyagarajan MM, Stracquatanio RP, Pronin AN, Evanko DS, Benovic JL, Wedegaertner PB (2004) A predicted amphipathic helix mediates plasma membrane localization of GRK5. J Biol Chem 279(17):17989–17995. https://doi.org/10.1074/jbc.M310738200

Thomsen ARB, Plouffe B, Cahill TJ 3rd, Shukla AK, Tarrasch JT, Dosey AM, Kahsai AW, Strachan RT, Pani B, Mahoney JP, Huang L, Breton B, Heydenreich FM, Sunahara RK, Skiniotis G, Bouvier M, Lefkowitz RJ (2016) GPCR-G protein-beta-Arrestin super-complex mediates sustained G protein signaling. Cell 166(4):907–919. https://doi.org/10.1016/j.cell.2016.07.004

Torii S, Kusakabe M, Yamamoto T, Maekawa M, Nishida E (2004) Sef is a spatial regulator for Ras/MAP kinase signaling. Dev Cell 7(1):33–44. https://doi.org/10.1016/j.devcel.2004.05.019

Touhara K, Inglese J, Pitcher JA, Shaw G, Lefkowitz RJ (1994) Binding of G protein beta gamma-subunits to pleckstrin homology domains. J Biol Chem 269(14):10217–10220

Tsvetanova NG, von Zastrow M (2014) Spatial encoding of cyclic AMP signaling specificity by GPCR endocytosis. Nat Chem Biol 10(12):1061–1065. https://doi.org/10.1038/nchembio.1665

Tsvetanova NG, Trester-Zedlitz M, Newton BW, Peng GE, Johnson JR, Jimenez-Morales D, Kurland AP, Krogan NJ, von Zastrow M (2021) Endosomal cAMP production broadly impacts the cellular phosphoproteome. J Biol Chem 297(1):100907. https://doi.org/10.1016/j.jbc.2021.100907

Turjanski AG, Vaque JP, Gutkind JS (2007) MAP kinases and the control of nuclear events. Oncogene 26(22):3240–3253. https://doi.org/10.1038/sj.onc.1210415

Valdehita A, Bajo AM, Fernandez-Martinez AB, Arenas MI, Vacas E, Valenzuela P, Ruiz-Villaespesa A, Prieto JC, Carmena MJ (2010) Nuclear localization of vasoactive intestinal peptide (VIP) receptors in human breast cancer. Peptides 31(11):2035–2045. https://doi.org/10.1016/j.peptides.2010.07.024

Valenzuela R, Costa-Besada MA, Iglesias-Gonzalez J, Perez-Costas E, Villar-Cheda B, Garrido-Gil P, Melendez-Ferro M, Soto-Otero R, Lanciego JL, Henrion D, Franco R, Labandeira-Garcia JL (2016) Mitochondrial angiotensin receptors in dopaminergic neurons. Role in cell protection and aging-related vulnerability to neurodegeneration. Cell Death Dis 7(10):e2427. https://doi.org/10.1038/cddis.2016.327

Vogler O, Bogatkewitsch GS, Wriske C, Krummenerl P, Jakobs KH, van Koppen CJ (1998) Receptor subtype-specific regulation of muscarinic acetylcholine receptor sequestration by dynamin. Distinct sequestration of m2 receptors. J Biol Chem 273(20):12155–12160. https://doi.org/10.1074/jbc.273.20.12155

Wainstein E, Seger R (2016) The dynamic subcellular localization of ERK: mechanisms of translocation and role in various organelles. Curr Opin Cell Biol 39:15–20. https://doi.org/10.1016/j.ceb.2016.01.007

Wei W, Smrcka A (2024) Internalized β2-adrenergic receptors inhibit subcellular phospholipase C-dependent cardiac hypertrophic signaling. Physiology 39(S1):1600. https://doi.org/10.1152/physiol.2024.39.S1.1600

Wolfe BL, Trejo J (2007) Clathrin-dependent mechanisms of G protein-coupled receptor endocytosis. Traffic 8(5):462–470. https://doi.org/10.1111/j.1600-0854.2007.00551.x

Wootten D, Christopoulos A, Marti-Solano M, Babu MM, Sexton PM (2018) Mechanisms of signalling and biased agonism in G protein-coupled receptors. Nat Rev Mol Cell Biol 19(10): 638–653. https://doi.org/10.1038/s41580-018-0049-3

Wright CD, Chen Q, Baye NL, Huang Y, Healy CL, Kasinathan S, O'Connell TD (2008) Nuclear alpha1-adrenergic receptors signal activated ERK localization to caveolae in adult cardiac myocytes. Circ Res 103(9):992–1000. https://doi.org/10.1161/CIRCRESAHA.108.176024

Wright CD, Wu SC, Dahl EF, Sazama AJ, O'Connell TD (2012) Nuclear localization drives alpha1-adrenergic receptor oligomerization and signaling in cardiac myocytes. Cell Signal 24(3):794–802. https://doi.org/10.1016/j.cellsig.2011.11.014

Wu SC, Dahl EF, Wright CD, Cypher AL, Healy CL, O'Connell TD (2014) Nuclear localization of a1A-adrenergic receptors is required for signaling in cardiac myocytes: an "inside-out" a1-AR signaling pathway. J Am Heart Assoc 3(2):e000145. https://doi.org/10.1161/jaha.113.000145

Yamamoto S, Kawamura K, James TN (1998) Intracellular distribution of adenylate cyclase in human cardiocytes determined by electron microscopic cytochemistry. Microsc Res Tech 40(6): 479–487. https://doi.org/10.1002/(SICI)1097-0029(19980301)40:6<479::AID-JEMT8>3.0.CO;2-K

Yang CF, Tsai WC (2022) Calmodulin: the switch button of calcium signaling. Tzu Chi Med J 34(1):15–22. https://doi.org/10.4103/tcmj.tcmj_285_20

Yarwood RE, Imlach WL, Lieu T, Veldhuis NA, Jensen DD, Klein Herenbrink C, Aurelio L, Cai Z, Christie MJ, Poole DP, Porter CJH, McLean P, Hicks GA, Geppetti P, Halls ML, Canals M, Bunnett NW (2017) Endosomal signaling of the receptor for calcitonin gene-related peptide mediates pain transmission. Proc Natl Acad Sci USA 114(46):12309–12314. https://doi.org/10.1073/pnas.1706656114

Zarca A, Perez C, van den Bor J, Bebelman JP, Heuninck J, de Jonker RJF, Durroux T, Vischer HF, Siderius M, Smit MJ (2021) Differential involvement of ACKR3 C-Tail in beta-Arrestin recruitment, trafficking and internalization. Cells 10(3). https://doi.org/10.3390/cells10030618

Zhan X, Kook S, Gurevich EV, Gurevich VV (2014) Arrestin-dependent activation of JNK family kinases. Handb Exp Pharmacol 219:259–280. https://doi.org/10.1007/978-3-642-41199-1_13

Zhang JH, Barr VA, Mo Y, Rojkova AM, Liu S, Simonds WF (2001) Nuclear localization of G protein beta 5 and regulator of G protein signaling 7 in neurons and brain. J Biol Chem 276(13): 10284–10289. https://doi.org/10.1074/jbc.M009247200

Zhang J, Liu W, Liu J, Xiao W, Liu L, Jiang C, Sun X, Liu P, Zhu Y, Zhang C, Chen Q (2010) G-protein β2 subunit interacts with mitofusin 1 to regulate mitochondrial fusion. Nat Commun 1(1):101. https://doi.org/10.1038/ncomms1099

Zhang L, Malik S, Pang J, Wang H, Park KM, Yule DI, Blaxall BC, Smrcka AV (2013) Phospholipase Cepsilon hydrolyzes perinuclear phosphatidylinositol 4-phosphate to regulate cardiac hypertrophy. Cell 153(1):216–227. https://doi.org/10.1016/j.cell.2013.02.047

Zhang JZ, Lu TW, Stolerman LM, Tenner B, Yang JR, Zhang JF, Falcke M, Rangamani P, Taylor SS, Mehta S, Zhang J (2020) Phase separation of a PKA regulatory subunit controls cAMP compartmentation and oncogenic signaling. Cell 182(6):1531–1544 e1515. https://doi.org/10.1016/j.cell.2020.07.043

Zhang X, Connelly J, Chao Y, Wang QJ (2021) Multifaceted functions of protein kinase D in pathological processes and human diseases. Biomolecules 11(3). https://doi.org/10.3390/biom11030483

Zhang M, Chen T, Lu X, Lan X, Chen Z, Lu S (2024) G protein-coupled receptors (GPCRs): advances in structures, mechanisms, and drug discovery. Signal Transduct Target Ther 9(1):88. https://doi.org/10.1038/s41392-024-01803-6

Zimber A, Nguyen QD, Gespach C (2004) Nuclear bodies and compartments: functional roles and cellular signalling in health and disease. Cell Signal 16(10):1085–1104. https://doi.org/10.1016/j.cellsig.2004.03.020

Zong Y, Li H, Liao P, Chen L, Pan Y, Zheng Y, Zhang C, Liu D, Zheng M, Gao J (2024) Mitochondrial dysfunction: mechanisms and advances in therapy. Signal Transduct Target Ther 9(1):124. https://doi.org/10.1038/s41392-024-01839-8

S-Nitrosylation of GPCR Regulatory Machinery as a Mechanism to Bias Signaling

Mingda Chen, Zachary W. Grimmett, Richard T. Premont, and Jonathan S. Stamler

Contents

Abstract

Upon stimulation by endogenous ligands, G protein-coupled receptors (GPCRs) activate downstream signaling pathways through multiple mechanisms, including G protein subtypes, β-arrestins, and receptor-specific partners. Synthetic ligands

M. Chen · Z. W. Grimmett
Institute for Transformative Molecular Medicine and Department of Medicine, Case Western Reserve University School of Medicine, Cleveland, OH, USA

R. T. Premont · J. S. Stamler (✉)
Institute for Transformative Molecular Medicine and Department of Medicine, Case Western Reserve University School of Medicine, Cleveland, OH, USA

Harrington Discovery Institute, University Hospitals Cleveland Medical Center, Cleveland, OH, USA
e-mail: jss156@case.edu

© The Author(s), under exclusive license to Springer Nature Switzerland AG 2025
Z. Li, K. Xiao (eds.), *Pharmacology of GPCRs Biased Signaling and Agonists*,
Handbook of Experimental Pharmacology 290, https://doi.org/10.1007/164_2025_765

may activate only a subset of these pathways, resulting in *functional selectivity* or *signaling bias*. Since not all signaling outputs are therapeutically desirable, there is pharmaceutical interest in exploiting biased signaling. Although much effort is focused on designing ligands to induce receptor conformations that result in signal bias, it is also true that cellular systems adapt dynamically in ways that tune receptor signaling, termed *system bias*. In this chapter, we provide evidence that posttranslational modification of receptor machinery by S-nitrosylation is an important regulator of system bias in GPCR signaling. S-nitrosylation has been reported to affect the function of multiple classes of GPCR signaling pathway components, including receptors, G proteins, G protein-coupled receptor kinases, β-arrestins, and others. Further, untargeted proteomic studies of S-nitrosylated proteins have identified over 60 GPCRs, most heterotrimeric G proteins, and numerous GPCR signaling components, hinting at a class effect and unifying mechanism to bias the functional repertoires of GPCRs in vivo. Thus, protein S-nitrosylation provides prototypic examples for how post-translational regulatory mechanisms bias GPCRs endogenously.

Keywords

Biased signaling · Functional selectivity · G protein-coupled receptor · S-nitrosothiol · S-nitrosylation · Systemic bias

1 Introduction: GPCRs, Signaling, and Bias

G protein-coupled receptors (GPCRs) regulate a wide array of biological processes, including vision, taste, olfaction, and much of endocrinology (Pierce et al. 2002). GPCRs share a seven membrane-spanning helix architecture, and canonically signal by activating GDP–GTP exchange on heterotrimeric G proteins that regulate intracellular messenger pathways (Pierce et al. 2002; Liu et al. 2024), but also through general GPCR partner proteins such as G protein-coupled receptor kinases (GRKs) and arrestins, and through receptor-specific partners (Hilger et al. 2018). With more than a third of all FDA-approved medications directed at GPCRs and their pathways, the ~800 human GPCRs represent the largest group of therapeutic targets (Hauser et al. 2018; Sriram and Insel 2018).

GPCR ligands exist on a continuum between full receptor activation and complete silencing. *Agonists* stabilize receptor conformations that result in the activation of downstream intracellular messenger systems. On the other hand, *antagonist* ligands bind to a receptor but fail to activate downstream signaling, thus preventing activation by native ligands. Because GPCRs can exhibit agonist-independent basal activity, *inverse agonists* reduce basal receptor signaling, whereas neutral antagonists do not. Ligands that partially activate GPCRs (*partial agonist*) are often leveraged for therapeutic use.

Since many GPCRs can initiate signals through multiple downstream signaling pathways (through one or more classes of heterotrimeric G proteins, arrestins, etc.),

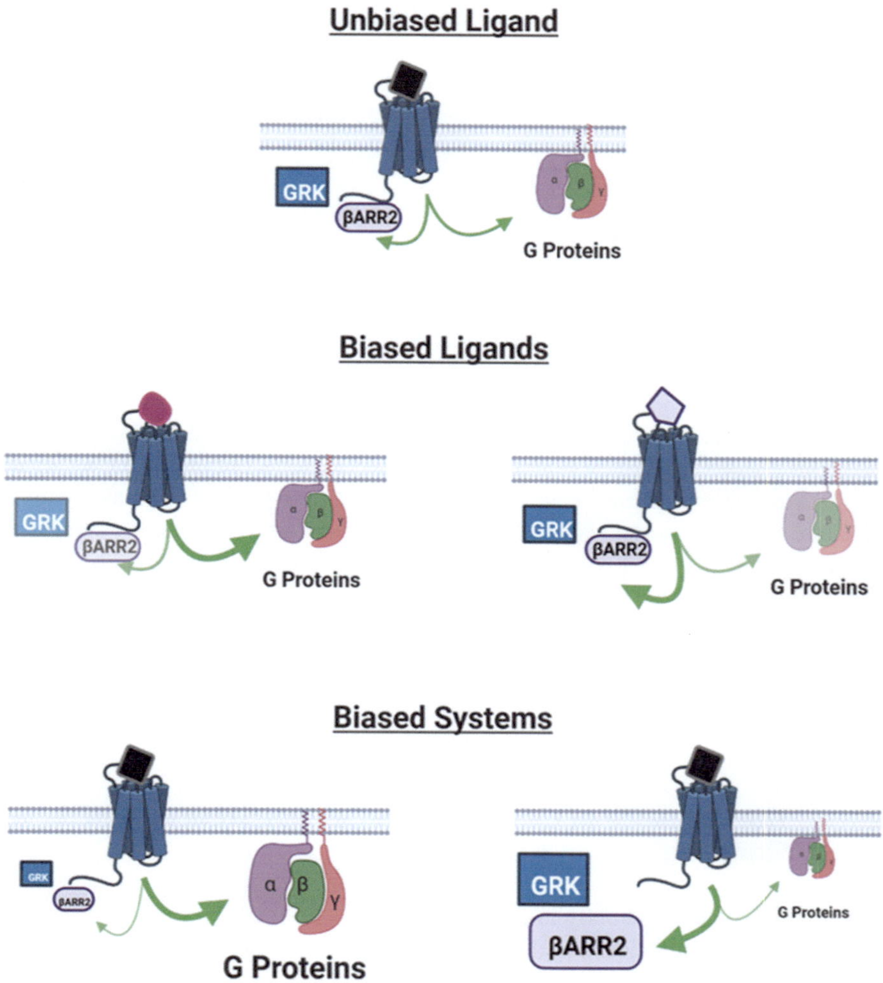

Fig. 1 Ligand bias and system bias of GPCR pathways. In ligand bias, activation of signaling pathways varies due to how the ligand interacts with the receptor to create distinct activated states. An unbiased/balanced GPCR ligand induces a receptor conformation that activates both G protein and GRK/arrestin pathways (top), whereas biased ligands induce receptor conformations that preferentially activate one or the other of these pathways (middle). In system bias, the functionality of downstream signaling elements is altered under specific cellular conditions so that the native (balanced) agonist produces different signaling outcomes (bottom). This can arise from changed expression level or regulation of the ability of signaling components to transmit signals (e.g., by post-translational modification). (Created with BioRender)

ligands are further considered *balanced* or *biased* depending on their degree of pathway selectivity compared to the endogenous ligand (Azzi et al. 2003; Wei et al. 2003) (Fig. 1). Mechanistically, a biased ligand stabilizes receptor conformations that preferentially activate only a subset of a receptor's downstream pathways (Smith et al. 2018; Tan et al. 2018; Seyedabadi et al. 2022). Biased agonism occurs when chemically distinct ligands activate the same receptor in different ways, and thus it is the ligand–receptor complex, not the receptor alone, that specifies the cellular response. The therapeutic promise of biased agonism lies in its ability to produce biological response patterns that cannot be obtained using conventional agonists or antagonists, and thus direct beneficial signals while avoiding detrimental signals.

There are two main conceptual mechanisms by which a GPCR system can exhibit biased signaling: due to a ligand that engenders a specific conformational state of the receptor to drive only a subset of signals (as described above) or due to alterations in the ability of receptors and their downstream signaling partners to signal. That is, just as the level of cell surface expression of a GPCR has a role in determining its activity, so too do the expression level, cellular localization, and functional state of G proteins, arrestins, and other signaling proteins in a cellular context (Fernandez et al. 2020; Mohammad Nezhady et al. 2020; Eiger et al. 2022; Li et al. 2023).

In this chapter, we briefly summarize existing paradigms of biased GPCR signaling and examine emerging evidence that protein S-nitrosylation acts as a global regulator that must be considered in the framework of biased signaling. S-nitrosylation plays a pivotal role in generating signaling bias through GPCRs and does so through myriad individual regulatory events that in aggregate alter cell responsivity, that is, the receptiveness of the cell to signaling through specific pathways. Further exploration of such state-dependent signaling bias will likely reveal novel mechanisms by which GPCR therapeutics can engender unique, biased functional profiles.

2 The Influence of Cell Type and Cellular State on GPCR Signaling

A receptor may act differently in different physiological settings, such as in distinct cell types and tissues (Zhou and Bohn 2014). Even in a single defined cell type, signaling is not constant. Rather, it is dynamically modulated by post-translational modifications (e.g., phosphorylation, ubiquitination, and as described here, S-nitrosylation) that regulate the activity of receptors and signaling components (Patwardhan et al. 2021). This is seen most readily through the phenomenon of desensitization, where previous activation of a receptor leads to reduced signaling through feedback regulation (Sun and Kim 2021). In a system where a given receptor can activate multiple downstream signaling pathways, feedback events affecting one pathway may leave other pathways intact, a form of signal bias. Feedback and signaling crosstalk events may also enhance signaling to achieve bias. Desensitization has traditionally been classified as *homologous* if a receptor agonist reduces future stimulation by that agonist alone, or *heterologous* if a receptor agonist also reduces future signaling ability by distinct receptor types. Heterologous desensitization occurs because receptor activation of intracellular messengers by one receptor can drive post-translational modification of distinct receptors and other signaling proteins to reduce signaling those other receptors. In this manner, the mix of downstream signaling pathways available to a specific GPCR is also dependent on the activation state of the cell.

System bias refers to the set and efficacy of signaling pathways available to a receptor in a specific cell type, resulting from the differential expression of signaling pathway elements. These can include the receptor itself, G proteins, GRKs, and β-arrestins, as well as expression of effector and amplification cascades distal to the receptor. As the limit case, if a critical element of a pathway is not present in a specific cell type, that pathway is unavailable to the receptor no matter what ligand stimulates it. GPCRs can also differ in signaling properties depending on the target tissue or organ system, and such system bias can result in different signaling properties (Urs et al. 2017). System bias may also differ between the same tissue type from different species, which is an important consideration in translational studies. To identify biased agonists with therapeutic potential, it is crucial to remove or account for the effects of system bias (Kenakin 2015).

Regulatory bias refers to the dynamic alteration of cellular signaling pathways in response to cellular conditions. Although not often explicitly presented as such, one major function of the GPCR regulatory apparatus (particularly the GRK/arrestin system) *is* to produce regulatory bias of receptors (e.g., reducing G protein signaling and enabling arrestin signaling). More broadly, any regulation of GPCR signaling is thus a potential contributor to receptor bias (Zheng et al. 2013; Anand et al. 2021).

Importantly, disease states may alter both signaling protein expression and regulatory machinery function through disrupted or overactive post-translational modifications, producing system and regulatory bias that changes GPCR signaling. Failure to account for such changes can result in the inability to produce the desired therapeutic effects.

2.1 S-Nitrosylation, a Post-translational Regulator

S-nitrosylation is the post-translational modification of cysteine thiol in a target protein by the covalent attachment of nitric oxide (NO) to form an S-nitrosothiol (SNO) (Seth et al. 2018) (Fig. 2). Protein S-nitrosylation typically begins with the production of NO. In mammals, three isoforms of nitric oxide synthase (NOS) produce NO from L-arginine: neuronal nNOS/NOS1, inducible iNOS/NOS2, and endothelial eNOS/NOS3 (Förstermann and Sessa 2012), but NO can also be generated by microbes (Seth et al. 2019) and produced from dietary nitrate and nitrite (Carlström et al. 2020), and perhaps nitrated fatty acids (Sanchez-Vicente et al. 2024). Importantly, nNOS and eNOS are coupled to multiple classes of receptors including GPCRs (Dudzinski and Michel 2007). Mechanistically, NO is formally redox-activated to NO^+ by transition metals, allowing it to bind cysteine residues (or other cellular thiols like glutathione or coenzyme A) to form SNO (Cys-S-N=O) (Stomberski et al. 2019) (Fig. 2).

Once thought to be a stochastic chemical reaction ("S-nitrosation"), S-nitrosylation is increasingly appreciated as a facile physiological process mediated by specific enzymes (Angelo et al. 2006; Hess and Stamler 2012; Seth et al. 2018;

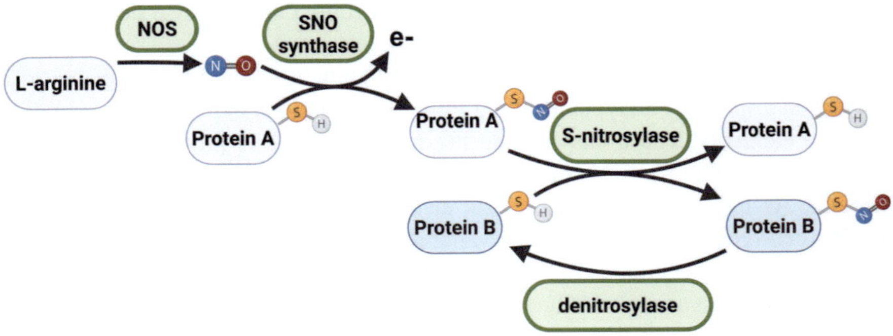

Fig. 2 Schematic overview of protein S-nitrosylation, transnitrosylation, and denitrosylation. NO produced by nitric oxide synthases (NOS) can be redox activated by SNO synthases to react with cysteine thiol on a protein to form protein S-nitrosothiol. Once formed, the S-nitrosothiol group can be transferred to another free thiol on a distinct protein (transnitrosylation) or degraded by denitrosylase enzymes such as thioredoxins (Trxs), SNO-glutathione reductases (GSNORs), or SNO-coenzyme A reductases (SCoRs). (Created with BioRender)

Zhou et al. 2023). NO production by NOS enzymes, in response to GPCRs or other signals, makes NO available to SNO synthases that fix NO into SNO. Once formed, SNOs can be transferred between thiol groups, defining a third class of enzymes, transnitrosylases (Hess and Stamler 2012; Seth et al. 2018; Stomberski et al. 2022; Zhou et al. 2023). Transnitrosylation reactions propagate SNO from one protein to another (Nakamura and Lipton 2013; Jia et al. 2014; Seth et al. 2018) to channel SNO signals and control the proteins modified by SNO. For instance, the SNO-CoA assisted nitrosylase (SCAN) regulates insulin signaling by selectively catalyzing the transfer of NO groups from SCAN to multiple proteins, including the insulin receptor (INSR) β-subunit and insulin receptor substrate 1 (IRS1) (Zhou et al. 2023); SCAN utilizes a co-factor, SNO-CoA, as a source of NO.

Denitrosylation is also controlled enzymatically by thioredoxin-related proteins and the SNO reductase enzymes (e.g., S-nitroso-glutathione reductases [GSNORs] and S-nitroso-coenzyme A reductases [SCoRs]) (Stomberski et al. 2019). Protein denitrosylases are considered to be basally active, but may be regulated by cell surface receptors, including members of the tumor necrosis factor family of receptors, GPCRs and receptor tyrosine kinases (Benhar et al. 2009).

S-nitrosylation is analogous to phosphorylation in the regulation of all classes of proteins (Benhar et al. 2008; Chen et al. 2016; Hara et al. 2005; Hess et al. 2005; Lipton et al. 1993; Stamler et al. 1992a, b, 2001; Uehara et al. 2006; Yao et al. 2004) but more similar to ubiquitination in utilizing a multi-stage enzymatic machinery to direct SNO to target proteins (Chaugule and Walden 2016) and to acylation in use of CoA cofactor (Trefely et al. 2020). As a general mechanism for controlling protein function, S-nitrosylation modifies active or allosteric sites to regulate protein activity, localization, stability, and/or protein-protein interactions (Stomberski et al. 2019). S-nitrosylation is ubiquitous, with over 10,000 SNO-proteins and 25,000 specific sites identified to date (Stomberski et al. 2019) and more than 70% of the proteome identified in predictive algorithms. Aberrant protein S-nitrosylation has been implicated in a broad range of human disease, including important roles in the cardiovascular, pulmonary, musculoskeletal, and nervous systems, as well as in tumor proliferation (Foster et al. 2009; Zhang et al. 2020).

3 GPCRs as Sources of NO

NO was discovered as a gasotransmitter downstream of GPCR activation in vascular endothelium. Initial focus was on signaling by eNOS-derived NO through guanylyl cyclase–cGMP–protein kinase G. In fact, many GPCRs activate eNOS or nNOS through pathways involving calcium, AKT, PKA, and Src (Kone et al. 2003; Siragusa and Fleming 2016), and co-localization of GPCRs and NOS within caveolae (Maniatis et al. 2006) was viewed through a prism of effective NO generation. However, later discovery of direct NOS binding to GPCRs (Marrero et al. 1999) and to receptor regulators/effectors (GRK, arrestins, etc.) (Liu et al. 2012, 2020; Siragusa and Fleming 2016), and of regulation of these proteins by S-nitrosylation, has generated interest in the role of NO on GPCR signaling.

Among different mechanisms by which biased signaling can occur after GPCR activation, it is important to acknowledge that receptor activation can stimulate NO production and thus potentially increase the S-nitrosylation of a large number of proteins. In other words, through NO and S-nitrosylation (as with phosphorylation) GPCR activation creates system bias in a ligand-dependent manner, hence *biased activation*. This can occur during activation of a single GCPR to tune its own signaling profile (akin to homologous desensitization), or via affecting the future signaling of distinct GPCRs (akin to heterologous desensitization). In the following sections, we present examples that highlight roles of S-nitrosylation in biasing signaling through GPCRs through regulation of specific receptor associated G proteins, GRKs, arrestins, and other signaling elements, but it important to keep in mind that these specific alterations occur in a background of more widespread changes to protein S-nitrosylation that remain to be fully characterized.

4 S-Nitrosylation as a Regulator of GPCR Signaling and Bias

4.1 Effects of NO Donors

Treatment of cells and intact animals with NO donors has been reported to generally alter GPCR activity and downstream signaling. NO inhibited β_2-adrenergic receptor (β_2AR)-stimulated cAMP production through the functional uncoupling of the β_2AR from G_s (Adam et al. 1999). Treatment with the NO donor S-nitrosoglutathione (GSNO) disrupted the coupling between bradykinin 2 receptor and G_i/G_q (Miyamoto et al. 1997) and inhibited serotonin-mediated pulmonary vasoconstriction via a cGMP-independent mechanism likely involving S-nitrosylation of its

GPCR system (Nozik-Grayck et al. 2006). Rat atrial membranes treated with NO donor sodium nitroprusside uncoupled M2 muscarinic receptor from G proteins (Aronstam et al. 1995), and cell treatment with the NO donor SIN-1 promoted cGMP-independent dissociation of endothelin from ET1 receptors consistent with G protein uncoupling (Goligorsky et al. 1994). Indeed, G protein coupling to several G_i-coupled receptors in brain slices was shown to be reduced following GSNO treatment (Kokkola et al. 2005). Treatment of lung or pulmonary artery with GSNO reduced the contractile effects of serotonin through the $5HT_2$ receptor (Nozik-Grayck et al. 2002) and to an α_1-adrenergic receptor agonist (Nozik-Grayck et al. 2006). For the μ-opioid receptor, continuous infusion of the NO donor S-nitroso-L-cysteine (CysSNO) in rats alleviated the respiratory depression elicited by opiate receptors after fentanyl injection (Getsy et al. 2022). Thus overall, studies with NO donors have shown inhibitory effects on GPCR coupling, but mechanisms are ill defined.

4.2 S-Nitrosylation of GPCRs

Evidence of direct S-nitrosylation of GPCRs has been gradually accumulating. Unbiased proteomic screens of S-nitrosylated proteins in various cells and tissues have identified 45 non-olfactory GPCRs as SNO-modified proteins. All receptors that couple to NOS are potentially subject to feedback regulation by agonist-dependent S-nitrosylation. Additionally, receptors that do not activate NOS themselves or that are not being activated at the moment still may be subject to crosstalk or heterologous regulation from cellular pathways that are activating NOS activity. Although the current understanding of how NO or S-nitrosylation influences signaling is still limited, some interesting details have begun to emerge.

AT1R. NO donor sodium nitroprusside (SNP) treatment of HEK293 cells expressing the angiotensin II type 1 (AT1) receptor reduced the ligand-binding affinity of the receptor without reducing receptor number, and this effect required Cys289 (Leclerc et al. 2006), suggesting direct S-nitrosylation. SNP or GSNO treatment of isolated rat middle cerebral artery inhibited AT1 receptor-mediated vasoconstriction in a cGMP-independent manner, and GSNO treatment caused direct AT1 receptor S-nitrosylation in receptor-transfected HEK293 cells (Bouressam et al. 2019). Agonist-dependent S-nitrosylation of AT1 receptor in receptor-transfected HEK293 cells was recently demonstrated, establishing physiological relevance (Fonseca et al. 2022).

β_1AR. The β_1-adrenergic receptor (β_1AR) was identified as a SNO-modified protein in mouse (Beigi et al. 2012) and human heart, where the level is increased in heart failure (Fonseca et al. 2022). Interestingly, the mixed β-receptor "antagonist" carvedilol was identified as a biased agonist ligand for the β_1AR, where it induced coupling to and activation of G_i rather than G_s (Wang et al. 2017). In a recent report, carvedilol stimulation of β_1AR in cardiomyocytes activated a G_i-dependent pathway leading to eNOS activity and cGMP signaling that promoted cardiac contractility (Wang et al. 2021), potentially explaining why carvedilol has better cardioprotective actions in the clinic than traditional β-receptor antagonists. S-nitrosylation is highly likely to be increased in carvedilol-stimulated cardiomyocytes and potentially lead to S-nitrosylation of β_1AR.

β_2AR. The β_2AR has been reported to be S-nitrosylated endogenously in mouse heart and lungs (Fonseca et al. 2022) and following NO donor infusion (Wanschel et al. 2014). The effect of S-nitrosylation of the human β_2AR has been characterized in detail, revealing that β_2AR is S-nitrosylated basally and SNO-β_2AR levels are increased following treatment with CysNO or in response to receptor activation (Fonseca et al. 2022). Three sites were identified by mass-spectroscopy: Cys265 in the third intracellular loop, and the carboxyl terminal Cys341 (the palmitoylation site) and Cys378 (Fonseca et al. 2022). Of these, Cys265 was identified as the predominant site. Mutation of Cys265 to Ser or Ala led to greatly prolonged signaling to cAMP and eNOS. Although Cys265-mutant β_2AR interacted normally with arrestins, receptor internalization from the cell surface was inhibited. Further, treatment of cells with CysNO led to β_2AR internalization in the absence of agonist, and agonist-stimulated internalization of wild-type receptor was inhibited by inhibition of eNOS (Fonseca et al. 2022). This NO-dependent internalization was blocked by inhibitors of caveolae and of protein kinase A-phosphorylation of the receptor (Fonseca et al. 2022). NO produced in response to β_2AR activation S-nitrosylates the β_2AR and protein kinase A R1 subunit to release active PKA that phosphorylates the β_2AR, and receptor S-nitrosylation and phosphorylation together drive receptor internalization through caveolae to desensitize receptor signaling (Fig. 3A). Thus, β_2AR S-nitrosylation reduces signaling output from the receptor through G proteins (G_s to cAMP and G_i to eNOS) and to a lesser degree through arrestins (to Erk), effectively biasing the system away from G protein signaling. In a knock-in mouse model of β_2AR-C265S, airway contractility to muscarinic agonist is reduced compared to wild-type due to constitutive cAMP and NO signaling and is restored by treatment of mice with inhibitors of G_i or eNOS. These mice with β_2AR unable to be S-nitrosylated are protected from allergic asthma, including airway hyperreactivity, immune infiltration, and lung remodeling (Fonseca et al. 2022).

P2Y_6R. A redox-mediated receptor internalization pathway was described for the P2Y_6 purinergic (UDP) receptor, whereby electrophilic modification of Cys220 by an isothiocyanate group promoted ubiquitin-dependent internalization and degradation of the receptor (Nishiyama et al. 2022). Treatment of cells with GSNO similarly promoted P2Y_6R internalization and degradation, but this was lost in the C220S mutant receptor (Nishiyama et al. 2022), suggesting that S-nitrosylation of this cysteine has the same function. While mice lacking P2Y_6R were protected compared to wild-type in a model of colitis, mice with the P2Y_6R C220S mutation exhibited worse outcomes (Nishiyama et al. 2022), implicating regulation at this site in pathophysiology, potentially by endogenous S-nitrosylation.

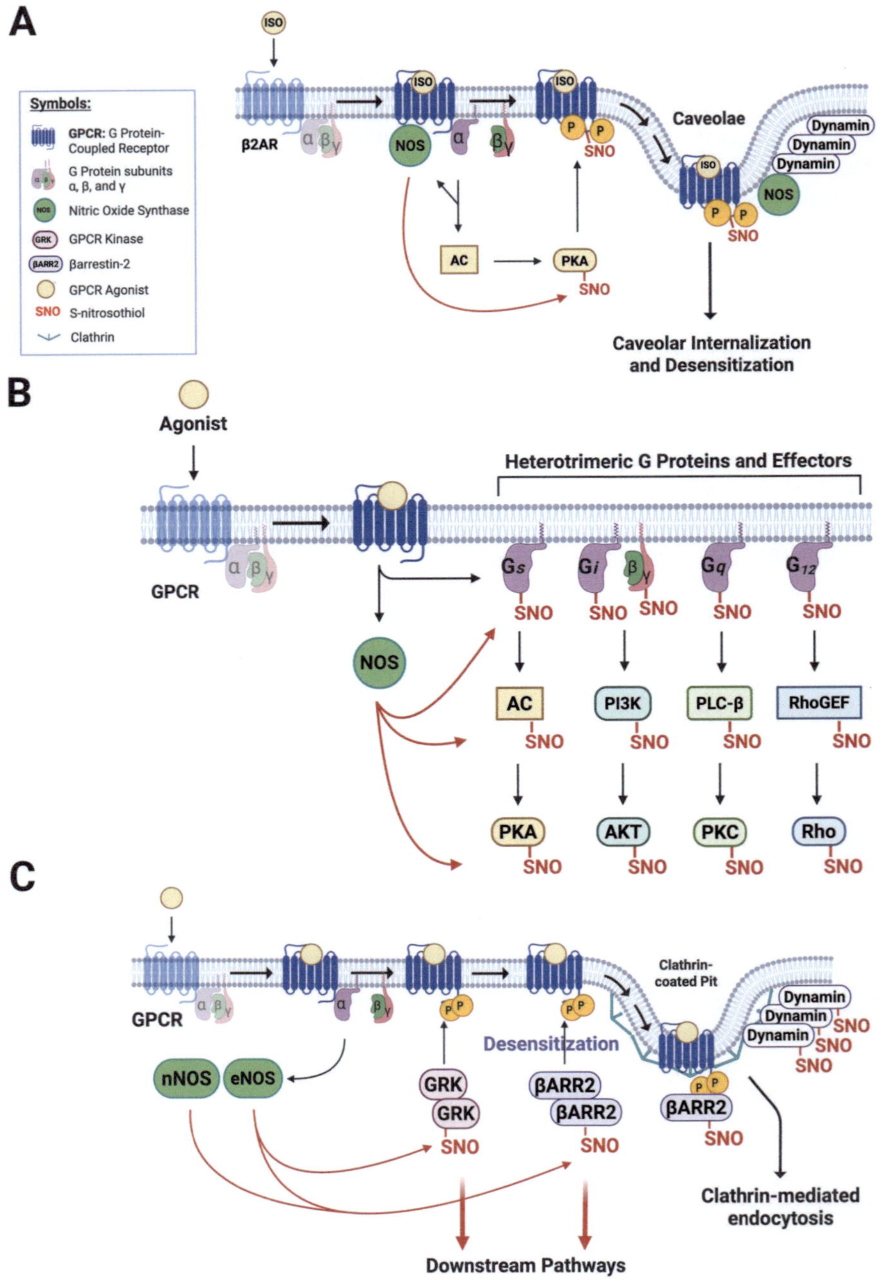

Fig. 3 S-nitrosylation alters GPCR signaling components to produce system bias. (**A**) β_2AR activation (by isoproterenol, ISO) leads to activation of downstream G protein signaling pathways (exemplified by adenylyl cyclase (AC) and subsequent activation of protein kinase A (PKA) to phosphorylate targets including the β_2AR itself) and also activates GRK/arrestins to promote signaling and β-arrestin-mediated desensitization and receptor endocytosis through the clathrin pathway (not depicted). Downstream signals include activation of eNOS to produce NO that elevates total intracellular protein S-nitrosylation (SNO). Feedback S-nitrosylation of the β_2AR at

4.3 G Protein S-Nitrosylation

Twelve distinct heterotrimeric G protein α-subunits and multiple G protein β- and γ-subunits have been identified as being SNO modified in proteomic screens. Although it seems likely that these modifications will alter G protein function (e.g., receptor coupling, GTPase activity/RGS regulation, or effector activation) to contribute to dynamic bias, few studies have yet addressed this. These include papers mentioned in Sect. 4.1, where NO donors affect GPCR-G protein coupling at an undefined locus (either receptor or G protein). Additionally, some groups have reported direct SNO-modification of G protein subunits and/or alterations in G protein activity (Fig. 3B). NO donor treatment was reported to increase the rate of GTP hydrolysis of G_s and G_i proteins (Lander et al. 1995), as it does small G protein activity (Lander et al. 1997). The brain G_o α-subunit protein was reported to be S-nitrosylated in synaptosome preparations exposed to NO, and this reduced the ability of pertussis toxin to ADP-ribosylate G_o (Hess et al. 1994) (suggesting the Cys ADP-ribosylation site in the carboxyl terminal as the site of modification). S-nitrosylated G_o and G_{i2} α-subunits have been identified in glomerular mesangial cells treated with NO donor (Kuncewicz et al. 2003).

BIAS. A recent report found that G_{i2} α-subunit was S-nitrosylated in diabetes-associated atherosclerosis (Chao et al. 2021). Treatment of human umbilical vein endothelial cells (HUVEC) with oxidized LDL (oxLDL) and high glucose was used to mimic disease conditions, and SNO-proteins were identified in an unbiased mass-spectroscopy screen; G_{i2}-α was a top hit. SNO-G_{i2} was elevated in coronary artery from diabetic atherosclerosis patients (vs healthy controls) and in aorta from LDL-knockout mice fed high fat diet and treated with streptozotocin, as well as in HUVEC and human aorta endothelial cells (HAEC) treated with glucose and oxidized LDL. G_{i1} and G_{i3} were not S-nitrosylated under these conditions. The site of glucose/oxLDL-dependent S-nitrosylation of G_{i2} was mapped to Cys66 (in a region where G_i isoforms differ). Expression of G_{i2} C66A reduced expression of adhesion molecules and chemokines, suggesting that SNO-G_{i2} promotes inflammatory cell interactions with vascular endothelial cells to augment atherosclerosis.

Fig. 3 (continued) Cys265 (along with PKA S-nitrosylation that increases kinase activity) reduces $β_2$AR signaling by promoting receptor internalization and desensitization through the caveolar pathway. (**B**) Heterotrimeric G protein subunits and their downstream effectors have been reported to be S-nitrosylated. These include G_s, adenylyl cyclase (AC) and protein kinase A (PKA); G_i (both α and βγ-subunits), phosphatidyl inositol 3-kinase-γ (PI3K), and the AKT protein kinase; G_q, phospholipase C-β (PLC-β), and protein kinase C (PKC); and G_{12}, Rho guanine nucleotide exchange factors (RhoGEF), and the RhoA small GTP-binding protein (Rho). The role of GPCR activation in promoting these S-nitrosylation events and the effects of these post-translational modifications on signaling remain almost entirely uncharacterized. (**C**) GPCR stimulation activates eNOS and/or nNOS to drive S-nitrosylation of GRKs, arrestins, and their downstream signaling and regulatory proteins (including dynamin) to produce system bias, as described in the text. (Created with BioRender)

Adeno-associated virus was used to overexpress G_{i2} wild-type or C66A in mouse endothelium, and LDL-knockout mice infected with C66A showed reduced atherosclerosis and macrophage infiltration following high fat diet plus streptozotocin. SNO-G_{i2} was driven by glucose/oxLDL-driven expression of iNOS (e.g., not by receptor activation). The effect of SNO-G_{i2} on receptor signaling was assessed using knockdown of each chemokine receptor in endothelial cells; CXCR5 was found to be the key functional GPCR. CXCR5 immunoprecipitated with G_{i2}, and treatment of cells with glucose/oxLDL increased this interaction, while C66A mutation abolished it. Thus, SNO-G_{i2} couples better to CXCR5 than does unmodified G_{i2}; that is, SNO-G_{i2} at Cys66 in this system increases bias toward G protein pathways.

4.4 SNO Modification of G Protein Effectors

Heterotrimeric G proteins mediate their physiological functions by binding to effector enzymes and ion channels (Wettschureck and Offermanns 2005), and the effect of their S-nitrosylation has been characterized for some as described below (Fig. 3B).

Adenylyl cyclase (AC) isoforms are stimulated by G_s family G proteins to generate cAMP and activate protein kinase A, but some isoforms are also inhibited by the G_i family of heterotrimeric G proteins (Khannpnavar et al. 2020). Adenylyl cyclase isoforms AC5 and AC6 have been reported to be inhibited by S-nitrosylation (McVey et al. 1999; Hill et al. 2000), resulting in bias away from cAMP signaling. In gut smooth muscle, iNOS induction promotes AC5 S-nitrosylation to result in reduced cAMP synthesis (Mahavadi et al. 2014). In a swine model of persistent pulmonary hypertension of the newborn, hypoxia results in increased SNO-AC6 and reduced cAMP synthesis (Sikarwar et al. 2018). Adenylyl cyclases produce cAMP that activates protein kinase A, and SNO-modification of the PKA type 1 regulatory R1 subunit leads to release of the catalytic subunit, promoting kinase activity in the absence of cAMP (Burgoyne and Eaton 2009). This regulation has the potential to produce PKA-dependent cell state alterations as if a G_s-coupled receptor had been activated, such as inducing PKA-dependent heterologous desensitization of GPCR-driven G protein pathways (Chuang et al. 1996).

Phospholipase C-β enzymes are stimulated by G_q family α-subunit proteins to cleave membrane PIP_2 into diacylglycerol and inositol tris-phosphate (IP3) to initiate intracellular calcium release and protein kinase C (PKC) signaling (Litosch 2016), and two PLC-β and seven PKC isoforms have been identified in SNO-proteomic screens. Purified PKC-α treated with NO donor exhibited reduced activity that was attributed to S-nitrosylation (Gopalakrishna et al. 1993). In cultured pulmonary artery endothelial cells exposed to NO, PKCs α, ε, and ζ, each displayed reduced activity, and this was reversed by exposure to dithiothreitol or the denitrosylase thioredoxin, suggesting a SNO-based mechanism (Kahlos et al. 2003). In isolated aorta contraction assays, treatment with NO donor or a denitrosylase inhibitor led to reduced ability of the PKC activator phorbol-12,13-dibutyrate to produce contraction (Choi et al. 2011). Dietary nitrite converted to S-nitrosothiol was reported to increase SNO-PKC-α in aorta, inhibiting its activation by angiotensin II through the ATR1 receptor (Pinheiro et al. 2021). In endothelial cells, TNF-α stimulated eNOS activity leads to SNO-PKC-ζ at Cys503 in the kinase domain and is associated with *elevated* PKC activity and increased leukocyte adhesion to endothelial cells (Aguilar et al. 2021). Thus, although SNO-PKC typically has reduced activity, which would bias signaling by GPCRs away from Gq-mediated effects, some PKC S-nitrosylation events appear to be activating.

Phosphoinosotide 3-kinase (PI3K) isoforms are effectors for G proteins and G protein-activated pathways (particularly PI3Kγ that is directly activated by Gβγ subunits). All PI3K isoforms are regulated indirectly by the PTEN phosphatase, which inactivates phosphoinositol-3,4,5-phosphate derived from PI3K enzymes by removing the 3-phosphate to inhibit PI3K-dependent signaling to Akt (Liu et al. 2022). PTEN is well known to be modified and inhibited by S-nitrosylation, thus amplifying signaling through PI3K (Carver et al. 2007; Lim and Clément 2007; Ding et al. 2021).

4.5 GRK S-Nitrosylation and Bias

GRKs play an essential role in GPCR regulation by phosphorylating agonist-occupied GPCRs to promote arrestin binding to receptor. This causes receptor uncoupling from G protein pathways and stimulation of arrestin signaling (i.e., arrestin bias), along with internalization and downregulation of the receptor (Pierce et al. 2002; Gurevich and Gurevich 2019) (Fig. 3C). There are seven mammalian GRKs in three structural and functional subclasses: the visual system GRKs 1 and 7, the two classes of widely expressed GRKs, GRKs 2 and 3, and GRKs 4/5/6 (Premont et al. 1995).

GRK2 S-nitrosylation at Cys340 increases following agonist stimulation of multiple GPCRs, which decreases GRK2 kinase activity and reduces both recruitment of β-arrestins to the receptor and agonist-dependent receptor internalization. The GRK2 C340S mutant loses this inhibition (Whalen et al. 2007). However, GRK2 S-nitrosylation spares G protein-mediated second messenger signaling (Whalen et al. 2007), but would be predicted to reduce GRK2-dependent β-arrestin signaling, thus biasing receptor signaling toward G protein pathways.

GRK2 S-nitrosylation is cardioprotective (Pfleger et al. 2019). eNOS activation inhibits GRK2 via S-nitrosylation, thereby maintaining cardiac function through preserving cAMP signaling by βARs (Whalen et al. 2007; Kayki-Mutlu and Koch 2021). Ischemic stress and heart failure are typified by increased abundance of GRK2, which counteracts cardioprotection by eNOS (Huang et al. 2013). The GRK2-C340S knock-in mouse exhibits loss of SNO inhibition and increased GRK2 desensitizing activity (Huang et al. 2013), and significantly more myocardial damage through resistance to NO-mediated cardioprotection after ischemic injury. By 12 months of age, GRK2-C340S mice develop significant vascular and myocardial pathology compared to age-matched wild-type controls (Lieu et al. 2020). In addition to desensitizing cardiac βAR signaling through G proteins and internalizing the receptors, augmented GRK2 activity should also promote β-arrestin signaling to generate bias away from G protein pathways, although this has not yet been explicitly demonstrated.

Studies in Parkinson's disease have shown that excessive S-nitrosylation (nitrosative stress) can contribute to pathogenesis (Chung and David 2010; Nakamura et al. 2015). In the α-synuclein-A53T transgenic mouse model of Parkinson's disease, GRK6 was shown to be S-nitrosylated to enhance its kinase activity toward phosphorylation of its non-GPCR substrate α-synuclein at Ser129 (Wu et al. 2020). This phosphorylation is strongly associated with neurodegenerative disease (Sato et al. 2013), suggesting that SNO-GRK6 may increase the risk and severity of Parkinson's disease. GRK6 S-nitrosylation would be predicted to promote receptor bias toward arrestins in Parkinson's disease, where GRK6 is already implicated (Gainetdinov et al. 2003; Managò et al. 2012; Ahmed et al. 2015).

4.6 Arrestin S-Nitrosylation and Bias

Arrestins are signaling scaffolding proteins that link activated GPCRs to specific signaling and trafficking pathways, while also interfering with GPCR coupling to G proteins (Black et al. 2016). There are two visual system arrestins, and two ubiquitous β-arrestin proteins, β-arrestin1 and β-arrestin2, that regulate GPCRs throughout the rest of the body (Black et al. 2016). β-arrestin signaling partners are known to regulate a number of post-translational signals, including phosphorylation, ubiquitination, and also S-nitrosylation (Fig. 3C). The stimulation of β_2AR, which activates eNOS, promotes both the formation of the β-arrestin2–eNOS complex and β-arrestin2 S-nitrosylation at Cys410 (Ozawa et al. 2008). β_2AR-induced S-nitrosylation of β-arrestin2 results in both its dissociation from eNOS and its association with the endocytic machinery (e.g., clathrin and β-adaptin/AP-2), thereby accelerating the rate of β_2AR internalization (Ozawa et al. 2008). Additionally, NO regulates clathrin-mediated endocytic vesicle budding and membrane fission through S-nitrosylation of dynamin family members (Fig. 3C). Notably S-nitrosylation of dynamin1 at Cys607 increases its GTPase activity, self-assembly, and membrane localization to increase receptor internalization (Wang et al. 2006). Along with dynamins, many other members of the endocytic machinery are also S-nitrosylated, including other clathrin isoforms and multiple subunits of adaptin protein complexes 1–4 (e.g., AP-1, AP-2, AP-3, AP-4).

S-nitrosylation of β-arrestins by nNOS and iNOS (β-arrestin1 at Cys251 and β-arrestin2 at cognate Cys253) suppresses the ligand-induced recruitment of β-arrestin1/2 to the β_2AR and receptor internalization, but leaves G protein-mediated signaling unaffected, thus generating bias toward G protein signaling (Hayashi et al. 2018). Heart failure may represent an important example where diminished GPCR–G protein coupling reflects the state of β-arrestin S-nitrosylation (Hayashi et al. 2018). S-nitrosylation of Cys251/253 also suppressed the rate of ligand-induced membrane recruitment of β-arrestin to angiotensin AT1a and bradykinin 1 receptors and increased interaction of β-arrestin2 with E3 ubiquitin ligase MDM2 (Hayashi et al. 2018). Thus, S-nitrosylation of β-arrestins alters their partner interaction profiles, providing a general mechanism for bias among arrestin-mediated signaling pathways themselves.

5 Pharmacological Implications

The pharmacological implications of SNO-biased GPCR signaling are numerous and profound. First, NO signaling in general and S-nitrosylation in particular are widely overlooked when considering the multiple signals emanating from a specific GPCR that could contribute to bias, so no biased compounds affecting signaling by any GPCR to NOS are yet known. Second, accumulating evidence indicates that S-nitrosylation is a target- and site-specific enzyme-mediated process, where nitrosylase and denitrosylase enzymes represent potential pharmacological targets (e.g., of small-molecule inhibitors). In combination with biased GPCR ligands, the systemic bias derived from SNO-enzyme regulation could be leveraged to design drugs with pathway-specific roles, minimizing off-target effects and enhancing therapeutic precision. For example, in acute kidney injury, drugs that inhibit the denitrosylase SCoR2 may be able to enhance the renoprotective effect of eNOS-derived NO and alleviate kidney damage. In the context of obesity, increased activity of the nitrosylase SCAN contributes to insulin resistance (i.e., receptor desenstitization) through hypernitrosylation of INSR and IRS1. Therefore, inhibitors of SCAN may prevent the development of insulin resistance while preserving normal insulin signaling, offering a strategic advantage for developing safer and more effective obesity drugs. Many such potential roles likely exist in GPCR signaling as well.

6 Concluding Remarks

In the context of GPCR signaling, S-nitrosylation is emerging as a key downstream signaling pathway in its own right as well as an important regulator of signal transduction. Notably, S-nitrosylation resulting from receptor-stimulated NOS activation influences cellular state to generate biased GPCR responses. Mechanisms by which S-nitrosylation can bias downstream receptor responses include direct modification of specific intracellular signaling components to affect receptor-effector coupling or by altering the available pool of active receptors, transducers, and effectors. Compared to traditional models of bias controlled through a specific ligand, the evidence we present here suggests a multi-layered view of biased GPCR signaling, where at the cellular level, ligands act in the context of a cellular system that is dynamically biased in response to cellular signals—including S-nitrosylation—in addition to traditional phosphorylation-based "desensitization."

It is suggested that system-based bias through post-translational modification of elements shared by all GPCRs (e.g., arrestins) is exploited by nature far more often than the ligand-specific model. Existing evidence demonstrates that S-nitrosylation can regulate universal responsiveness of GPCR signaling systems in this manner, as well as modify the responsiveness of specific signaling components. Beyond several well-studied examples, there are a large number of GPCR pathway proteins reported to be SNO-modified in unbiased screens that remain uncharacterized, suggesting that nearly all GPCR signaling pathway components are regulated by SNO (e.g., 65 GPCRs, 12 G protein α-subunits, numerous intracellular messenger effector enzymes). These also include mechanisms we have not discussed here, including S-nitrosylation of multiple RGS proteins, arrestin partners including Src kinases (Tang et al. 2012) and MAP kinases, many small GTPases (Lander et al. 1995), and myriad other GPCR regulated pathways (e.g., all 4 G_{12}-regulated RhoGEFs). Much future work will be required to fill this knowledge gap by first characterizing the effects of individual S-nitrosylation events to regulate single proteins and their specific pathways, then by developing a systems-level understanding of the effects of simultaneous or temporally overlapping regulation of multiple GPCR signaling components by S-nitrosylation in concert with other mechanisms such as phosphorylation.

In the broader scope of cellular signaling, the advent of SNO-biased GPCR signaling highlights S-nitrosylation both as a signal downstream of GPCR activation (via stimulation of eNOS or nNOS) and as a mechanism for feedback regulation of these pathways by NO/SNO. Given that NOS is an effector for many GPCRs, SNO-mediated regulation as a mechanism to bias the cellular context (state/structure of the ligand, receptor, effectors, availability of signaling components) is likely to be widespread. Ultimately, S-nitrosylation of key signaling proteins under specific conditions (in health and disease) can be used to manipulate cellular state to generate systemic signaling bias that may be targeted by functionally selective and more efficacious pharmacotherapies.

Acknowledgments Funded by NIH grants HL075443, HL128192, HL158507, and HL157151.

References

Adam L, Bouvier M, Jones TLZ (1999) Nitric oxide modulates β2-adrenergic receptor Palmitoylation and signaling. J Biol Chem 274:26337–26343. https://doi.org/10.1074/jbc.274.37.26337

Aguilar G, Córdova F, Koning T et al (2021) TNF-α-activated eNOS signaling increases leukocyte adhesion through the S-nitrosylation pathway. Am J Phys Heart Circ Phys 321:H1083–H1095. https://doi.org/10.1152/ajpheart.00065.2021

Ahmed MR, Bychkov E, Kook S, Zurkovsky L, Dalby KN, Gurevich EV (2015) Overexpression of GRK6 rescues l-DOPA-induced signaling abnormalities in the dopamine-depleted striatum of hemiparkinsonian rats. Exp Neurol 266:42–54. https://doi.org/10.1016/j.expneurol.2015.02.008

Anand P, Norton C, JoAnn T (2021) Post-translational modifications of G protein–coupled receptors control cellular signaling dynamics in space and time. Pharmacol Rev 73:120. https://doi.org/10.1124/pharmrev.120.000082

Angelo M, Singel DJ, Stamler JS (2006) An S-nitrosothiol (SNO) synthase function of hemoglobin that utilizes nitrite as a substrate. Proc Natl Acad Sci USA 103:8366–8371. https://doi.org/10.1073/pnas.0600942103

Aronstam RS, Martin DC, Dennison RL, Cooley HG (1995) S-Nitrosylation of m2 muscarinic receptor thiols disrupts receptor-G-protein Couplinga. Ann N Y Acad Sci 757:215–217. https://doi.org/10.1111/j.1749-6632.1995.tb17477.x

Azzi M, Charest PG, Angers S, Rousseau G, Kohout T, Bouvier M, Piñeyro G (2003) Beta-arrestin-mediated activation of MAPK by inverse agonists reveals distinct active conformations for G protein-coupled receptors. Proc Natl Acad Sci USA 100:11406–11411. https://doi.org/10.1073/pnas.1936664100

Beigi F, Gonzalez DR, Minhas KM et al (2012) Dynamic denitrosylation via S-nitrosoglutathione reductase regulates cardiovascular function. Proc Natl Acad Sci USA 109:4314–4319. https://doi.org/10.1073/pnas.1113319109

Benhar M, Forrester MT, Hess DT, Stamler JS (2008) Regulated protein denitrosylation by cytosolic and mitochondrial thioredoxins. Science 320:1050–1054. https://doi.org/10.1126/science.1158265

Benhar M, Forrester MT, Stamler JS (2009) Protein denitrosylation: enzymatic mechanisms and cellular functions. Nat Rev Mol Cell Biol 10:721–732. https://doi.org/10.1038/nrm2764

Black JB, Premont RT, Daaka Y (2016) Feedback regulation of G protein-coupled receptor signaling by GRKs and arrestins. Semin Cell Dev Biol 50:95–104. https://doi.org/10.1016/j.semcdb.2015.12.015

Bouressam M-L, Lecat S, Raoul A, Gaucher C, Perrin-Sarrado C, Lartaud I, Dupuis F (2019) S-nitrosoglutathione inhibits cerebrovascular angiotensin II-dependent and -independent AT1 receptor responses: a possible role of S-nitrosation. Br J Pharmacol 176:2049–2062. https://doi.org/10.1111/bph.14644

Burgoyne JR, Eaton P (2009) Transnitrosylating nitric oxide species directly activate type I protein kinase a, providing a novel adenylate cyclase-independent cross-talk to beta-adrenergic-like signaling. J Biol Chem 284:29260–29268. https://doi.org/10.1074/jbc.M109.046722

Carlström M, Moretti CH, Weitzberg E, Lundberg JO (2020) Microbiota, diet and the generation of reactive nitrogen compounds. Free Radic Biol Med 161:321–325. https://doi.org/10.1016/j.freeradbiomed.2020.10.025

Carver DJ, Gaston B, deRonde K, Palmer LA (2007) Akt-Mediated activation of HIF-1 in pulmonary vascular endothelial cells by S-Nitrosoglutathione. Am J Respir Cell Mol Biol 37: 255–263. https://doi.org/10.1165/rcmb.2006-0289SM

Chao ML, Luo S, Zhang C et al (2021) S-nitrosylation-mediated coupling of G-protein alpha-2 with CXCR5 induces Hippo/YAP-dependent diabetes-accelerated atherosclerosis. Nat Commun 12: 4452. https://doi.org/10.1038/s41467-021-24736-y

Chaugule VK, Walden H (2016) Specificity and disease in the ubiquitin system. Biochem Soc Trans 44:212–227. https://doi.org/10.1042/BST20150209

Chen LN, Shi Q, Zhang BY et al (2016) Proteomic analyses for the global S-Nitrosylated proteins in the brain tissues of different human prion diseases. Mol Neurobiol 53:5079–5096. https://doi.org/10.1007/s12035-015-9440-7

Choi H, Tostes RC, Webb RC (2011) S-nitrosylation Inhibits protein kinase C-mediated contraction in mouse aorta. J Cardiovasc Pharmacol 57:65–71. https://doi.org/10.1097/FJC.0b013e3181fef9cb

Chuang TT, Iacovelli L, Sallese M, De Blasi A (1996) G protein-coupled receptors: heterologous regulation of homologous desensitization and its implications. Trends Pharmacol Sci 17:416–421. https://doi.org/10.1016/S0165-6147(96)10048-1

Chung KK, David KK (2010) Emerging roles of nitric oxide in neurodegeneration. Nitric Oxide 22: 290–295. https://doi.org/10.1016/j.niox.2010.02.002

Ding Z, Ogata D, Roszik J et al (2021) iNOS associates with poor survival in melanoma: a role for nitric oxide in the PI3K-AKT pathway stimulation and PTEN S-Nitrosylation. Front Oncol 11: 631766

Dudzinski DM, Michel T (2007) Life history of eNOS: partners and pathways. Cardiovasc Res 75: 247–260. https://doi.org/10.1016/j.cardiores.2007.03.023

Eiger DS, Pham U, Gardner J, Hicks C, Rajagopal S (2022) GPCR systems pharmacology: a different perspective on the development of biased therapeutics. Am J Phys Cell Phys 322: C887–C895. https://doi.org/10.1152/ajpcell.00449.2021

Fernandez TJ, De Maria M, Lobingier BT (2020) A cellular perspective of bias at G protein-coupled receptors. Protein Sci 29:1345–1354. https://doi.org/10.1002/pro.3872

Fonseca FV, Raffay TM, Xiao K et al (2022) S-nitrosylation is required for β2AR desensitization and experimental asthma. Mol Cell 82. https://doi.org/10.1016/j.molcel.2022.06.033

Förstermann U, Sessa WC (2012) Nitric oxide synthases: regulation and function. Eur Heart J 33: 829–837, 837a–837d. https://doi.org/10.1093/eurheartj/ehr304

Foster MW, Hess DT, Stamler JS (2009) Protein S-nitrosylation in health and disease: a current perspective. Trends Mol Med 15:391–404. https://doi.org/10.1016/j.molmed.2009.06.007

Gainetdinov RR, Bohn LM, Sotnikova TD et al (2003) Dopaminergic Supersensitivity in G protein-coupled receptor kinase 6-deficient mice. Neuron 38:291–303. https://doi.org/10.1016/S0896-6273(03)00192-2

Getsy PM, Baby SM, Gruber RB et al (2022) S-Nitroso-L-cysteine Stereoselectively blunts the deleterious effects of fentanyl on breathing while augmenting Antinociception in freely-moving rats. Front Pharmacol 13:892307. https://doi.org/10.3389/fphar.2022.892307

Goligorsky MS, Tsukahara H, Magazine H, Andersen TT, Malik AB, Bahou WF (1994) Termination of endothelin signaling: role of nitric oxide. J Cell Physiol 158:485–494. https://doi.org/10.1002/jcp.1041580313

Gopalakrishna R, Chen ZH, Gundimeda U (1993) Nitric oxide and nitric oxide-generating agents induce a reversible inactivation of protein kinase C activity and phorbol ester binding. J Biol Chem 268:27180–27185. https://doi.org/10.1016/S0021-9258(19)74235-5

Gurevich VV, Gurevich EV (2019) GPCR signaling regulation: the role of GRKs and Arrestins. Front Pharmacol 10:125. https://doi.org/10.3389/fphar.2019.00125

Hara MR, Agrawal N, Kim SF et al (2005) S-nitrosylated GAPDH initiates apoptotic cell death by nuclear translocation following Siah1 binding. Nat Cell Biol 7:665–674. https://doi.org/10.1038/ncb1268

Hauser AS, Chavali S, Masuho I, Jahn LJ, Martemyanov KA, Gloriam DE, Babu MM (2018) Pharmacogenomics of GPCR drug targets. Cell 172(41–54):e19. https://doi.org/10.1016/j.cell.2017.11.033

Hayashi H, Hess DT, Zhang R et al (2018) S-Nitrosylation of β-Arrestins biases receptor signaling and confers ligand Independence. Mol Cell 70:473–487.e476. https://doi.org/10.1016/j.molcel.2018.03.034

Hess DT, Stamler JS (2012) Regulation by S-nitrosylation of protein post-translational modification. J Biol Chem 287:4411–4418. https://doi.org/10.1074/jbc.R111.285742

Hess DT, Lin L-H, Freeman JA, Norden JJ (1994) Modification of cysteine residues within go and other neuronal proteins by exposure to nitric oxide. Neuropharmacology 33:1283–1292. https://doi.org/10.1016/0028-3908(94)90028-0

Hess DT, Matsumoto A, Kim SO, Marshall HE, Stamler JS (2005) Protein S-nitrosylation: purview and parameters. Nat Rev Mol Cell Biol 6:150–166. https://doi.org/10.1038/nrm1569

Hilger D, Masureel M, Kobilka BK (2018) Structure and dynamics of GPCR signaling complexes. Nat Struct Mol Biol 25:4–12. https://doi.org/10.1038/s41594-017-0011-7

Hill J, Howlett A, Klein C (2000) Nitric oxide selectively inhibits adenylyl cyclase isoforms 5 and 6. Cell Signal 12:233–237. https://doi.org/10.1016/s0898-6568(99)00082-0

Huang ZM, Gao E, Fonseca FV et al (2013) Convergence of G protein-coupled receptor and S-nitrosylation signaling determines the outcome to cardiac ischemic injury. Sci Signal 6:ra95. https://doi.org/10.1126/scisignal.2004225

Jia J, Arif A, Terenzi F, Willard B, Plow EF, Hazen SL, Fox PL (2014) Target-selective protein S-nitrosylation by sequence motif recognition. Cell 159:623–634. https://doi.org/10.1016/j.cell.2014.09.032

Kahlos K, Zhang J, Block ER, Patel JM (2003) Thioredoxin restores nitric oxide-induced inhibition of protein kinase C activity in lung endothelial cells. Mol Cell Biochem 254:47–54. https://doi.org/10.1023/A:1027380828645

Kayki-Mutlu G, Koch WJ (2021) Nitric oxide and S-Nitrosylation in cardiac regulation: G protein-coupled receptor Kinase-2 and β-Arrestins as targets. Int J Mol Sci 22. https://doi.org/10.3390/ijms22020521

Kenakin T (2015) The effective application of biased signaling to new drug discovery. Mol Pharmacol 88:1055–1061. https://doi.org/10.1124/mol.115.099770

Khannpnavar B, Mehta V, Qi C, Korkhov V (2020) Structure and function of adenylyl cyclases, key enzymes in cellular signaling. Curr Opin Struct Biol 63:34–41. https://doi.org/10.1016/j.sbi.2020.03.003

Kokkola T, Savinainen JR, Mönkkönen KS, Retamal MD, Laitinen JT (2005) S-nitrosothiols modulate G protein-coupled receptor signaling in a reversible and highly receptor-specific manner. BMC Cell Biol 6:21. https://doi.org/10.1186/1471-2121-6-21

Kone BC, Kuncewicz T, Zhang W, Yu Z-Y (2003) Protein interactions with nitric oxide synthases: controlling the right time, the right place, and the right amount of nitric oxide. Am J Physiol Renal Physiol 285:F178–F190. https://doi.org/10.1152/ajprenal.00048.2003

Kuncewicz T, Sheta EA, Goldknopf IL, Kone BC (2003) Proteomic analysis of S-Nitrosylated proteins in mesangial cells*. Mol Cell Proteomics 2:156–163. https://doi.org/10.1074/mcp.M300003-MCP200

Lander HM, Ogiste JS, Pearce SF, Levi R, Novogrodsky A (1995) Nitric oxide-stimulated guanine nucleotide exchange on p21ras. J Biol Chem 270:7017–7020. https://doi.org/10.1074/jbc.270.13.7017

Lander HM, Hajjar DP, Hempstead BL, Mirza UA, Chait BT, Campbell S, Quilliam LA (1997) A molecular redox switch on p21ras: structural basis for the nitric oxide-p21ras interaction*. J Biol Chem 272:4323–4326. https://doi.org/10.1074/jbc.272.7.4323

Leclerc PC, Lanctot PM, Auger-Messier M, Escher E, Leduc R, Guillemette G (2006) S-nitrosylation of cysteine 289 of the AT1 receptor decreases its binding affinity for angiotensin II. Br J Pharmacol 148:306–313. https://doi.org/10.1038/sj.bjp.0706725

Li A, Liu S, Huang R, Ahn S, Lefkowitz RJ (2023) Loss of biased signaling at a G protein-coupled receptor in overexpressed systems. PLoS One 18:e0283477. https://doi.org/10.1371/journal.pone.0283477

Lieu M, Traynham CJ, de Lucia C et al (2020) Loss of dynamic regulation of G protein-coupled receptor kinase 2 by nitric oxide leads to cardiovascular dysfunction with aging. Am J Phys Heart Circ Phys 318:H1162–H1175. https://doi.org/10.1152/ajpheart.00094.2020

Lim S, Clément M-V (2007) Phosphorylation of the survival kinase Akt by superoxide is dependent on an ascorbate-reversible oxidation of PTEN. Free Radic Biol Med 42:1178–1192. https://doi.org/10.1016/j.freeradbiomed.2007.01.013

Lipton SA, Choi YB, Pan ZH et al (1993) A redox-based mechanism for the neuroprotective and neurodestructive effects of nitric oxide and related nitroso-compounds. Nature 364:626–632. https://doi.org/10.1038/364626a0

Litosch I (2016) Decoding Gαq signaling. Life Sci 152:99–106. https://doi.org/10.1016/j.lfs.2016.03.037

Liu S, Premont RT, Rockey DC (2012) G-protein-coupled receptor kinase interactor-1 (GIT1) is a new endothelial nitric-oxide synthase (eNOS) interactor with functional effects on vascular homeostasis. J Biol Chem 287:12309–12320. https://doi.org/10.1074/jbc.M111.320465

Liu S, Luttrell LM, Premont RT, Rockey DC (2020) β-Arrestin2 is a critical component of the GPCR-eNOS signalosome. Proc Natl Acad Sci USA 117:11483–11492. https://doi.org/10.1073/pnas.1922608117

Liu A, Zhu Y, Chen W, Merlino G, Yu Y (2022) PTEN dual lipid- and protein-phosphatase function in tumor progression. Cancer 14. https://doi.org/10.3390/cancers14153666

Liu S, Anderson PJ, Rajagopal S, Lefkowitz RJ, Rockman HA (2024) G protein-coupled receptors: a century of research and discovery. Circ Res 135:174–197. https://doi.org/10.1161/CIRCRESAHA.124.323067

Mahavadi S, Nalli AD, Kumar DP, Hu W, Kuemmerle JF, Grider JR, Murthy KS (2014) Cytokine-induced iNOS and ERK1/2 inhibit adenylyl cyclase type 5/6 activity and stimulate phosphodiesterase 4D5 activity in intestinal longitudinal smooth muscle. Am J Physiol Cell Physiol 307: C402–C411. https://doi.org/10.1152/ajpcell.00123.2014

Managò F, Espinoza S, Salahpour A, Sotnikova TD, Caron MG, Premont RT, Gainetdinov RR (2012) The role of GRK6 in animal models of Parkinson's disease and L-DOPA treatment. Sci Rep 2:301. https://doi.org/10.1038/srep00301

Maniatis NA, Brovkovych V, Allen SE et al (2006) Novel mechanism of endothelial nitric oxide synthase activation mediated by caveolae internalization in endothelial cells. Circ Res 99:870–877. https://doi.org/10.1161/01.Res.0000245187.08026.47

Marrero MB, Venema VJ, Ju H, He H, Liang H, Caldwell RB, Venema RC (1999) Endothelial nitric oxide synthase interactions with G-protein-coupled receptors. Biochem J 343:335–340. https://doi.org/10.1042/bj3430335

McVey M, Hill J, Howlett A, Klein C (1999) Adenylyl cyclase, a coincidence detector for nitric oxide. J Biol Chem 274:18887–18892. https://doi.org/10.1074/jbc.274.27.18887

Miyamoto A, Laufs U, Pardo C, Liao JK (1997) Modulation of bradykinin receptor ligand binding affinity and its coupled G-proteins by nitric oxide. J Biol Chem 272:19601–19608. https://doi.org/10.1074/jbc.272.31.19601

Mohammad Nezhady MA, Rivera JC, Chemtob S (2020) Location bias as emerging paradigm in GPCR biology and drug discovery. iScience 23:101643. https://doi.org/10.1016/j.isci.2020.101643

Nakamura T, Lipton SA (2013) Emerging role of protein-protein transnitrosylation in cell signaling pathways. Antioxid Redox Signal 18:239–249. https://doi.org/10.1089/ars.2012.4703

Nakamura T, Prikhodko OA, Pirie E et al (2015) Aberrant protein S-nitrosylation contributes to the pathophysiology of neurodegenerative diseases. Neurobiol Dis 84:99–108. https://doi.org/10.1016/j.nbd.2015.03.017

Nishiyama K, Nishimura A, Shimoda K et al (2022) Redox-dependent internalization of the purinergic P2Y6 receptor limits colitis progression. Sci Signal 15:eabj0644. https://doi.org/10.1126/scisignal.abj0644

Nozik-Grayck E, McMahon TJ, Huang YC, Dieterle CS, Stamler JS, Piantadosi CA (2002) Pulmonary vasoconstriction by serotonin is inhibited by S-nitrosoglutathione. Am J Physiol Lung Cell Mol Physiol 282:L1057–L1065. https://doi.org/10.1152/ajplung.00081.2001

Nozik-Grayck E, Whalen EJ, Stamler JS, McMahon TJ, Chitano P, Piantadosi CA (2006) S-nitrosoglutathione inhibits α1-adrenergic receptor-mediated vasoconstriction and ligand binding in pulmonary artery. Am J Phys Lung Cell Mol Phys 290:L136–L143. https://doi.org/10.1152/ajplung.00230.2005

Ozawa K, Whalen EJ, Nelson CD, Mu Y, Hess DT, Lefkowitz RJ, Stamler JS (2008) S-nitrosylation of beta-arrestin regulates beta-adrenergic receptor trafficking. Mol Cell 31: 395–405. https://doi.org/10.1016/j.molcel.2008.05.024

Patwardhan A, Cheng N, Trejo J (2021) Post-translational modifications of G protein–coupled receptors control cellular signaling dynamics in space and time. Pharmacol Rev 73:120. https://doi.org/10.1124/pharmrev.120.000082

Pfleger J, Gresham K, Koch WJ (2019) G protein-coupled receptor kinases as therapeutic targets in the heart. Nat Rev Cardiol 16:612–622. https://doi.org/10.1038/s41569-019-0220-3

Pierce KL, Premont RT, Lefkowitz RJ (2002) Seven-transmembrane receptors. Nat Rev Mol Cell Biol 3:639–650. https://doi.org/10.1038/nrm908

Pinheiro LC, Oliveira-Paula GH, Ferreira GC, Dal-Cin de Paula T, Duarte DA, Costa-Neto CM, Tanus-Santos JE (2021) Oral nitrite treatment increases S-nitrosylation of vascular protein kinase C and attenuates the responses to angiotensin II. Redox Biol 38:101769. https://doi.org/10.1016/j.redox.2020.101769

Premont RT, Inglese J, Lefkowitz RJ (1995) Protein kinases that phosphorylate activated G protein-coupled receptors. FASEB J 9:175–182. https://doi.org/10.1096/fasebj.9.2.7781920

Sanchez-Vicente I, Albertos P, Sanz C et al (2024) Reversible S-nitrosylation of bZIP67 by peroxiredoxin IIE activity and nitro-fatty acids regulates the plant lipid profile. Cell Rep 43: 114091. https://doi.org/10.1016/j.celrep.2024.114091

Sato H, Kato T, Arawaka S (2013) The role of Ser129 phosphorylation of α-synuclein in neurodegeneration of Parkinson's disease: a review of in vivo models. Rev Neurosci 24:115–123. https://doi.org/10.1515/revneuro-2012-0071

Seth D, Hess DT, Hausladen A, Wang L, Wang YJ, Stamler JS (2018) A multiplex enzymatic machinery for cellular protein S-nitrosylation. Mol Cell 69:451–464.e456. https://doi.org/10.1016/j.molcel.2017.12.025

Seth P, Hsieh PN, Jamal S et al (2019) Regulation of MicroRNA machinery and development by interspecies S-Nitrosylation. Cell 176:1014–1025.e1012. https://doi.org/10.1016/j.cell.2019.01.037

Seyedabadi M, Gharghabi M, Gurevich EV, Gurevich VV (2022) Structural basis of GPCR coupling to distinct signal transducers: implications for biased signaling. Trends Biochem Sci 47:570–581. https://doi.org/10.1016/j.tibs.2022.03.009

Sikarwar AS, Hinton M, Santhosh KT, Dhanaraj P, Talabis M, Chelikani P, Dakshinamurti S (2018) Hypoxia inhibits adenylyl cyclase catalytic activity in a porcine model of persistent pulmonary hypertension of the newborn. Am J Physiol Lung Cell Mol Physiol 315:L933–l944. https://doi.org/10.1152/ajplung.00130.2018

Siragusa M, Fleming I (2016) The eNOS signalosome and its link to endothelial dysfunction. Pflugers Arch – Eur J Physiol 468:1125–1137. https://doi.org/10.1007/s00424-016-1839-0

Smith JS, Lefkowitz RJ, Rajagopal S (2018) Biased signalling: from simple switches to allosteric microprocessors. Nat Rev Drug Discov 17:243–260. https://doi.org/10.1038/nrd.2017.229

Sriram K, Insel PA (2018) G protein-coupled receptors as targets for approved drugs: how many targets and how many drugs? Mol Pharmacol 93:251–258. https://doi.org/10.1124/mol.117.111062

Stamler JS, Simon DI, Jaraki O et al (1992a) S-nitrosylation of tissue-type plasminogen activator confers vasodilatory and antiplatelet properties on the enzyme. Proc Natl Acad Sci USA 89: 8087–8091. https://doi.org/10.1073/pnas.89.17.8087

Stamler JS, Simon DI, Osborne JA et al (1992b) S-nitrosylation of proteins with nitric oxide: synthesis and characterization of biologically active compounds. Proc Natl Acad Sci USA 89: 444–448. https://doi.org/10.1073/pnas.89.1.444

Stamler JS, Lamas S, Fang FC (2001) Nitrosylation. The prototypic redox-based signaling mechanism. Cell 106:675–683. https://doi.org/10.1016/s0092-8674(01)00495-0

Stomberski CT, Hess DT, Stamler JS (2019) Protein S-Nitrosylation: determinants of specificity and enzymatic regulation of S-Nitrosothiol-based signaling. Antioxid Redox Signal 30:1331–1351. https://doi.org/10.1089/ars.2017.7403

Stomberski CT, Venetos NM, Zhou HL et al (2022) A multienzyme S-nitrosylation cascade regulates cholesterol homeostasis. Cell Rep 41:111538. https://doi.org/10.1016/j.celrep.2022.111538

Sun N, Kim K-M (2021) Mechanistic diversity involved in the desensitization of G protein-coupled receptors. Arch Pharm Res 44:342–353. https://doi.org/10.1007/s12272-021-01320-y

Tan L, Yan W, McCorvy JD, Cheng J (2018) Biased ligands of G Protein-Coupled Receptors (GPCRs): Structure–Functional Selectivity Relationships (SFSRs) and therapeutic potential. J Med Chem 61:9841–9878. https://doi.org/10.1021/acs.jmedchem.8b00435

Tang LJ, Li C, Hu SQ et al (2012) S-nitrosylation of c-Src via NMDAR-nNOS module promotes c-Src activation and NR2A phosphorylation in cerebral ischemia/reperfusion. Mol Cell Biochem 365:363–377. https://doi.org/10.1007/s11010-012-1280-4

Trefely S, Lovell CD, Snyder NW, Wellen KE (2020) Compartmentalised acyl-CoA metabolism and roles in chromatin regulation. Mol Metab 38:100941. https://doi.org/10.1016/j.molmet.2020.01.005

Uehara T, Nakamura T, Yao D et al (2006) S-nitrosylated protein-disulphide isomerase links protein misfolding to neurodegeneration. Nature 441:513–517. https://doi.org/10.1038/nature04782

Urs NM, Peterson SM, Caron MG (2017) New concepts in dopamine D(2) receptor biased signaling and implications for schizophrenia therapy. Biol Psychiatry 81:78–85. https://doi.org/10.1016/j.biopsych.2016.10.011

Wang G, Moniri NH, Ozawa K, Stamler JS, Daaka Y (2006) Nitric oxide regulates endocytosis by S-nitrosylation of dynamin. Proc Natl Acad Sci USA 103:1295–1300. https://doi.org/10.1073/pnas.0508354103

Wang J, Hanada K, Staus DP et al (2017) Gαi is required for carvedilol-induced β1 adrenergic receptor β-arrestin biased signaling. Nat Commun 8:1706. https://doi.org/10.1038/s41467-017-01855-z

Wang Q, Wang Y, West TM et al (2021) Carvedilol induces biased β1 adrenergic receptor-nitric oxide synthase 3-cyclic guanylyl monophosphate signalling to promote cardiac contractility. Cardiovasc Res 117:2237–2251. https://doi.org/10.1093/cvr/cvaa266

Wanschel AC, Caceres VM, Moretti AI et al (2014) Cardioprotective mechanism of S-nitroso-N-acetylcysteine via S-nitrosated betadrenoceptor-2 in the LDLr-/- mice. Nitric Oxide 36:58–66. https://doi.org/10.1016/j.niox.2013.12.003

Wei H, Ahn S, Shenoy SK, Karnik SS, Hunyady L, Luttrell LM, Lefkowitz RJ (2003) Independent beta-arrestin 2 and G protein-mediated pathways for angiotensin II activation of extracellular signal-regulated kinases 1 and 2. Proc Natl Acad Sci USA 100:10782–10787. https://doi.org/10.1073/pnas.1834556100

Wettschureck N, Offermanns S (2005) Mammalian G proteins and their cell type specific functions. Physiol Rev 85:1159–1204. https://doi.org/10.1152/physrev.00003.2005

Whalen EJ, Foster MW, Matsumoto A et al (2007) Regulation of β-adrenergic receptor signaling by S-Nitrosylation of G-protein-coupled receptor kinase 2. Cell 129:511–522. https://doi.org/10.1016/j.cell.2007.02.046

Wu W, Sung CC, Yu P, Li J, Chung KKK (2020) S-Nitrosylation of G protein-coupled receptor kinase 6 and casein kinase 2 alpha modulates their kinase activity toward alpha-synuclein phosphorylation in an animal model of Parkinson's disease. PLoS One 15:e0232019. https://doi.org/10.1371/journal.pone.0232019

Yao D, Gu Z, Nakamura T et al (2004) Nitrosative stress linked to sporadic Parkinson's disease: S-nitrosylation of parkin regulates its E3 ubiquitin ligase activity. Proc Natl Acad Sci USA 101:10810–10814. https://doi.org/10.1073/pnas.0404161101

Zhang Y, Deng Y, Yang X, Xue H, Lang Y (2020) The relationship between protein S-Nitrosylation and human diseases: a review. Neurochem Res 45:2815–2827. https://doi.org/10.1007/s11064-020-03136-6

Zheng H, Loh HH, Law P-Y (2013) Posttranslation modification of G protein-coupled receptor in relationship to biased Agonism. In: Conn PM (ed) Methods in enzymology. Academic, pp 391–408

Zhou L, Bohn LM (2014) Functional selectivity of GPCR signaling in animals. Curr Opin Cell Biol 27:102–108. https://doi.org/10.1016/j.ceb.2013.11.010

Zhou HL, Grimmett ZW, Venetos NM et al (2023) An enzyme that selectively S-nitrosylates proteins to regulate insulin signaling. Cell 186. https://doi.org/10.1016/j.cell.2023.11.009

KCTD Family: Emerging Regulators of GPCR Biased Signaling

Wentong Jiang and Sanduo Zheng

Contents

Abstract

G protein-coupled receptors (GPCRs) engage multiple transducers to regulate distinct physiological processes. These transducers include various G proteins subtypes, GPCR kinases (GRKs), and β-arrestins. In addition to promoting receptor desensitization, β-arrestins serve as scaffolds for signaling via non-G

W. Jiang
National Institute of Biological Sciences, Beijing, China

S. Zheng (✉)
National Institute of Biological Sciences, Beijing, China

Tsinghua Institute of Multidisciplinary Biomedical Research, Tsinghua University, Beijing, China
e-mail: zhengsanduo@nibs.ac.cn

© The Author(s), under exclusive license to Springer Nature Switzerland AG 2025
Z. Li, K. Xiao (eds.), *Pharmacology of GPCRs Biased Signaling and Agonists*,
Handbook of Experimental Pharmacology 290, https://doi.org/10.1007/164_2025_766

protein pathways. Biased signaling enables GPCRs to selectively engage specific transducers, typically through different conformational states of GPCRs. While significant focus has been placed on developing biased ligands that preferentially activate specific G proteins or β-arrestins, the strategy focused on modulating particular G protein subunits (Gα versus βγ) remains underexplored. Recently, members of the KCTD (potassium channel tetramerization domain-containing) family have emerged as critical regulators of GPCR signaling, particularly through their roles in mediating Gβγ degradation or uncoupling Gβγ from downstream effectors. This ability positions the KCTD family as potential targets for selectively modulating Gβγ signaling with minimal impact on Gα-mediated pathways. In this chapter, we introduce the KCTD family, summarize current knowledge of their role in GPCR signaling regulation, and highlight unsolved questions in existing models, along with directions for future research.

Keywords

GPCR desensitization · Gβγ · KCTD family · Ubiquitination

1 GPCR-Biased Signaling

G protein-coupled receptors (GPCRs) represent the largest family of membrane receptors and play a critical role in mediating cellular responses to a vast array of extracellular signals. These signals encompass light, odors, ions, small molecules, peptides, and proteins (Hilger et al. 2018; Liu et al. 2024; Wacker et al. 2017), and GPCRs are essential in regulating diverse physiological processes, including sensory perception, immune response, and neurotransmission. Upon ligand binding, GPCRs initiate signaling through two major pathways: the G protein pathway and the β-arrestin pathway.

In the classical G protein signaling pathway, receptor activation results in the dissociation of heterotrimeric G proteins into their constituent Gα and Gβγ subunits. Gα is classified into four subfamilies—$G\alpha_s$, $G\alpha_{i/o}$, $G\alpha_{q/11}$, and $G\alpha_{12/13}$—and each subunit engages distinct downstream effectors to propagate signals (Wilkie et al. 1992) (Fig. 1). For example, Gαs activates adenylyl cyclases (Northup et al. 1980), promoting the synthesis of cAMP, while Gβγ subunits interact with effectors such as the G protein-coupled inwardly rectifying potassium (GIRK) channels, voltage-gated calcium channel (Cav), phosphoinositide 3 kinase, and adenylyl cyclase (Smrcka 2008). In parallel to G protein signaling, activated GPCRs recruit β-arrestins (Attramadal et al. 1992; Lohse et al. 1990), which mediate receptor internalization, and prevent sustained G protein activation (Laporte et al. 1999; Luttrell and Lefkowitz 2002). Additionally, β-arrestins serve as scaffolds for the initiation of distinct signaling cascades (Beaulieu et al. 2005; Luttrell et al. 1999), such as the Raf–MEK–ERK pathway, collectively termed the β-arrestin pathway. These two major signaling modes—G protein-mediated and β-arrestin-mediated—underscore the remarkable versatility of GPCRs in regulating cellular responses.

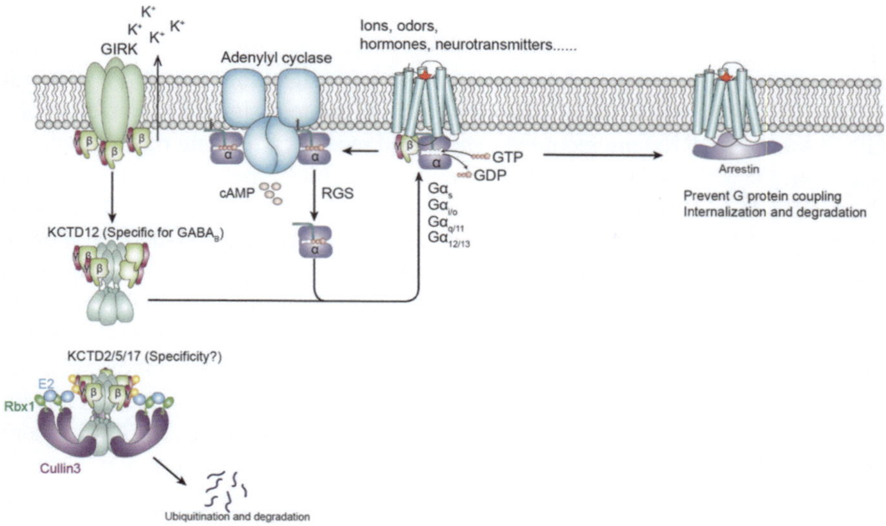

Fig. 1 GPCR signaling pathway. Ligand-induced conformational changes in GPCRs facilitate the recruitment of heterotrimeric G proteins, which consist of four major subtypes. G protein activation by GPCRs triggers nucleotide exchange in the Gα subunit, leading to the dissociation of Gα from Gβγ. Both Gα and Gβγ independently regulate distinct downstream effectors. For instance, the GTP-bound Gαs activates the adenylyl cyclase, resulting in the production of cAMP. When dissociated from $G\alpha_{i/o}$, Gβγ can activate G protein-regulated inwardly rectifying potassium (GIRK) channels. Under prolonged or repeated agonist stimulation, nature has evolved several mechanisms to induce receptor desensitization. One such mechanism involves the phosphorylation of the activated receptors, which facilitates arrestin binding. The coupling prevents further interaction with G proteins and promotes receptor internalization and degradation. To terminate G proteins signaling, RGSs enhance the GTPase activity of Gα, driving the hydrolysis of GTP to GDP and the subsequent reassociation of Gα with Gβγ. Moreover, KCTD12 that specifically interacts with the $GABA_B$ receptor scavenges Gβγ from GIRK following $GABA_B$ activation, resulting in rapid desensitization. KCTD2, KCTD5, and KCTD17 interact with five copies of free Gβγ, initiating their ubiquitination and degradation. However, it is unclear which GPCRs are regulated by these KCTDs

A notable feature of GPCRs is their ability to adopt multiple active states, which allows them to interact with various signaling partners, including different G protein subtypes and β-arrestins (Weis and Kobilka 2018; Wootten et al. 2018). This functional plasticity enables GPCRs to mediate diverse biological effects depending on the nature of the ligand and the cellular context. The concept of biased signaling has emerged, where ligands selectively activate particular signaling pathways, preferentially engaging either G protein or β-arrestin-mediated pathways (Rajagopal et al. 2010; Smith et al. 2018). Biased ligands have the potential to induce specific conformational changes in GPCRs, promoting the activation of desired signaling cascades while minimizing unwanted side effects. Given that Gα and Gβγ subunits activate distinct downstream effectors, leading to divergent physiological outcomes, biased signaling that selectively activates specific G protein subunits (Gα versus Gβγ) represents an intriguing yet largely unexplored area of research. While the development of ligands for the receptors that inherently favor signaling through specific G protein subunits presents challenges, such selectivity may be achievable by specifically modulating particular G protein signaling pathways. Several mechanisms have been identified to modulate G protein signaling. For example, GPCR kinases (GRKs) are recruited to activated receptors, forming tight complexes with both the activated Gα and Gβγ subunits to inhibit further G protein activation (Lodowski et al. 2003; Raveh et al. 2010). Moreover, regulators of G protein signaling (RGS) proteins function as GTPase-activating proteins (GAPs), promoting the hydrolysis of GTP to GDP on Gα subunits, thus returning them to their inactive state in complex with Gβγ (Ross and Wilkie 2000; Watson et al. 1996). Notably, certain RGS proteins display a preference for specific Gα subtypes, further enhancing the specificity of G protein regulation (Masuho et al. 2020). Recent research has also identified KCTD proteins as novel regulators of GPCR signaling, specifically targeting Gβγ subunits or adenylyl cyclases (Brockmann et al. 2017; Liao and Muntean 2024; Schwenk et al. 2010) (Fig. 1). These findings add a new layer of complexity to the already intricate GPCR signaling machinery, highlighting the dynamic and multifaceted nature of this system. While GRKs simultaneously terminate signaling through both Gα and Gβγ subunits, the KCTD family acts selectively on Gβγ signaling, with minimal impact on Gα-mediated pathways. Therefore, the KCTD family could serve as potential targets for the development of biased ligands that selectively promote or suppress Gβγ signaling.

2 KCTD Proteins Regulate GPCR Signaling by Directly Targeting the Central Components of the Signaling Axis

2.1 The Structural Characteristics of the KCTD Family Proteins

The KCTD family, short for potassium channel tetramerization domain containing proteins, consists of 25 members encoded in the human genome (Teng et al. 2019). KCTD proteins are characterized by the presence of at least one BTB domain (Bric-a-brac, Tramtrack, and Broad Complex/Poxvirus Zinc Finger) at the N-terminus and a C-terminal domain (CTD) that exhibits minimal sequence homology to known protein families. Sequence alignment of the KCTD family has revealed eight main clades (Clade A-H), with paralogs within each clade sharing high sequence similarity (Fig. 2a). The BTB domains in KCTD proteins are most homologous to those found in voltage-gated potassium channels (VGKCs), which tetramerize to form functional ion channels within the membrane. Like VGKCs, KCTD proteins also form homo-oligomers, predominantly pentamers in solution, except for KCTD10 and KCTD13, which form tetramers similar to VGKCs (Ji et al. 2016; Pinkas et al. 2017). Notably, KCTD proteins do not contain features of transmembrane domains or exhibit potassium channel activity. In addition to oligomerization, BTB domains are known to bind Cullin-3, an E3 ligase within the Cullin-RING ligase family (Zimmerman et al. 2010). Many KCTD proteins but not all KCTD members function as substrate adaptors for Cullin-3 (Smaldone et al. 2015), facilitating the recruitment

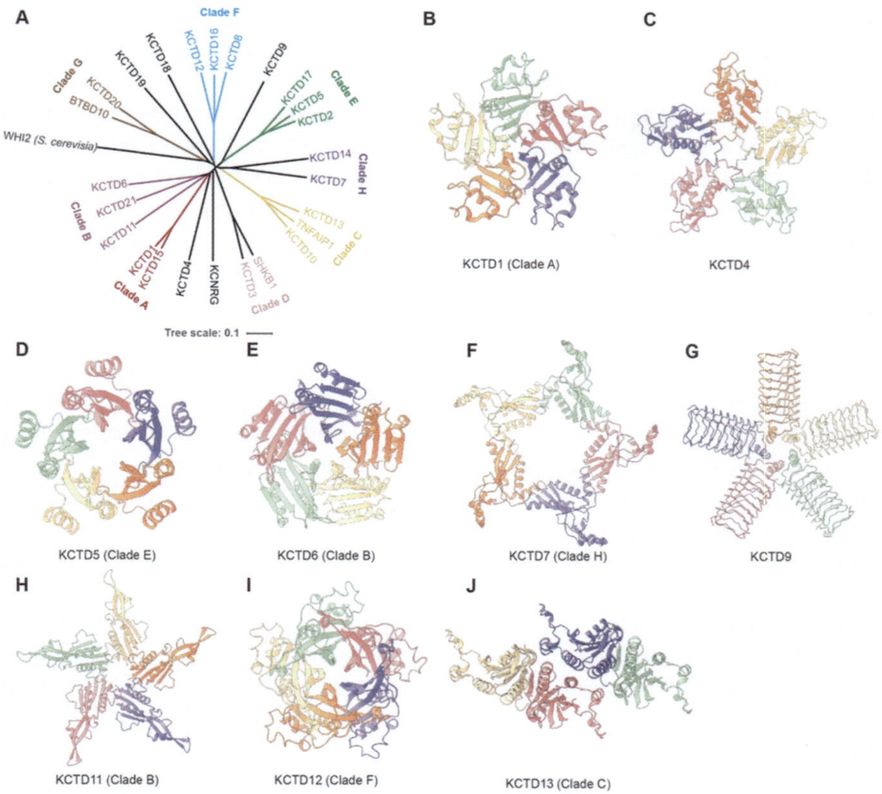

Fig. 2 Classification of the KCTD family members. (**a**) Phylogenetic trees. (**b–j**) Alphafold-predicted oligomeric structures of the CTD domains of KCTD1 (**b**), KCTD4 (**c**), KCTD5 (**d**), KCTD6 (**e**), KCTD7 (**f**), KCTD9 (**g**), KCTD11 (**h**), KCTD12, (**i**) and KCTD13 (**j**) from different clades

of substrates for ubiquitination. In contrast, the CTDs of KCTD members exhibit high structural variability across clades, suggesting they possibly recruit different substrates for ubiquitination (Fig. 2b–j).

2.2 KCTDs Are Frequently Associated with Neurodevelopmental and Neural Psychiatric Disorders

One of the most striking features of the KCTD family is their frequent association with neural developmental and neuropsychiatric disorders. For instance, genome-wide association studies have identified *kctd2* as a risk factor of Alzheimer's disease (Boada et al. 2014), while its paralog, *kctd17,* has been implicated as a potential causal gene for childhood early-onset hyperkinetic movement disorder and autosomal dominant myoclonus-dystonia (Mencacci et al. 2015). Similarly, missense mutation or frameshift has been found on *kctd3* in several families with neurocognitive disorders, where affected individuals exhibited developmental delay, seizure, and cerebellar hypoplasia (Faqeih et al. 2018). A single mutation in *kctd10* has been linked to schizophrenia, and its paralog (Mu et al. 2024), *kctd13*, has been frequently implicated as a major contributor to neuropsychiatric disorders associated with copy-number variants of chromosome 16p11.2 region (Escamilla et al. 2017; Golzio et al. 2012; Lin et al. 2015). Furthermore, loss-of-function mutations in *kctd7* are known to cause early-onset progressive myoclonic epilepsy (PME), with missense mutations, frameshift, and early stop mutations identified in PME families (Blumkin et al. 2012; Dai et al. 2019; Farhan et al. 2014; Kousi et al. 2012; Van Bogaert 2016). *kctd1* and *kctd15* have been shown in animal models and in vitro studies to regulate neural crest formation. Other members of the KCTD family have also been sporadically linked to different neural developmental disorders, as summarized in detail in recent studies (Teng et al. 2019).

Despite high clinical relevance of KCTD family members, the molecular mechanisms underlying their roles in these disorders remain largely unclear. For most KCTD members, the connection between human genetic evidence and their biochemical and cellular functions is not well understood. Future research is required to clarify the disease-causing mechanisms of these mutations and provide insights for potential therapeutic strategies. Interestingly, recent findings have begun to uncover a unifying theme in the cellular and biochemical functions of several KCTD family members: they serve as key regulators of GPCR signaling. These members include KCTD2, 5, 17 from Clade E and KCTD8,12 and 16 from Clade F.

2.3 KCTD2/5/17 of Clade E Targets Target-Free Gβγ Subunits for Ubiquitination-Based Degradation

KCTD5 was initially identified in *Drosophila melanogaster* (referred to as *insomniac* or *inc*) during a forward genetic screen for genes involved in regulation of sleep behavior (Pfeiffenberger and Allada 2012; Stavropoulos and Young 2011). Loss of *kctd5* gene in flies significantly reduces total sleep time and disrupts homeostatic sleep rebound. KCTD5 serves as substrate adaptor protein for the E3 ligase Cullin-3, and it was further shown that knocking out Cullin-3 produced similar sleep defect as KCTD5 knockout, suggesting Cullin-3/KCTD5 E3 ligase complex and its potential substrate proteins as crucial regulators of sleep behavior. More recently, another genetic screen in flies revealed that following acute blockade of glutamine receptors at synapse, Cullin-3 and KCTD5 accumulate in the post-synaptic compartment, where they are necessary for the production of retrograde homeostatic signaling (Kikuma et al. 2019). These findings highlight important regulatory roles of KCTD5 in the neuronal system. However, the specific substrates targeted by the Cullin-3/KCTD5 complex that may be responsible for these processes remained unclear.

In mammals, *kctd5* shares over 80% sequence homology with its drosophila ortholog *inc* in drosophila. Proteome and ubiquitin-proteome analysis have revealed that the absence of human KCTD5 in cells leads to significant accumulation of G protein βγ subunits with a corresponding reduction in their ubiquitination levels

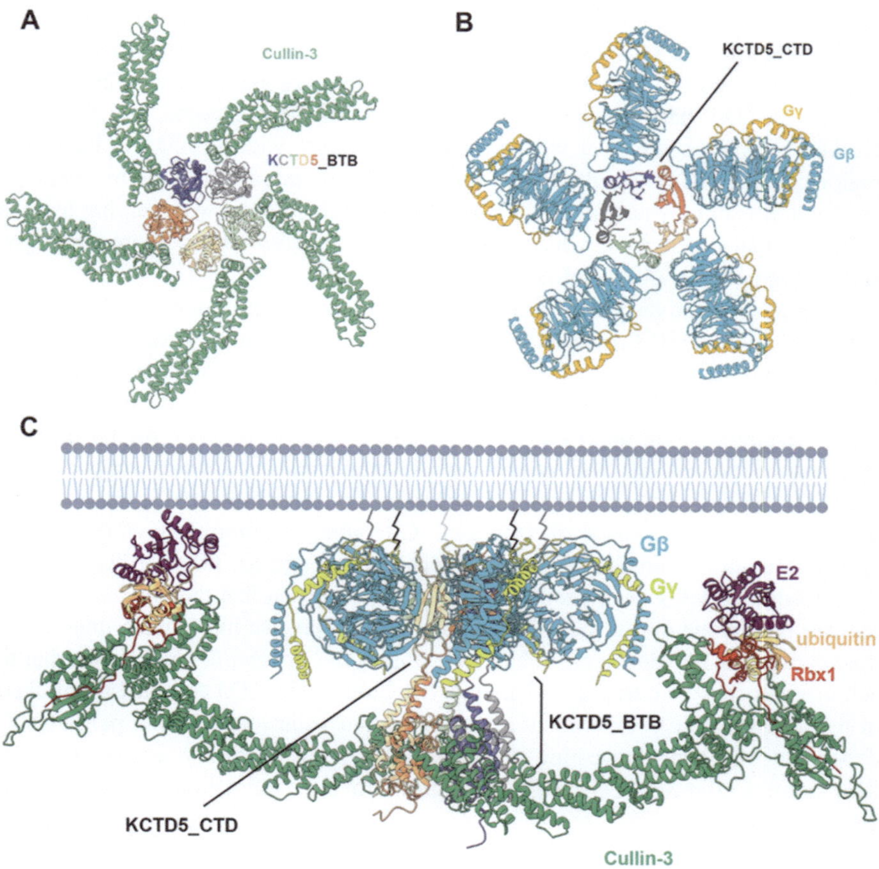

Fig. 3 Mechanisms of Gβγ ubiquitination by KCTD5. (**a**) Structural model of the BTB domain of KCTD5 bound to Cullin-3 generated based on the cryo-EM structure of KCTD7 and Cullin-3 complex. (**b**) Cryo-EM structure of the CTD of KCTD5 in complex with five copies of Gβγ. (**c**) Structural model of KCTD5-Cullin3-Rbx1 E3 ligase complex, along with E2-ubiquitin and the substrate Gβγ

(Brockmann et al. 2017; Young et al. 2021). Subsequent cellular, biochemical, and structural studies have since demonstrated that KCTD5 forms pentamers and recruits five copies of Cullin-3 through its N terminal BTB domains (Balasco et al. 2014; Jiang et al. 2023; Nguyen et al. 2024). The arch-shaped Cullin-3 proteins dock around the BTB of KCTD5, bending backward to bring E2-ubiquitin in proximity to the CTD (Fig. 3a–c). This arrangement creates five reactive centers around the CTD. Upon GPCR activation, KCTD5 captures one to five copies of free Gβγ subunits and catalyzes the transfer of ubiquitin to the N-terminal lysine residues of Gβ or Gγ subunits (Jiang et al. 2023; Nguyen et al. 2024). The ubiquitinated Gβγ are targeted for degradation via proteasome. These findings establish KCTD5 as a key regulator of GPCR signaling by directly modulating Gβγ activity. KCTD5 desensitizes GPCR signaling by degrading excessively activated Gβγ proteins. Remarkably, the *Drosophila* homolog of KCTD5 can recruit both mammalian Gβγ and their *Drosophila* counterparts, indicating a highly conserved regulatory mechanism (Jiang et al. 2023). KCTD5 has two paralogs in the mammalian genome, KCTD2 and KCTD17, which share over 90% sequence homology with KCTD5 in their core regions. While KCTD2 and KCTD5 are functionally redundant at the biochemical level in terms of Gβγ targeting, KCTD17 has several isoforms with varying lengths of C-terminal extensions, which significantly impair its ability to recruit Gβγ, suggesting potential dominant negative effects.

Despite these advances, several discrepancies and gaps remain in the current model of KCTD2/5/17-mediated Gβγ regulation. For instance, although KCTD2, KCTD5, and the short isoform of KCTD17 are functionally redundant in recruiting Gβγ, the absence of any of these genes is sufficient to cause Gβγ accumulation and cAMP overproduction upon GPCR activation, at least in primary striatal neurons (Muntean et al. 2022). Furthermore, while biochemical evidence supports that KCTD2/5/17 only ubiquitinates and degrades free Gβγ potentially upon GPCR activation, direct evidence of increased Gβγ ubiquitination following specific GPCR activation remains lacking. Additionally, although KCTD2/5/17 are primarily cytosolic proteins, their proposed mechanisms suggest that they are recruited to the cell membrane during GPCR signaling, yet the precise mechanism underlying this recruitment remains unclear. Notably, studies in *Drosophila* have shown that to achieve homeostatic retrograde signaling, the Cullin-3/KCTD5 complex is enriched in the post synaptic compartment of the neuro-muscular junction in a peflin/Ca^{2+}-dependent manner, suggesting the involvement of auxiliary components in facilitating Cullin-3/KCDT2/5/17 recruitment to Gβγ for action (Kikuma et al. 2019).

2.4 KCTD8/12/16 Modulate the Pharmacology and Kinetics of $GABA_B$ Signaling by Serving as the Auxiliary Subunits

The metabotropic $GABA_B$ receptors mediate the effects of the major inhibitory neurotransmitter GABA by activating the Gi/o pathway. $GABA_B$ functions as an obligatory heterodimer composed of two principal subunits, $GABA_{B1}$ and $GABA_{B2}$. Upon activation, $GABA_B$ causes the dissociation of the Gα subunit from Gβγ. Presynaptic GABAB inhibits voltage-gate calcium channel via Gβγ, thereby inhibiting neurotransmitter release, whereas the postsynaptic receptor generates slow inhibitory postsynaptic potentials through activation of GIRK by Gβγ (Bettler et al. 2004). KCTD8, 12, 12b, and 16 have been identified as auxiliary subunits of $GABA_B$ receptors through affinity purification and mass spectrometry analysis of the native $GABA_{B1/2}$ receptor signaling complex (Schwenk et al. 2010, 2016). Among these, KCTD12 plays a dual role: it accelerates the activation of receptor-induced GIRK currents by preassembling Gβγ at the receptor and induces rapid desensitization by scavenging Gβγ from the channel (Fritzius et al. 2024; Turecek et al. 2014).

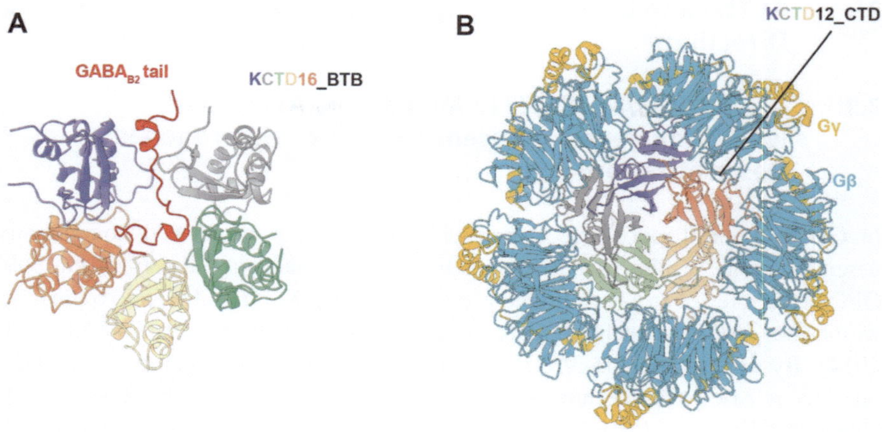

Fig. 4 Molecular mechanisms of KCTD-mediated desensitization of the $GABA_B$ receptor. **(a)** Crystal structure of the BTB domain of KCTD16 in complex with a C-terminal peptide derived from the $GABA_{B2}$ subunit (PDB: 6M8R). **(b)** Crystal structure of the CTD of KCTD12 in complex with five copies of Gβγ (PDB: 6M8S)

Mechanistically, unlike other KCTDs, whose BTB domains oligomerize into pentamers with C5 symmetry, the N terminal BTB domains of KCTD8, 12, and 16 form an unusual open pentamer structure. This configuration allows the C-terminal peptide of $GABA_{B2}$ receptor to insert into the center of the BTB pentamer, forming a tight complex that anchors KCTDs to the membrane (Fig. 4a) (Zheng et al. 2019; Zuo et al. 2019). The CTD of KCTD12, also named the H1 domain, symmetrically interacts with five copies of Gβγ in a highly cooperative manner (Fig. 4b). In contrast, KCTD8 and KCTD16 lack the ability to induce rapid desensitization of GIRK currents due to an additional H2 domain that sterically blocks the interaction between the H1 domain and Gβγ (Seddik et al. 2012). These auxiliary subunits contribute to the functional diversity of $GABA_B$ receptor signaling. Intriguingly, while $GABA_B$ receptors are primarily known for mediating inhibitory neurotransmission in the brain, they exert strong presynaptic excitation in habenula cholinergic neurons (Zhang et al. 2016). This excitatory effect may be attributed to the presence of KCTD8 and KCTD12, which facilitate axonal localization of $GABA_B$ receptors (Ren et al. 2022). These findings highlight the unique roles of KCTD8, KCTD12, and KCTD16 as auxiliary subunits that modulate the pharmacology and kinetics of $GABA_B$ receptor signaling. Their ability to influence receptor localization, agonist potency, and signaling dynamics underscores their importance in shaping the functional diversity of $GABA_B$ receptor-mediated responses.

3 KCTDs and GPCR Signaling: Unsolved Problems and Future Directions

3.1 Are Cullin-3/KCTD2/5/17 Modulators Associated with Homogeneous Desensitization or Heterogeneous Desensitization?

In GPCR desensitization, receptor-specific mechanisms are termed homologous desensitization, while global desensitization mechanisms affecting multiple GPCRs are referred to as heterologous desensitization. KCTD8, 12, and 16 function within the $GABA_B$ receptor complex in a receptor-specific manner (Turecek et al. 2014). By contrast, Cullin-3/KCTD2/5/17 appears to act by capturing free Gβγ proteins released from heterotrimeric Gαβγ complexes upon GPCR activation. Given that KCTD2/5/17 biochemically recognize Gβ1–4 of five subtypes of Gβ, they may regulate Gβγ signaling broadly, independent of the specific GPCR or agonist involved. If so, KCTD2/5/17 would be categorized as mediators of heterologous desensitization, influencing all downstream signaling events involving Gβγ. However, direct evidence for such global regulation is lacking. It remains unclear whether KCTD2/5/17 regulate Gβγ signaling following activation of any GPCR or if additional factors recruit or confine their activity to specific receptors or contexts. Physiological conditions may involve auxiliary components within the Cullin-3/KCTD2/5/17 complex that enable membrane localization and receptor-specific targeting.

KCTD-mediated GPCR regulation also differs fundamentally from known mechanisms involving β-arrestins, GRKs, or RGS proteins, raising critical questions about its functional dynamics. For example, under what circumstances—such as specific agonists, receptor types, signaling pathways, or timescales—does KCTD-mediated regulation dominate, and how does it interact with other regulatory mechanisms? Answering these questions will illuminate the unique contributions of KCTD proteins to GPCR desensitization and signaling specificity.

3.2 The KCTD Family Can Be Leveraged to Develop Biased Ligands That Selectively Prolong or Inhibit Gβγ Signaling

A genome-wide association study of bipolar I disorder has identified single-nucleotide polymorphisms (SNP) in the KCTD12 gene (Lee et al. 2011). Moreover, altered KCTD12 expression has been observed in patients with major depressive disorder and schizophrenia (Glatt et al. 2005; Sibille et al. 2009). In mouse models, KCTD12 influences emotionality, behavioral activity, and neuronal excitability (Cathomas et al. 2015). Although the $GABA_B$ receptor is considered a potential drug target for conditions such as anxiety, addition, depression, and neuropathic pain, the most notable approved drug targeting the $GABA_B$ receptor is baclofen used as a muscle relaxant and antispastic agent (Nieto et al. 2022). Unlike glutamate receptors, the $GABA_B$ receptor lacks distinct subtypes and also fails to activate the other pathways such as β-arrestins (Fairfax et al. 2004; Perroy et al. 2003; Sudo et al. 2012), making it difficult to separate therapeutic effects from side effects. This limitation poses a challenge to drug development targeting this receptor. Therefore, modulating the function of KCTD12 represents a novel strategy for targeting $GABA_B$-related neuropsychiatric disorders, with the potential to offer therapeutic benefits while reducing unwanted side effects. Recently, a highly potent peptide-based inhibitor has been developed to disrupt the KCTD and $GABA_B$ receptor complex, effectively slowing desensitization and prolonging Gβγ signaling (Sereikaite et al. 2019). Conversely, since the binding interface of KCTD5 and Gβγ creates a ligand binding pocket (Jiang et al. 2023), molecular glues that stabilize KCTD5/Gβγ complex can induce rapid degradation of Gβγ, possibly mitigating side effects associated with Gβγ signaling. However, further research is necessary to understand the physiological and pathological outcomes of different G protein pathways linked to these receptors.

References

Attramadal H, Arriza JL, Aoki C, Dawson TM, Codina J, Kwatra MM, Snyder SH, Caron MG, Lefkowitz RJ (1992) Beta-arrestin2, a novel member of the arrestin/beta-arrestin gene family. J Biol Chem 267:17882–17890

Balasco N, Pirone L, Smaldone G, Di Gaetano S, Esposito L, Pedone EM, Vitagliano L (2014) Molecular recognition of Cullin3 by KCTDs: insights from experimental and computational investigations. Biochim Biophys Acta 1844:1289–1298. https://doi.org/10.1016/j.bbapap.2014.04.006

Beaulieu JM, Sotnikova TD, Marion S, Lefkowitz RJ, Gainetdinov RR, Caron MG (2005) An Akt/beta-arrestin 2/PP2A signaling complex mediates dopaminergic neurotransmission and behavior. Cell 122:261–273. https://doi.org/10.1016/j.cell.2005.05.012

Bettler B, Kaupmann K, Mosbacher J, Gassmann M (2004) Molecular structure and physiological functions of GABA(B) receptors. Physiol Rev 84:835–867. https://doi.org/10.1152/physrev.00036.2003

Blumkin L, Kivity S, Lev D, Cohen S, Shomrat R, Lerman-Sagie T, Leshinsky-Silver E (2012) A compound heterozygous missense mutation and a large deletion in the KCTD7 gene presenting as an opsoclonus-myoclonus ataxia-like syndrome. J Neurol 259:2590–2598. https://doi.org/10.1007/s00415-012-6545-z

Boada M, Antunez C, Ramirez-Lorca R, DeStefano AL, Gonzalez-Perez A, Gayan J, Lopez-Arrieta J, Ikram MA, Hernandez I, Marin J, Galan JJ, Bis JC, Mauleon A, Rosende-Roca M, Moreno-Rey C, Gudnasson V, Moron FJ, Velasco J, Carrasco JM, Alegret M, Espinosa A, Vinyes G, Lafuente A, Vargas L, Fitzpatrick AL, Alzheimer's Disease Neuroimaging I, Launer LJ, Saez ME, Vazquez E, Becker JT, Lopez OL, Serrano-Rios M, Tarraga L, van Duijn CM, Real LM, Seshadri S, Ruiz A (2014) ATP5H/KCTD2 locus is associated with Alzheimer's disease risk. Mol Psychiatry 19:682–687. https://doi.org/10.1038/mp.2013.86

Brockmann M, Blomen VA, Nieuwenhuis J, Stickel E, Raaben M, Bleijerveld OB, Altelaar AFM, Jae LT, Brummelkamp TR (2017) Genetic wiring maps of single-cell protein states reveal an off-switch for GPCR signalling. Nature 546:307–311. https://doi.org/10.1038/nature22376

Cathomas F, Stegen M, Sigrist H, Schmid L, Seifritz E, Gassmann M, Bettler B, Pryce CR (2015) Altered emotionality and neuronal excitability in mice lacking KCTD12, an auxiliary subunit of GABAB receptors associated with mood disorders. Transl Psychiatry 5:e510. https://doi.org/10.1038/tp.2015.8

Dai L, Ding C, Fang F (2019) Two Chinese siblings with two novel KCTD7 mutations have dystonia or seizures and epileptic discharge on electroencephalograms. Seizure 70:27–29. https://doi.org/10.1016/j.seizure.2019.06.007

Escamilla CO, Filonova I, Walker AK, Xuan ZX, Holehonnur R, Espinosa F, Liu S, Thyme SB, Lopez-Garcia IA, Mendoza DB, Usui N, Ellegood J, Eisch AJ, Konopka G, Lerch JP, Schier AF, Speed HE, Powell CM (2017) Kctd13 deletion reduces synaptic transmission via increased RhoA. Nature 551:227–231. https://doi.org/10.1038/nature24470

Fairfax BP, Pitcher JA, Scott MG, Calver AR, Pangalos MN, Moss SJ, Couve A (2004) Phosphorylation and chronic agonist treatment atypically modulate GABAB receptor cell surface stability. J Biol Chem 279:12565–12573. https://doi.org/10.1074/jbc.M311389200

Faqeih EA, Almannai M, Saleh MM, AlWadei AH, Samman MM, Alkuraya FS (2018) Phenotypic characterization of KCTD3-related developmental epileptic encephalopathy. Clin Genet 93: 1081–1086. https://doi.org/10.1111/cge.13227

Farhan SM, Murphy LM, Robinson JF, Wang J, Siu VM, Rupar CA, Prasad AN, Consortium FC, Hegele RA (2014) Linkage analysis and exome sequencing identify a novel mutation in KCTD7 in patients with progressive myoclonus epilepsy with ataxia. Epilepsia 55:e106-11. https://doi.org/10.1111/epi.12730

Fritzius T, Turecek R, Fernandez-Fernandez D, Isogai S, Rem PD, Kralikova M, Gassmann M, Bettler B (2024) Preassembly of specific Gbetagamma subunits at GABA(B) receptors through auxiliary KCTD proteins accelerates channel gating. Biochem Pharmacol 228:116176. https://doi.org/10.1016/j.bcp.2024.116176

Glatt SJ, Everall IP, Kremen WS, Corbeil J, Sasik R, Khanlou N, Han M, Liew CC, Tsuang MT (2005) Comparative gene expression analysis of blood and brain provides concurrent validation of SELENBP1 up-regulation in schizophrenia. Proc Natl Acad Sci USA 102:15533–15538. https://doi.org/10.1073/pnas.0507666102

Golzio C, Willer J, Talkowski ME, Oh EC, Taniguchi Y, Jacquemont S, Reymond A, Sun M, Sawa A, Gusella JF, Kamiya A, Beckmann JS, Katsanis N (2012) KCTD13 is a major driver of mirrored neuroanatomical phenotypes of the 16p11.2 copy number variant. Nature 485:363–367. https://doi.org/10.1038/nature11091

Hilger D, Masureel M, Kobilka BK (2018) Structure and dynamics of GPCR signaling complexes. Nat Struct Mol Biol 25:4–12. https://doi.org/10.1038/s41594-017-0011-7

Ji AX, Chu A, Nielsen TK, Benlekbir S, Rubinstein JL, Prive GG (2016) Structural insights into KCTD protein assembly and Cullin3 recognition. J Mol Biol 428:92–107. https://doi.org/10.1016/j.jmb.2015.08.019

Jiang W, Wang W, Kong Y, Zheng S (2023) Structural basis for the ubiquitination of G protein betagamma subunits by KCTD5/Cullin3 E3 ligase. Sci Adv 9:eadg8369. https://doi.org/10.1126/sciadv.adg8369

Kikuma K, Li X, Perry S, Li Q, Goel P, Chen C, Kim D, Stavropoulos N, Dickman D (2019) Cul3 and insomniac are required for rapid ubiquitination of postsynaptic targets and retrograde homeostatic signaling. Nat Commun 10:2998. https://doi.org/10.1038/s41467-019-10992-6

Kousi M, Anttila V, Schulz A, Calafato S, Jakkula E, Riesch E, Myllykangas L, Kalimo H, Topcu M, Gokben S, Alehan F, Lemke JR, Alber M, Palotie A, Kopra O, Lehesjoki AE (2012) Novel mutations consolidate KCTD7 as a progressive myoclonus epilepsy gene. J Med Genet 49:391–399. https://doi.org/10.1136/jmedgenet-2012-100859

Laporte SA, Oakley RH, Zhang J, Holt JA, Ferguson SS, Caron MG, Barak LS (1999) The beta2-adrenergic receptor/betaarrestin complex recruits the clathrin adaptor AP-2 during endocytosis. Proc Natl Acad Sci USA 96:3712–3717. https://doi.org/10.1073/pnas.96.7.3712

Lee MT, Chen CH, Lee CS, Chen CC, Chong MY, Ouyang WC, Chiu NY, Chuo LJ, Chen CY, Tan HK, Lane HY, Chang TJ, Lin CH, Jou SH, Hou YM, Feng J, Lai TJ, Tung CL, Chen TJ, Chang CJ, Lung FW, Chen CK, Shiah IS, Liu CY, Teng PR, Chen KH, Shen LJ, Cheng CS, Chang TP, Li CF, Chou CH, Chen CY, Wang KH, Fann CS, Wu JY, Chen YT, Cheng AT (2011) Genome-wide association study of bipolar I disorder in the Han Chinese population. Mol Psychiatry 16: 548–556. https://doi.org/10.1038/mp.2010.43

Liao Y, Muntean BS (2024) KCTD1 regulation of adenylyl cyclase type 5 adjusts striatal cAMP signaling. Proc Natl Acad Sci USA 121:e2406686121. https://doi.org/10.1073/pnas.2406686121

Lin GN, Corominas R, Lemmens I, Yang X, Tavernier J, Hill DE, Vidal M, Sebat J, Iakoucheva LM (2015) Spatiotemporal 16p11.2 protein network implicates cortical late mid-fetal brain development and KCTD13-Cul3-RhoA pathway in psychiatric diseases. Neuron 85:742–754. https://doi.org/10.1016/j.neuron.2015.01.010

Liu S, Anderson PJ, Rajagopal S, Lefkowitz RJ, Rockman HA (2024) G protein-coupled receptors: a century of research and discovery. Circ Res 135:174–197. https://doi.org/10.1161/CIRCRESAHA.124.323067

Lodowski DT, Pitcher JA, Capel WD, Lefkowitz RJ, Tesmer JJ (2003) Keeping G proteins at bay: a complex between G protein-coupled receptor kinase 2 and Gbetagamma. Science 300:1256–1262. https://doi.org/10.1126/science.1082348

Lohse MJ, Benovic JL, Codina J, Caron MG, Lefkowitz RJ (1990) Beta-Arrestin: a protein that regulates beta-adrenergic receptor function. Science 248:1547–1550. https://doi.org/10.1126/science.2163110

Luttrell LM, Lefkowitz RJ (2002) The role of beta-arrestins in the termination and transduction of G-protein-coupled receptor signals. J Cell Sci 115:455–465. https://doi.org/10.1242/jcs.115.3.455

Luttrell LM, Ferguson SS, Daaka Y, Miller WE, Maudsley S, Della Rocca GJ, Lin F, Kawakatsu H, Owada K, Luttrell DK, Caron MG, Lefkowitz RJ (1999) Beta-arrestin-dependent formation of beta2 adrenergic receptor-Src protein kinase complexes. Science 283:655–661. https://doi.org/10.1126/science.283.5402.655

Masuho I, Balaji S, Muntean BS, Skamangas NK, Chavali S, Tesmer JJG, Babu MM, Martemyanov KA (2020) A global map of G protein signaling regulation by RGS proteins. Cell 183(503–521):e19. https://doi.org/10.1016/j.cell.2020.08.052

Mencacci NE, Rubio-Agusti I, Zdebik A, Asmus F, Ludtmann MH, Ryten M, Plagnol V, Hauser AK, Bandres-Ciga S, Bettencourt C, Forabosco P, Hughes D, Soutar MM, Peall K, Morris HR, Trabzuni D, Tekman M, Stanescu HC, Kleta R, Carecchio M, Zorzi G, Nardocci N, Garavaglia B, Lohmann E, Weissbach A, Klein C, Hardy J, Pittman AM, Foltynie T, Abramov AY, Gasser T, Bhatia KP, Wood NW (2015) A missense mutation in KCTD17 causes autosomal dominant myoclonus-dystonia. Am J Hum Genet 96:938–947. https://doi.org/10.1016/j.ajhg.2015.04.008

Mu C, Liu P, Liu L, Wang Y, Liu K, Li X, Li G, Cheng J, Bu M, Chen H, Tang M, Yao Y, Guan J, Ma T, Zhou Z, Wu Q, Li J, Guo H, Xia K, Hu Z, Peng X, Lang B, Li F, Chen XW, Xu Z, Yuan L (2024) KCTD10 p.C124W variant contributes to schizophrenia by attenuating LLPS-mediated synapse formation. Proc Natl Acad Sci USA 121:e2400464121. https://doi.org/10.1073/pnas.2400464121

Muntean BS, Marwari S, Li X, Sloan DC, Young BD, Wohlschlegel JA, Martemyanov KA (2022) Members of the KCTD family are major regulators of cAMP signaling. Proc Natl Acad Sci USA 119. https://doi.org/10.1073/pnas.2119237119

Nguyen DM, Rath DH, Devost D, Petrin D, Rizk R, Ji AX, Narayanan N, Yong D, Zhai A, Kuntz DA, Mian MUQ, Pomroy NC, Keszei AFA, Benlekbir S, Mazhab-Jafari MT, Rubinstein JL, Hebert TE, Prive GG (2024) Structure and dynamics of a pentameric KCTD5/CUL3/Gbetagamma E3 ubiquitin ligase complex. Proc Natl Acad Sci USA 121:e2315018121. https://doi.org/10.1073/pnas.2315018121

Nieto A, Bailey T, Kaczanowska K, McDonald P (2022) GABA(B) receptor chemistry and pharmacology: agonists, antagonists, and allosteric modulators. Curr Top Behav Neurosci 52: 81–118. https://doi.org/10.1007/7854_2021_232

Northup JK, Sternweis PC, Smigel MD, Schleifer LS, Ross EM, Gilman AG (1980) Purification of the regulatory component of adenylate cyclase. Proc Natl Acad Sci USA 77:6516–6520. https://doi.org/10.1073/pnas.77.11.6516

Perroy J, Adam L, Qanbar R, Chenier S, Bouvier M (2003) Phosphorylation-independent desensitization of GABA(B) receptor by GRK4. EMBO J 22:3816–3824. https://doi.org/10.1093/emboj/cdg383

Pfeiffenberger C, Allada R (2012) Cul3 and the BTB adaptor insomniac are key regulators of sleep homeostasis and a dopamine arousal pathway in drosophila. PLoS Genet 8:e1003003. https://doi.org/10.1371/journal.pgen.1003003

Pinkas DM, Sanvitale CE, Bufton JC, Sorrell FJ, Solcan N, Chalk R, Doutch J, Bullock AN (2017) Structural complexity in the KCTD family of Cullin3-dependent E3 ubiquitin ligases. Biochem J 474:3747–3761. https://doi.org/10.1042/BCJ20170527

Rajagopal S, Rajagopal K, Lefkowitz RJ (2010) Teaching old receptors new tricks: biasing seven-transmembrane receptors. Nat Rev Drug Discov 9:373–386. https://doi.org/10.1038/nrd3024

Raveh A, Cooper A, Guy-David L, Reuveny E (2010) Nonenzymatic rapid control of GIRK channel function by a G protein-coupled receptor kinase. Cell 143:750–760. https://doi.org/10.1016/j.cell.2010.10.018

Ren Y, Liu Y, Zheng S, Luo M (2022) KCTD8 and KCTD12 facilitate axonal expression of GABA (B) receptors in Habenula cholinergic neurons. J Neurosci 42:1648–1665. https://doi.org/10.1523/JNEUROSCI.1676-21.2021

Ross EM, Wilkie TM (2000) GTPase-activating proteins for heterotrimeric G proteins: regulators of G protein signaling (RGS) and RGS-like proteins. Annu Rev Biochem 69:795–827. https://doi.org/10.1146/annurev.biochem.69.1.795

Schwenk J, Metz M, Zolles G, Turecek R, Fritzius T, Bildl W, Tarusawa E, Kulik A, Unger A, Ivankova K, Seddik R, Tiao JY, Rajalu M, Trojanova J, Rohde V, Gassmann M, Schulte U, Fakler B, Bettler B (2010) Native GABA(B) receptors are heteromultimers with a family of auxiliary subunits. Nature 465:231–235. https://doi.org/10.1038/nature08964

Schwenk J, Perez-Garci E, Schneider A, Kollewe A, Gauthier-Kemper A, Fritzius T, Raveh A, Dinamarca MC, Hanuschkin A, Bildl W, Klingauf J, Gassmann M, Schulte U, Bettler B, Fakler B (2016) Modular composition and dynamics of native GABAB receptors identified by high-resolution proteomics. Nat Neurosci 19:233–242. https://doi.org/10.1038/nn.4198

Seddik R, Jungblut SP, Silander OK, Rajalu M, Fritzius T, Besseyrias V, Jacquier V, Fakler B, Gassmann M, Bettler B (2012) Opposite effects of KCTD subunit domains on GABA (B) receptor-mediated desensitization. J Biol Chem 287:39869–39877. https://doi.org/10.1074/jbc.M112.412767

Sereikaite V, Fritzius T, Kasaragod VB, Bader N, Maric HM, Schindelin H, Bettler B, Stromgaard K (2019) Targeting the gamma-aminobutyric acid type B (GABA(B)) receptor complex: development of inhibitors targeting the K(+) channel Tetramerization domain (KCTD) containing proteins/GABA(B) receptor protein-protein interaction. J Med Chem 62:8819–8830. https://doi.org/10.1021/acs.jmedchem.9b01087

Sibille E, Wang Y, Joeyen-Waldorf J, Gaiteri C, Surget A, Oh S, Belzung C, Tseng GC, Lewis DA (2009) A molecular signature of depression in the amygdala. Am J Psychiatry 166:1011–1024. https://doi.org/10.1176/appi.ajp.2009.08121760

Smaldone G, Pirone L, Balasco N, Di Gaetano S, Pedone EM, Vitagliano L (2015) Cullin 3 recognition is not a universal property among KCTD proteins. PLoS One 10:e0126808. https://doi.org/10.1371/journal.pone.0126808

Smith JS, Lefkowitz RJ, Rajagopal S (2018) Biased signalling: from simple switches to allosteric microprocessors. Nat Rev Drug Discov 17:243–260. https://doi.org/10.1038/nrd.2017.229

Smrcka AV (2008) G protein betagamma subunits: central mediators of G protein-coupled receptor signaling. Cell Mol Life Sci 65:2191–2214. https://doi.org/10.1007/s00018-008-8006-5

Stavropoulos N, Young MW (2011) Insomniac and Cullin-3 regulate sleep and wakefulness in drosophila. Neuron 72:964–976. https://doi.org/10.1016/j.neuron.2011.12.003

Sudo Y, Hojo M, Ando Y, Takada M, Murata H, Kurata S, Nishida N, Uezono Y (2012) GABA (B) receptors do not internalize after baclofen treatment, possibly due to a lack of beta-arrestin association: study with a real-time visualizing assay. Synapse 66:759–769. https://doi.org/10.1002/syn.21565

Teng X, Aouacheria A, Lionnard L, Metz KA, Soane L, Kamiya A, Hardwick JM (2019) KCTD: A new gene family involved in neurodevelopmental and neuropsychiatric disorders. CNS Neurosci Ther 25: 887–902. https://doi.org/10.1111/cns.13156

Turecek R, Schwenk J, Fritzius T, Ivankova K, Zolles G, Adelfinger L, Jacquier V, Besseyrias V, Gassmann M, Schulte U, Fakler B, Bettler B (2014) Auxiliary GABAB receptor subunits uncouple G protein betagamma subunits from effector channels to induce desensitization. Neuron 82:1032–1044. https://doi.org/10.1016/j.neuron.2014.04.015

Van Bogaert P (2016) KCTD7-related progressive myoclonus epilepsy. Epileptic Disord 18:115–119. https://doi.org/10.1684/epd.2016.0856

Wacker D, Stevens RC, Roth BL (2017) How ligands illuminate GPCR molecular pharmacology. Cell 170:414–427. https://doi.org/10.1016/j.cell.2017.07.009

Watson N, Linder ME, Druey KM, Kehrl JH, Blumer KJ (1996) RGS family members: GTPase-activating proteins for heterotrimeric G-protein alpha-subunits. Nature 383:172–175. https://doi.org/10.1038/383172a0

Weis WI, Kobilka BK (2018) The molecular basis of G protein-coupled receptor activation. Annu Rev Biochem 87:897–919. https://doi.org/10.1146/annurev-biochem-060614-033910

Wilkie TM, Gilbert DJ, Olsen AS, Chen XN, Amatruda TT, Korenberg JR, Trask BJ, de Jong P, Reed RR, Simon MI et al (1992) Evolution of the mammalian G protein alpha subunit multigene family. Nat Genet 1:85–91. https://doi.org/10.1038/ng0592-85

Wootten D, Christopoulos A, Marti-Solano M, Babu MM, Sexton PM (2018) Mechanisms of signalling and biased agonism in G protein-coupled receptors. Nat Rev Mol Cell Biol 19:638–653. https://doi.org/10.1038/s41580-018-0049-3

Young BD, Sha J, Vashisht AA, Wohlschlegel JA (2021) Human multisubunit E3 ubiquitin ligase required for heterotrimeric G-protein beta-subunit ubiquitination and downstream signaling. J Proteome Res 20:4318–4330. https://doi.org/10.1021/acs.jproteome.1c00292

Zhang J, Tan L, Ren Y, Liang J, Lin R, Feng Q, Zhou J, Hu F, Ren J, Wei C, Yu T, Zhuang Y, Bettler B, Wang F, Luo M (2016) Presynaptic excitation via GABAB receptors in Habenula cholinergic neurons regulates fear memory expression. Cell 166:716–728. https://doi.org/10.1016/j.cell.2016.06.026

Zheng S, Abreu N, Levitz J, Kruse AC (2019) Structural basis for KCTD-mediated rapid desensitization of GABAB signalling. Nature 567:127–131. https://doi.org/10.1038/s41586-019-0990-0

Zimmerman ES, Schulman BA, Zheng N (2010) Structural assembly of cullin-RING ubiquitin ligase complexes. Curr Opin Struct Biol 20:714–721. https://doi.org/10.1016/j.sbi.2010.08.010

Zuo H, Glaaser I, Zhao Y, Kurinov I, Mosyak L, Wang H, Liu J, Park J, Frangaj A, Sturchler E, Zhou M, McDonald P, Geng Y, Slesinger PA, Fan QR (2019) Structural basis for auxiliary subunit KCTD16 regulation of the GABA(B) receptor. Proc Natl Acad Sci USA 116:8370–8379. https://doi.org/10.1073/pnas.1903024116

Part II

The Structural Basis of GPCR Biased Signaling and Ligands

Structural Perspectives on Biased Allostery of GPCR Signaling

Chang Zhao, Siyuan Shen, Chao Wu, Renxuan Luo, Wei Yan, and Zhenhua Shao

Contents

Abstract

G protein-coupled receptors (GPCRs) are highly dynamic membrane receptors with numerous subtypes and complex signal transduction pathways. Precise regulation of GPCR signaling is closely related to disease treatment but presents significant challenges with classical orthosteric ligands. Allosteric modulators, a

Authors Chang Zhao, Siyuan Shen, Chao Wu and Renxuan Luo have equally contributed to this chapter.

C. Zhao · C. Wu · Z. Shao (✉)
Division of Nephrology and Kidney Research Institute, State Key Laboratory of Biotherapy and Cancer Center, West China Hospital, Sichuan University, Chengdu, China

Tianfu Jincheng Laboratory, Chengdu, China
e-mail: zhenhuashao@scu.edu.cn

S. Shen · R. Luo · W. Yan (✉)
Division of Nephrology and Kidney Research Institute, State Key Laboratory of Biotherapy and Cancer Center, West China Hospital, Sichuan University, Chengdu, China
e-mail: weiyan2018@scu.edu.cn

© The Author(s), under exclusive license to Springer Nature Switzerland AG 2025
Z. Li, K. Xiao (eds.), *Pharmacology of GPCRs Biased Signaling and Agonists*, Handbook of Experimental Pharmacology 290, https://doi.org/10.1007/164_2025_767

class of emerging drug candidates, can selectively bind to the allosteric sites located outside the conserved orthosteric pocket. In particular, biased allosteric modulators (BAMs) can stabilize specific conformations of GPCRs to harness signal transduction with high selectivity and specificity, offering a novel approach to modulate GPCR pharmacology and develop safer therapeutic agents. In recent years, significant progress has been made in the study of GPCR allosteric modulation due to advancements in structural biology. However, knowledge about GPCR-biased allostery is still in its infancy. In this chapter, we present the most recent breakthroughs in the discovery of BAM binding site in GPCRs and provide structural insights into biased allostery of GPCR signaling.

Keywords

Allosteric modulator · Biased allostery · Biased signaling · Molecular mechanism · Pharmacology

Abbreviations

GPCRs	G protein-coupled receptors
BAMs	Biased allosteric modulators
NAMs	Negative allosteric modulators
cryo-EM	Cryogenic electron microscopy
TM	Transmembrane
ECL	Extracellular loop
BSA	Buried surface area
GRK2	GPCR kinase 2
NTS	Neurotensin
CUD	Cannabis use disorders
NMR	Nuclear magnetic resonance

1 Introduction

G protein-coupled receptors (GPCRs) constitute the largest family of receptors encoded by the human genome and play a crucial role in mediating a diverse array of biological functions. These receptors exhibit remarkable functional versatility, orchestrating cellular responses by engaging multiple effectors, including G proteins (e.g., Gs/olf, Gi/o, Gq/11, G12/13), β-arrestins, and others (Campbell and Smrcka 2018). Due to their pivotal roles in human physiology and pathology, GPCRs have become prime targets for FDA-approved drugs (Hauser et al. 2017; Isberg et al. 2016; Pandy-Szekeres et al. 2023). To date, a total of 516 approved drugs have been developed against GPCRs, representing 36% of all approved therapeutics and targeting 121 distinct GPCRs (Lorente et al. 2025). Despite the success of GPCR-targeted therapies, only a small fraction of these receptors have synthetic ligands available for clinical use, and many GPCRs still lack highly selective modulators. Most approved GPCR drugs target orthosteric sites, making it difficult to achieve subtype selectivity. Additionally, although extensive research has focused on the mechanism of orthosteric ligand-receptor interaction, managing both off-target and on-target effects remains challenging due to the diverse subtypes and complex signaling pathways of GPCRs (Cheng et al. 2023b). A deeper understanding of these mechanisms is crucial for the development of more selective and effective lead compounds (Hauser et al. 2017; Santos et al. 2017). Notably, allosteric regulation has emerged as a promising strategy to overcome these limitations (Conn et al. 2009; Conn et al. 2014; Foster and Conn 2017; Slosky et al. 2021; Wootten et al. 2013).

Biased signaling, also referred to as functional selectivity or ligand-directed signaling, entails the preferential engagement of specific signaling pathways by ligands, thereby eliciting biased physiological responses (Caroli et al. 2023; Smith et al. 2018; Tan et al. 2018). Biased allosteric modulators (BAMs) are a new category of GPCR ligands that interact with less conserved sites outside the classical orthosteric binding pocket and modulate receptor signaling in a pathway-specific manner (Shen et al. 2024; Slosky et al. 2021; Zhao et al. 2023). This distinctive ability of BAMs to modulate receptor activity opens up possibilities for more precise control of physiological responses. Consequently, BAMs hold promise for the development of safer and more selective therapeutic agents.

BAMs combine the advantages of both allosteric and biased ligands, offering several benefits over classical orthosteric ligands (Conn et al. 2009; Conn et al. 2014). First, BAMs can function synergistically with endogenous agonists, thereby preserving the spatiotemporal dynamics of physiological signaling. Second, BAMs exhibit a ceiling effect, enabling precise modulation of physiological responses in both positive and negative directions and reducing the risk of overdose (Krumm et al. 2023). Third, BAMs exert disproportionate effects on distinct downstream signaling pathways, thereby modifying the receptor's natural output (Ahn et al. 2023; Shen et al. 2024). Fourth, BAMs can selectively modulate specific ligands without uniformly impacting others (Kenakin 2021; Valant et al. 2012). Finally, allosteric modulators facilitate receptor subtype selectivity and provide an opportunity to target "undruggable" GPCRs (Burger et al. 2018).

Allosteric modulation of GPCR signaling has garnered significant interest and has seen substantial progress over recent years (Draper-Joyce et al. 2021; Liu et al. 2017, 2020a; O'Brien et al. 2024). Nevertheless, the field of GPCR-biased allostery remains in its nascent stages. Table 1 provides an overview of some selected BAMs and explores therapeutic applications where ligand bias may confer advantages. Developing allosteric modulators for GPCRs remains challenging, partly due to limitations in detecting allosteric behavior. For instance, negative allosteric modulators (NAMs) may attenuate the binding or activation of an endogenous ligand, resembling a competitor or antagonist. BPTU, initially unrecognized as an allosteric modulator for P2RY1 until the elucidation of its complex structure (PDB code: 4XNV), illustrates this challenge (Zhang et al. 2015). The integration of

Table 1 Overview of selected BAMs

BAMs	Conditions	GPCR Target	Agonist probes	Signaling bias[a]	References
CB-02	Pain	CB1	CP55940	Gi1 > Gi2 > Gz ~ Gob ~ Goa > Gi3 Gi>β-arrestin2	Shen et al. (2024)
CB-05	Pain	CB1	CP55940	Gi1 > Gi2 > Gz Gi>β-arrestin2	Shen et al. (2024)
GAT1601	Anti-glaucoma	CB1	CP55940	Gi>β-arrestin	Garai et al. (2021)
Cmpd-3	Alzheimer's disease, heart failure	α_{1A}AR	Norepinephrine	Gs>Gq	Papay et al. (2023)
Cmpd-6	High blood pressure, heart failure	β1AR	Carvedilol	β-arrestin>Gs	Wang et al. (2021)
Difluorophenyl quinazoline (DFPQ)	Asthma	β2AR	Isoproterenol	β-arrestin>Gs	Ippolito et al. (2023)
ICL1–9	Myocardial infarction, heart failure, cardiac ischemia	β2AR	ICYP	β-arrestin>Gs	Grisanti et al. (2018)
Compound 9n	Inflammation	HCAR2	Niacin, MMF, BHB, MK-6892	Gi>β-arrestin1	Cheng et al. (2023a), Zhao et al. (2023)
SBI-553	Psychostimulant abuse, drug abuse	NTSR1	NTS	β-arrestin>Gq > G15 > Gi	Krumm et al. (2023)
ML314	Addiction, psychiatric disorders	NTSR1	NTS	β-arrestin>Gq/Ca^{2+}	Peddibhotla et al. (2013)
Oxytocin	Pain	κ-opioid receptor	U50488, dynorphin A, morphine	Gi>β-arrestin	Miyano et al. (2021)
Boronic acid 14	Autoimmune disease, cancer, vascular disease, transplant rejection	CXCR3	CXCL11	β-arrestin2>G protein	Bernat et al. (2014)
ATI-2341	HIV, leukeamias	CXCR4	SDF-1	Gi >β-arrestin, GRK2, GRK3≫G13	Quoyer et al. (2013)
AZD8797	Atherosclerosis, metabolic disorders	CX_3CR1	CX_3CL1	β-arrestin>Gi	Cederblad et al. (2016)

PDC113.824	Preterm labor	PGF2α receptor	PGF2α	Gq>G12	Goupil et al. (2010)
AZ1729	Metabolic disorders	FFAR2	C3	Gi>Gq/11	Simonsen (1989)
BMS 986187	Pain, depression	δ-opioid receptor	Leu-enkephalin, SNC80, TAN67	Gi >β-arrestin2	Stanczyk et al. (2019)
COMP	Cardiovascular diseases	AT1R	AngII	β-arrestin2>Gq/Gi	Fu et al. (2021)

[a]The ">" symbol indicates that the BAMs bias signal transduction to the left signaling pathway over the right signaling pathway; The "~" symbol indicates that BAMs have similar effects on signaling pathways on the left and right sides

molecular dynamics simulations, cryogenic electron microscopy (cryo-EM), and artificial intelligence methods provides a synergistic framework to systematically uncover cryptic allosteric sites and accelerate the discovery of BAMs with tailored signaling bias, thereby advancing next-generation GPCR-targeted therapeutics.

2 Structural Basis of Biased Allosteric Modulation of GPCR

Allosteric modulators bind to sites topographically distinct from orthosteric ligands, stabilizing GPCRs in specific conformations and potentially resulting in G protein or β-arrestin signal bias (Slosky et al. 2021; Smith et al. 2018). Recent advances in structural biology have enabled the identification of a growing number of allosteric sites in GPCRs (Pandy-Szekeres et al. 2023), such as those in the dopamine receptor DRD1, cannabinoid receptor CB1, bile acid receptor GPBAR, γ-aminobutyric acid (GABA) receptor $GABA_B$, and adrenergic receptor β_2AR (Liu et al. 2019, 2020b; Shao et al. 2019; Shen et al. 2021; Xiao et al. 2021; Yang et al. 2020, 2022). These allosteric sites, located in various regions of GPCRs, play crucial roles in regulating GPCR signal transduction (Shen et al. 2023; Thal et al. 2018; van der Westhuizen et al. 2020).

However, despite increasing research interest, BAMs have been identified for only a limited subset of GPCRs (Table 1), and the detailed structural basis underlying their biased signaling remains poorly understood. Among these, HCAR2, CB1, and NTSR1 represent pharmacologically and structurally diverse receptors for which biased allosteric modulation has been characterized. HCAR2 is primarily expressed in the peripheral system and contributes to anti-inflammatory and lipid-lowering effects (Blad et al. 2011; Graff et al. 2016; Kang et al. 2024), whereas CB1 and NTSR1 are widely distributed in the central nervous system and are involved in analgesia and attenuation of drug addiction, respectively (Anthony et al. 2020; Slosky et al. 2020). However, the development of orthosteric drugs targeting these receptors has been hampered by undesirable on-target or off-target side effects. For instance, orthosteric agonists targeting CB1 are often associated with addiction and catalepsy (Connor et al. 2021; Nguyen et al. 2017). In contrast, biased allosteric modulation—G protein-biased for HCAR2 and CB1, and β-arrestin-biased for NTSR1—offers a promising strategy for developing safer and more effective therapeutics. These receptors thus serve as model systems for understanding the structural basis of biased allosteric modulation and offer insights for structure-guided drug design.

2.1 G Protein-Biased Allostery

2.1.1 HCAR2

Hydroxycarboxylic acid receptor HCAR2, also known as the niacin receptor, represents a promising target against inflammatory diseases and dyslipidemia. HCAR2 mediates distinct physiological and pathophysiological processes through

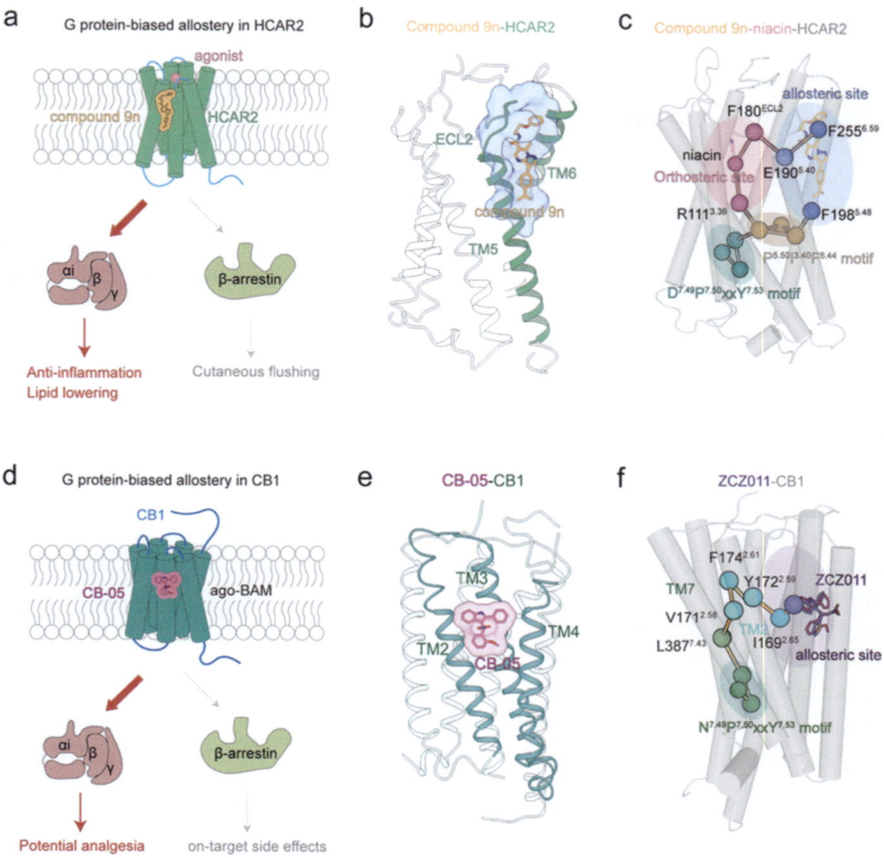

Fig. 1 Structural insights into the G protein-biased allostery in HCAR2 and CB1. (**a**) Schematic diagram of compound 9n-induced HCAR2-Gi-biased signaling and pharmacological effects. (**b**) The allosteric binding site of compound 9n in HCAR2(PDB ID: 8JII). (**c**) The biased allosteric regulation path in the structure of HCAR2. (**d**) Schematic diagram of ago-BAM CB-05-induced CB1-Gi-biased signaling and pharmacological effects. (**e**) The allosteric binding site of CB-05 in CB1 (PDB ID: 8IKH). (**f**) The biased allosteric regulation path in the structure of CB1. The structural figures were prepared with UCSF ChimeraX (Pettersen et al. 2021) and PyMOL (https://pymol.org/2/) software

the activation of Gi protein and β-arrestins. Activation of HCAR2-β-arrestin1 pathway is associated with on-target side effect of cutaneous flushing, which limits patient compliance (Walters et al. 2009). Conversely, the Gi-mediated signaling is required for disease treatment (Chen et al. 2018; Walters et al. 2009) (Fig. 1a). Accordingly, the discovery of Gi-biased ligands targeting HCAR2 is imperative.

Although the Gi-biased orthosteric agonist MK-0354 was developed by Merck & Co. in 2008, it was terminated in Phase II clinical trials, possibly due to the low efficacy and potency (Lai et al. 2008; Semple et al. 2008). Recently, compound 9n has been identified as a potent Gi-BAM of HCAR2, showing great potential in anti-inflammatory pharmacology (Cheng et al. 2023a; Zhao et al. 2023). Compound 9n preferentially augments the Gi signaling pathway over β-arrestin recruitment, either when cooperating with diverse orthosteric agonists or acting alone (Cheng et al. 2023a; Zhao et al. 2023) (Fig. 1a).

To gain insights into the molecular details of compound 9n, the structures of HCAR2-Gi signaling complex bound to compound 9n alone, to niacin, and to compound 9n together with niacin simultaneously were determined (Mao et al. 2023; Zhao et al. 2023). Structural analysis revealed that compound 9n is exposed to a lipidic environment and situated in the extracellular cleft formed by TM5, TM6, and ECL2 (Mao et al. 2023; Zhao et al. 2023), covering approximately 390 $Å^2$ of the buried surface area (BSA) (Fig. 1b). Compound 9n appears to mediate biased signaling through a dual allosteric regulatory pathway.

Firstly, compound 9n drives the allosteric sites toward the orthosteric site through direct contacts (Fig. 1c), thereby reshaping the orthosteric site and agonist-receptor contact network. In particular, $F180^{ECL2}$ in the orthosteric site functions as a transmitter, conveying the biased signal from the $F255^{6.59}$-$E190^{5.40}$ site to $R111^{3.36}$ (Fig. 1c), a key residue responsible for ligand recognition and Gi recruitment. This interaction triggers the rearrangement of the $P^{5.50}I^{3.40}F^{6.44}$ motif, a critical microswitch in the connector region regulating G protein signaling (Cheng et al. 2023b; Latorraca et al. 2017).

Additionally, the isopropylbenzene group of compound 9n extends into a shallow pocket and interacts with $F198^{5.48}$, an aromatic residue adjacent to the $P^{5.50}I^{3.40}F^{6.44}$ motif (Fig. 1c). Mutagenesis studies revealed that $F198^{5.48}$ significantly contributes to Gi-biased signaling. The downstream $D^{7.49}P^{7.50}xxY^{7.53}$ motif, together with the allosteric site, orthosteric site and PIF motif, constitute a finely tuned network for biased allostery (Fig. 1c). Compared to the BAM-free HCAR2-Gi complex, the binding of compound 9n leads to an increase in the total BSA between HCAR2 and Gi from 871.7 $Å^2$ to 912.2 $Å^2$, thus contributing to Gi-biased signaling transduction.

2.1.2 CB1

The opioid crisis and the increasing prevalence of chronic pain have sparked an urgent need for non-opioid analgesics (Volkow and McLellan 2016). Marijuana from the plant *Cannabis sativa L* has been used for pain relief dating back to ancient China (Pain 2015) and is also the third commonly used psychoactive drug globally (Lemberger 1980; Tan et al. 2018). The cannabinoid receptor CB1, one of the most highly expressed GPCRs in the central nervous system, is involved in various physiological functions such as pain, memory, cognition, and motor coordination (Anthony et al. 2020; Elliott et al. 2020; Schulz et al. 2021; van den Hoogen et al. 2021). Previous studies have shown that plant-derived cannabinoids such as Δ9-THC and synthetic cannabinoids (CP55940 and WIN55212–2) exhibit analgesic activity in preclinical pain models (Alves et al. 2020; Banister et al. 2019; Fagan and Campbell 2014; Maldonado et al. 2016; Pryce and Baker 2012). Unfortunately, these effective analgesic ligands targeting the CB1 orthosteric site often induce undesirable cannabimimetic effects, including addiction, catalepsy, hypothermia, cardiovascular diseases, and memory impairment, limiting their clinical application

(Cooper and Haney 2009; Hampson and Deadwyler 2000; Hutcheson et al. 1998; Justinova et al. 2003; Moreno-Rius 2019; Thomas et al. 2014; Wei et al. 2022).

The discovery of the endogenous allosteric ligand LXA4 for CB1 in 2012 opened the door to the development of allosteric modulators (Pamplona et al. 2012). Since then, numerous CB1 allosteric modulators have been identified, providing new strategies for selectively modulating receptor activity. For instance, ZCZ011 have shown analgesic property (Ignatowska-Jankowska et al. 2015; Slivicki et al. 2018; Tseng et al. 2019). However, as a balanced allosteric modulator, ZCZ011 can simultaneously activate G protein pathways and β-arrestin signaling pathways of CB1 (Shen et al. 2024; Yang et al. 2022). Studies suggest that selectively activating the G protein pathway of the CB1 receptor while inhibiting β-arrestin signaling has better analgesic effects with fewer side effects (Nguyen et al. 2012). Recent clinical data emphasize the therapeutic effects of the allosteric modulator AEF0117 in treating cannabis use disorders (CUD) by selectively inhibiting β-arrestin signaling via the CB1 receptor (Haney et al. 2023). Therefore, the design of G protein-biased allosteric drugs targeting CB1 allosteric sites offers the potential for the development of novel analgesics with long-lasting efficacy and fewer side effects (Fig. 1d).

Shen et al. conducted structure-based design to identify G protein-biased ago-PAMs (agonist-BAMs) (Shen et al. 2024) (Fig. 1e). CB-02 and CB-05 were identified to have specific effects on the G protein pathway. Subsequently, they determined the cryo-EM structures of the CB1-Gi1 complex bound with ago-BAMs CB-02 or CB-05, respectively. Through pharmacological analysis and molecular dynamics simulations, they deciphered the molecular determinants of CB1-mediated G protein and β-arrestin2 signaling responses to ago-PAMs. Structural analysis revealed that $I245^{4.54}$ in TM4 of CB1 are key residues involved in G protein signal transduction (Shen et al. 2024).

Additionally, they identified key residues involved in β-arrestin signaling. In detail, the methyl group of ago-PAM ZCZ011 induces significant conformational changes, affecting residues like $I169^{2.65}$, $F170^{2.57}$, $F174^{2.61}$, and $Y172^{2.59}$, resulting in a large displacement of TM2 (Fig. 1f). Notably, $V171^{2.58}$ in TM2 and $L387^{7.43}$ in TM7 show slight movements due to van der Waals interaction. The conformational change in TM7 caused by $L387^{7.43}$ is linked to the $N^{7.49}P^{7.50}xxY^{7.53}$ motif and participates in the signaling transmission of β-arrestin signaling (Fig. 1f), consistent with previous studies on TM7 in 5-HT2BR, β1AR, or NTSR1, which play important roles in β-arrestin recruitment (Cao et al. 2022; Huang et al. 2020; Lee et al. 2020).

2.2 β-Arrestin-Biased Allostery

2.2.1 NTSR1

In addition to G protein-biased allostery, some allosteric modulators can also induce β-arrestin-biased signaling. SBI-553 has been identified as a β-arrestin-BAM of neurotensin receptor NTSR1, selectively promoting GPCR kinase 2 (GRK2) recruitment and subsequent β-arrestin signaling, while antagonizing a broad spectrum of G protein (Gq > G15 > Gi) signaling stimulated by the endogenous agonist

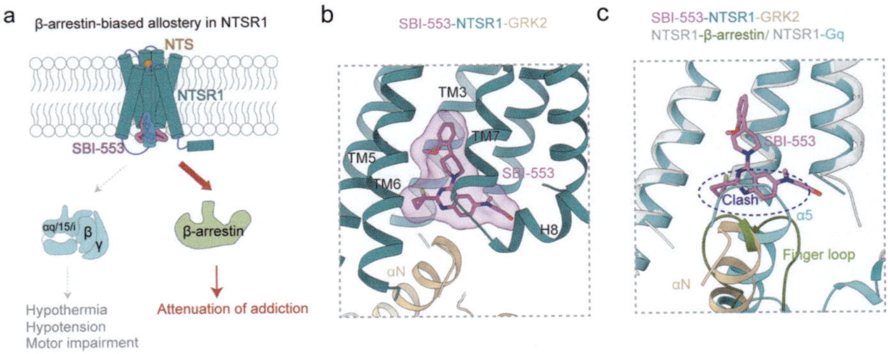

Fig. 2 Structural insights into the β-arrestin-biased allostery in NTSR1. (**a**) Schematic diagram of SBI-553-induced NTSR1-β-arrestin-biased signaling and pharmacological effects. (**b**) The allosteric binding site of SBI-553 in NTSR1-GRK2 complex (PDB ID: 8jpb). SBI-553 contacts both NTSR1 and GRK2. (**c**) Structural superposition of SBI-553-NTSR1-GRK2 (PDB ID: 8jpb) with NTSR1-β-arrestin (PDB ID: 6up7) and NTSR1-Gq (PDB ID: 8fmz). The superposition was based on the NTSR1 receptor. The structural figures were prepared with UCSF ChimeraX software (Pettersen et al. 2021)

neurotensin (NTS) (Krumm et al. 2023; Slosky et al. 2020) (Fig. 2a). Pharmacologically, SBI-553 shows promise in treating psychostimulant addictions without inducing typical G-protein-mediated adverse effects such as hypothermia, hypotension, and motor impairment (Fig. 2a).

To elucidate the structural basis of BAM activity, Krumm et al. and Duan et al. independently identified the binding site of SBI-553 in NTSR1 by using single-particle cryo-EM method (Duan et al. 2023; Krumm et al. 2023). Unlike the binding mode of compound 9n in HCAR2 or CB-02 in CB1, SBI-553 inserts into the cytoplasmic pocket of NTSR1 formed by TM2, TM3, TM5, TM6, TM7, and H8 (Duan et al. 2023; Krumm et al. 2023) (Fig. 2b). Besides, SBI-553 directly engages with the N terminal α-helix (αN) of GRK2, thereby stabilizing the active state of both the receptor and GRK2 transducer (Fig. 2b). Structural superposition of the SBI-553-bound NTSR1-GRK2 complex with the NTSR1-β-arrestin and NTSR1-Gq complexes reveals that SBI-553 is spatially compatible with the finger loop of β-arrestin but sterically clash with the α5 helix of Gαq (Fig. 2c). These structural insights provide a direct explanation for the β-arrestin-biased allosteric modulation property of SBI-553.

3 Conclusions

BAMs represent a promising new class of GPCR-targeting ligands that combine the pathway specificity of biased agonists with the spatial selectivity of allosteric modulators. The structural perspectives on biased allostery of GPCR signaling constitute a pivotal area of research that has garnered significant attention in recent years (Shen et al. 2023; Thal et al. 2018). In this section, we summarized several representative receptor systems—HCAR2, CB1, and NTSR1—highlighting their distinct but converging mechanisms of biased allosteric regulation.

Although these BAMs act on different receptors and binding sites, they consistently stabilize receptor conformations that preferentially engage specific intracellular effectors while disfavoring others. For instance, in both HCAR2 and CB1, Gi-BAMs binds within inter-helical crevices located at the receptor-lipid interface, facilitating subtle yet functionally decisive conformational shifts. The biased modulation frequently involves allosteric networks that bridge orthosteric binding pockets, key activation motifs, and intracellular effector coupling regions, effectively redirecting receptor signaling output. In contrast, the β-arrestin-BAM SBI-553 targeting NTSR1 functions more like molecular glue, simultaneously engaging the receptor and intracellular effectors such as β-arrestin or GRKs while preventing G proteins coupling. Interestingly, a similar mechanism has been observed in parathyroid hormone 1 receptor (PTH1R), where the Gs-biased agonist PCO371 binds at the receptor-G protein interface to selectively induce G protein signaling while blocking β-arrestin engagement (Kobayashi et al. 2023). These examples underscore the emerging strategy of designing BAMs that target receptor-transducer interfaces to achieve signaling bias.

The discovery and mechanistic elucidation of these allosteric sites offer a structural and conceptual foundation for rational BAM drug design. As technological advances deepen our understanding of receptor dynamics and signaling selectivity, BAMs hold significant promise for precision therapeutics that maximize efficacy and minimize side effects.

4 Current Research Gaps and Future Directions

Despite the advances discussed above, several critical gaps remain in harnessing GPCR-biased allostery for drug discovery.

(1) Challenges in allosteric site identification

Allosteric sites are typically diverse, often buried in lipid-exposed regions of receptors, making them difficult to identify. Differentiating electron densities corresponding to small-molecule modulators from those of surrounding lipids and accurately determining the ligand conformation remain significant challenges. Furthermore, currently available BAM-bound GPCR structures are limited to class A and class B receptors, thereby constraining our comprehensive understanding of allosteric modulation across the GPCR superfamily. Additionally, structural techniques typically capture static snapshots, limiting insight into transient or metastable allosteric pockets. Emerging computational approaches offer promise in this area. For example, a residue-intuitive hybrid machine learning (RHML) model coupled with molecular dynamics (MD) simulation pipeline has been developed to mine large conformational ensembles and identify transient allosteric pockets and key residues of GPCRs (Chen et al. 2024). Using such a pipeline, a novel allosteric site on β2-adrenergic receptor (β2AR) was identified, enabling virtual screening of potential BAM ZINC5042 with biased negative modulation properties (Chen et al. 2024).

(2) The complexity of GPCR signaling pathways

Traditionally, GPCR signaling has been categorized into G protein-dependent and β-arrestin-dependent pathways. However, accumulating evidence suggests that these pathways are interconnected and can influence each other's activity (Jean-Charles et al. 2017; Tilley 2011). As research delves deeper into GPCR signal transduction, it becomes evident that GPCRs possess complex signaling networks. GPCRs can activate different subtypes of heterotrimeric G proteins, including Gs, Gi/o, Gq/11, and G12/13 (Syrovatkina et al. 2016). Each G protein subtype comprises various isoforms with distinct signaling properties (Kamato et al. 2015). GPCRs interact with multiple signaling pathways simultaneously, leading to intricate crosstalk and feedback mechanisms within cellular signaling networks. An increasing number of studies are focusing on the impact of biased allosteric compounds on different subtypes of G protein signaling (Che and Roth 2023). Disentangling the specific contributions of biased signaling pathways amidst this complexity presents a significant challenge. Future research must employ systems biology approaches to comprehensively characterize the interconnectedness of signaling pathways and elucidate the functional consequences of biased signaling events within the broader cellular context.

(3) Need for in vivo validation and clinical translation

While many BAMs show promise in vitro or in preclinical models, few have progressed to clinical trials. Bridging this gap will require optimization of pharmacokinetic and safety profiles, better animal models, and rigorous in vivo validation of signaling bias. While structural and computational methods have greatly enhanced our mechanistic understanding, verifying biased signaling events in physiologically relevant systems remains difficult. Future research must prioritize the development of robust in vivo assays and experimental platforms to validate computational predictions and translate findings into therapeutic applications. Advancements in structural biology, pharmacology, live-cell imaging, nuclear magnetic resonance (NMR), computational modeling, and translational medicine will be critical to this effort (Morales-Pastor et al. 2022; Thal et al. 2018). High-resolution structural elucidation can reveal molecular mechanisms underlying biased signaling, while advanced imaging techniques help uncover context-dependent effects in live systems. Computational modeling, in turn, enable the prediction of BAM-induced GPCR dynamics. Through a multidisciplinary approach, new strategies and insights will emerge for developing biased allosteric drugs targeting GPCRs.

Acknowledgments The authors were supported by the Ministry of Technology Department of China grant (2024YFA1107500 to Z.S.), the National Natural Science Foundation of China (T2221004 to Z.S., 32371288 to W.Y., 323B2038 to C.Z., and 823B2101 to C.W.), Frontiers Medical Center, Tianfu Jincheng Laboratory Foundation (TFJC2023010010 to Z.S., 2025ZH021 to C.Z., 2025ZH039 to C.W.), 1.3.5 Project for Disciplines of Excellence, West China Hospital, Sichuan University (ZYYC23022 to Z.S.), the China Postdoctoral Science Foundation (2023 M732474 and GZB20230480 to S.S.), and Science and Technology Department of Sichuan Province (2024NSFJQ0052 to Z.S. and 24NSFSC5396 to S.S.).

Competing Interests The authors have no conflicts of interest to declare that are relevant to the content of this chapter.

References

Ahn S, Maarsingh H, Walker JK, Liu S, Hegde A, Sumajit HC, Kahsai AW, Lefkowitz RJ (2023) Allosteric modulator potentiates beta2AR agonist-promoted bronchoprotection in asthma models. J Clin Invest 133. https://doi.org/10.1172/JCI167337

Alves P, Amaral C, Teixeira N, Correia-da-Silva G (2020) Cannabis sativa: much more beyond Delta(9)-tetrahydrocannabinol. Pharmacol Res 157:104822. https://doi.org/10.1016/j.phrs.2020.104822

Anthony AT, Rahmat S, Sangle P, Sandhu O, Khan S (2020) Cannabinoid receptors and their relationship with chronic Pain: a narrative review. Cureus 12:e10436. https://doi.org/10.7759/cureus.10436

Banister SD, Krishna Kumar K, Kumar V, Kobilka BK, Malhotra SV (2019) Selective modulation of the cannabinoid type 1 (CB(1)) receptor as an emerging platform for the treatment of neuropathic pain. Medchemcomm 10:647–659. https://doi.org/10.1039/c8md00595h

Bernat V, Admas TH, Brox R, Heinemann FW, Tschammer N (2014) Boronic acids as probes for investigation of allosteric modulation of the chemokine receptor CXCR3. ACS Chem Biol 9: 2664–2677. https://doi.org/10.1021/cb500678c

Blad CC, Ahmed K, AP IJ Offermanns S (2011) Biological and pharmacological roles of HCA receptors. Adv Pharmacol 62:219–250. https://doi.org/10.1016/B978-0-12-385952-5.00005-1

Burger WAC, Sexton PM, Christopoulos A, Thal DM (2018) Toward an understanding of the structural basis of allostery in muscarinic acetylcholine receptors. J Gen Physiol 150:1360–1372. https://doi.org/10.1085/jgp.201711979

Campbell AP, Smrcka AV (2018) Targeting G protein-coupled receptor signalling by blocking G proteins. Nat Rev Drug Discov 17:789–803. https://doi.org/10.1038/nrd.2018.135

Cao C, Barros-Alvarez X, Zhang S, Kim K, Damgen MA, Panova O, Suomivuori CM, Fay JF, Zhong X, Krumm BE, Gumpper RH, Seven AB, Robertson MJ, Krogan NJ, Huttenhain R, Nichols DE, Dror RO, Skiniotis G, Roth BL (2022) Signaling snapshots of a serotonin receptor activated by the prototypical psychedelic LSD. Neuron 110:3154–3167 e7. https://doi.org/10.1016/j.neuron.2022.08.006

Caroli J, Mamyrbekov A, Harpsoe K, Gardizi S, Dorries L, Ghosh E, Hauser AS, Kooistra AJ, Gloriam DE (2023) A community biased signaling atlas. Nat Chem Biol 19:531–535. https://doi.org/10.1038/s41589-023-01292-8

Cederblad L, Rosengren B, Ryberg E, Hermansson NO (2016) AZD8797 is an allosteric non-competitive modulator of the human CX3CR1 receptor. Biochem J 473:641–649. https://doi.org/10.1042/BJ20150520

Che T, Roth BL (2023) Molecular basis of opioid receptor signaling. Cell 186:5203–5219. https://doi.org/10.1016/j.cell.2023.10.029

Chen Y, Ouyang X, Hoque R, Garcia-Martinez I, Yousaf MN, Tonack S, Offermanns S, Dubuquoy L, Louvet A, Mathurin P, Massey V, Schnabl B, Bataller RA, Mehal WZ (2018)

Beta-Hydroxybutyrate protects from alcohol-induced liver injury via a Hcar2-cAMP dependent pathway. J Hepatol 69:687–696. https://doi.org/10.1016/j.jhep.2018.04.004

Chen X, Wang K, Chen J, Wu C, Mao J, Song Y, Liu Y, Shao Z, Pu X (2024) Integrative residue-intuitive machine learning and MD Approach to Unveil Allosteric Site and Mechanism for beta2AR. Nat Commun 15:8130. https://doi.org/10.1038/s41467-024-52399-y

Cheng L, Sun S, Wang H, Zhao C, Tian X, Liu Y, Fu P, Shao Z, Chai R, Yan W (2023a) Orthosteric ligand selectivity and allosteric probe dependence at Hydroxycarboxylic acid receptor HCAR2. Signal Transduct Target Ther 8:364. https://doi.org/10.1038/s41392-023-01625-y

Cheng L, Xia F, Li Z, Shen C, Yang Z, Hou H, Sun S, Feng Y, Yong X, Tian X, Qin H, Yan W, Shao Z (2023b) Structure, function and drug discovery of GPCR signaling. Mol Biomed 4:46. https://doi.org/10.1186/s43556-023-00156-w

Conn PJ, Christopoulos A, Lindsley CW (2009) Allosteric modulators of GPCRs: a novel approach for the treatment of CNS disorders. Nat Rev Drug Discov 8:41–54. https://doi.org/10.1038/nrd2760

Conn PJ, Lindsley CW, Meiler J, Niswender CM (2014) Opportunities and challenges in the discovery of allosteric modulators of GPCRs for treating CNS disorders. Nat Rev Drug Discov 13:692–708. https://doi.org/10.1038/nrd4308

Connor JP, Stjepanovic D, Le Foll B, Hoch E, Budney AJ, Hall WD (2021) Cannabis use and cannabis use disorder. Nat Rev Dis Primers 7:16. https://doi.org/10.1038/s41572-021-00247-4

Cooper ZD, Haney M (2009) Actions of delta-9-tetrahydrocannabinol in cannabis: relation to use, abuse, dependence. Int Rev Psychiatry 21:104–112. https://doi.org/10.1080/09540260902782752

Draper-Joyce CJ, Bhola R, Wang J, Bhattarai A, Nguyen ATN, Cowie-Kent I, O'Sullivan K, Chia LY, Venugopal H, Valant C, Thal DM, Wootten D, Panel N, Carlsson J, Christie MJ, White PJ, Scammells P, May LT, Sexton PM, Danev R, Miao Y, Glukhova A, Imlach WL, Christopoulos A (2021) Positive allosteric mechanisms of adenosine A(1) receptor-mediated analgesia. Nature 597:571–576. https://doi.org/10.1038/s41586-021-03897-2

Duan J, Liu H, Zhao F, Yuan Q, Ji Y, Cai X, He X, Li X, Li J, Wu K, Gao T, Zhu S, Lin S, Wang MW, Cheng X, Yin W, Jiang Y, Yang D, Xu HE (2023) GPCR activation and GRK2 assembly by a biased intracellular agonist. Nature 620:676–681. https://doi.org/10.1038/s41586-023-06395-9

Elliott J, DeJean D, Clifford T, Coyle D, Potter BK, Skidmore B, Alexander C, Repetski AE, Shukla V, McCoy B, Wells GA (2020) Cannabis-based products for pediatric epilepsy: an updated systematic review. Seizure 75:18–22. https://doi.org/10.1016/j.seizure.2019.12.006

Fagan SG, Campbell VA (2014) The influence of cannabinoids on generic traits of neurodegeneration. Br J Pharmacol 171:1347–1360. https://doi.org/10.1111/bph.12492

Foster DJ, Conn PJ (2017) Allosteric modulation of GPCRs: new insights and potential utility for treatment of schizophrenia and other CNS disorders. Neuron 94:431–446. https://doi.org/10.1016/j.neuron.2017.03.016

Fu Y, Huang Y, Yang Z, Chen Y, Zheng J, Mao C, Li Z, Liu Z, Yu B, Li T, Wang M, Xu C, Zhou Y, Zhao G, Jia Y, Guo W, Jia X, Zhang T, Li L, Liu Z, Guo S, Ma M, Zhang H, Liu B, Du J, Wang W, Tang C, Gao P, Xu Q, Wang X, Liu J, Sun J, Kong W (2021) Cartilage oligomeric matrix protein is an endogenous beta-arrestin-2-selective allosteric modulator of AT1 receptor counteracting vascular injury. Cell Res 31:773–790. https://doi.org/10.1038/s41422-020-00464-8

Garai S, Leo LM, Szczesniak AM, Hurst DP, Schaffer PC, Zagzoog A, Black T, Deschamps JR, Miess E, Schulz S, Janero DR, Straiker A, Pertwee RG, Abood ME, Kelly MEM, Reggio PH, Laprairie RB, Thakur GA (2021) Discovery of a biased allosteric modulator for cannabinoid 1 receptor: preclinical anti-glaucoma efficacy. J Med Chem 64:8104–8126. https://doi.org/10.1021/acs.jmedchem.1c00040

Goupil E, Tassy D, Bourguet C, Quiniou C, Wisehart V, Petrin D, Le Gouill C, Devost D, Zingg HH, Bouvier M, Saragovi HU, Chemtob S, Lubell WD, Claing A, Hebert TE, Laporte SA (2010) A novel biased allosteric compound inhibitor of parturition selectively impedes the prostaglandin F2alpha-mediated rho/ROCK signaling pathway. J Biol Chem 285:25624–25636. https://doi.org/10.1074/jbc.M110.115196

Graff EC, Fang H, Wanders D, Judd RL (2016) Anti-inflammatory effects of the hydroxycarboxylic acid receptor 2. Metabolism 65:102–113. https://doi.org/10.1016/j.metabol.2015.10.001

Grisanti LA, Thomas TP, Carter RL, de Lucia C, Gao E, Koch WJ, Benovic JL, Tilley DG (2018) Pepducin-mediated cardioprotection via beta-arrestin-biased beta2-adrenergic receptor-specific signaling. Theranostics 8:4664–4678. https://doi.org/10.7150/thno.26619

Hampson RE, Deadwyler SA (2000) Cannabinoids reveal the necessity of hippocampal neural encoding for short-term memory in rats. J Neurosci 20:8932–8942. https://doi.org/10.1523/JNEUROSCI.20-23-08932.2000

Haney M, Vallee M, Fabre S, Collins Reed S, Zanese M, Campistron G, Arout CA, Foltin RW, Cooper ZD, Kearney-Ramos T, Metna M, Justinova Z, Schindler C, Hebert-Chatelain E, Bellocchio L, Cathala A, Bari A, Serrat R, Finlay DB, Caraci F, Redon B, Martin-Garcia E, Busquets-Garcia A, Matias I, Levin FR, Felpin FX, Simon N, Cota D, Spampinato U, Maldonado R, Shaham Y, Glass M, Thomsen LL, Mengel H, Marsicano G, Monlezun S, Revest JM, Piazza PV (2023) Signaling-specific inhibition of the CB(1) receptor for cannabis use disorder: phase 1 and phase 2a randomized trials. Nat Med 29:1487–1499. https://doi.org/10.1038/s41591-023-02381-w

Hauser AS, Attwood MM, Rask-Andersen M, Schioth HB, Gloriam DE (2017) Trends in GPCR drug discovery: new agents, targets and indications. Nat Rev Drug Discov 16:829–842. https://doi.org/10.1038/nrd.2017.178

Huang W, Masureel M, Qu Q, Janetzko J, Inoue A, Kato HE, Robertson MJ, Nguyen KC, Glenn JS, Skiniotis G, Kobilka BK (2020) Structure of the neurotensin receptor 1 in complex with beta-arrestin 1. Nature 579:303–308. https://doi.org/10.1038/s41586-020-1953-1

Hutcheson DM, Tzavara ET, Smadja C, Valjent E, Roques BP, Hanoune J, Maldonado R (1998) Behavioural and biochemical evidence for signs of abstinence in mice chronically treated with delta-9-tetrahydrocannabinol. Br J Pharmacol 125:1567–1577. https://doi.org/10.1038/sj.bjp.0702228

Ignatowska-Jankowska BM, Baillie GL, Kinsey S, Crowe M, Ghosh S, Owens RA, Damaj IM, Poklis J, Wiley JL, Zanda M, Zanato C, Greig IR, Lichtman AH, Ross RA (2015) A cannabinoid CB1 receptor-positive allosteric modulator reduces neuropathic Pain in the mouse with no psychoactive effects. Neuropsychopharmacology 40:2948–2959. https://doi.org/10.1038/npp.2015.148

Ippolito M, De Pascali F, Hopfinger N, Komolov KE, Laurinavichyute D, Reddy PAN, Sakkal LA, Rajkowski KZ, Nayak AP, Lee J, Lee J, Cao G, Donover PS, Reichman M, An SS, Salvino JM, Penn RB, Armen RS, Scott CP, Benovic JL (2023) Identification of a beta-arrestin-biased negative allosteric modulator for the beta(2)-adrenergic receptor. Proc Natl Acad Sci USA 120:e2302668120. https://doi.org/10.1073/pnas.2302668120

Isberg V, Mordalski S, Munk C, Rataj K, Harpsoe K, Hauser AS, Vroling B, Bojarski AJ, Vriend G, Gloriam DE (2016) GPCRdb: an information system for G protein-coupled receptors. Nucleic Acids Res 44:D356–D364. https://doi.org/10.1093/nar/gkv1178

Jean-Charles PY, Kaur S, Shenoy SK (2017) G protein-coupled receptor signaling through beta-Arrestin-dependent mechanisms. J Cardiovasc Pharmacol 70:142–158. https://doi.org/10.1097/FJC.0000000000000482

Justinova Z, Tanda G, Redhi GH, Goldberg SR (2003) Self-administration of delta9-tetrahydrocannabinol (THC) by drug naive squirrel monkeys. Psychopharmacology 169:135–140. https://doi.org/10.1007/s00213-003-1484-0

Kamato D, Thach L, Bernard R, Chan V, Zheng W, Kaur H, Brimble M, Osman N, Little PJ (2015) Structure, function, pharmacology, and therapeutic potential of the G protein, Galpha/q,11. Front Cardiovasc Med 2:14. https://doi.org/10.3389/fcvm.2015.00014

Kang HJ, Krumm BE, Tassou A, Geron M, DiBerto JF, Kapolka NJ, Gumpper RH, Sakamoto K, Dewran Kocak D, Olsen RHJ, Huang XP, Zhang S, Huang KL, Zaidi SA, Nguyen MT, Jo MJ, Katritch V, Fay JF, Scherrer G, Roth BL (2024) Structure-guided design of a peripherally restricted chemogenetic system. Cell 187:7433–7449 e20. https://doi.org/10.1016/j.cell.2024.11.001

Kenakin T (2021) Biased signaling as allosteric probe dependence. Cell Signal 79:109844. https://doi.org/10.1016/j.cellsig.2020.109844

Kobayashi K, Kawakami K, Kusakizako T, Tomita A, Nishimura M, Sawada K, Okamoto HH, Hiratsuka S, Nakamura G, Kuwabara R, Noda H, Muramatsu H, Shimizu M, Taguchi T, Inoue A, Murata T, Nureki O (2023) Class B1 GPCR activation by an intracellular agonist. Nature 618:1085–1093. https://doi.org/10.1038/s41586-023-06169-3

Krumm BE, DiBerto JF, Olsen RHJ, Kang HJ, Slocum ST, Zhang S, Strachan RT, Huang XP, Slosky LM, Pinkerton AB, Barak LS, Caron MG, Kenakin T, Fay JF, Roth BL (2023) Neurotensin receptor Allosterism revealed in complex with a biased allosteric modulator. Biochemistry 62:1233–1248. https://doi.org/10.1021/acs.biochem.3c00029

Lai E, Waters MG, Tata JR, Radziszewski W, Perevozskaya I, Zheng W, Wenning L, Connolly DT, Semple G, Johnson-Levonas AO, Wagner JA, Mitchel Y, Paolini JF (2008) Effects of a niacin receptor partial agonist, MK-0354, on plasma free fatty acids, lipids, and cutaneous flushing in humans. J Clin Lipidol 2:375–383. https://doi.org/10.1016/j.jacl.2008.08.445

Latorraca NR, Venkatakrishnan AJ, Dror RO (2017) GPCR dynamics: structures in motion. Chem Rev 117:139–155. https://doi.org/10.1021/acs.chemrev.6b00177

Lee Y, Warne T, Nehme R, Pandey S, Dwivedi-Agnihotri H, Chaturvedi M, Edwards PC, Garcia-Nafria J, Leslie AGW, Shukla AK, Tate CG (2020) Molecular basis of beta-arrestin coupling to formoterol-bound beta(1)-adrenoceptor. Nature 583:862–866. https://doi.org/10.1038/s41586-020-2419-1

Lemberger L (1980) Potential therapeutic usefulness of marijuana. Annu Rev Pharmacol Toxicol 20:151–172. https://doi.org/10.1146/annurev.pa.20.040180.001055

Liu J, Zhang Z, Moreno-Delgado D, Dalton JA, Rovira X, Trapero A, Goudet C, Llebaria A, Giraldo J, Yuan Q, Rondard P, Huang S, Liu J, Pin JP (2017) Allosteric control of an asymmetric transduction in a G protein-coupled receptor heterodimer. elife 6. https://doi.org/10.7554/eLife.26985

Liu X, Masoudi A, Kahsai AW, Huang LY, Pani B, Staus DP, Shim PJ, Hirata K, Simhal RK, Schwalb AM, Rambarat PK, Ahn S, Lefkowitz RJ, Kobilka B (2019) Mechanism of beta(2)AR regulation by an intracellular positive allosteric modulator. Science 364:1283–1287. https://doi.org/10.1126/science.aaw8981

Liu H, Yi P, Zhao W, Wu Y, Acher F, Pin JP, Liu J, Rondard P (2020a) Illuminating the allosteric modulation of the calcium-sensing receptor. Proc Natl Acad Sci USA 117:21711–21722. https://doi.org/10.1073/pnas.1922231117

Liu X, Kaindl J, Korczynska M, Stossel A, Dengler D, Stanek M, Hubner H, Clark MJ, Mahoney J, Matt RA, Xu X, Hirata K, Shoichet BK, Sunahara RK, Kobilka BK, Gmeiner P (2020b) An allosteric modulator binds to a conformational hub in the beta(2) adrenergic receptor. Nat Chem Biol 16:749–755. https://doi.org/10.1038/s41589-020-0549-2

Lorente JS, Sokolov AV, Ferguson G, Schioth HB, Hauser AS, Gloriam DE (2025) GPCR drug discovery: new agents, targets and indications. Nat Rev Drug Discov 24. https://doi.org/10.1038/s41573-025-01139-y

Maldonado R, Banos JE, Cabanero D (2016) The endocannabinoid system and neuropathic pain. Pain 157(Suppl 1):S23–S32. https://doi.org/10.1097/j.pain.0000000000000428

Mao C, Gao M, Zang SK, Zhu Y, Shen DD, Chen LN, Yang L, Wang Z, Zhang H, Wang WW, Shen Q, Lu Y, Ma X, Zhang Y (2023) Orthosteric and allosteric modulation of human HCAR2 signaling complex. Nat Commun 14:7620. https://doi.org/10.1038/s41467-023-43537-z

Miyano K, Yoshida Y, Hirayama S, Takahashi H, Ono H, Meguro Y, Manabe S, Komatsu A, Nonaka M, Mizuguchi T, Fujii H, Higami Y, Narita M, Uezono Y (2021) Oxytocin is a positive allosteric modulator of kappa-opioid receptors but not delta-opioid receptors in the G protein signaling pathway. Cells 10. https://doi.org/10.3390/cells10102651

Morales-Pastor A, Nerin-Fonz F, Aranda-Garcia D, Dieguez-Eceolaza M, Medel-Lacruz B, Torrens-Fontanals M, Peralta-Garcia A, Selent J (2022) In Silico study of allosteric communication networks in GPCR signaling bias. Int J Mol Sci 23. https://doi.org/10.3390/ijms23147809

Moreno-Rius J (2019) The cerebellum, THC, and cannabis addiction: findings from animal and human studies. Cerebellum 18:593–604. https://doi.org/10.1007/s12311-018-0993-7

Nguyen PT, Schmid CL, Raehal KM, Selley DE, Bohn LM, Sim-Selley LJ (2012) Beta-arrestin2 regulates cannabinoid CB1 receptor signaling and adaptation in a central nervous system region-dependent manner. Biol Psychiatry 71:714–724. https://doi.org/10.1016/j.biopsych.2011.11.027

Nguyen T, Li JX, Thomas BF, Wiley JL, Kenakin TP, Zhang Y (2017) Allosteric modulation: An alternate approach targeting the cannabinoid CB1 receptor. Med Res Rev 37:441–474. https://doi.org/10.1002/med.21418

O'Brien ES, Rangari VA, El Daibani A, Eans SO, Hammond HR, White E, Wang H, Shiimura Y, Krishna Kumar K, Jiang Q, Appourchaux K, Huang W, Zhang C, Kennedy BJ, Mathiesen JM, Che T, McLaughlin JP, Majumdar S, Kobilka BK (2024) A micro-opioid receptor modulator that works cooperatively with naloxone. Nature 631:686–693. https://doi.org/10.1038/s41586-024-07587-7

Pain S (2015) A potted history. Nature 525:S10–S11. https://doi.org/10.1038/525S10a

Pamplona FA, Ferreira J, Menezes de Lima O Jr, Duarte FS, Bento AF, Forner S, Villarinho JG, Bellocchio L, Wotjak CT, Lerner R, Monory K, Lutz B, Canetti C, Matias I, Calixto JB, Marsicano G, Guimaraes MZ, Takahashi RN (2012) Anti-inflammatory lipoxin A4 is an endogenous allosteric enhancer of CB1 cannabinoid receptor. Proc Natl Acad Sci USA 109:21134–21139. https://doi.org/10.1073/pnas.1202906109

Pandy-Szekeres G, Caroli J, Mamyrbekov A, Kermani AA, Keseru GM, Kooistra AJ, Gloriam DE (2023) GPCRdb in 2023: state-specific structure models using AlphaFold2 and new ligand resources. Nucleic Acids Res 51:D395–D402. https://doi.org/10.1093/nar/gkac1013

Papay RS, Macdonald JD, Stauffer SR, Perez DM (2023) Characterization of a novel positive allosteric modulator of the alpha(1A)-Adrenergic receptor. Curr Res Pharmacol Drug Discov 4:100142. https://doi.org/10.1016/j.crphar.2022.100142

Peddibhotla S, Hedrick MP, Hershberger P, Maloney PR, Li Y, Milewski M, Gosalia P, Gray W, Mehta A, Sugarman E, Hood B, Suyama E, Nguyen K, Heynen-Genel S, Vasile S, Salaniwal S, Stonich D, Su Y, Mangravita-Novo A, Vicchiarelli M, Roth GP, Smith LH, Chung TD, Hanson GR, Thomas JB, Caron MG, Barak LS, Pinkerton AB (2013) Discovery of ML314, a brain penetrant non-Peptidic beta-Arrestin biased agonist of the Neurotensin NTR1 receptor. ACS Med Chem Lett 4:846–851. https://doi.org/10.1021/ml400176n

Pettersen EF, Goddard TD, Huang CC, Meng EC, Couch GS, Croll TI, Morris JH, Ferrin TE (2021) UCSF ChimeraX: structure visualization for researchers, educators, and developers. Protein Sci 30:70–82. https://doi.org/10.1002/pro.3943

Pryce G, Baker D (2012) Potential control of multiple sclerosis by cannabis and the endocannabinoid system. CNS Neurol Disord Drug Targets 11:624–641. https://doi.org/10.2174/187152712801661310

Quoyer J, Janz JM, Luo J, Ren Y, Armando S, Lukashova V, Benovic JL, Carlson KE, Hunt SW 3rd, Bouvier M (2013) Pepducin targeting the C-X-C chemokine receptor type 4 acts as a biased agonist favoring activation of the inhibitory G protein. Proc Natl Acad Sci USA 110:E5088–E5097. https://doi.org/10.1073/pnas.1312515110

Santos R, Ursu O, Gaulton A, Bento AP, Donadi RS, Bologa CG, Karlsson A, Al-Lazikani B, Hersey A, Oprea TI, Overington JP (2017) A comprehensive map of molecular drug targets. Nat Rev Drug Discov 16:19–34. https://doi.org/10.1038/nrd.2016.230

Schulz P, Hryhorowicz S, Rychter AM, Zawada A, Slomski R, Dobrowolska A, Krela-Kazmierczak I (2021) What role does the endocannabinoid system play in the pathogenesis of obesity? Nutrients 13. https://doi.org/10.3390/nu13020373

Semple G, Skinner PJ, Gharbaoui T, Shin YJ, Jung JK, Cherrier MC, Webb PJ, Tamura SY, Boatman PD, Sage CR, Schrader TO, Chen R, Colletti SL, Tata JR, Waters MG, Cheng K, Taggart AK, Cai TQ, Carballo-Jane E, Behan DP, Connolly DT, Richman JG (2008)

3-(1H-tetrazol-5-yl)-1,4,5,6-tetrahydro-cyclopentapyrazole (MK-0354): a partial agonist of the nicotinic acid receptor, G-protein coupled receptor 109a, with antilipolytic but no vasodilatory activity in mice. J Med Chem 51:5101–5108. https://doi.org/10.1021/jm800258p

Shao Z, Yan W, Chapman K, Ramesh K, Ferrell AJ, Yin J, Wang X, Xu Q, Rosenbaum DM (2019) Structure of an allosteric modulator bound to the CB1 cannabinoid receptor. Nat Chem Biol 15: 1199–1205. https://doi.org/10.1038/s41589-019-0387-2

Shen C, Mao C, Xu C, Jin N, Zhang H, Shen DD, Shen Q, Wang X, Hou T, Chen Z, Rondard P, Pin JP, Zhang Y, Liu J (2021) Structural basis of GABA(B) receptor-G(i) protein coupling. Nature 594:594–598. https://doi.org/10.1038/s41586-021-03507-1

Shen S, Zhao C, Wu C, Sun S, Li Z, Yan W, Shao Z (2023) Allosteric modulation of G protein-coupled receptor signaling. Front Endocrinol (Lausanne) 14:1137604. https://doi.org/10.3389/fendo.2023.1137604

Shen S, Wu C, Lin G, Yang X, Zhou Y, Zhao C, Miao Z, Tian X, Wang K, Yang Z, Liu Z, Guo N, Li Y, Xia A, Zhou P, Liu J, Yan W, Ke B, Yang S, Shao Z (2024) Structure-based identification of a G protein-biased allosteric modulator of cannabinoid receptor CB1. Proc Natl Acad Sci USA 121:e2321532121. https://doi.org/10.1073/pnas.2321532121

Simonsen J (1989) Discussion of "An unusual, deep lingual hemorrhage as a consequence of ligature strangulation". J Forensic Sci 34:529–531

Slivicki RA, Xu Z, Kulkarni PM, Pertwee RG, Mackie K, Thakur GA, Hohmann AG (2018) Positive allosteric modulation of cannabinoid receptor type 1 suppresses pathological Pain without producing tolerance or dependence. Biol Psychiatry 84:722–733. https://doi.org/10.1016/j.biopsych.2017.06.032

Slosky LM, Bai Y, Toth K, Ray C, Rochelle LK, Badea A, Chandrasekhar R, Pogorelov VM, Abraham DM, Atluri N, Peddibhotla S, Hedrick MP, Hershberger P, Maloney P, Yuan H, Li Z, Wetsel WC, Pinkerton AB, Barak LS, Caron MG (2020) Beta-Arrestin-biased allosteric modulator of NTSR1 selectively attenuates addictive behaviors. Cell 181:1364–1379 e14. https://doi.org/10.1016/j.cell.2020.04.053

Slosky LM, Caron MG, Barak LS (2021) Biased allosteric modulators: new Frontiers in GPCR drug discovery. Trends Pharmacol Sci 42:283–299. https://doi.org/10.1016/j.tips.2020.12.005

Smith JS, Lefkowitz RJ, Rajagopal S (2018) Biased signalling: from simple switches to allosteric microprocessors. Nat Rev Drug Discov 17:243–260. https://doi.org/10.1038/nrd.2017.229

Stanczyk MA, Livingston KE, Chang L, Weinberg ZY, Puthenveedu MA, Traynor JR (2019) The delta-opioid receptor positive allosteric modulator BMS 986187 is a G-protein-biased allosteric agonist. Br J Pharmacol 176:1649–1663. https://doi.org/10.1111/bph.14602

Syrovatkina V, Alegre KO, Dey R, Huang XY (2016) Regulation, signaling, and physiological functions of G-proteins. J Mol Biol 428:3850–3868. https://doi.org/10.1016/j.jmb.2016.08.002

Tan L, Yan W, McCorvy JD, Cheng J (2018) Biased ligands of G protein-coupled receptors (GPCRs): structure-functional selectivity relationships (SFSRs) and therapeutic potential. J Med Chem 61:9841–9878. https://doi.org/10.1021/acs.jmedchem.8b00435

Thal DM, Glukhova A, Sexton PM, Christopoulos A (2018) Structural insights into G-protein-coupled receptor allostery. Nature 559:45–53. https://doi.org/10.1038/s41586-018-0259-z

Thomas G, Kloner RA, Rezkalla S (2014) Adverse cardiovascular, cerebrovascular, and peripheral vascular effects of marijuana inhalation: what cardiologists need to know. Am J Cardiol 113: 187–190. https://doi.org/10.1016/j.amjcard.2013.09.042

Tilley DG (2011) G protein-dependent and G protein-independent signaling pathways and their impact on cardiac function. Circ Res 109:217–230. https://doi.org/10.1161/CIRCRESAHA.110.231225

Tseng CC, Baillie G, Donvito G, Mustafa MA, Juola SE, Zanato C, Massarenti C, Dall'Angelo S, Harrison WTA, Lichtman AH, Ross RA, Zanda M, Greig IR (2019) The Trifluoromethyl group as a bioisosteric replacement of the aliphatic nitro group in CB(1) receptor positive allosteric modulators. J Med Chem 62:5049–5062. https://doi.org/10.1021/acs.jmedchem.9b00252

Valant C, Felder CC, Sexton PM, Christopoulos A (2012) Probe dependence in the allosteric modulation of a G protein-coupled receptor: implications for detection and validation of allosteric ligand effects. Mol Pharmacol 81:41–52. https://doi.org/10.1124/mol.111.074872

van den Hoogen NJ, Harding EK, Davidson CED, Trang T (2021) Cannabinoids in chronic Pain: therapeutic potential through microglia modulation. Front Neural Circuits 15:816747. https://doi.org/10.3389/fncir.2021.816747

van der Westhuizen ET, Choy KHC, Valant C, McKenzie-Nickson S, Bradley SJ, Tobin AB, Sexton PM, Christopoulos A (2020) Fine tuning muscarinic acetylcholine receptor signaling through Allostery and bias. Front Pharmacol 11:606656. https://doi.org/10.3389/fphar.2020.606656

Volkow ND, McLellan AT (2016) Opioid abuse in chronic pain–misconceptions and mitigation strategies. N Engl J Med 374:1253–1263. https://doi.org/10.1056/NEJMra1507771

Walters RW, Shukla AK, Kovacs JJ, Violin JD, DeWire SM, Lam CM, Chen JR, Muehlbauer MJ, Whalen EJ, Lefkowitz RJ (2009) Beta-Arrestin1 mediates nicotinic acid-induced flushing, but not its antilipolytic effect, in mice. J Clin Invest 119:1312–1321. https://doi.org/10.1172/JCI36806

Wang J, Pani B, Gokhan I, Xiong X, Kahsai AW, Jiang H, Ahn S, Lefkowitz RJ, Rockman HA (2021) Beta-Arrestin-biased allosteric modulator potentiates carvedilol-stimulated beta adrenergic receptor Cardioprotection. Mol Pharmacol 100:568–579. https://doi.org/10.1124/molpharm.121.000359

Wei TT, Chandy M, Nishiga M, Zhang A, Kumar KK, Thomas D, Manhas A, Rhee S, Justesen JM, Chen IY, Wo HT, Khanamiri S, Yang JY, Seidl FJ, Burns NZ, Liu C, Sayed N, Shie JJ, Yeh CF, Yang KC, Lau E, Lynch KL, Rivas M, Kobilka BK, Wu JC (2022) Cannabinoid receptor 1 antagonist genistein attenuates marijuana-induced vascular inflammation. Cell 185:1676–1693 e23. https://doi.org/10.1016/j.cell.2022.04.005

Wootten D, Christopoulos A, Sexton PM (2013) Emerging paradigms in GPCR allostery: implications for drug discovery. Nat Rev Drug Discov 12:630–644. https://doi.org/10.1038/nrd4052

Xiao P, Yan W, Gou L, Zhong YN, Kong L, Wu C, Wen X, Yuan Y, Cao S, Qu C, Yang X, Yang CC, Xia A, Hu Z, Zhang Q, He YH, Zhang DL, Zhang C, Hou GH, Liu H, Zhu L, Fu P, Yang S, Rosenbaum DM, Sun JP, Du Y, Zhang L, Yu X, Shao Z (2021) Ligand recognition and allosteric regulation of DRD1-Gs signaling complexes. Cell 184:943–956 e18. https://doi.org/10.1016/j.cell.2021.01.028

Yang F, Mao C, Guo L, Lin J, Ming Q, Xiao P, Wu X, Shen Q, Guo S, Shen DD, Lu R, Zhang L, Huang S, Ping Y, Zhang C, Ma C, Zhang K, Liang X, Shen Y, Nan F, Yi F, Luca VC, Zhou J, Jiang C, Sun JP, Xie X, Yu X, Zhang Y (2020) Structural basis of GPBAR activation and bile acid recognition. Nature 587:499–504. https://doi.org/10.1038/s41586-020-2569-1

Yang X, Wang X, Xu Z, Wu C, Zhou Y, Wang Y, Lin G, Li K, Wu M, Xia A, Liu J, Cheng L, Zou J, Yan W, Shao Z, Yang S (2022) Molecular mechanism of allosteric modulation for the cannabinoid receptor CB1. Nat Chem Biol 18:831–840. https://doi.org/10.1038/s41589-022-01038-y

Zhang D, Gao ZG, Zhang K, Kiselev E, Crane S, Wang J, Paoletta S, Yi C, Ma L, Zhang W, Han GW, Liu H, Cherezov V, Katritch V, Jiang H, Stevens RC, Jacobson KA, Zhao Q, Wu B (2015) Two disparate ligand-binding sites in the human P2Y1 receptor. Nature 520:317–321. https://doi.org/10.1038/nature14287

Zhao C, Wang H, Liu Y, Cheng L, Wang B, Tian X, Fu H, Wu C, Li Z, Shen C, Yu J, Yang S, Hu H, Fu P, Ma L, Wang C, Yan W, Shao Z (2023) Biased allosteric activation of ketone body receptor HCAR2 suppresses inflammatio. Mol Cell 83:3171–3187 e7. https://doi.org/10.1016/j.molcel.2023.07.030

Structural Basis of GPCR-Biased Modulation

Yan Zhang

Contents

Abstract

G protein-coupled receptors (GPCRs) constitute the largest superfamily of membrane receptors in humans and serve as crucial targets for drug development. These receptors engage multiple downstream signaling pathways, including various G-proteins and arrestins, each of which can elicit distinct physiological and pathological responses. Understanding the mechanisms of biased signaling among these pathways is vital for designing more effective drugs with reduced side effects. In this chapter, we summarize the current understanding of how GPCRs selectively couple to different signaling proteins. We delve into the structural insights derived from recent studies, which reveal how ligands can stabilize specific receptor conformations, thereby favoring particular signaling pathways over others. Furthermore, we highlight various biased ligands and their mechanisms of action, emphasizing their therapeutic potential. These findings

Y. Zhang (✉)
Zhejiang University, Hangzhou, China
e-mail: zhang_yan@zju.edu.cn

© The Author(s), under exclusive license to Springer Nature Switzerland AG 2025
Z. Li, K. Xiao (eds.), *Pharmacology of GPCRs Biased Signaling and Agonists*,
Handbook of Experimental Pharmacology 290, https://doi.org/10.1007/164_2025_768

provide a critical structural foundation for future drug discovery and optimization efforts, paving the way for more targeted and safer pharmacological interventions. Through a deeper comprehension of biased signaling mechanisms, we aim to enhance the efficacy and safety profiles of new therapeutic agents.

Keywords

Biased signaling · G protein · GPCR · Ligand modulation · Selectivity · StructureArrestin

1 Introduction

G protein-coupled receptors (GPCRs) represent the largest and most diverse family of membrane receptors in the human genome, playing critical roles in various physiological processes, including sensory perception, neurotransmission, hormone action, and immune response (Yang et al. 2021). Their significance as drug targets is underscored by their involvement in numerous pathologies, making GPCRs essential for pharmaceutical interventions. The complexity of GPCR signaling arises from their ability to couple with multiple downstream pathways, notably different G proteins and β-arrestins, each of which can elicit distinct physiological and pathological responses. Understanding the intricate mechanisms governing GPCR signaling is therefore crucial. Recent advancements in cryo-electron microscopy (cryo-EM) have greatly enhanced our understanding of GPCRs, particularly regarding biased signaling mechanisms. Cryo-EM enables the visualization of GPCRs in their native conformations when bound to various ligands, yielding structural insights that were previously unattainable (Zhang et al. 2024). By elucidating the interactions between GPCRs and their signaling partners, cryo-EM has facilitated a deeper comprehension of biased signaling, in which a single receptor preferentially activates specific downstream pathways while downregulating others (Tóth et al. 2024). This selective activation is vital for developing drugs that maximize therapeutic benefits while minimizing adverse effects.

In this chapter, we provide a comprehensive overview of the current knowledge regarding the mechanisms underlying biased signaling in GPCRs. We explore how distinct conformational states of GPCRs, stabilized by specific ligands, influence interactions with G proteins and β-arrestins. Biased ligands can shift the equilibrium of receptor conformations, promoting pathways that yield beneficial physiological outcomes while mitigating those leading to adverse effects. This nuanced modulation of GPCR signaling holds significant potential for designing targeted therapies for conditions such as heart disease, chronic pain, and neurodegenerative disorders. We also review several reported biased ligands and their mechanisms of action. For instance, ligands designed for the angiotensin II type 1 receptor (AT1R) selectively activate β-arrestin-mediated signaling pathways, conferring cardioprotective benefits while minimizing harmful G protein-dependent effects (Wingler et al. 2020). Similarly, biased agonists for the mu-opioid receptor (μOR), such as oliceridine (also named TRV130), illustrate the potential for reducing side effects in pain management (Miyano et al. 2020). These examples highlight how structural insights can inform drug design, leading to therapeutics that enhance efficacy with lower toxicity.

The heterogeneity of biased signaling pathways among different GPCRs further emphasizes the need for a tailored approach in drug development. Structural studies reveal that even within the same GPCR class, mechanisms of biased signaling can vary significantly, enriching our understanding of GPCR biology while posing challenges in developing universally effective biased ligands (Wootten et al. 2018). As we move forward, integrating cryo-EM with other advanced biophysical techniques will be essential for unraveling the complexities of GPCR signaling (Zhang et al. 2023). The knowledge gained from these studies will be invaluable for designing next-generation therapeutics. The exploration of GPCRs and their biased signaling mechanisms represents a promising frontier in pharmacology, offering potential for precise therapeutic agents that address numerous health challenges as our understanding of GPCR structure-function relationships continues to evolve.

2 GPCR Activation and Downstream Transducer Coupling

2.1 G Protein Coupling and Selectivity

GPCRs play a crucial role in cellular signaling. Upon ligand binding, GPCRs undergo a conformational change that activates associated G proteins by facilitating the exchange of GDP for GTP on the Gα subunit. This activation results in the dissociation of the Gα and G$\beta\gamma$ subunits, which subsequently interact with various downstream effectors, such as adenylate cyclase and phospholipase C, leading to the production of second messengers like cAMP and IP3 (Inoue et al. 2019). Moreover, activated GPCRs can recruit arrestin proteins, which are essential for receptor desensitization and internalization (Fig. 1a). Arrestins not only terminate G protein signaling but also initiate alternative signaling pathways, including mitogen-activated protein kinase (MAPK) cascades, thereby diversifying the cellular response. The balance between G protein and arrestin pathways ultimately dictates the overall signaling outcome, enabling cells to respond dynamically to extracellular stimuli (Flock et al. 2017).

GPCRs exhibit a complex interplay between selectivity and promiscuity in their interactions with G proteins. They can bind multiple G protein subtypes, such as Gs, Gi/o, Gq/11, and G12/13, but GPCRs usually show a preference for one subtype while maintaining weaker affinities for others (Fig. 1b). This selectivity is influenced by the GPCR dynamic, which modulates the stability and affinity of GPCR-G protein interactions (Glukhova et al. 2018). Molecular dynamic (MD) simulations and other techniques have demonstrated that GPCRs undergo dynamic conformational changes over time and space, which affects the frequency and duration of interactions between GPCR residues and G protein subunits. Specific residues on the intracellular surface of GPCRs interact with multiple G protein subtypes, exhibiting

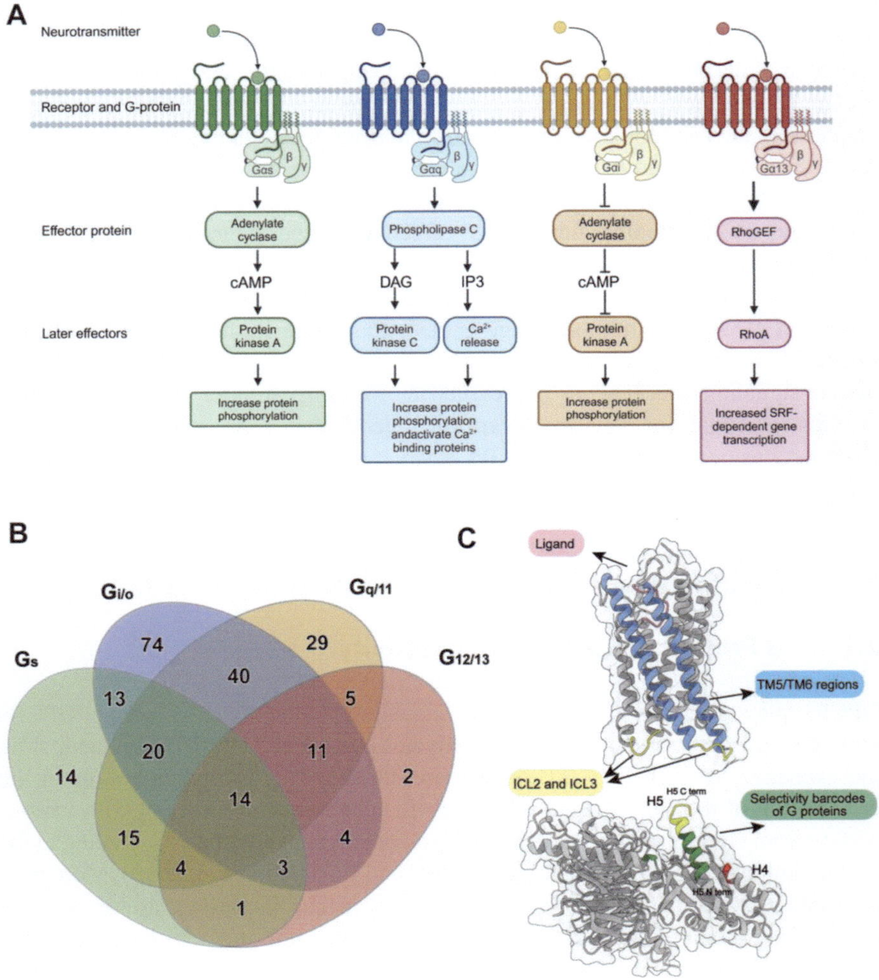

Fig. 1 An overview of current understanding of GPCR-G protein selectivity. (**a**) Schematic representation of how signaling through G protein pathways can regulate systemic functions. (**b**) The distribution of GPCRs (across all classes) that interact with various (combinations of) G proteins. (**c**) The interaction network of amino acids at the APJ-Gαi interface (PDB identifier 8XZI). Amino acids belonging to different clusters (as described in the Methods section) are colored in pink, blue, green, red, and yellow. To the right: a meta-network illustrating the interconnections among the clusters, with the size of the nodes representing the quantity of connections

varying degrees of the interaction duration that collectively contribute to the receptor's overall selectivity (Sandhu et al. 2022; Anantakrishnan and Naganathan 2023). Residues located at the periphery of the GPCR-G protein interface often engage in specific interactions with particular G protein subtypes, playing a crucial role in determining receptor specificity. Thus, the dynamic regulation of GPCR structures enables selective coupling with G proteins, orchestrating precise cellular signaling responses (Anantakrishnan and Naganathan 2023). Nonetheless, elucidating the molecular basis of G protein selectivity remains a significant challenge in GPCR research. Recent advancements in cryo-EM have significantly enhanced our understanding of GPCR-G protein complexes, providing critical insights into the molecular mechanisms governing G protein selectivity. Structural analyses reveal that the C-terminal helix of Gα subunits inserts into the cytosolic transmembrane cavity of GPCRs, establishing a common mode of recognition (Glukhova et al. 2018). However, the specific interactions between GPCRs and Gα subunits vary considerably across different complexes, contributing to the diversity of G protein selectivity profiles (Fig. 1c). This section delves into the groundbreaking findings from cryo-EM studies, emphasizing the intricate mechanisms that regulate G protein selectivity and how these interactions shape diverse signaling outcomes.

GPCRs selectively couple to specific G proteins to initiate distinct signaling pathways, and this selectivity is mediated by several key mechanisms. First, the ligand selectivity of GPCRs is closely linked to their ability to engage selectively with different G proteins. For example, researchers employed a bioluminescence resonance energy transfer (BRET) assay to study the activation of TAAR1 by various biologically active amines, including β-PEA, T1AM, and others. The cellular assays demonstrated that β-PEA and T1AM selectively activated the Gs subtype, whereas cyclohexylamine (CHA) and isoamylamine (IAA) served as specific agonists for TAAR1-Gq signaling, and cadaverine (CAD) uniquely activated Gi signaling. In the TAAR1-Gs ligand complex, Ser107$^{3.36}$ and Tyr294$^{7.43}$ are essential for the selective activation of Gs proteins. Mutations in these residues markedly decrease the Gs activity induced by (S)-AMPH and RO-6889450, with only a minimal impact on Gi or Gq activity. This suggests that these residues are critical for the specific recognition and activation of Gs proteins. In contrast, the residue Ile225$^{5.72}$ in TM5 is key for the activation of Gq proteins, indicating that the mechanism of Gq activation diverges from that of Gs and Gi. Residues within the transmembrane bundle that links the ligand-binding pocket to the receptor-G protein interface, such as I111$^{3.40}$, R121$^{3.50}$, F260$^{6.44}$, and Y304$^{7.53}$, are indispensable for Gs protein signaling. Mutations in these residues significantly impair Gs protein signaling, while mutations in Leu114$^{3.43}$, Thr252$^{6.36}$, Leu253$^{6.37}$, and Phe307$^{7.56}$ have a notable effect on Gi activity (Xu et al. 2023). Second, the transmembrane helices TM5 and TM6 are crucial in determining GPCR-G protein selectivity. For instance, histamine receptors such as H2R and H3R selectively couple with Gs and Gi proteins, respectively, resulting in distinct downstream signaling pathways. The structural geometries of TM5 and TM6 in GPCRs serve as determinants for primary G-protein signaling selectivity, potentially aiding in engineering GPCR selectivity for specific G-protein interactions. CryoEM studies have elucidated the structural basis of various GPCR-G protein complexes, identifying the length, tilt angle, and outward movement of TM5 and TM6 as critical determinants of selectivity across the GPCR family (Shen et al. 2024). Similarly, the structures of 5-HT receptors with Gs and Gi complexes provide clear examples of these mechanisms; for the 5-HT4 receptor, the lengths of TM5 and TM6 influence the differential insertion angles of the Gα helix, creating unique binding pockets for Gs distinct from Gi. Third, variations in the interactions between intracellular loops 2 and 3 (ICL2 and ICL3) and the Gα subunit are vital for determining G protein coupling specificity (Huang et al. 2022). For instance, in 2024, cryo-EM structures of activated PAR1, bound to its tethered agonist and either Gq or Gi heterotrimers, demonstrated that ICL2 and ICL3 of PAR1 have distinct roles in mediating Gq and Gi coupling. Mutations in specific residues, such as S306 in ICL3, significantly affected Gq signaling, while mutations in ICL2 impacted Gq efficacy without altering Gi binding, underscoring the differential mechanisms of G protein selectivity (Guo et al. 2024). Furthermore, each G protein possesses a "selectivity barcode," a unique arrangement of amino acids that distinguishes it from other G proteins. This barcode interacts with specific residues on the GPCR, facilitating selective binding through non-covalent interactions. Cryo-EM studies have illustrated this concept in various complexes, such as Gαi1 and Gαq in the GPR120-Gi and GPR120-Giq complexes, where the presence of charged residues in the barcode leads to electrostatic interactions and preferential coupling to Gαi, while the absence of charged residues in the barcode of Gαq promotes hydrophobic interactions and coupling to Gαq. Additionally, the specific geometry of the GPCR ligand-binding pocket and the conformational changes induced by ligand binding further contribute to the selectivity of G protein coupling. For example, the presence of aromatic residues in the ligand-binding pocket of GPR120 allows it to recognize specific double bonds in unsaturated fatty acids, leading to biased signaling toward Gs activation (Mao et al. 2023) with specific G proteins. Collectively, these findings highlight the intricate interplay of structural features and molecular interactions that govern GPCR selectivity for different G protein subtypes.

The mechanism of selectivity in GPCR signaling can be vividly illustrated through the metaphor of keys and locks. In this analogy, GPCRs serve as keys, while G proteins function as locks that open various doors, each representing distinct signaling pathways. Some GPCRs, akin to master keys, can activate multiple locks—such as promiscuous receptors like GPR4 and Lpar4—while others, like chemokine and odorant receptors, are designed to fit only one specific lock. This specificity is encoded in the key's "cut pattern," which corresponds to the GPCR-G protein interface's structural features, including grooves and ridges. Different strategies can be employed to design keys that fit the same lock by varying the arrangement or presence of specific "ridges." This concept is particularly evident among different GPCR subfamilies, where interface positions undergo positive and negative selection around a conserved center to effectively couple with specific G proteins. Additionally, since there are over 800 GPCRs in the human genome compared to only four major G protein subtypes (Gs, Gi, Gq, G11), evolutionary pressure has led G protein subtypes to develop distinct "lock" patterns to accommodate a wide variety of GPCRs (Fig. 1b).

2.2 Arrestin Function and Coupling

Arrestins are multifunctional adapter proteins that play crucial roles in regulating various signaling pathways. There are four major isoforms: two retinal forms (visual arrestin and cone arrestin) and two ubiquitous forms (β-arrestin1 and β-arrestin2) (Lohse and Hoffmann 2014). Despite their structural similarities, they exhibit distinct functions (Fig. 1). Arrestins adopt diverse conformations in different cellular pools, enabling interaction with numerous cargo proteins and activated GPCRs (Cahill 3rd et al. 2017; Kumari et al. 2017). Without stimulation, arrestins remain in inactive state, sequestering specific proteins in the cytosol or binding to microtubules, which dampens basal signaling activities. Upon GPCR activation, arrestins are recruited to the plasma membrane after phosphorylation by GPCR kinases (GRKs) (Latorraca et al. 2018). Arrestins mediate the receptor desensitization by sterically hindering GPCR-G protein coupling and scaffolding signaling complexes, such as Raf-MEK-ERK. Arrestins also facilitate GPCR internalization and regulate receptor trafficking, influencing whether receptors are recycled or degraded. This modulation is vital for preventing overstimulation and potential cellular damage during prolonged hormonal or neurotransmitter signaling (Ahn et al. 2020).

Arrestins significantly impact cell growth and survival by activating key pathways, including ERK, AKT, and NFκB (Reiter and Lefkowitz 2006). They promote ERK activation through interactions with nonreceptor tyrosine kinases and scaffold complexes, inhibiting apoptosis. In the AKT pathway, arrestins regulate PI3K and PTEN, affecting protein translation and cell cycle progression. They stabilize IκBα, thereby reducing NFκB activity. Additionally, arrestins enhance cytoskeletal dynamics by interacting with proteins such as filamin-A and cofilin, promoting actin rearrangement and cell migration (Fig. 2). Notably, β-arrestin1 can translocate to the nucleus, where it interacts with transcription factors, influencing gene expression and transcriptional regulation. Overall, arrestins are multifunctional proteins that regulate diverse cellular processes, including receptor desensitization, signaling, cytoskeletal dynamics, and transcriptional activity.

Distinct conformational complexes are formed between GPCRs and arrestins, which are primarily categorized into three types. The first type, referred to as "tail interactions" or the hanging model, is characterized by the interaction between arrestin and the phosphorylated C-terminal tail of the receptor. The second type involves a fully engaged "tight" interaction, where arrestin's finger loop and C loop engage with the receptor's transmembrane core (Shukla et al. 2014). The third type, known as the megaplex, involves the coexistence of arrestin and G protein within the same complex (Nguyen et al. 2019; Thomsen et al. 2016). In tail interactions, arrestin binds to phosphorylated serine and threonine residues on the receptor's C-terminal tail through phosphate-binding residues like arginine and lysine. This initial contact is highly specific, serving as a recognition code for arrestin recruitment. These interactions are critical for the selectivity of arrestin binding, as different phosphorylation patterns can dictate preferences for specific arrestin subtypes and the subsequent activation of signaling pathways. Arrestin is stabilized in a

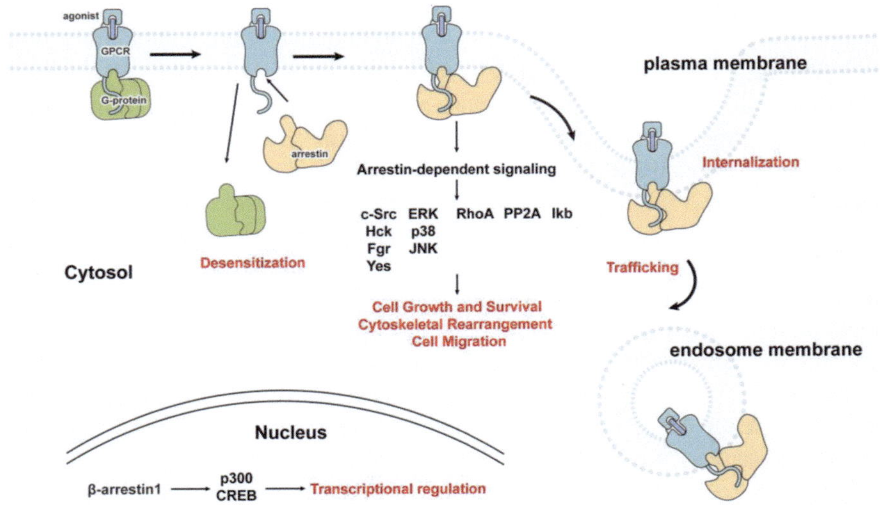

Fig. 2 An overview of the arrestin-mediated GPCR signaling functions and biological activities. Upon agonist stimulation of a GPCR, arrestin are recruited and activated. They subsequently activate or inhibit various signaling pathways. β-arrestin signaling is important for chemotaxis and antiapoptosis. In addition, arrestin can translocate to the nucleus and regulate the expression of various genes through reorganization of chromatin

pre-activated state by tail interactions, facilitating further engagement with receptor core elements. Core interactions between arrestins and GPCRs occur when arrestins engage with the receptor's transmembrane regions. Following the establishment of tail interactions, arrestins undergo significant conformational changes, allowing them to interface with key transmembrane domains of the GPCR. This engagement involves the penetration of the finger loop and C loop into the receptor's cytoplasmic cavity. These contacts result in stabilization of the arrestin–receptor complex and occlusion of the G protein coupling site on the GPCR, thereby promoting receptor desensitization. The structural basis of this interaction has been elucidated by high-resolution structures of GPCR–arrestin complexes, including structures of the rhodopsin–arrestin (Kang et al. 2015), β1AR–arrestin (Lee et al. 2020), M2R–arrestin (Staus et al. 2020), V2R–arrestin (Bous et al. 2022), NTSR1–arrestin (Yin et al. 2019), 5-HT1B–arrestin (Cao et al. 2022a), CB1–arrestin (Liao et al. 2023), and GCGR–arrestin complexes (Chen et al. 2023). In most of these complexes, tight binding between arrestin and the receptor is facilitated by hydrophobic interactions involving the finger loop. The finger loop has been observed to adopt two conformations—a loop or a helix—in these structures. Notably, the angle at which NTSR1 binds to arrestin differs significantly from that of other receptors, indicating a unique mode of interaction (Yin et al. 2019). In the GCGR–arrestin complex, helix 8 of the receptor contributes significantly to the binding interface (Chen et al. 2023). A sophisticated aspect of GPCR-arrestin interactions is the formation of a megaplex, characterized by the simultaneous binding of arrestin to both the GPCR and G protein. However, the precise structural basis for the formation of this GPCR-G protein-arrestin megaplex remains elusive due to a lack of high-resolution structural information.

2.3 Similarities and Differences in Arrestin and G Protein Coupling to GPCRs

Arrestins and G proteins are both primary downstream signaling molecules activated by GPCRs. Upon stimulation by extracellular signals, GPCRs undergo conformational changes that enable interactions with various G proteins and arrestins, triggering multiple downstream pathways that regulate diverse physiological functions (Zhang et al. 2024). Both G proteins and arrestins directly interact with activated GPCRs. When a GPCR binds an extracellular ligand, it experiences conformational shifts involving conserved motifs. Specifically, TM5 and TM6 move away from the receptor core for the monomeric GPCRs, creating binding sites for both G proteins and arrestins (Fig. 3) (Rose et al. 2014; Zhou et al. 2019). Upon activation, the α5 helix of the Gα protein inserts into the cytoplasmic pocket of the GPCR, while the finger loop of arrestin extends into the same region, sharing an (E/D)x(I/L)xxxGL motif with G proteins (Szczepek et al. 2014). This shared binding pocket is crucial for the desensitization of G protein-dependent signaling (Shenoy and Lefkowitz 2011). For example, structural comparisons between the CB1-G_i complex and CB1-β-arrestin1 complex demonstrate that the CB1 receptor adopts an active conformation (Liao et al. 2023; Krishna Kumar et al. 2019), as indicated by the significant outward shifts in TM5 and TM6 when compared to the inactive state of CB1 (Fig. 3c) (Hua et al. 2016).

However, the receptor conformation differs slightly depending on whether G proteins or arrestins are bound. We will also take CB1 as an example. To achieve the active conformation, a series of rearrangements in conserved motifs are undergone by CB1, including the $C^{6.47}W^{6.48}xP^{6.50}$, $L^{5.50}V^{3.40}L^{6.44}$, $D^{3.49}R^{3.50}Y^{3.51}$, and $N^{7.49}P^{7.50}xxY^{7.53}$ motifs. Nevertheless, distinct intracellular cavity conformations are resulted from the divergence of the side chains of these crucial residues between two structures. Additionally, the finger loop of β-arrestin1 occupies an analogous position to that of the a5 helix of Gi protein, both of which are inserted into the receptor core cavity. Moreover, β-arrestin-1 has a larger buried surface area with the CB1 receptor, resulting in a more pronounced outward movement of TM6 (Hua et al. 2016).

G proteins and arrestins interact with GPCRs, and subsequent to their activation, they elicit distinct downstream signaling cascades. G protein pathways are typically associated with rapid, transient responses, such as stimulating adenylyl cyclase, which alters cAMP levels and activates protein kinase A (PKA). Immediate physiological responses, including neurotransmission and hormone secretion, are often driven by these pathways. In contrast, arrestin binds to GPCRs after their activation and subsequent phosphorylation by GRKs (Shukla et al. 2013). This phosphorylation targets arrestin to the receptor, terminating G protein signaling and initiating

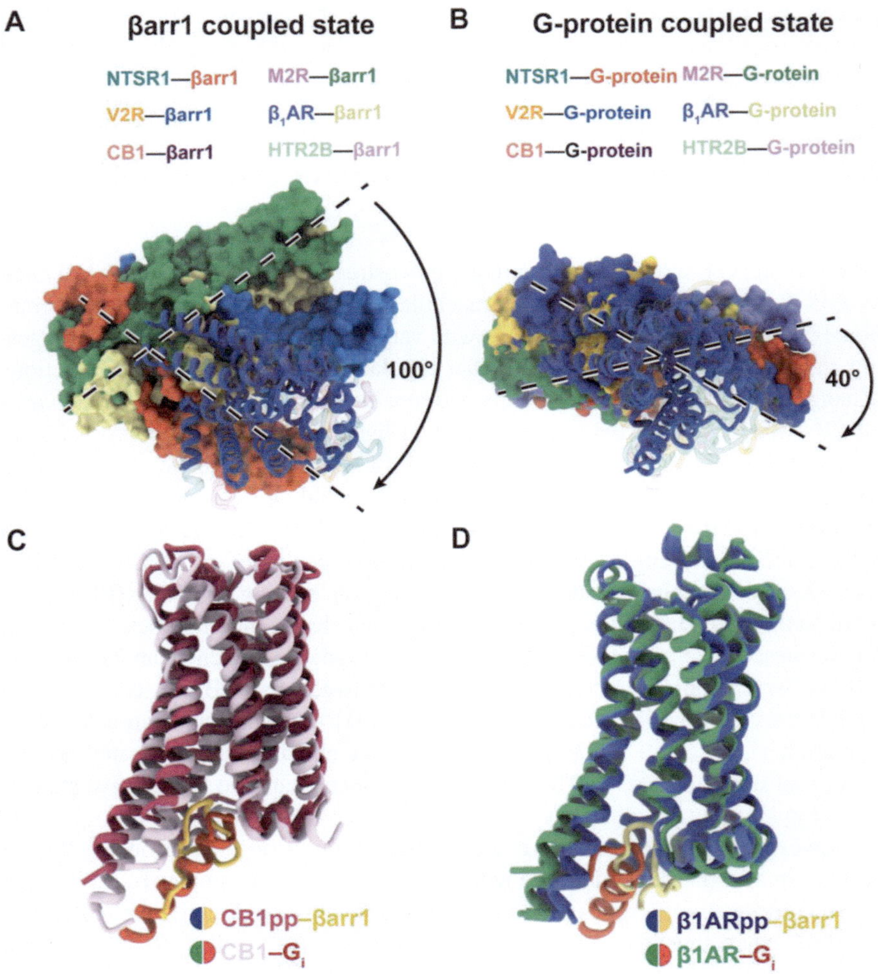

Fig. 3 Structural comparison of the binding mode of G protein and β-arrestin1 to GPCR. (**a**) Overlay of the β1AR-β-arrestin1 (PDB: 6TKO) structure with V2R-β-arrestin1 (PDB: 7R0C), NTSR1-β-arrestin1 (PDB: 6UP7), HTR2B-β-arrestin1 (PDB: 7SRS), CB1pp-β-arrestin1 (PDB: 8WRZ), and M2R-β-arrestin1 (PDB: 6U1N) structures on the basis of alignment of the receptor chains, viewed from the extracellular space. (**b**) Overlay of the β1AR-G_s structure with V2R-G_s (PDB: 7BB7), M2R-G_o (PDB: 6OIK), NTSR1-G_i (PDB: 6OS9), HTR2B-miniG_q (PDB: 7SRR) structures on the basis of alignment of the receptor chains, viewed from the extracellular space. (**c**) Superposed structures of the CB1pp-β-arrestin1(PDB: 8WRZ) and CB1-Gi complexes (PDB: 6N4B) aligned by CB1. (**d**) Superposed structures of the β1AR-β-arrestin1 (PDB: 6TKO) and β1AR-β-arrestin1-Gs complexes (PDB: 7JJO) aligned by β1AR

arrestin-dependent pathways. More prolonged responses, including the activation of MAPKs and Src family kinases, are generally resulted from arrestin signaling, potentially influencing gene expression and cellular reorganization (Yang et al. 2013). Furthermore, extended processes such as receptor desensitization, internalization, and tissue remodeling are often linked to arrestin pathways (Ahn et al. 2020).. In summary, arrestin and G protein pathways represent two distinct modalities through which GPCRs regulate cellular signaling. The differences in their activation, downstream signaling, and physiological effects enhance the complexity and adaptability of GPCR-mediated signal transduction, enabling cells to respond dynamically to a broad range of extracellular stimuli.

3 Mechanisms of Biased Modulation

3.1 Representative-Biased Ligands

Biased signaling—sometimes referred to as functional selectivity or biased agonism—occurs when a ligand preferentially activates either the β-arrestin or G-protein pathway of a GPCR, producing distinct functional outcomes (Fig. 4a). In drug discovery, there is significant interest in understanding the mechanisms of biased signaling and designing biased modulators. Recent advancements in GPCR structures have enabled researchers to visualize how agonists induce signal bias by stabilizing specific receptor conformations. This insight provides a solid theoretical foundation for the precise design and optimization of biased modulators. Here, we summarize the structural basis for ligand recognition by GPCRs exhibiting diverse signaling profiles, delve into the mechanisms of signal transduction, and discuss innovative drug design targeting specific pathways, highlighting key advancements from the past 5 years.

The exploration of biased signaling mechanisms was initially driven by the undesirable side effects associated with critical drug targets. For instance, Angiotensin II Receptor Blockers (ARBs), commonly used for cardiovascular disease treatment, are designed to inhibit harmful cardiovascular events like myocardial hypertrophy induced by Angiotensin II (AngII). Activation of the AT1R through Gq protein interactions can lead to detrimental cardiac effects, whereas β-arrestin signaling offers cardioprotective benefits. This challenge has spurred interest in designing agonists that selectively activate the β-arrestin signaling pathway. TRV027, one of the first biased agonists developed, blocks AngII-induced vasoconstriction while promoting beneficial cardiac effects through β-arrestin signaling (Violin et al. 2014). Most notable is oliceridine, an analgesic that targets μOR, which currently stands as the sole FDA approved that has been developed based on the concept of G protein bias (Miyano et al. 2020). Additionally, many promising molecules with tailored signaling profiles have been developed to enhance therapeutic outcomes (Table 1). Including biased agonists for apelin receptor (anti-cardiac hypertrophy), S1P receptor (multiple sclerosis), kappa receptor (uremic pruritus), 5HT2A receptor (antidepressant), α2A receptor (labor pain), PTH receptor (anti-hypoparathyroidism and anti-osteoporosis), and NTS receptor (treating addictive behavior).

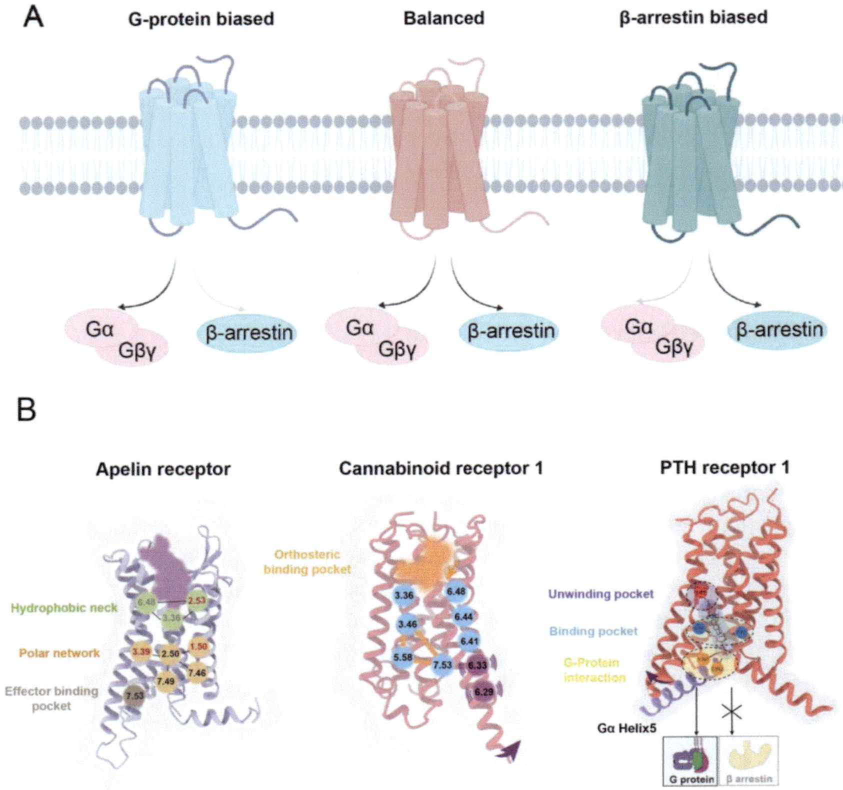

Fig. 4 A schematic representation of GPCR signaling bias. (**a**) Illustration of the signaling mechanisms of three types of GPCR agonists: G protein-biased, balanced, and β-arrestin biased. G protein biased ligands primarily activate G proteins (Gα and Gβγ), while β-arrestin-biased ligands primarily activate β-arrestin. Balanced ligands activate both G protein and β-arrestin. Schematic depiction showing the biased signaling transduction at specific important positions of APLNR, CB1, and PTH1R. (**b**) Schematic depiction showing the biased signaling transduction at specific important positions of APLNR, CB1, and PTH1R. Schematic depiction showing the biased signaling transduction at specific important positions of APLNR, CB1, and PTH1R

3.2 Structural Evidence of Biased Modulation

Recent advances in structural biology have substantially deepened our understanding of the mechanisms of GPCR-biased signaling. Most designed GPCR-biased ligands currently target the orthosteric pocket, adopting binding poses that differ from those of balanced agonists (Fig. 4b and Table 1). We take several typical Class A GPCRs as examples. Apelin receptor is regarded as a promising therapeutic target for cardiovascular disease. However, adverse effects through the β-arrestin pathway limit its pharmacological use. Researchers identified "twin hotspots" in APLNR as key determinants for signaling bias by comparing APLNR-Gi1 complexes bound to three agonists with divergent signaling profiles. They successfully designed absolute

Table 1 Structural insights into receptor bias mechanisms across GPCRs

Agonists	Receptor	Bias	Binding site	Mechanism of bias signaling
TRV023, TRV026	AT1R	β-arrestin	Orthosteric pocket	Polar network in the receptor core act as a biased signaling switch (Wingler et al. 2020; Suomivuori et al. 2020)
TRV130	μOR	G protein	Orthosteric pocket	The interaction between ligand and TM6/7 is crucial for maintaining β-arrestin activity (Zhuang et al. 2022)
Nalfurafine/ WMS-X600	KOR	G protein /β-arrestin	Orthosteric pocket	Interactions with the extracellular helices and loops restrict the conformational changes and thus affect G protein or arrestin signaling (El Daibani et al. 2023)
WN561, MM07, CMF019	APLNR	G protein	Orthosteric pocket	Twin hotspots in APLNR are key determinants forsignaling bias (Wang et al. 2024)
/	CB1	G protein	Orthosteric pocket	The balanced agonist Fub inserts deeper in theβ-arrestin1-coupled CB1 than G protein-coupled and the "toggle switch" motif fine-tunes CB1 to recruit particular effector proteins (Liao et al. 2023)
IHCH-7113	5-HT2AR	β-arrestin	Extended binding pocket (EBP)	Ligand recognition in the EBP, specifically at $L362^{7.35}$, Affects ligand bias (Cao et al. 2022b)
FTY720-P, BAF312	S1PR1	β-arrestin	Orthosteric pocket	The intermediate flipping of $W269^{6.48}$and the retained interaction between $F265^{6.44}$and $N307^{7.49}$are the key features of the β-arrestin bias (Xu et al. 2022a)
OXY	α2AR	G protein	Orthosteric pocket	$Y431^{7.43}$, $S215^{5.42}$, and particularly $Y409^{6.55}$, that may lead to a signaling bias of OXY (Xu et al. 2022b)
SBI-553 (PAM)	NTSR1	β-arrestin	Intercellular binding pocket	The binding of SBI-553 is compatible with β-arrestin binding but would clash with Gq binding (Huang et al. 2020; Duan et al. 2023)
PCO371	PTH1R	G protein	Intercellular binding pocket	PCO371 binds to an unanticipated agonist-binding site, which act as a G protein-biased ligand that is incapable of β-arrestin recruitment (Kobayashi et al. 2023; Zhao et al. 2023)
CCL15S	CCR1	G protein	Orthosteric pocket	The conformational change of $Y291^{7.43}$ that triggered its polar network rearrangement in the orthosteric binding pocket and allosterically regulated the activation of β-arrestin signaling (Shao et al. 2022)

G protein-biased agonists based on the analysis of the "twin hotspots." The design principle involved reducing the interaction between the ligand and amino acids that are crucial for β-arrestin activity, while enhancing the interaction with amino acids that are vital for G protein activity. Further analysis of the signaling transmission mechanism revealed that conformational changes in the ligand pocket led to rearrangement of the machine pocket, disrupting the polar interaction between $N^{1.50}$ and $D^{2.50}$, which they regard it's crucial for β-arrestin signaling, resulting in a receptor conformation that favors G protein binding (Wang et al. 2024). Similarly, the structural characteristics of μOR agonists, which activate the receptor and its downstream signaling complexes in diverse ways, have facilitated the design of absolute signaling-biased agonists. Structural alignment of μOR–oliceridine and μOR–fentanyl complexes shows that G protein-biased agonists preferentially interact with the TM3 side of the ligand-binding pocket rather than the TM6/7 side (Zhuang et al. 2022).

The structural insights into the GPCR-β-arrestin complex have significantly contributed to deciphering the mechanisms underlying biased signaling. Exemplified by CB1, the same ligand (FUB) adopts a different pose in the Gi-coupled and β-arrestin-coupled states. This induces rearrangement of the twin toggle switch, resulting in distinct conformations to interact with different effector proteins, thereby providing a structural basis for drug design (Liao et al. 2023). Specifically, the displacement of the Gi α5 helix by the bulkier finger loop of βarr1 leads to the steric hindrance between $L341^{6.33}$ and $M337^{6.29}$ of TM6 and βarr1. This significant steric clash effectively triggers pronounced conformational alterations in TM6, characterized by an enhanced outward displacement and an on-axis clockwise rotation, which in turn forms a cytoplasmic cavity to accommodate the β-arrestin1 finger loop. Subsequently, the movement of $L349^{6.41}$ toward $Y294^{5.58}$ results in a steric clash that propels $Y294^{5.58}$ to shift upward, engaging in polar interactions with $T210^{3.46}$ on TM3 and $Y397^{7.53}$ on TM7. This interaction pattern establishes the $T^{3.46}Y^{5.58}Y^{7.53}$ triad polar network, underscoring the pivotal role of $T^{3.46}$ in the $T^{3.46}Y^{5.58}Y^{7.53}$ triad motif for stabilizing the TM core of the CB1 receptor in a conformation that preferentially couples with β-arrestin1 (Fig. 4b and Table 1). The above information indicates that, even within Class A GPCRs, the pathways of biased signal transduction exhibit considerable heterogeneity. The structure details of biased mechanism of other class A GPCRs are shown in Table 1, including kappa receptor, S1P receptor, CCR1 and α2A receptor. This observation underscores the imperative need for comprehensive structural data pertaining to the diverse configurations of GPCR signaling transduction complexes.

Additionally, biased ligands may occupy intracellular allosteric sites, influencing receptor conformations that interact with effector proteins, as seen with PTH1R (Fig. 4 and Table 1). With reference to PTH, PCO371 is a G protein-biased ligand that is incapable of β-arrestin recruitment. The structure reveals that PCO371-binding site is within the transmembrane domain (TMD) at the interface with the G protein and contacts with G protein (Kobayashi et al. 2023; Zhao et al. 2023). This binding mode rearranges the intracellular region toward the active conformation without extracellularly induced allosteric signal propagation. Compare to the peptide-bound active PTH1R structures, an approximately 2.4 Å inward shift at the cytoplasmic end of TM6 and a 2.7 Å outward shift at the cytoplasmic end of TM7, to couple preferentially with the G protein. Their modeling and receptor activation studies indicate that a pocket resembling PCO371 is likely to be preserved across the majority of class B GPCRs. Consequently, the identification of this conserved intracellular agonist-binding pocket introduces a new strategy for developing biased agonists.

Biased agonists have demonstrated favorable therapeutic outcomes with significantly reduced side effects in animal models, indicating their promising potential for future clinical applications. However, the complex physiological environment in vivo necessitates extensive clinical research to accurately predict and confirm the physiological effects of these compounds. Despite these challenges, biased drugs represent a significant advancement in modern drug design, paving the way for more targeted and safer therapeutic interventions. The field of biased signaling within GPCR drug design is at the forefront of therapeutic innovation. As we better understand the structural and mechanistic basis of biased signaling, we can develop more precise therapeutics that maximize efficacy and minimize side effects. The continued application of cryo-EM and other advanced technologies will be crucial in unlocking the full potential of biased drug development.

4 Concluding Remarks

The study of GPCR signaling has evolved to include the concept of biased signaling, where specific ligands preferentially activate distinct downstream pathways, resulting in varied physiological responses (Zhou et al. 2017). Understanding this nuanced signaling mechanism is crucial for developing more effective and safer therapeutic agents (Hauser et al. 2017). Recent advancements in structure biology provide high-resolution structural insights that elucidate how different ligands stabilize specific conformations of GPCRs (Yang et al. 2021; Hauser et al. 2021). This capability has enhanced our understanding of the complex interactions between GPCRs and their downstream signaling partners, allowing researchers to identify conformational states associated with biased signaling. Such insights are fundamental for designing drugs that selectively engage beneficial signaling pathways while avoiding those that lead to adverse effects.

The therapeutic implications of biased signaling are significant. For example, biased ligands have been developed for receptors like the AT1R (Wingler et al. 2020; Suomivuori et al. 2020) and the mu-opioid receptor (Zhuang et al. 2022). These biased agonists can selectively activate pathways that confer therapeutic benefits, such as cardioprotection or analgesia, while minimizing the harmful side effects typically associated with conventional receptor activation (Wingler et al. 2020; Zhuang et al. 2022; Suomivuori et al. 2020). Exploring biased signaling pathways not only enhances our understanding of GPCR biology but also underscores the necessity for a tailored approach in drug design (Rankovic et al. 2016). As structural studies reveal the heterogeneity of biased signaling mechanisms across different GPCRs, it becomes evident that one-size-fits-all solutions may be inadequate. Future research should focus on the intricate details of GPCR-ligand interactions and how these dynamics can be manipulated to develop more selective therapeutics.

Looking ahead, integrating cryo-EM with other advanced techniques, such as MD simulations and functional assays, will be pivotal in further elucidating the complexities of GPCR signaling (Shen et al. 2024; Zhou et al. 2017). These multifaceted approaches can facilitate the identification of novel biased ligands and deepen our understanding of how specific receptor conformations influence downstream signaling pathways. Ultimately, ongoing research into GPCR-biased signaling mechanisms holds immense promise for drug development. By leveraging this knowledge, scientists can create precision therapeutics that not only improve efficacy but also reduce unwanted side effects. The future of GPCR research is poised to significantly advance the field of pharmacology, leading to the next generation of targeted drugs that can address a wide range of health challenges more effectively and safely. As our understanding of these complex signaling mechanisms deepens, so too does our capacity to design innovative solutions that improve patient outcomes.

References

Ahn S, Shenoy SK, Luttrell LM, Lefkowitz RJ (2020) SnapShot: beta-Arrestin functions. Cell 182: 1362–1362 e1361. https://doi.org/10.1016/j.cell.2020.07.034

Anantakrishnan S, Naganathan AN (2023) Thermodynamic architecture and conformational plasticity of GPCRs. Nat Commun 14:128. https://doi.org/10.1038/s41467-023-35790-z

Bous J, Fouillen A, Orcel H, Trapani S, Cong X, Fontanel S, Saint-Paul J, Lai-Kee-Him J, Urbach S, Sibille N et al (2022) Structure of the vasopressin hormone-V2 receptor-beta-arrestin1 ternary complex. Sci Adv 8:eabo7761. https://doi.org/10.1126/sciadv.abo7761

Cahill TJ 3rd, Thomsen AR, Tarrasch JT, Plouffe B, Nguyen AH, Yang F, Huang LY, Kahsai AW, Bassoni DL, Gavino BJ et al (2017) Distinct conformations of GPCR-beta-arrestin complexes mediate desensitization, signaling, and endocytosis. Proc Natl Acad Sci USA 114:2562–2567. https://doi.org/10.1073/pnas.1701529114

Cao C, Barros-Álvarez X, Zhang S, Kim K, Dämgen MA, Panova O, Suomivuori CM, Fay JF, Zhong X, Krumm BE et al (2022a) Signaling snapshots of a serotonin receptor activated by the prototypical psychedelic LSD. Neuron 110:3154–3167.e3157. https://doi.org/10.1016/j.neuron.2022.08.006

Cao D, Yu J, Wang H, Luo Z, Liu X, He L, Qi J, Fan L, Tang L, Chen Z et al (2022b) Structure-based discovery of nonhallucinogenic psychedelic analogs. Science 375:403–411. https://doi.org/10.1126/science.abl8615

Chen K, Zhang C, Lin S, Yan X, Cai H, Yi C, Ma L, Chu X, Liu Y, Zhu Y et al (2023) Tail engagement of arrestin at the glucagon receptor. Nature 620:904–910. https://doi.org/10.1038/s41586-023-06420-x

Duan J, Liu H, Zhao F, Yuan Q, Ji Y, Cai X, He X, Li X, Li J, Wu K et al (2023) GPCR activation and GRK2 assembly by a biased intracellular agonist. Nature 620:676–681. https://doi.org/10.1038/s41586-023-06395-9

El Daibani A, Paggi JM, Kim K, Laloudakis YD, Popov P, Bernhard SM, Krumm BE, Olsen RHJ, Diberto J, Carroll FI et al (2023) Molecular mechanism of biased signaling at the kappa opioid receptor. Nat Commun 14:1338. https://doi.org/10.1038/s41467-023-37041-7

Flock T, Hauser AS, Lund N, Gloriam DE, Balaji S, Babu MM (2017) Selectivity determinants of GPCR-G-protein binding. Nature 545:317–322. https://doi.org/10.1038/nature22070
Glukhova A, Draper-Joyce CJ, Sunahara RK, Christopoulos A, Wootten D, Sexton PM (2018) Rules of engagement: GPCRs and G proteins. ACS Pharmacol Transl Sci 1:73–83. https://doi.org/10.1021/acsptsci.8b00026
Guo J, Zhou YL, Yang Y, Guo S, You E, Xie X, Jiang Y, Mao C, Xu HE, Zhang Y (2024) Structural basis of tethered agonism and G protein coupling of protease-activated receptors. Cell Res 34:725–734. https://doi.org/10.1038/s41422-024-00997-2
Hauser AS, Attwood MM, Rask-Andersen M, Schioth HB, Gloriam DE (2017) Trends in GPCR drug discovery: new agents, targets and indications. Nat Rev Drug Discov 16:829–842. https://doi.org/10.1038/nrd.2017.178
Hauser AS, Kooistra AJ, Munk C, Heydenreich FM, Veprintsev DB, Bouvier M, Babu MM, Gloriam DE (2021) GPCR activation mechanisms across classes and macro/microscales. Nat Struct Mol Biol 28:879–888. https://doi.org/10.1038/s41594-021-00674-7
Hua T, Vemuri K, Pu M, Qu L, Han GW, Wu Y, Zhao S, Shui W, Li S, Korde A et al (2016) Crystal structure of the human cannabinoid receptor CB(1). Cell 167:750–762.e714. https://doi.org/10.1016/j.cell.2016.10.004
Huang W, Masureel M, Qu Q, Janetzko J, Inoue A, Kato HE, Robertson MJ, Nguyen KC, Glenn JS, Skiniotis G, Kobilka BK (2020) Structure of the neurotensin receptor 1 in complex with beta-arrestin 1. Nature 579:303–308. https://doi.org/10.1038/s41586-020-1953-1
Huang S, Xu P, Shen DD, Simon IA, Mao C, Tan Y, Zhang H, Harpsoe K, Li H, Zhang Y et al (2022) GPCRs steer G(i) and G(s) selectivity via TM5-TM6 switches as revealed by structures of serotonin receptors. Mol Cell 82:2681–2695 e2686. https://doi.org/10.1016/j.molcel.2022.05.031
Inoue A, Raimondi F, Kadji FMN, Singh G, Kishi T, Uwamizu A, Ono Y, Shinjo Y, Ishida S, Arang N et al (2019) Illuminating G-protein-coupling selectivity of GPCRs. Cell 177:1933–1947 e1925. https://doi.org/10.1016/j.cell.2019.04.044
Kang Y, Zhou XE, Gao X, He Y, Liu W, Ishchenko A, Barty A, White TA, Yefanov O, Han GW et al (2015) Crystal structure of rhodopsin bound to arrestin by femtosecond X-ray laser. Nature 523:561–567. https://doi.org/10.1038/nature14656
Kobayashi K, Kawakami K, Kusakizako T, Tomita A, Nishimura M, Sawada K, Okamoto HH, Hiratsuka S, Nakamura G, Kuwabara R et al (2023) Class B1 GPCR activation by an intracellular agonist. Nature 618:1085–1093. https://doi.org/10.1038/s41586-023-06169-3
Krishna Kumar K, Shalev-Benami M, Robertson MJ, Hu H, Banister SD, Hollingsworth SA, Latorraca NR, Kato HE, Hilger D, Maeda S et al (2019) Structure of a signaling cannabinoid receptor 1-G protein complex. Cell 176:448–458.e412. https://doi.org/10.1016/j.cell.2018.11.040
Kumari P, Srivastava A, Ghosh E, Ranjan R, Dogra S, Yadav PN, Shukla AK (2017) Core engagement with beta-arrestin is dispensable for agonist-induced vasopressin receptor endocytosis and ERK activation. Mol Biol Cell 28:1003–1010. https://doi.org/10.1091/mbc.E16-12-0818
Latorraca NR, Wang JK, Bauer B, Townshend RJL, Hollingsworth SA, Olivieri JE, Xu HE, Sommer ME, Dror RO (2018) Molecular mechanism of GPCR-mediated arrestin activation. Nature 557:452–456. https://doi.org/10.1038/s41586-018-0077-3
Lee Y, Warne T, Nehmé R, Pandey S, Dwivedi-Agnihotri H, Chaturvedi M, Edwards PC, García-Nafría J, Leslie AGW, Shukla AK, Tate CG (2020) Molecular basis of β-arrestin coupling to formoterol-bound β(1)-adrenoceptor. Nature 583:862–866. https://doi.org/10.1038/s41586-020-2419-1
Liao YY, Zhang H, Shen Q, Cai C, Ding Y, Shen DD, Guo J, Qin J, Dong Y, Zhang Y, Li XM (2023) Snapshot of the cannabinoid receptor 1-arrestin complex unravels the biased signaling mechanism. Cell 186:5784–5797.e5717. https://doi.org/10.1016/j.cell.2023.11.017
Lohse MJ, Hoffmann C (2014) Arrestin interactions with G protein-coupled receptors. Handb Exp Pharmacol 219:15–56. https://doi.org/10.1007/978-3-642-41199-1_2

Lv X, Gao K, Nie J, Zhang X, Zhang S, Ren Y, Sun X, Li Q, Huang J, Liu L et al (2023) Structures of human prostaglandin F(2alpha) receptor reveal the mechanism of ligand and G protein selectivity. Nat Commun 14:8136. https://doi.org/10.1038/s41467-023-43922-8

Mao, C et al. (2023) Unsaturated bond recognition leads to biased signal in a fatty acid receptor. Science (New York, N.Y.) vol. 380, 6640 (2023):eadd6220. https://doi.org/10.1126/science.add6220

Miyano K, Manabe S, Komatsu A, Fujii Y, Mizobuchi Y, Uezono E, Ohshima K, Nonaka M, Kuroda Y, Narita M, Uezono Y (2020) The G protein signal-biased compound TRV130; structures, its site of action and clinical studies. Curr Top Med Chem 20:2822–2829. https://doi.org/10.2174/1568026620999201027224229

Nguyen AH, Thomsen ARB, Cahill TJ 3rd, Huang R, Huang LY, Marcink T, Clarke OB, Heissel S, Masoudi A, Ben-Hail D et al (2019) Structure of an endosomal signaling GPCR-G protein-β-arrestin megacomplex. Nat Struct Mol Biol 26:1123–1131. https://doi.org/10.1038/s41594-019-0330-y

Rankovic Z, Brust TF, Bohn LM (2016) Biased agonism: an emerging paradigm in GPCR drug discovery. Bioorg Med Chem Lett 26:241–250. https://doi.org/10.1016/j.bmcl.2015.12.024

Reiter E, Lefkowitz RJ (2006) GRKs and beta-arrestins: roles in receptor silencing, trafficking and signaling. Trends Endocrinol Metab 17:159–165. https://doi.org/10.1016/j.tem.2006.03.008

Rose AS, Elgeti M, Zachariae U, Grubmüller H, Hofmann KP, Scheerer P, Hildebrand PW (2014) Position of transmembrane helix 6 determines receptor G protein coupling specificity. J Am Chem Soc 136:11244–11247. https://doi.org/10.1021/ja5055109

Sandhu M, Cho A, Ma N, Mukhaleva E, Namkung Y, Lee S, Ghosh S, Lee JH, Gloriam DE, Laporte SA et al (2022) Dynamic spatiotemporal determinants modulate GPCR:G protein coupling selectivity and promiscuity. Nat Commun 13:7428. https://doi.org/10.1038/s41467-022-34055-5

Shao Z, Shen Q, Yao B, Mao C, Chen LN, Zhang H, Shen DD, Zhang C, Li W, Du X et al (2022) Identification and mechanism of G protein-biased ligands for chemokine receptor CCR1. Nat Chem Biol 18:264–271. https://doi.org/10.1038/s41589-021-00918-z

Shen Q, Tang X, Wen X, Cheng S, Xiao P, Zang SK, Shen DD, Jiang L, Zheng Y, Zhang H et al (2024) Molecular determinant underlying selective coupling of primary G-protein by class A GPCRs. Adv Sci (Weinh) 11:e2310120. https://doi.org/10.1002/advs.202310120

Shenoy SK, Lefkowitz RJ (2011) β-Arrestin-mediated receptor trafficking and signal transduction. Trends Pharmacol Sci 32:521–533. https://doi.org/10.1016/j.tips.2011.05.002

Shukla AK, Manglik A, Kruse AC, Xiao K, Reis RI, Tseng WC, Staus DP, Hilger D, Uysal S, Huang LY et al (2013) Structure of active β-arrestin-1 bound to a G-protein-coupled receptor phosphopeptide. Nature 497:137–141. https://doi.org/10.1038/nature12120

Shukla AK, Westfield GH, Xiao K, Reis RI, Huang LY, Tripathi-Shukla P, Qian J, Li S, Blanc A, Oleskie AN et al (2014) Visualization of arrestin recruitment by a G-protein-coupled receptor. Nature 512:218–222. https://doi.org/10.1038/nature13430

Staus DP, Hu H, Robertson MJ, Kleinhenz ALW, Wingler LM, Capel WD, Latorraca NR, Lefkowitz RJ, Skiniotis G (2020) Structure of the M2 muscarinic receptor-beta-arrestin complex in a lipid nanodisc. Nature 579:297–302. https://doi.org/10.1038/s41586-020-1954-0

Suomivuori CM, Latorraca NR, Wingler LM, Eismann S, King MC, Kleinhenz ALW, Skiba MA, Staus DP, Kruse AC, Lefkowitz RJ, Dror RO (2020) Molecular mechanism of biased signaling in a prototypical G protein-coupled receptor. Science 367:881–887. https://doi.org/10.1126/science.aaz0326

Szczepek M, Beyrière F, Hofmann KP, Elgeti M, Kazmin R, Rose A, Bartl FJ, von Stetten D, Heck M, Sommer ME et al (2014) Crystal structure of a common GPCR-binding interface for G protein and arrestin. Nat Commun 5:4801. https://doi.org/10.1038/ncomms5801

Thomsen ARB, Plouffe B, Cahill TJ 3rd, Shukla AK, Tarrasch JT, Dosey AM, Kahsai AW, Strachan RT, Pani B, Mahoney JP et al (2016) GPCR-G protein-β-Arrestin super-complex mediates sustained G protein signaling. Cell 166:907–919. https://doi.org/10.1016/j.cell.2016.07.004

Tóth AD, Turu G, Hunyady L (2024) Functional consequences of spatial, temporal and ligand bias of G protein-coupled receptors. Nat Rev Nephrol. https://doi.org/10.1038/s41581-024-00869-3

Violin JD, Crombie AL, Soergel DG, Lark MW (2014) Biased ligands at G-protein-coupled receptors: promise and progress. Trends Pharmacol Sci 35:308–316. https://doi.org/10.1016/j.tips.2014.04.007

Wang WW, Ji SY, Zhang W, Zhang J, Cai C, Hu R, Zang SK, Miao L, Xu H, Chen LN et al (2024) Structure-based design of non-hypertrophic apelin receptor modulator. Cell 187:1460–1475.e1420. https://doi.org/10.1016/j.cell.2024.02.004

Wingler LM, Skiba MA, McMahon C, Staus DP, Kleinhenz ALW, Suomivuori CM, Latorraca NR, Dror RO, Lefkowitz RJ, Kruse AC (2020) Angiotensin and biased analogs induce structurally distinct active conformations within a GPCR. Science (New York, NY) 367:888–892. https://doi.org/10.1126/science.aay9813

Wootten D, Christopoulos A, Marti-Solano M, Babu MM, Sexton PM (2018) Mechanisms of signalling and biased agonism in G protein-coupled receptors. Nat Rev Mol Cell Biol 19:638–653. https://doi.org/10.1038/s41580-018-0049-3

Xu Z, Ikuta T, Kawakami K, Kise R, Qian Y, Xia R, Sun MX, Zhang A, Guo C, Cai XH et al (2022a) Structural basis of sphingosine-1-phosphate receptor 1 activation and biased agonism. Nat Chem Biol 18:281–288. https://doi.org/10.1038/s41589-021-00930-3

Xu J, Cao S, Hübner H, Weikert D, Chen G, Lu Q, Yuan D, Gmeiner P, Liu Z, Du Y (2022b) Structural insights into ligand recognition, activation, and signaling of the α(2A) adrenergic receptor. Sci Adv 8:eabj5347. https://doi.org/10.1126/sciadv.abj5347

Xu Z, Guo L, Yu J, Shen S, Wu C, Zhang W, Zhao C, Deng Y, Tian X, Feng Y et al (2023) Ligand recognition and G-protein coupling of trace amine receptor TAAR1. Nature 624:672–681. https://doi.org/10.1038/s41586-023-06804-z

Yang SH, Sharrocks AD, Whitmarsh AJ (2013) MAP kinase signalling cascades and transcriptional regulation. Gene 513:1–13. https://doi.org/10.1016/j.gene.2012.10.033

Yang D, Zhou Q, Labroska V, Qin S, Darbalaei S, Wu Y, Yuliantie E, Xie L, Tao H, Cheng J et al (2021) G protein-coupled receptors: structure- and function-based drug discovery. Signal Transduct Target Ther 6:7. https://doi.org/10.1038/s41392-020-00435-w

Yin W, Li Z, Jin M, Yin YL, de Waal PW, Pal K, Yin Y, Gao X, He Y, Gao J et al (2019) A complex structure of arrestin-2 bound to a G protein-coupled receptor. Cell Res 29:971–983. https://doi.org/10.1038/s41422-019-0256-2

Zhang L, Mobbs JI, May LT, Glukhova A, Thal DM (2023) The impact of cryo-EM on determining allosteric modulator-bound structures of G protein-coupled receptors. Curr Opin Struct Biol 79: 102560. https://doi.org/10.1016/j.sbi.2023.102560

Zhang M, Chen T, Lu X, Lan X, Chen Z, Lu S (2024) G protein-coupled receptors (GPCRs): advances in structures, mechanisms, and drug discovery. Signal Transduct Target Ther 9:88. https://doi.org/10.1038/s41392-024-01803-6

Zhao LH, He Q, Yuan Q, Gu Y, He X, Shan H, Li J, Wang K, Li Y, Hu W et al (2023) Conserved class B GPCR activation by a biased intracellular agonist. Nature 621:635–641. https://doi.org/10.1038/s41586-023-06467-w

Zhou XE, Melcher K, Xu HE (2017) Understanding the GPCR biased signaling through G protein and arrestin complex structures. Curr Opin Struct Biol 45:150–159. https://doi.org/10.1016/j.sbi.2017.05.004

Zhou Q, Yang D, Wu M, Guo Y, Guo W, Zhong L, Cai X, Dai A, Jang W, Shakhnovich EI et al (2019) Common activation mechanism of class a GPCRs. eLife 8. https://doi.org/10.7554/eLife.50279

Zhuang Y, Wang Y, He B, He X, Zhou XE, Guo S, Rao Q, Yang J, Liu J, Zhou Q et al (2022) Molecular recognition of morphine and fentanyl by the human mu-opioid receptor. Cell 185: 4361–4375 e4319. https://doi.org/10.1016/j.cell.2022.09.041

Part III

Drug Discovery and Development of Biased Ligands

Biased Agonism at β-Adrenoceptor Subtypes: A Drug Development Perspective

Martin C. Michel and Ongun Onaran

Contents

Abstract

Selectivity of a drug for a desired response as compared to undesirable responses (side effect) is a key goal of drug development. Early concepts to achieve such selectivity were based on selectivity for a molecular target as compared to others, pharmacokinetic factors to achieve high concentrations in the target tissue as compared to low concentrations in others, differential efficacy in the target vs. others tissues, and leveraging the concept of cell type and tissue differences in expression levels of receptors and their related signaling molecules, which can be further complicated by alterations of such ratios in disease. Biased agonism occurs when one response is activated preferentially over another after accounting for the above other factors. Thus, assessment of ligand bias is not always easy. β-Adrenoceptors have played a relevant role in our understanding of

M. C. Michel (✉)
Department of Pharmacology, University Medical Center, Johannes Gutenberg University, Mainz, Germany
e-mail: marmiche@uni-mainz.de

O. Onaran
Department of Pharmacology, School of Medicine, Ankara University, Ankara, Türkiye

© The Author(s), under exclusive license to Springer Nature Switzerland AG 2025
Z. Li, K. Xiao (eds.), *Pharmacology of GPCRs Biased Signaling and Agonists*,
Handbook of Experimental Pharmacology 290, https://doi.org/10.1007/164_2025_769

the phenomenon of biased agonism. Several clinically used β-adrenoceptor ligands were proposed to exhibit biased agonism, but the findings often are inconclusive, at least partly based on the overall complexity of assessment of biased signaling. These complexities also make it challenging to determine the desired biased profile of a ligand at the start of a drug research and development project, particularly for innovative applications. Thus, biased agonism has potential to contribute to functional target selectivity, but its prospective use remains challenging.

Keywords

Biased agonism · Drug development · β_1-adrenoceptor · β_2-adrenoceptor · β_3-adrenoceptor

Abbreviations

AR	adrenoceptor
CHO	Chinese hamster ovary
ECAR	extracellular acidification rate
EPAC	exchange proteins directly activated by cAMP
ERK	extracellular signal-regulated kinase
GPCR	G protein-coupled receptor
HEK	human embryonic kidney
MAPK	mitogen-activated protein kinase
PTX	pertussis toxin

1 Introduction

Adrenoceptors (ARs) mediate the effects of the endogenous catecholamines adrenaline and noradrenaline, including positive inotropic, chronotropic, dromotropic, and lusitropic effects on the heart; modulation of smooth muscle tone, e.g., of blood vessels, airways, prostate and urinary bladder; and modulation of glucose homeostasis by acting on glycogenolysis, thermogenesis, and pancreatic insulin release, and of brain function including ocular function. This wide range of physiological functions led to the development of a plethora of drugs. Many of these AR-ligands have become standard of care in therapeutic areas including the cardiovascular system, respiratory medicine, urogenital conditions, migraine, or ocular disease. As research on this receptor class started more than a century ago, ARs, particularly the β_2-AR, have become prototypes for our understanding of the action of G protein-coupled receptors (GPCRs) (Michel 2024).

Achieving a good *efficacy/tolerability profile* requires selecting a drug candidate that causes the desired effect with as little as possible undesired effects. This can be achieved in multiple, not mutually exclusive ways (Box 1). Firstly, it is possible to design compounds that interact with the desired molecular target selectively as compared to other molecules, such as subtype-selective receptor ligands. This is the oldest approach obtaining a favorable efficacy/tolerability profile in AR research. Following the initial proposal to subdivide AR into the subtypes α and β (Ahlquist 1948), further subdivision into α_1 and α_2 (Langer 1974; Starke 1987) and β_1 and β_2 emerged (Lands et al. 1967). However, shortly thereafter it became clear that even that was insufficient (Harms et al. 1977). Following the availability of more selective tool compounds and the cloning of AR subtypes, it ultimately became accepted that the AR family consists of three subfamilies (α_1, α_2 and β) including three subtypes each (α_{1A}, α_{1B}, α_{1D}, α_{2A}, α_{2B}, α_{2C}, β_1, β_2, and β_3) (Bylund et al. 1994; Hieble et al. 1995). The selective targeting of AR subfamilies or subtypes proved to be a very successful strategy in the design and development of novel drugs that are efficacious and have limited side effects. Examples are β_1-AR antagonists in cardiovascular indications (Bond et al. 2022), β_2-AR agonists in obstructive lung disease (Kume et al. 2015), or β_3-AR agonists in the treatment of the overactive bladder syndrome (He et al. 2023). The pioneering work in the development of selective β-AR antagonists was honored with a Nobel prize to Sir James Black (1989).

Box 1: Means to Achieve Selectivity for a Targeted Drug Response

- Selectivity for molecular target
- Enrichment in or exclusion of tissue on pharmacokinetic grounds
- Degree of agonism/inverse agonism
- Cell type/tissue specific stochiometry of molecular target and associated signaling molecules
- Biased agonism at the receptor level

A second approach to improve the efficacy/tolerability ratio of AR ligands was the identification of compounds with particular pharmacokinetic properties that enrich in the target as compared to other tissues (Michel 2010) or the opposite, i.e., the sparing of the brain by drug candidates that exhibit limited penetration through the blood-brain barrier (Callegari et al. 2011). Other than exploiting inherent target tissue selectivity of a drug, this can also be achieved by local administration, for instance, in the administration of β_2-AR agonists by inhalation in the treatment of obstructive lung disease (Kume et al. 2015).

A third approach relies on the observation that ligands can exhibit different degrees of *efficacy* at the molecular target. While original concept of drug action on ARs dichotomized ligands as activators (agonists) or inhibitors (antagonists) of the receptor, it turned out that efficacy covers a continuous spectrum from full agonists (e.g., isoprenaline for β-AR) to antagonists, with partial agonists in between (Jasper and Insel 1992; Clarke and Bond 1998). Finally, this spectrum has been extended beyond the competitive antagonism to include inverse agonists with negative efficacy, i.e., ligands that can reduce the constitutive activity of GPCRs, including ARs in the absence of agonist (Schütz and Freissmuth 1992; Michel et al.

2020). Of note, although efficacy represents an invariant quantity encoded in the chemical identity of ligand, receptor, and transducer, its manifestation in the observed response may differ among cell types, most likely due to the differential expression of signaling molecules mediating a response (Michel et al. 2020). Thus, *inverse agonism* is easier to detect in systems with high receptor expression, such as those often achieved after transfection of the receptor. Depending on the degree of expression of a receptor and/or associated signaling molecules, occupation of as little as 5% of the receptors may be sufficient to reach a close to maximal response, as in the case of positive inotropic effects of β-AR agonists in the rat heart (Brown et al. 1992). This phenomenon is sometimes referred to as receptor reserve, which arise from the nonlinearity of receptor-effector coupling. Thus, a weak partial agonist may be desirable if the target cell type or tissue exhibits a large receptor reserve whereas tissues mediating side effects exhibit little or no receptor reserve.

A fourth approach can also be based on the fact that the efficiency of stimulus-response coupling depends on the relative expression levels of signaling molecules involved in the relevant pathways. This may provide additional means of selectivity when we consider the fact that a signal starting from a single receptor type can lead to multiple responses via branching signaling pathways. In case of β-AR, for example, the receptor can activate multiple G proteins, adenylyl cyclases, arrestins, protein kinase A, mitogen-activated protein kinases (MAPK), or exchange proteins directly activated by cAMP (*EPAC*s). The magnitudes of such responses depend on the relative concentrations of these players in a cell type (Ostrom et al. 2000). This may lead to a single receptor subtype preferentially activating response X in one cell type, where signaling molecules involved in this response are highly expressed. On the other hand, preferential activation of response Y may occur in cases where signaling molecules involved in that response are highly expressed. This phenomenon is called cellular or tissue bias and does not necessarily involve biased agonism inherent to a ligand. Of note, subtypes of β-AR exhibit intrinsically divergent affinity and efficacy in coupling to G_s and to arrestins, which may make ligands acting on both partner molecules look as being biased, whereas this may reflect system bias (see below) and not biased signaling by the ligand (Casella et al. 2011).

Another level of complexity occurs when some signaling molecules undergo regulation in disease or upon drug treatment. For instance, heart failure may lead to redistribution of β_1- and β_2-ARs (Nikolaev et al. 2010), upregulation of β_3-ARs (Dal Monte et al. 2020), downregulation of $G_{\alpha s}$, and upregulation of $G_{\alpha i}$ proteins in the heart (Lohse et al. 2003). The expression level of β_2-AR affects interaction with the GRK/arrestin pathway in transgenic mice (Dorn II et al. 1999). Prolonged exposure to a β-AR agonist may lead not only to changes in receptor and G protein expression but also to a diminished activity of adenylyl cyclase (Okeke et al. 2019), thereby altering the relative concentrations of the signaling molecules involved in a response. This phenomenon has been called "*dynamic bias*" (Michel et al. 2014).

A fifth possibility to achieve the selective activation of a desired response came from the observation that the rank order of agonists to elicit one response via a single AR subtype may differ from that eliciting another response, if this phenomenon cannot be explained by any of the above factors (Nagi and Onaran 2021). This fifth dimension of selectivity has been described by various names including functional selectivity, agonist-directed trafficking, protean agonism, or ligand-directed signaling (Michel and Alewijnse 2007) but is now generally referred to as biased agonism (Kenakin and Miller 2010). While early conceptual work on biased agonism involved several GPCRs including opioid receptors and angiotensin II type 1 receptors, β-AR were important prototypes for our understanding of biased agonism (Ippolito and Benovic 2021). For instance, *propranolol* and ICI 118,551 are antagonists for G_s-mediated β-AR signaling but can promote the phosphorylation/activation of *extracellular signal-regulated kinase* (ERK) via arrestin, independent of G_s or $G_{i/o}$ proteins (Azzi et al. 2003; Baker et al. 2003; Shenoy et al. 2006). Interestingly, biased agonism can not only be elicited by small molecules but also by nanobodies (Staus et al. 2014). Pioneering work on biased agonism at β-AR particularly came from the groups of Terry P. Kenakin at Glaxo Research Laboratories (Kenakin and Morgan 1989) and Roger Summers at Monash University (Evans et al. 2013).

In the following, we will first discuss conceptual issues with the assessment of biased agonism at β-ARs, then review the evidence for biased agonism at each of the three β-AR subtypes, followed by a discussion of the implications of biased agonism for translational research, drug research and development, and clinical medicine. We explicitly acknowledge informative previous reviews in this area (Evans et al. 2010; Patel et al. 2010; Baker et al. 2011; Reiter et al. 2012; Ippolito and Benovic 2021).

2 What Constitutes Biased Agonism?

A rank order of potency and/or efficacy of two ligands, that is, A > B for response X but B > A for response Y, can point to the presence of biased agonism inherent to a ligand but may potentially also be explained by the four other determinants of selectivity mentioned above, particularly if responses X and Y are measured in different cell types or even different tissues (cell/tissue bias). These alternative explanations include molecular target/receptor subtype selectivity, tissue selectivity, degree of agonism, cell/tissue bias, or dynamic bias (Box 1). It follows from this complexity that biased signaling of ligands cannot easily be evaluated when the ligands being compared are tested in different cell types/tissues. Moreover, biased agonism inherently is a drug property relative to a reference compound. Even minor chemical changes within a molecule can markedly affect its biased signaling; for instance, 12 stereoisomers of *fenoterol* exhibited distinct biased profiles across six molecular and cellular assays (Reinartz et al. 2015). Thus, conclusive statements on ligand bias should be based on a direct comparison of two or more ligands within a cell type (Onaran et al. 2014; Kenakin 2015; Kolb et al. 2022). Computational methods to quantify ligand bias have been reported (Rajagopal et al. 2011; Reinartz et al. 2015).

True ligand bias is based on the interaction between a biological and a chemical phenomenon. Biologically, a given β-AR subtype may not only couple to α-subunits of G_s, which is its prototypical signaling pathway (Alexander et al. 2023), but also to those of other G proteins including forms of G_i and G_q, to βγ-subunits of G proteins, and even to non-G protein targets such as arrestins (Wenzel-Seifert and Seifert 2000; Lefkowitz and Shenoy 2005; Stallaert et al. 2012; Wess et al. 2023). The degree of coupling to multiple pathways may partly differ between β-AR subtypes; for instance, β_2-ARs may be more prone to couple to G_i proteins than β_1-ARs (Abramson et al. 1988; Xiao et al. 1995), and β_3-ARs may exhibit an even greater affinity for G_i proteins (Cao et al. 2000). Chemically, based on their molecular interaction with the receptor, some ligands inherently favor/induce conformational states that couple to one as compared to another signaling pathway present in substantial quantity in a cell (Bokoch et al. 2010; Kahsai et al. 2011). To further complicate the matter, the degree of intrinsic efficacy for the activation of individual signaling pathways may differ between ligands.

3 Methodological Challenges in the Assessment of Bias at β-Adrenoceptor Subtypes

Several approaches are used to explore biased signaling at β-ARs. This includes the *extracellular acidification rate* (ECAR) (Hutchinson et al. 2005), GPCR kinase phosphorylation and receptor trafficking (De Pascali et al. 2022), and impedance responses (and integrated indicator of multiple signaling pathways) (Stallaert et al. 2012). However, the most frequently used comparator to cAMP formation is the phosphorylation (as proxy for activation) of ERK and other MAPKs; however, ERK/MAPK phosphorylation/activation is a complex response. Thus, other than arrestin, cAMP itself can lead to ERK phosphorylation (Vossler et al. 1997; Stork and Schmitt 2002), G_i may be involved in the ERK phosphorylation response even for primarily G_s-coupled receptors (Daaka et al. 1997; Galandrin et al. 2008), and Src can contribute with or without the involvement of arrestin (Luttrell et al. 1999; Ma et al. 2000; Sun et al. 2007; Galandrin et al. 2008). Moreover, such contributions are not only cell-dependent (Qiu et al. 2000; Lefkowitz et al. 2002) but may also depend on the state of the same cell clone (Kaya et al. 2012). Therefore, the fact that ERK phosphorylation is a complex response possibly involving multiple mechanisms should be kept in mind when interpreting the phosphorylation data. Similarly, glucose uptake into mouse soleus muscle can be stimulated by multiple ligands including BRL 37344 and clenbuterol, but this may involve distinct signaling G_s- and G_i-mediated pathways (Evans et al. 2013; Ngala et al. 2013).

Off-target effects can obscure the detection of true biased agonism (van der Westhuizen et al. 2014). For example, the clinically used β-AR antagonist carvedilol has been proposed to be a biased agonist based on its ability to stimulate arrestin signaling (Wisler et al. 2007); this appears to be mediated by a G_i protein when acting on β_1-ARs, but not when acting on β_2-ARs (Wang et al. 2017). Moreover, carvedilol has additional actions not shared by most other β-AR antagonists. It has been reported to be an antagonist at α_1-AR, exhibit antioxidative effects and clash with NO production (Yoshioka et al. 2000; Afonso et al. 2006), inhibit endothelin production (Saijonmaa et al. 1997; Ohlstein et al. 1998), and at least in high concentrations block voltage-operated Ca^{2+} channels (Ruffolo et al. 1990). Another example of this problem is the β_1-selective antagonist *nebivolol* that can also stimulate arrestin signaling (Erickson et al. 2013). It has also been proposed to exhibit α_1-AR antagonism, antioxidative effects, and stimulating effects on *NO production* through activation of NO synthase; the latter was proposed to occur through β_3-AR agonism (Rozec et al. 2006), but others found no evidence for nebivolol being a β_3-AR agonist in transfected cell lines or rat bladder tissue (Frazier et al. 2011). Linking observed effects, particularly in vivo, to biased agonism is close to impossible with such "dirty" ligands as the observed effect may be due to any of these effects or any combination thereof.

Another level of complexity comes from the general observation that 50% or more of reported findings in biology are not robust (Vollert et al. 2022). For instance, controversial data on biased agonism of *fenoterol* and *salmeterol* at β_2-AR have been reported (see below). Thus, the presence of ligand bias of many if not most known adrenergic agonists remains undecidable for the moment (Onaran et al. 2017). Thus, it seems impossible to associate confidently the therapeutic advantage of some bronchodilators (like salmeterol) with bias. Very few if any β-AR ligands exhibit a robustly proven bias for a signaling pathway, e.g., compound C1-S apparently favoring G_s over arrestin when acting on β_2-AR (Kim et al. 2021). Finally, allosteric modulators may affect signaling. Thus, compound-6 was reported to be a positive allosteric modulator enhancing agonism at β_2-AR; among a panel of structurally diverse β-AR antagonists, compound-6 potentiated arrestin but not Gs-mediated effects of *carvedilol*, including activation of ERK, receptor endocytosis, or receptor trafficking to lysosomes (Pani et al. 2021), implying that biased signaling may in some cases depend on allosteric modulation.

4 Biased Signaling via β_1-Adrenoceptors

Given the widespread use of β_1-AR, specifically antagonists in more than 30 indications (Bond et al. 2022), studies concerning biased agonism at this subtype are surprisingly sparse. A study using transfected human embryonic kidney (HEK) cells compared isoprenaline, bucindolol, and propranolol for their effects on ERK activation, which are full, partial, and inverse agonists, respectively, for cAMP formation (Galandrin et al. 2008). Despite their differential effectiveness for cAMP formation, all activated ERK to a similar extent. This was dependent on Src for the three ligands; for bucindolol and propranolol, in contrast to isoprenaline, this was independent of G protein activation.

The β_1-selective antagonist nebivolol was reported to stimulate arrestin signaling (Erickson et al. 2013). However, based on multiple other effects of nebivolol, perhaps including those on β_1-AR (Rozec et al. 2006; Frazier et al. 2011), it remained difficult to determine whether this represents biased agonism. Metoprolol induced an interaction between the β_1-AR and arrestin-2 but not arrestin-1; accordingly, metoprolol-induced cardiac fibrosis was abolished in arrestin-2 knockout mice (Nakaya et al. 2012). Carvedilol was reported to activate the cGMP pathway in the murine heart in concentrations having little effect on the cAMP pathway (Wang et al. 2021). This is unlikely to represent a system bias as it was shared by nebivolol but not by other β-blockers such as metoprolol, propranolol, or sotalol.

5 Biased Signaling via β_2-Adrenoceptors

Some groups have examined large panels of ligands for potential biased agonism at β_2-AR. The group of Michel Bouvier from Montrèal tested 14 ligands in HEK cells and various transfected variants thereof in assays for cAMP accumulation, ERK activation, cell impedance assay, or Ca^{2+} elevation (Stallaert et al. 2012). Based on their findings, they categorized ligands into five groups. Group I ligands (isoprenaline, adrenaline) similarly stimulated cAMP accumulation and ERK phosphorylation. Group II ligands (*salbutamol, salmeterol*) strongly activated cAMP accumulation but were weak partial agonists for ERK phosphorylation. Group III ligands (alprenolol, bucindolol, labetolol, pindolol) were weak partial agonists for cAMP and ERK responses. Group IV ligands (propranolol, carvedilol) were very weak partial agonists in both assays. Finally, group V ligands (atenolol, ICI 118,551, metoprolol, timolol) were inverse agonists for the cAMP and the ERK responses. A follow-up study from the same group tested 19 (mostly clinically used) β_2-AR ligands for cAMP production, ERK activation, Ca^{2+} elevation, and receptor endocytosis (van der Westhuizen et al. 2014). This data supported the clustering into five groups. While apparent biased signaling of nine compounds could be explained by off-target effects, the clustering into five groups was confirmed with the remaining 10 compounds. Calculation of relative effectiveness within a pathway and of bias factors between pathways for each compound using an operational model of agonism showed a global signaling signature of all compounds relative to isoprenaline with most being biased toward ERK activation relative to the other pathways. Finally, a collaboration between German, Japanese, and US investigators tested 65 β_2-AR ligands (40 classically considered as agonists and 25 as antagonists) in HEK cells for their ability to recruit β-arrestin 1 and 2 to the β_2-AR (Littmann et al. 2015). Many agonists showed only weak partial agonism for arrestin recruitment with potency and/or efficacy increasing depending on the number of chirality centers in (R) configuration; no (S)-configured enantiomer was more effective in arrestin recruitment than the eutomer. Generally, β-arrestin 2 was recruited more effectively than β-arrestin 1. Several agonists showed strong bias for activation of Gαs relative to arrestin recruitment. Compounds classically considered as antagonists did not promote arrestin recruitment.

Other groups looked at smaller numbers of compounds, typically focusing on a single molecule relative to one or more reference compounds (in most cases isoprenaline). However, findings across groups were inconsistent. For instance, the β_2-AR agonist fenoterol was proposed to be G_s-biased (over G_i) by some investigators (Reinartz et al. 2015), but others did not confirm that (Onaran et al. 2017; De Pascali et al. 2022).

Similarly, some investigators found the β_2-AR agonist salmeterol to be G_s-biased but not providing state-of-the-art bias analysis (Carter and Hill 2005; Gimenez et al. 2015), whereas others found it to be arrestin-biased (Rajagopal et al. 2011); salmeterol is not biased at all according to others (De Pascali et al. 2022) or in our hands (unpublished data). At the end, the bias status of most known adrenergic agonists remains undecidable for the moment (Onaran et al. 2017).

Finally, the β-AR antagonist carvedilol, clinically used in the treatment of heart failure, was reported to be an inverse agonist for cAMP formation but a partial agonist for β_2-AR ERK receptor phosphorylation, arresting binding, ERK activation, and receptor internalization (Wisler et al. 2007). Within a panel including acebutolol, alprenolol, atenolol, bisoprolol, betaxolol, carvedilol, ICI 118,551, labetalol, metoprolol, nadolol, oxprenolol, pindolol, propranolol, sotalol, and timolol, carvedilol was the only inverse agonist for cAMP that activated ERK.

6 Biased Signaling via β_3-Adrenoceptors

In contrast to the many indications of β_1- and β_2-AR ligands (Bond et al. 2022), the only approved use for β_3-AR agonists is the overactive bladder syndrome (Michel et al. 2023). Nonetheless, β_3-AR ligands have intensively been investigated for biased agonism. An early study reported, based on Chinese hamster ovary (CHO) cells transfected with human β_3-AR, that agonists stimulated ERK activation but not that of the related MAPKs, JNK, and p38 (Gerhardt et al. 1999). In a limited panel of compounds, adrenaline and noradrenaline preferentially activated cAMP formation, whereas BRL 37,344 preferentially stimulated ERK. The latter response was sensitive to PTX, indicating an effect on G_i proteins, and the phosphatidylinositol-3 kinase inhibitors wortmannin and LY 294002.

More detailed studies on biased agonism at β_3-ARs came from a series of studies by the group of Roger Summers in Melbourne. Their initial study was performed in CHO cells transfected with cloned murine β_3-ARs, in murine 3 T3-F442 adipocytes, and in murine ileum and was based on a comparison of SR 59,230 and CL 316,243 (Hutchinson et al. 2005). The efficacy of the partial agonist SR 59,230 for stimulating cAMP formation increased with increasing levels of β_3-AR expression in the CHO cells. On the other hand, SR 59,230 was a full agonist for the ECAR response at all expression levels, an observation that could potentially be explained as by a greater receptor reserve for the ECAR as compared to the cAMP response. In 3T3-F442A cells, SR 59,230, in contrast to CL 316,243, had no agonist effects, an observation that could potentially be explained by low expression of the β_3-AR and/or by a less effective effector coupling in these cells. However, SR 59,230 had greater efficacy than CL 316,243 in the ECAR assay in 3T3-F442A cells, i.e., there was a reversal in order of efficacy that cannot be explained easily by a receptor reserve. Relaxation responses in mouse ileum were evoked by SR 59,230 in concentrations where it did not affect cAMP levels.

In a follow-up study in CHO cells transfected with the human β_3-AR, zinterol and L 755,507 caused robust, concentration-dependent increases in cAMP whereas L

748,337 had low efficacy (Sato et al. 2008). The cAMP responses to zinterol and L 755,507 were increased after pre-treatment with PTX, indicating that the β_3-AR concomitantly coupled to G_s and $G_{i/o}$ proteins in the CHO cells. However, both L 755,507 and L 748,337 stimulated the phosphorylation of ERK and, with much lower potency, of p38 MAPK. PTX fully blocked activation of ERK and of p38 MAPK by L 748,337, whereas the p38 phosphorylation stimulated by L 755,507 was not inhibited by PTX and that of ERK phosphorylation by only about 30%. The ECAR response was elicited with similar efficacy by all three agonists. Taken together these observations were interpreted that L 755,507 couples to both G_s and $G_{i/o}$ proteins whereas L 748,337 coupled predominantly to $G_{i/o}$ proteins.

We have studied the desensitization of cAMP responses elicited via human β_3-ARs transfected into HEK cells at near physiological density (Okeke et al. 2019). Ligands stimulated cAMP formation with a numerical rank order of isoprenaline $\geq$ L 755,507 $\geq$ CL 316,243 $>$ solabegron $>$ SR 59,230 $>$ L 748,337, an observation in line with the findings of others (Hutchinson et al. 2005; Sato et al. 2008). Except for the weakest agonist, L 748,337, pretreatment with any ligand reduced cAMP responses to freshly added isoprenaline or forskolin to a similar extent, indicating that the ability to cause desensitization of the β_3-AR did not depend on cAMP formation. On the other hand, we were unable to detect ERK phosphorylation despite testing a wide variation of conditions. In a follow-up study in transfected CHO cells, cAMP formation was stimulated with an agonist order of efficacy of isoprenaline (255% of control) $\approx$ L755,507 (247%) $>$ CL316,243 (209%) $>$ L748,337 (120%) $\approx$ SR59,230 (108%), whereas the order of efficacy for ERK phosphorylation was L755,507 (151%) $\approx$ CL316,243 (149%) $\approx$ isoprenaline (148%) $>$ SR59,230 (137%) $>$ L748,337 (122%) (Okeke et al. 2018). In these cells, desensitization of cAMP formation was caused by all ligands except for L 748,337, whereas L 748,337, but not isoprenaline, reduced ERK phosphorylation relative to a lowered baseline. Taken together, these findings demonstrate the presence of biased agonism at murine and human β_3-ARs.

7 Conclusions and Perspectives

It emerges from the above that studies of biased agonism are inherently complex because multiple factors other than biased agonism can be explained by different cellular, tissue, and in vivo responses when comparing two or more ligands. The possible role of allosteric modulators and frequent inconsistencies in the assessment of biased agonism across laboratories make robust conclusions on specific compounds difficult in most cases. Considering the limited robustness of reported findings, it can generally be concluded that distinguishing biased from partial agonism is challenging unless bias is extreme. That many studies in the field provided initial evidence for bias but few quantified it (Rajagopal et al. 2011; Reinartz et al. 2015) makes interpretation challenging. If we cannot/do not quantify bias relative to other drug properties such as partial agonism, rational selection of developmental candidates based on properties such as biased agonism becomes difficult. This is exemplified by the discrepancy between high expectations and limited clinical success in other fields such as opioid receptor activation (Kelly 2013; Schmid et al. 2017; Gillis et al. 2020; Conibear et al. 2024).

This has sparked intensive discussions about whether the existence of biased agonism opens attractive avenues for *drug research and development*. On the one hand, it is tempting to exploit biased agonism as another path to achieve selective activation of a desired as compared to an undesirable response (Woo et al. 2015; Kenakin 2018). On the other hand, signaling heterogeneity across cells/tissues and across species within tissues as well as their changes under pathophysiological conditions can make predictions on human target tissue in a given disease close to impossible (Li et al. 2023). The roles of allosteric modulators (Pani et al. 2021) and of auxiliary signaling molecules including RGSs (De Vries et al. 2000) and AGSs (Lanier 2004) may additionally blur the picture. Similarly, the efficiency of receptor-arrestin coupling may depend on the expression levels of GRKs (Winpenny et al. 2016). Therefore, it was argued that predicting the desirable biased agonism profile at the start of a research and development project is close to impossible, unless a large body of evidence for a drug target already exists (Michel and Charlton 2018; Onaran and Costa 2021). However, drug targets with a large body of existing evidence and often many approved medicines acting on those targets have become unpopular in the pharmaceutical industry for commercial reasons. Thus, no compounds designed to be biased agonists have reached late-stage clinical development or even became marketed drugs at present.

References

Abramson SN, Martin MW, Hughes AR, Harden TK, Neve KA, Barrett DA, Molinoff PB (1988) Interaction of beta-adrenergic receptors with the inhibitory guanine nucleotide-binding protein of adenylate cyclase in membranes prepared from cyc-S49 lymphoma cells. Biochem Pharmacol 37:4289–4297. https://doi.org/10.1016/0006-2952(88)90609-0

Afonso RA, Patarrao RS, Macedo MP, Carmo MM (2006) Carvedilol action is dependent on endogenous production of nitric oxide*. Am J Hypertens 19:419–425. https://doi.org/10.1016/j.amjhyper.2005.11.011

Ahlquist RP (1948) A study of the adrenotropic receptors. Am J Phys 153:586–600

Alexander SPH, Christopoulos A, Davenport AP, Kelly E, Mathie AA, Peters JA, Veale EL, Armstrong JF, Faccenda E, Harding SD, Davies JA, Abbracchio MP, Abraham G, Agoulnik A, Alexander W, Al-Hosaini K, Bäck M, Baker JG, Barnes NM, Bathgate R, Beaulieu JM, Beck-Sickinger AG, Behrens M, Bernstein KE, Bettler B, Birdsall NJM, Blaho V, Boulay F, Bousquet C, Bräuner-Osborne H, Burnstock G, Caló G, Castaño JP, Catt KJ, Ceruti S, Chazot P, Chiang N, Chini B, Chun J, Cianciulli A, Civelli O, Clapp LH, Couture R, Cox HM, Csaba Z, Dahlgren C, Dent G, Douglas SD, Dournaud P, Eguchi S, Escher E, Filardo EJ, Fong T, Fumagalli M, Gainetdinov RR, Garelja ML, de Gasparo M, Gerard C, Gershengorn M, Gobeil F, Goodfriend TL, Goudet C, Grätz L, Gregory KJ, Gundlach AL, Hamann J, Hanson J, Hauger RL, Hay DL, Heinemann A, Herr D, Hollenberg MD, Holliday ND, Horiuchi M, Hoyer D, Hunyady L, Husain A, AP IJ, Inagami T, Jacobson KA, Jensen RT, Jockers R, Jonnalagadda D, Karnik S, Kaupmann K, Kemp J, Kennedy C, Kihara Y, Kitazawa T, Kozielewicz P, Kreienkamp HJ, Kukkonen JP, Langenhan T, Larhammar D, Leach K, Lecca D, Lee JD, Leeman SE, Leprince J, Li XX, Lolait SJ, Lupp A, Macrae R,

Maguire J, Malfacini D, Mazella J, McArdle CA, Melmed S, Michel MC, Miller LJ, Mitolo V, Mouillac B, Müller CE, Murphy PM, Nahon JL, Ngo T, Norel X, Nyimanu D, O'Carroll AM, Offermanns S, Panaro MA, Parmentier M, Pertwee RG, Pin JP, Prossnitz ER, Quinn M, Ramachandran R, Ray M, Reinscheid RK, Rondard P, Rovati GE, Ruzza C, Sanger GJ, Schöneberg T, Schulte G, Schulz S, Segaloff DL, Serhan CN, Singh KD, Smith CM, Stoddart LA, Sugimoto Y, Summers R, Tan VP, Thal D, Thomas WW, Timmermans P, Tirupula K, Toll L, Tulipano G, Unal H, Unger T, Valant C, Vanderheyden P, Vaudry D, Vaudry H, Vilardaga JP, Walker CS, Wang JM, Ward DT, Wester HJ, Willars GB, Williams TL, Woodruff TM, Yao C, Ye RD (2023) The Concise Guide to PHARMACOLOGY 2023/24: G protein-coupled receptors. Br J Pharmacol 180(Suppl 2):S23–s144. https://doi.org/10.1111/bph.16177

Azzi M, Charest PG, Angers S, Rousseau G, Kohout T, Bouvier M, Pineyro G (2003) Beta-arrestin-mediated activation of MAPK by inverse agonists reveals distinct active conformations for G protein-coupled receptors. Proc Natl Acad Sci USA 100:11406–11411. https://doi.org/10.1073/pnas.1936664100

Baker JG, Hall IP, Hill SJ (2003) Agonist and inverse agonist actions of β-blockers at the human β2-Adrenoceptor provide evidence for agonist-directed signaling. Mol Pharmacol 64:1357–1369. https://doi.org/10.1124/mol.64.6.1357

Baker JG, Hill SJ, Summers RJ (2011) Evolution of β-blockers: from anti-anginal drugs to ligand-directed signalling. Trends Pharmacol Sci 32:227–234. https://doi.org/10.1016/j.tips.2011.02.010

Black J (1989) Drugs from emasculated hormones: the principle of syntopic antagonism. Science 245:486–493

Bokoch MP, Zou Y, Rasmussen SGF, Liu CW, Nygaard R, Rosenbaum DM, Fung JJ, Choi HJ, Thian FS, Kobilka TS, Puglisi JD, Weis WI, Pardo L, Prosser RS, Mueller L, Kobilka BK (2010) Ligand-specific regulation of the extracellular surface of a G-protein-coupled receptor. Nature 463:108–112. https://doi.org/10.1038/nature08650

Bond RA, Michel MC, Parra S (2022) ß-Adrenoceptor antagonists. In: Michel MC (ed) Cardiovascular, hematopoietic, urinary and respiratory pharmacology. Elsevier, Amsterdam, pp 497–506

Brown L, Deighton NM, Bals S, Söhlmann W, Zerkowski HR, Michel MC, Brodde OE (1992) Spare receptors for ß-adrenoceptor-mediated positive inotropic effects of catecholamines in the human heart. J Cardiovasc Pharmacol 19:222–232. https://doi.org/10.1097/00005344-199202000-00011

Bylund DB, Eikenberg DC, Hieble JP, Langer SZ, Lefkowitz RJ, Minneman KP, Molinoff PB, Ruffolo RR Jr, Trendelenburg U (1994) IV. International Union of Pharmacology Nomenclature of Adrenoceptors. Pharmacol Rev 46:121–136

Callegari E, Malhotra B, Bungay PJ, Webster R, Fenner KS, Kempshhall S, LaPerle JL, Michel MC, Kay GG (2011) A comprehensive nonclinical evaluation of the CNS penetration potential of antimuscarinic agents for the treatment of overactive bladder. Br J Clin Pharmacol 72:235–246. https://doi.org/10.1111/j.1365-2125.2011.03961.x

Cao W, Luttrell LM, Medvedev AV, Pierce KL, Daniel KW, Dixon TM, Lefkowitz RJ, Collins S (2000) Direct binding of activated c-src to the $ß_3$-adrenergic receptor is required for MAP kinase activation. J Biol Chem 275:38131–38134. https://doi.org/10.1074/jbc.C000592200

Carter AA, Hill SJ (2005) Characterization of isoprenaline- and salmeterol-stimulated interactions between $ß_2$-adrenoceptors and ß-arrestin 2 using ß-galactosidase complementation in C2C12 cells. J Pharmacol Exp Ther 315:839–848. https://doi.org/10.1124/jpet.105.088914

Casella I, Ambrosio C, Grò Maria C, Molinari P, Costa T (2011) Divergent agonist selectivity in activating β1- and β2-adrenoceptors for G-protein and arrestin coupling. Biochem J 438:191–202. https://doi.org/10.1042/BJ20110374

Clarke WP, Bond RA (1998) The elusive nature of intrinsic efficacy. Trends Pharmacol Sci 19:270–276

Conibear A, Bailey CP, Kelly E (2024) Biased signalling in analgesic research and development. Curr Opin Pharmacol 76:102465. https://doi.org/10.1016/j.coph.2024.102465

Daaka Y, Luttrell LM, Lefkowitz RJ (1997) Switching of the coupling of the β2-adrenergic receptor to different G proteins by protein kinase A. Nature 390:88–91. https://doi.org/10.1038/36362

Dal Monte M, Evans BA, Arioglu-Inan E, Michel MC (2020) Upregulation of β_3-adrenoceptors—a general marker of and protective mechanism against hypoxia? Naunyn Schmiedeberg's Arch Pharmacol 393:141–146. https://doi.org/10.1007/s00210-019-01780-6

De Pascali F, Ippolito M, Wolfe E, Komolov KE, Hopfinger N, Lemenze D, Kim N, Armen RS, An SS, Scott CP, Benovic JL (2022) β_2-Adrenoceptor agonist profiling reveals biased signalling phenotypes for the β_2-adrenoceptor with possible implications for the treatment of asthma. Br J Pharmacol 179:4692–4708. https://doi.org/10.1111/bph.15900

De Vries L, Zheng B, Fischer T, Elenko E, Farquhar MG (2000) The regulator of G protein signaling family. Annu Rev Pharmacol Toxicol 40:235–271. https://doi.org/10.1146/annurev.pharmtox.40.1.235

Dorn GW II, Tepe NM, Lorenz JN, Koch WJ, Liggett SB (1999) Low- and high-level transgenic expression of β_2-adrenergic receptors differentially affect cardiac hypertrophy and function in Gαq-overexpressing mice. Proc Natl Acad Sci 96:6400–6405. https://doi.org/10.1073/pnas.96.11.6400

Erickson CE, Gul R, Blessing CP, Nguyen J, Liu T, Pulakat L, Bastepe M, Jackson EK, Andresen BT (2013) The ß-blocker nebivolol is a GRK/ß-arrestin biased agonist. PLoS One 8:e71980. https://doi.org/10.1371/journal.pone.0071980

Evans BA, Sato M, Sarwar M, Hutchinson DS, Summers RJ (2010) Ligand-directed signalling at ß-adrenoceptors. Br J Pharmacol 159:1022–1038. https://doi.org/10.1111/j.1476-5381.2009.00602.x

Evans BA, Hutchinson DS, Summers RJ (2013) β_2-Adrenoceptor-mediated regulation of glucose uptake in skeletal muscle – ligand-idrected signalling or a reflection of system complexity? Naunyn Schmiedeberg's Arch Pharmacol 386:757–760. https://doi.org/10.1007/s00210-013-0879-7

Frazier EP, Michel-Reher MB, van Loenen P, Sand C, Schneider T, Peters SLM, Michel MC (2011) Lack of evidence that nebivolol is a β_3-adrenoceptor agonist. Eur J Pharmacol 654:86–91. https://doi.org/10.1016/j.ejphar.2010.11.036

Galandrin S, Oligny-Longpré G, Bonin H, Ogawa K, Galés C, Bouvier M (2008) Conformational rearrangements and signaling cascades involved in ligand-biased mitogen-activated protein kinase signaling through the ß1-adrenergic receptor. Mol Pharmacol 74:162–172. https://doi.org/10.1124/mol.107.043893

Gerhardt CC, Gros J, Strosberg AD, Issad T (1999) Stimulation of the extracellular signal-regulated kinase 1/2 pathway by human beta-3 adrenergic receptor: new pharmacological profile and mechanism of action. Mol Pharmacol 55:255–262. https://doi.org/10.1124/mol.55.2.255

Gillis A, Gondin AB, Kliewer A, Sanchez J, Lim HD, Alamein C, Manandhar P, Santiago M, Fritzwanker S, Schmiedel F, Katte TA, Reekie T, Grimsey NL, Kassiou M, Kellam B, Krasel C, Halls ML, Connor M, Lane JR, Schulz S, Christie MJ, Canals M (2020) Low intrinsic efficacy for G protein activation can explain the improved side effect profiles of new opioid agonists. Sci Signal 13:eaaz3140. https://doi.org/10.1126/scisignal.aaz3140

Gimenez LE, Baameur F, Vayttaden SJ, Clark RB (2015) Salmeterol efficacy and bias in the activation and kinase-mediated desensitization of β2-adrenergic receptors. Mol Pharmacol 87:954–964. https://doi.org/10.1124/mol.114.096800

Harms HH, Zaagsma J, de Vente J (1977) Differentiation of ß-adrenoceptors in right atrium, diaphragm and adipose tissue of the rat, using stereoisomers of propranolol, alprenolol, nifenalol and practolol. Life Sci 21:123–128

He W, Zhang Y, Huang G, Tian Y, Sun Q, Liu X (2023) Efficacy and safety of vibegron compared with mirabegron for overactive bladder: a systematic review and network meta-analysis. Low Urin Tract Symptoms. https://doi.org/10.1111/luts.12475

Hieble JP, Bylund DB, Clarke DE, Eikenburg DC, Langer SZ, Lefkowitz RJ, Minneman KP, Ruffolo RR Jr (1995) International Union of Pharmacology X. Recommendation for nomenclature of α_1-adrenoceptors: consensus update. Pharmacol Rev 47:267–270

Hutchinson DS, Sato M, Evans BA, Christopoulos A, Summers RJ (2005) Evidence for pleiotropic signaling at the mouse ß$_3$-adrenoceptor revealed by SR59230A [3-(2-ethylphenoxy)-1-[(1,S)-1,2,3,4-tetrahydronapth-1-ylamino]-2S-2-propanol oxalate]. J Pharmacol Exp Ther 312: 1064–1074. https://doi.org/10.1124/jpet.104.076901

Ippolito M, Benovic JL (2021) Biased agonism at β-adrenergic receptors. Cell Signal 80:109905. https://doi.org/10.1016/j.cellsig.2020.109905

Jasper JR, Insel PA (1992) Evolving concepts of partial agonism. The ß-adrenergic receptor as a paradigm. Biochem Pharmacol 43:119–130

Kahsai AW, Xiao K, Rajagopal S, Ahn S, Shukla AK, Sun J, Oas TG, Lefkowitz RJ (2011) Multiple ligand-specific conformations of the ß$_2$-adrenergic receptor. Nat Chem Biol 7:692–700. https://doi.org/10.1038/nchembio.634

Kaya AI, Onaran HO, Ozcan G, Ambrosio C, Costa T, Balli S, Ugur O (2012) Cell contact-dependent functional selectivity of beta2-adrenergic receptor ligands in stimulating cAMP accumulation and extracellular signal-regulated kinase phosphorylation. J Biol Chem 287: 6362–6374. https://doi.org/10.1074/jbc.M111.301820

Kelly E (2013) Efficacy and ligand bias at the μ-opioid receptor. Br J Pharmacol 169:1430–1446. https://doi.org/10.1111/bph.12222

Kenakin T (2015) Gaddum Memorial Lecture 2014: receptors as an evolving concept: from switches to biased microprocessors. Br J Pharmacol 172:4238–4253. https://doi.org/10.1111/bph.13217

Kenakin T (2018) Is the quest for signaling bias worth the effort? Mol Pharmacol 93:266–269. https://doi.org/10.1124/mol.117.111187

Kenakin T, Miller LJ (2010) Seven transmembrane receptors as shapeshifting proteins: the impact of allosteric modulation and functional selectivity on new drug discovery. Pharmacol Rev 62: 265–304. https://doi.org/10.1124/pr.108.000992

Kenakin TP, Morgan PH (1989) Theoretical effects of single and multiple transducer receptor coupling proteins on estimates of the relative potency of agonists. Mol Pharmacol 35:214–222

Kim D, Tokmakova A, Lujan LK, Strzelinski HR, Kim N, Najari Beidokhti M, Giulianotti MA, Mafi A, Woo J-AA, An SS, Goddard WA, Liggett SB (2021) Identification and characterization of an atypical Gαs-biased β2AR agonist that fails to evoke airway smooth muscle cell tachyphylaxis. Proc Natl Acad Sci 118:e2026668118. https://doi.org/10.1073/pnas.2026668118

Kolb P, Kenakin T, Alexander SPH, Bermudez M, Bohn LM, Breinholt CS, Bouvier M, Hill SJ, Kostenis E, Martemyanov KA, Neubig RR, Onaran HO, Rajagopal S, Roth BL, Selent J, Shukla AK, Sommer ME, Gloriam DE (2022) Community guidelines for GPCR ligand bias: IUPHAR review 32. Br J Pharmacol 179:3651–3674. https://doi.org/10.1111/bph.15811

Kume H, Fukunaga K, Oguma T (2015) Research and development of bronchodilators for asthma and COPD with a focus on G protein/K_{Ca} channel linkage and ß$_2$-adrenergic intrinsic efficacy. Pharmacol Ther 156:75–89. https://doi.org/10.1016/j.pharmthera.2015.09.004

Lands AM, Arnold A, McAuliff JP, Luduena FP, Brown TG (1967) Differentiation of receptor systems activated by sympathetic amines. Nature 214:597–598

Langer SZ (1974) Presynaptic regulation of catecholamine release. Biochem Pharmacol 23:1793–1800. https://doi.org/10.1016/0006-2952(74)90187-7

Lanier SM (2004) AGS proteins, GPR motifs and the signals processed by heterotrimeric G proteins. Biol Cell 96:369–372. https://doi.org/10.1016/j.biolcel.2004.03.012

Lefkowitz RJ, Shenoy SK (2005) Transduction of receptor signals by β-Arrestins. Science 308: 512–517. https://doi.org/10.1126/science.1109237

Lefkowitz RJ, Pierce KL, Luttrell LM (2002) Dancing with different partners: protein kinase a phosphorylation of seven membrane-spanning receptors regulates their G protein-coupling specificity. Mol Pharmacol 62:971. https://doi.org/10.1124/mol.62.5.971

Li A, Liu S, Huang R, Ahn S, Lefkowitz RJ (2023) Loss of biased signaling at a G protein-coupled receptor in overexpressed systems. PLoS One 18:e0283477. https://doi.org/10.1371/journal.pone.0283477

Littmann T, Göttle M, Reinartz MT, Kälble S, Wainer IW, Ozawa T, Seifert R (2015) Recruitment of ß-arrestins 1 and 2 to the $ß_2$-adrenoceptor: analysis of 65 ligands. J Pharmacol Exp Ther 355: 183–190. https://doi.org/10.1124/jpet.115.227959

Lohse MJ, Engelhardt S, Eschenhagen T (2003) What is the role of β-adrenergic signaling in heart failure? Circ Res 93:896–906. https://doi.org/10.1161/01.RES.0000102042.83024.CA

Luttrell LM, Ferguson SSG, Daaka Y, Miller WE, Maudsley S, Della Rocca GJ, Lin FT, Kawakatsu H, Owada K, Luttrell DK, Caron MG, Lefkowitz RJ (1999) β-Arrestin-dependent formation of β2 adrenergic receptor-Src protein kinase complexes. Science 283:655–661. https://doi.org/10.1126/science.283.5402.655

Ma Y-C, Huang J, Ali S, Lowry W, Huang X-Y (2000) Src tyrosine kinase is a novel direct effector of G proteins. Cell 102:635–646. https://doi.org/10.1016/S0092-8674(00)00086-6

Michel MC (2010) The forefront of novel therapeutic agents based on the pathophysiology of lower urinary tract dysfunction: α-blockers in the treatment of male voiding dysfunction – how do they work and why do they differ in tolerability? J Pharmacol Sci 112:151–157. https://doi.org/10.1254/jphs.09R15FM

Michel MC (2024) Introduction: a short history of sdrenoceptor research. Handb Exp Pharmacol 285:1–12. https://doi.org/10.1007/164_2024_718

Michel MC, Alewijnse AE (2007) Ligand-directed signaling: 50 ways to find a lover. Mol Pharmacol 72:1097–1099. https://doi.org/10.1124/mol.107.040923

Michel MC, Charlton SJ (2018) Biased Agonism in drug discovery—is it too soon to choose a path? Mol Pharmacol 93:259–265. https://doi.org/10.1124/mol.117.110890

Michel MC, Seifert R, Bond RA (2014) Dynamic bias and its implications for GPCR drug discovery. Nat Rev Drug Discov 13:869–870. https://doi.org/10.1038/nrd3954-c3

Michel MC, Michel-Reher MB, Hein P (2020) A systematic review of inverse agonism at adrenoceptor subtypes. Cells 9:1923. https://doi.org/10.3390/cells9091923

Michel MC, Cardozo L, Chermansky CJ, Cruz F, Igawa Y, Lee KS, Sahai A, Wein AJ, Andersson KE (2023) Current and emerging pharmacological targets and treatments of urinary incontinence and related disorders. Pharmacol Rev 75:554–674. https://doi.org/10.1124/pharmrev.121.000523

Nagi K, Onaran HO (2021) Biased agonism at G protein-coupled receptors. Cell Signal 83:109981. https://doi.org/10.1016/j.cellsig.2021.109981

Nakaya M, Chikura S, Watari K, Mizuno N, Mochinaga K, Mangmool S, Koyanagi S, Ohdo S, Sato Y, Ide T, Nishida M, Kurose H (2012) Induction of cardiac fibrosis by β-blocker in G protein-independent and G protein-coupled receptor kinase 5/β-arrestin2-dependent signaling pathways. J Biol Chem 287:35669–35677. https://doi.org/10.1074/jbc.M112.357871

Ngala RA, O'Dowd JF, Stocker CJ, Cawthorne MA, Arch JRS (2013) $ß_2$-Adrenoceptor agonists can both stimulate and inhibit glucose uptake in mouse soleus muscle through ligand-directed signalling. Naunyn Schmiedeberg's Arch Pharmacol 386:761–773. https://doi.org/10.1007/s00210-013-0860-5

Nikolaev VO, Moshkov A, Lyon AR, Miragoli M, Novak P, Paur H, Lohse MJ, Korchev YE, Harding SE, Gorelik J (2010) β2-adrenergic receptor redistribution in heart failure changes cAMP compartmentation. Science 327:1653–1657. https://doi.org/10.1126/science.1185988

Ohlstein EH, Arleth AJ, Storer B, Romanic AM (1998) Carvedilol inhibits Endothelin-1 biosynthesis in cultured human coronary artery endothelial cells. J Mol Cell Cardiol 30:167–173. https://doi.org/10.1006/jmcc.1997.0582

Okeke K, Michel-Reher M, Michel MC (2018) b_3-Adrenoceptor desensitisation in CHO cells: comparison of cAMP and ERK signalling. pA2 Online 18:017

Okeke K, Michel-Reher MB, Gravas S, Michel MC (2019) Desensitization of cAMP accumulation via human b_3-adrenoceptors expressed in human embryonic kidney cells by full, partial, and biased agonists. Front Pharmacol 10:596

Onaran HO, Costa T (2021) Conceptual and experimental issues in biased agonism. Cell Signal 82: 109955. https://doi.org/10.1016/j.cellsig.2021.109955

Onaran HO, Rajagopal S, Costa T (2014) What is biased efficacy? Defining the relationship between intrinsic efficacy and free energy coupling. Trends Pharmacol Sci 35:639–647. https://doi.org/10.1016/j.tips.2014.09.010

Onaran HO, Ambrosio C, Uğur Ö, Madaras Koncz E, Grò MC, Vezzi V, Rajagopal S, Costa T (2017) Systematic errors in detecting biased agonism: analysis of current methods and development of a new model-free approach. Sci Rep 7:44247. https://doi.org/10.1038/srep44247

Ostrom RS, Post SR, Insel PA (2000) Stoichiometry and compartmentation in G protein-coupled receptor signaling: implications for therapeutic interventions involving G_s. J Pharmacol Exp Ther 294:407–412

Pani B, Ahn S, Rambarat PK, Vege S, Kahsai AW, Liu A, Valan BN, Staus DP, Costa T, Lefkowitz RJ (2021) Unique positive cooperativity between the β-arrestin–niased β-blocker carvedilol and a small molecule positive allosteric modulator of the β2-adrenergic receptor. Mol Pharmacol 100:513–525. https://doi.org/10.1124/molpharm.121.000363

Patel CB, Noor N, Rockman HA (2010) Functional selectivity in adrenergic and angiotensin signaling systems. Mol Pharmacol 78:983–992. https://doi.org/10.1124/mol.110.067066

Qiu W, Zhuang S, von Lintig FC, Boss GR, Pilz RB (2000) Cell type-specific regulation of B-Raf kinase by cAMP and 14-3-3 proteins*. J Biol Chem 275:31921–31929. https://doi.org/10.1074/jbc.M003327200

Rajagopal S, Ahn S, Rominger DH, Gowen-MacDonald W, Lam CM, DeWire SM, Violin JD, Lefkowitz RJ (2011) Quantifying ligand bias at seven-transmembrane receptors. Mol Pharmacol 80:367–377. https://doi.org/10.1124/mol.111.072801

Reinartz MT, Kälble S, Littmann T, Ozawa T, Dove S, Kaever V, Wainer IW, Seifert R (2015) Structure-bias relationships for fenoterol stereoisomers in six molecular and cellular assays at the $ß_2$-adrenoceptor. Naunyn Schmiedeberg's Arch Pharmacol 388:51–65. https://doi.org/10.1007/s00210-014-1054-5

Reiter E, Ahn S, Shukla AK, Lefkowitz RJ (2012) Molecular mechanism of ß-arrestin-biased agonism at seven-transmembrane receptors. Annu Rev Pharmacol Toxicol 52:179–197. https://doi.org/10.1146/annurev.pharmtox.010909.105800

Rozec B, Quang TT, Noireaud J, Gauthier C (2006) Mixed β3-adrenoceptor agonist and α1-adrenoceptor antagonist properties of nebivolol in rat thoracic aorta. Br J Pharmacol 147:699–706. https://doi.org/10.1038/sj.bjp.0706648

Ruffolo RR, Gellai M, Hieble JP, Willette RN, Nichols AJ (1990) The pharmacology of carvedilol. Eur J Clin Pharmacol 38:S82–S88. https://doi.org/10.1007/BF01409471

Saijonmaa O, Metsärinne K, Fyhrquist F (1997) Carvedilol and its metabolites suppress Endothelin-1 production in human endothelial cell culture. Blood Press 6:24–28. https://doi.org/10.3109/08037059709086442

Sato M, Hutchinson DS, Evans BA, Summers RJ (2008) The $ß_3$-adrenoceptor agonist 4-[[(hexylamino)carbonyl]amino]-N-[4-[2-[[(2S)-2-hydroxy-3-(4-hydroxyphenoxy)propyl]amino]ethyl]-phenyl]-benzenesulfonamide (L755507) and antagonist (S)-N-[4-[2-[[3-[3-(acetamidomethyl)phenoxy]-2-hydroxypropyl]amino]-ethyl]phenyl]benzenesulfonamide (L748337) activate different signaling pathways in Chinese hamster ovary-K1 cells stably expressing the human $ß_3$-adrenoceptor. Mol Pharmacol 74:1417–1428

Schmid CL, Kennedy NM, Ross NC, Lovell KM, Yue Z, Morgenweck J, Cameron MD, Bannister TD, Bohn LM (2017) Bias factor and therapeutic window correlate to predict safer opioid analgesics. Cell 171:1165–1175.e1113. https://doi.org/10.1016/j.cell.2017.10.035

Schütz W, Freissmuth M (1992) Reverse intrinsic activity of antagonists on G protein-coupled receptors. Trends Pharmacol Sci 13:376–380. https://doi.org/10.1016/0165-6147(92)90116-n

Shenoy SK, Drake MT, Nelson CD, Houtz DA, Xiao K, Madabushi S, Reiter E, Premont RT, Lichtarge O, Lefkowitz RJ (2006) Beta-arrestin-dependent, G protein-independent ERK1/2 activation by the beta2 adrenergic receptor. J Biol Chem 281:1261–1273. https://doi.org/10.1074/jbc.M506576200

Stallaert W, Dorn JF, van der Westhuizen E, Audet M, Bouvier M (2012) Impedance responses reveal $ß_2$-adrenergic receptor signaling pluridimensionality and allow classification of ligands

with distinct signaling profiles. PLoS One 7:e29420. https://doi.org/10.1371/journal.pone.0029420
Starke K (1987) Presynaptic α-autoreceptors. Rev Physiol Biochem Pharmacol 107:74–146
Staus DP, Wingler LM, Strachan RT, Rasmussen SGF, Pardon E, Ahn S, Steyaert J, Kobilka BK, Lefkowitz RJ (2014) Regulation of beta-2-adrenergic receptor function by conformationally selective single-domain antibodies. Mol Pharmacol 85:472–481. https://doi.org/10.1124/mol.113.089516
Stork PJS, Schmitt JM (2002) Crosstalk between cAMP and MAP kinase signaling in the regulation of cell proliferation. Trends Cell Biol 12:258–266. https://doi.org/10.1016/S0962-8924(02)02294-8
Sun Y, Huang J, Xiang Y, Bastepe M, Jüppner H, Kobilka BK, Zhang JJ, Huang XY (2007) Dosage-dependent switch from G protein-coupled to G protein-independent signaling by a GPCR. EMBO J 26:53-64-64. https://doi.org/10.1038/sj.emboj.7601502
van der Westhuizen ET, Breton B, Christopoulos A, Bouvier M (2014) Quantification of ligand bias for clinically relevant $ß_2$-adrenergic receptor ligands: implications for drug taxonomy. Mol Pharmacol 85:492–509. https://doi.org/10.1124/mol.113.088880
Vollert J, Macleod M, Dirnagl U, Kas MJ, Michel MC, Potschka H, Riedel G, Wever KE, Würbel H, Steckler T, Rice ASC (2022) The EQIPD framework for rigor in the design, conduct, analysis and documentation of animal experiments. Nat Methods 19:1334–1337. https://doi.org/10.1038/s41592-022-01615-y
Vossler MR, Yao H, York RD, Pan M-G, Rim CS, Stork PJS (1997) cAMP activates MAP kinase and Elk-1 through a B-Raf- and Rap1-dependent pathway. Cell 89:73–82. https://doi.org/10.1016/S0092-8674(00)80184-1
Wang J, Hanada K, Staus DP, Makara MA, Dahal GR, Chen Q, Ahles A, Engelhardt S, Rockman HA (2017) Gαi is required for carvedilol-induced β1 adrenergic receptor β-arrestin biased signaling. Nat Commun 8:1706. https://doi.org/10.1038/s41467-017-01855-z
Wang Q, Wang Y, West TM, Liu Y, Reddy GR, Barbagallo F, Xu B, Shi Q, Deng B, Wei W, Xiang YK (2021) Carvedilol induces biased β1 adrenergic receptor-nitric oxide synthase 3-cyclic guanylyl monophosphate signalling to promote cardiac contractility. Cardiovasc Res 117:2237–2251. https://doi.org/10.1093/cvr/cvaa266
Wenzel-Seifert K, Seifert R (2000) Molecular analysis of $ß_2$-adrenoceptor coupling to G_s-, G_i-, and G_q-proteins. Mol Pharmacol 58:954–966
Wess J, Oteng A-B, Rivera-Gonzalez O, Gurevich EV, Gurevich VV (2023) β-Arrestins: structure, function, physiology, and pharmacological perspectives. Pharmacol Rev 75:854–884. https://doi.org/10.1124/pharmrev.121.000302
Winpenny D, Clark M, Cawkill D (2016) Biased ligand quantification in drug discovery: from theory to high throughput screening to identify new biased μ opioid receptor agonists. Br J Pharmacol 173:1393–1403. https://doi.org/10.1111/bph.13441
Wisler JW, DeWire SM, Whalen EJ, Violin JD, Drake MT, Ahn S, Shenov SK, Lefkowitz RJ (2007) A unique mechanism of ß-blocker action: carvedilol stimulates ß-arrestin. Proc Natl Acad Sci 104:16657–16662. https://doi.org/10.1073/pnas.0707936104
Woo AYH, Song Y, Xiao RP, Zhu W (2015) Biased $ß_2$-adrenoceptor signalling in heart failure: pathophysiology and drug discovery. Br J Pharmacol 172:5444–5456. https://doi.org/10.1111/bph.12965
Xiao RP, Ji X, Lakatta EG (1995) Functional coupling of the $ß_2$-adrenoceptor to a pertussis toxin-sensitive G protein in cardiac myocytes. Mol Pharmacol 47:322–329
Yoshioka T, Iwamoto N, Tsukahara F, Irie K, Urakawa I, Muraki T (2000) Anti-NO action of carvedilol in cell-free system and in vascular endothelial cells. Br J Pharmacol 129:1530–1535. https://doi.org/10.1038/sj.bjp.0703241

Agonism and Biased Signaling

Terry Kenakin

Contents

Abstract

This chapter considers biased signaling as a natural function of G protein-coupled receptors (GPCRs) in the form of probe dependence. Thus, any ligand that changes the conformation of the receptor (agonist, antagonist, or allosteric modulator) has the potential to change the natural signaling of the receptor through unequal conformational alterations in the receptor structure. This gives an added dimension to agonist selectivity beyond extracellular recognition, namely the ability of agonists to emphasize certain signaling pathways in the cell at the expense of others. Given this, selectivity is discussed in terms of varying intrinsic efficacy and selective stabilization of receptor states with methods to detect and measure these effects. Last, the translation of in vitro to complex in vivo systems will be considered.

T. Kenakin (✉)
Department of Pharmacology, School of Medicine, Chapel Hill, NC, USA
e-mail: kenakin@email.unc.edu

© The Author(s), under exclusive license to Springer Nature Switzerland AG 2025

Z. Li, K. Xiao (eds.), *Pharmacology of GPCRs Biased Signaling and Agonists*,
Handbook of Experimental Pharmacology 290, https://doi.org/10.1007/164_2025_770

1 Introduction

G protein-coupled receptors (GPCRs) are nature's prototypic allosteric protein and probably the most ubiquitous signaling proteins in all of physiology. Long since considered the 'low hanging fruit' for drug discovery (by virtue of the fact that GPCRs are on the cell membrane and control a myriad of cellular processes), a general view that this target class was 'mined out' emerged by the late 1980s with the realization that no new GPCR subtypes became available to yield selective signaling. This view radically changed with the discovery of biased signaling. With this concept, GPCRs became revitalized as drug targets (Kenakin 2015) and continue to be an ever-expanding source of potential drug therapeutics.

2 Agonism: State of the Art Before Bias

Pharmacologists almost always work in systems they do not fully understand. This being the case, the null method is the mainstay of receptor theory, i.e., a system is perturbed by an agonist, then a single change is made to the system and the agonism repeated. Under these conditions, it is assumed that the only change that has taken place is the designed change in the system. This approach treats the receptor as a control switch that binds agonist and then transfers a signal to the cell, which then reports the outcome. The signal imparted by the agonist is a stabilization of another protein conformation, which then activates signaling components in the cell; this new conformation is given the name 'active state'. Occam's razor (keep it simple) dictates that the minimal requirements of physiology are that there is a single active state. Under these circumstances, the only graded differences between agonists would be the magnitude of the signal; this is governed by the efficacy of the agonist and the sensitivity of the system.

This theoretical framework provided an important tool in the drug discovery of new therapeutic agonists, namely the agonist potency ratio. Since observed agonism is the result of the activated receptor interacting with cell surface receptors and the biochemical stimulus-response reactions in the cell cytosol, cell agonism is a system dependent parameter, i.e., the potency of a given agonist will be unique to the agonist and the cell type. This being the case, it is not possible to use the observed potency of an agonist as a predictor of response in other cell types since the components interacting with the activated receptor will be different. Since the in vivo profiles of agonists result from the interactions of agonists with different cell types, an in vitro agonist potency is a poor index of agonist efficacy for therapeutic application. However, if two agonists are compared in a single in vitro system and their activity expressed as a ratio of effect (usually a ratio of EC_{50} values, molar concentrations producing 50% maximal effect), then, since the agonists utilize the same cellular machinery to transform efficacy into response, the resulting ratio of EC_{50} values (potency ratio, PR) becomes a system independent measure of relative agonist efficacy transferable between any physiological systems. The prevailing information at the time suggested this to be a viable approach to the classifications of agonists, but it should be considered that the cellular response systems available to measure agonism were limited, i.e., mainly second messenger effects due to cyclic AMP or calcium. However, even then, there were sporadic reports of failures of the constant PR approach to agonism with changing cell types and/or measuring systems (Christmanson et al. 1994; Peters and Scott 2009; Peters et al. 2007) thus challenging this simplistic mechanism (Roth and Chuang 1987). With time and increasing new technology (i.e., the availability of new ways to measure agonist response), these 'exceptions' became the rule, and it became clear that agonism dependence on a single receptor active state was incapable of furnishing useful predictive data. Thus, the availability of new functional response assays and new ideas describing receptor mechanisms derived from molecule dynamics transformed the field and furnished new ideas to describe efficacy and agonism. This wave of change is given a general moniker of 'biased signaling'.

3 Biased Signaling Negates the Single Active State Model

The ability to measure the strength of more than one signal emanating from a single GPCR in response to the binding of an agonist unveiled the fact that different agonists produce different mixtures of signals to cells. These data are incompatible with a single receptor active state resulting from both agonists and compelled the idea that different agonists stabilize different receptor active states (Kenakin 1995). Experimental evidence for this has been obtained by the existence of 'protean agonists', which clearly stabilize a receptor active state that is different from the native constitutively formed receptor active state (Kenakin 1997a, b; Chidiac et al. 1996). In addition, theoretical analyses of receptors interacting with multiple signaling couplers (i.e., G Proteins) predict that different receptor conformations can yield different G Protein activations (Kenakin and Morgan 1989).

Historically agonism was described by so-called 'linkage models' whereby the protein species involved are linked together through pathways of equal energy (Kenakin 2016). A problem with these models is the need to predefine the protein species and if multiple agonists produce multiple different active states (to accommodate biased signaling), models cannot be constructed that are predictive of agonist effect. Specifically, how can biased signaling, which is the result of multiple receptor active states, adequately be characterized with models that require prior identification of unspecified states? However, models depicting multiple receptor conformations are consistent with molecular dynamics. GPCRs have a high degree of conformational flexibility (Frauenfelder et al. 1979; Tang and Dill 1998; Williams et al. 2007; Liapakis et al. 2012) and thus can form a vast array of tertiary conformations. It is postulated that GPCRs exist in collections of slightly different conformations of similar free energy and that agonists have varying affinities for these states to stabilize collections referred to as 'ensembles' (Dror et al. 2010, 2013; Park 2012; Nygaard et al. 2013; Motlagh et al. 2014) thus creating dynamic systems (Vardy and Roth 2013; Manglik and Kobilka 2014; Manglik et al. 2015). Agonist binding is not a passive property but rather necessarily will alter the energetics of the dynamics of the ensemble (Kenakin and Onaran 2002). In general, molecular dynamics furnishes the theoretical background to understand biased signaling.

In terms of molecular dynamics, the model for agonism has the agonist-bound receptor rolling on what is described as an 'energy landscape' comprising numerous 'wells' (depicting favored states) representing stabilized states. An important prediction of this model is that there need not be linearity of efficacy in GPCR systems as was assumed previously. Specifically, certain linear reactions were assumed to prevail in receptor function such as agonist binding leading to receptor activation further leading to receptor phosphorylation and finally receptor internalization. In this scheme, receptor internalization could not occur without receptor activation, but this was in fact disproved experimentally by the finding that some antagonists that did not produce receptor activation do, however, produce active receptor internalization (Roettger et al. 1997; Gray and Roth 2001). This can be explained in terms of dynamics with pathways on the energy landscape that linked wells for receptor binding and internalization but not activation (Kenakin 2005).

4 The Prevalence of Biased Signaling

Biased signaling was not discussed in the literature until decades after agonist pharmacology was a standard tool in drug discovery, and with that chronology, it is considered to be a new phenomenon. However, this is a misconception as bias signaling is simply the result of standard allosteric protein dependence always practiced by GPCRs. Probe dependence means that different molecules interacting with the receptor can be affected by an allosteric change in the protein differently, especially if those molecules bind to separate sites on the receptor. For example, the allosteric modulator alcuronium binds to the muscarinic receptor to increase the binding of the antagonist ^{3}H-atropine but decrease the binding of the antagonist ^{3}H-QNB (Hejnova et al. 1995). Probe dependence is the result of the fact that GPCR conformation changes throughout the protein are expressed in various ways, and the changes are not concerted or connected. Therefore, the allosteric conformational change in one locus of the protein will differ from another, and different molecules interacting with those loci will be affected in a different manner. Therefore, if two signaling proteins (i.e., G-protein and β-arrestin) interact with a GPCR, an allosteric change (such as that produced by agonist binding) will differentially affect those pathways and one may be emphasized at the expense of the other. Before separate methods to assess these pathways were available, there was no way to know that these differentials were occurring but with the advent of selective assays for different signaling pathways, the differences were discovered. The outcome is illustrated dramatically by TRV120, an angiotensin Gq-protein antagonist for angiotensin II receptors. As shown in Fig. 1, while angiotensin produces activation of Gq-protein and β-arrestin, TRV120 produces only activation of β-arrestin but not Gq protein (in fact, it functions as a competitive antagonist of angiotensin-mediated Gq protein response (Violin et al. 2006, 2010).

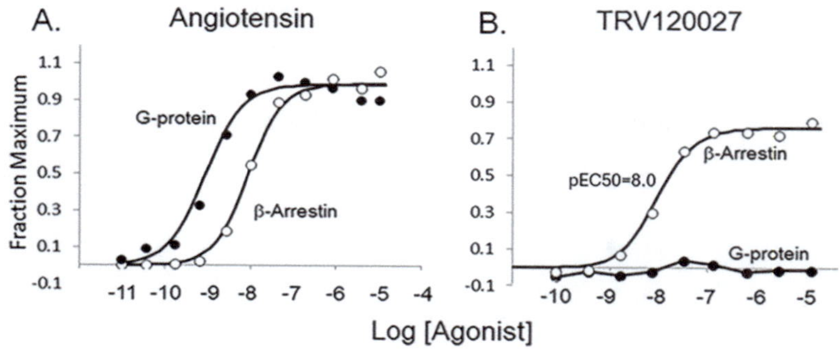

Fig. 1 Agonist responses to (**a**) angiotensin and (**b**) TRV120027. Signals for Gαq (filled circles) and β-arrestin (open circles). (Data from Violin et al. 2010)

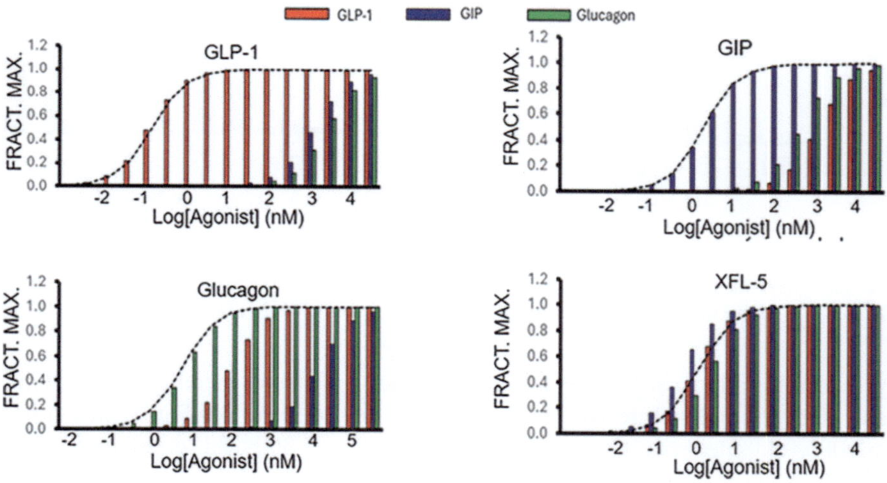

Fig. 2 Receptor selectivity for incretin agonists. Concentration-response curves to GLP-1 (red bars), GIP (blue bars), and glucagon (green bars). Dotted line shows the response to the primary agonist. (Data from Cui et al. 2020)

Agonist bias is a form of agonist selectivity operable on intracellular signaling mechanisms, but it differs from extracellular agonist selectivity where an agonist interacts with two separate receptor populations on the cell membrane. With receptor selectivity, the relative agonist effects on the different receptor types depend on the affinity and efficacy of the agonist for each receptor type and also the relative receptor density (and efficiency of receptor coupling to response mechanisms) of the respective receptor populations in cells. Thus, a physical separation in concentration can be imparted to the various receptor responses depending on these factors, i.e., a selective agonist may produce a selective response through one receptor type but no response in other subtypes until higher concentrations, which allows interaction with these secondary receptor types. Figure 2 shows the relative concentrations of incretin agonists for various incretin receptors; it can be seen that nature has

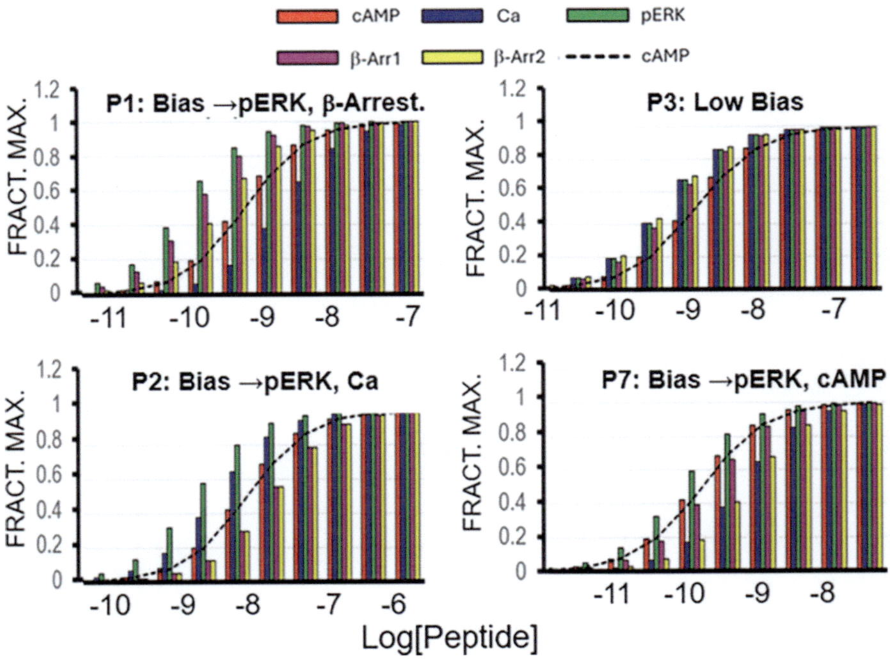

Fig. 3 Receptor bias for GLP-1 agonists. Concentration-response curves to cAMP (red bars), calcium (blue bars), pERK (green bars), β-arrestin1 (magenta bars), β-arrestin2 (yellow bars). Dotted line shows the responses for cAMP. (Data from Hager et al. 2017)

provided for a large separation of effect between the natural incretins GLP-1, GIP, and glucagon and their respective receptors. As can be seen from Fig. 2, GLP-1 has >3,000-fold selectivity for GLP-1 receptors, GIP has >300-fold selectivity for GIP receptors and Glucagon has >30-fold selectivity for glucagon receptors (Cui et al. 2020). In keeping with recent efforts to produce tri-receptor active peptides for diabetes and obesity treatment (Morissette and Mulvihill 2024), the peptide XFL-5 has comparable potency on all three incretin receptors. In contrast, biased signals begin uniformly when the agonist binds to the receptor but at different intensities. Figure 3 shows the relative signaling responses of four peptides on GLP-1 receptors (Hager et al. 2017); note that the responses are initiated at similar concentrations but with different magnitudes.

It can be seen from Fig. 3 that bias values can be relatively small (three to fivefold), and this raises the question as to what bias will have an impact on normal physiology. While clearly this may depend on the particular physiological pathway being explored, it is useful to note some known values of allosteric potentiation and how those values impact physiology. One example is the allosteric potentiation of GLP-1 response for the postprandial release of insulin in diabetes. A physiologically relevant change in GLP-1 effect can be gained from the blockade of metabolism of naturally released GLP-1 by inhibition of DPP-4, the enzyme that metabolizes GLP. Specifically, this typically produces a twofold increase in endogenous GLP-1, which nevertheless leads to favorable therapy (Brunton 2014), suggesting that this modest potentiation of GLP-1 (or signaling bias for the relevant signal to GLP-1 agonism) is sufficient to produce a therapeutically useful effect. This also sets a limit for maximal allosteric and/or bias effect as excess GLP-1 effect is known to produce nausea in some patients (Filippatos et al. 2014). Another example of a seemingly modest but actually powerful effect is seen with diazepam, which produces a limited potentiation of GABA (2.4-fold, Skerrit and MacDonald 1984) in in vitro studies but has profound CNS activity.

Given that synthetic agonists will practice bias through natural allostery, it is incumbent on agonist programs to determine which new agonists bias toward which pathways, i.e., to ignore such data would be to possibly lose valuable positive or negative information. At this point, it is useful to discuss the various methods that are available to detect and quantify signaling bias.

5 Detecting and Measuring Bias

Several models and approaches have been proposed to detect and finally quantify signaling bias; these are described in literature (Onaran et al. 2017; Kenakin 2019). These models quantify bias and yield parameters that gauge the extent of the effect to enable comparison of compounds for structure-activity relationships. However, the most simple way to detect signaling bias does not involve mathematical models at all but rather simply compares two signaling responses to an agonist to yield what is referred to as a 'bias plot'. As shown in Fig. 4, two signals from two agonists are shown in concentration-response curves (Fig. 4a), which can be compared to each other (Fig. 4b) to yield bias plots. These usually will be curved due to the differing stimulus-response characteristics of the pathways in the cells; this curvature is system bias and will be unique to the particular in vitro conditions under which the measurements are made and do not reflect differences in agonist-receptor active states. These effects will not be transferable to other systems (and thus will not be useful for therapeutic prediction). However, if one of the agonists produces a unique receptor active state, the observed bias will depart from the system bias observed for other agonists. This will indicate true receptor-based bias that will transfer to other systems and possibly be of value therapeutically. This may not be immediately obvious in the agonist concentration-response curves (Fig. 4c) but will emerge as a different curvature in the bias plot (Fig. 4d). This identifies a biased agonist.

While this is a convenient way to identify bias, it does not quantify it on a scale that allows comparison of agonists. A method to do this should be:

- Sensitive, system-independent
- Quantifiable (have a scale)
- Theoretically sound
- High-throughput
- Statistically bound and verifiable

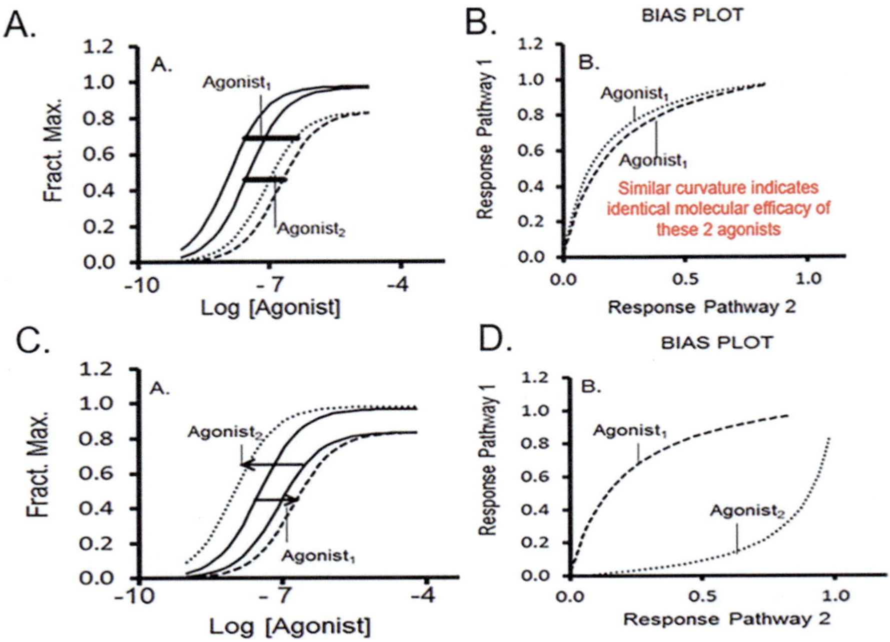

Fig. 4 Bias plots. Panel A shows concentration-response curves for two agonists for two signaling pathways in a cell (solid and broken lines respectively). Panel B shows the regression of responses to response pathway 1 as a function of the magnitude of responses to pathway 2 for the two agonists; these are bias plots indicating the system bias for the assays (differences in efficiency of receptor coupling). Panel C shows concentration-response curves to two different agonists for two pathways. Panel D shows the bias plot for the curves shown in panel C. In this case, agonist2 is biased toward pathway2 while agonist1 is biased toward pathway 1 as shown by the difference in curvature of the bias plots

A method that qualifies on all criteria above utilizes log(τ_A/K_A) values (where K_A is the equilibrium dissociation constant of the agonist-receptor complex, τ_A is the efficacy of the agonist (denoted by $\tau_A = [R_T]/K_E$ with $[R_T]$ being the receptor density on the membrane, and K_E the transduction constant for a saturable relationship between agonist-activated receptor and cell response). The advantage of the log (τ_A/K_A) scale is that it is linear for all ranges of agonist sensitivity from full to partial agonism (Kenakin et al. 2012) (unlike agonist potency ratios, which are not). Thus log(τ_A/K_A) functions as a single number identifier of agonist power, which can be used to scale the relative ability of a set of agonists to activate one signaling pathway through Δlog(τ_A/K_A) values (where all agonists are compared to an identified reference agonist). Once the agonists are ranked to each other within a signaling pathway, these Δlog(τ_A/K_A) values then can be subtracted across pathways to yield $\Delta\Delta$log(τ_A/K_A) values, which are the logarithms of bias. This procedure provides a number for the relative strength of signal by an agonist for two pathways compared to that of a reference agonist. If the reference agonist is the natural neurotransmitter or hormone for the receptor, then the bias number will provide a scale to denote the

Table 1 GLP-1 agonist signaling bias

cAMP								Ca
Agonist	Log(max/EC)*	Δlog(max/EC)	ΔΔLog(max/EC)	Bias→cAMP	Bias→Ca	Δlog(max/EC)	Log(max/EC)	Agonists
GLP-1	9.89	0.00	0.00	1.00	1.00	0.00	7.40	GLP-1
P1	8.80	-1.09	-0.52	0.30	3.31	-0.57	6.83	P1
P2	8.07	-1.82	0.11	1.28	0.78	-1.92	5.48	P2
P3	8.14	-1.75	-0.85	0.14	7.14	-0.90	6.50	P3
P5	9.89	0.00	-0.53	0.29	3.43	0.54	7.94	P5
P6	9.74	-0.15	-0.51	0.31	3.25	0.36	7.76	P6
P7	9.44	-0.45	-0.01	0.98	1.03	-0.44	6.96	P7
P8	8.31	-1.58	-0.92	0.12	8.25	-0.67	6.73	P8
P9	7.62	-2.27	-1.14	0.07	13.69	-1.14	6.26	P9

* max = maximal response / EC = EC_{50} for response

GLP-1 HAEGTSDVSYLEGQAKEFIAWLVGR-NH_2

P1	HAEGTFTSDVSSYLEGQAAXEFIXWLVZGRG-NH_2
P2	HAEGTFTSDVSSYLEXQAAXEFIXWLVZGRG-NH_2
P3	HAEGTFTSDVSXYLEXQAAXEFIXWLVZGRG-NH_2
P5	HAEGTFTSDASSYLEGQAAKEFIAWLVKGRG-NH_2
P6	HAEGTFTSDASSYLEGQAAKEFIAWLVKGRG-NH_2
P7	HAEGTFTSDVSXYLEGQAAKEFIAWLVKGRG-NH_2
P8	HAEGTFTSDVSXYLEXQAAXEFIAWLVKGRG-NH_2
P9	HAEGTFTSDVSXYLEXQAAXEFIXWLVKGRG-NH_2

Agonists	Bias →Ca	No Bias
GLP-1		
P1	●	
P2		●
P3	●	
P5	●	
P6	●	
P7		●
P8	●	
P9	●	

Data from Hager et al. (2017)

difference in agonist efficacy imparted by the synthetic agonist compared to natural agonism (Kenakin et al. 2012). It should be noted that if the slopes of the concentration-response curves for the agonists are not significantly different from unity, log(max/EC_{50}) values (where max is the maximal response to the agonist and EC_{50} the molar concentration of agonist producing 50% maximal response to that agonist) can be substituted for log(τ_A/K_A) values (Kenakin 2017). The description of agonism with a single number facilitates statistical analysis of bias differences. An example of a bias calculation utilizing log(max/EC50) values for incretin agonists is shown in Table 1.

6 Putting Bias into Context

While physiological bias clearly relates to relative strengths of signals, a scale must be established, i.e., bias in itself is not meaningful unless it is compared to a standard which is the reference agonist response. As noted, the natural agonist usually fulfills this task of being a standard and then all new agonists are compared to that standard. Physiology constructs systems to yield signaling patterns that are required for life therefore there is no such thing as ‘no bias’, i.e., non sensical terms for agonists such as ‘neutral’ agonists, ‘unbiased’, ‘balanced’ agonists, or ‘non-biased’ agonists. Such apparently unbiased profiles usually mean that the bias of a new agonist is not different from the natural physiological bias of the natural agonist. Without comparison to standard signaling, bias measurements simply would reflect the sensitivity of the various systems used to measure signaling in vitro, i.e., second messenger assays are more efficiently coupled than β-arrestin assays, and these effects must be canceled by the bias procedures outlined in this chapter to yield true agonist bias rooted in receptor conformational changes.

Agonists that produce signals in one signaling pathway but no response in another (in the assays used to assess the response) have erroneously been termed to have 'perfect bias'. This implies that the agonist will not produce response in that signaling system under any circumstances. However, testing such perfectly biased ligands as antagonists reveals that they do indeed bind to the receptor but that the stimulus-response machinery of the cells is incapable of generating a response to agonist-binding. An example of this is seen with TRV120, an angiotensin partial agonist for β-arrestin ($pEC_{50} = 8.0$; 75% maximal response) that produces no response to Gq-protein signaling. However, TRV120 blocks the receptor-mediated Gαq response to angiotensin with a pK_B, as shown by Schild analysis, of $pK_B = 8.0$ (Violin et al. 2010). It is important to identify perfect bias effects due to inadequate cellular sensitivity because these ligands may, in more sensitive cellular systems, actually show responses, i.e., not be perfectly biased. Selectively low efficacy can be a useful property in the design of biased agonists as in the case of the biased opioid analgesic oliceridine (Singleton et al. 2021).

Finally, it should be noted that a high level of bias does not mean that the agonist will produce a strong agonist response to that pathway; this still lies within the realm of efficacy. While bias only dictates the relative strength of two signals when the efficacy is sufficient for both responses to be produced and when the system is sensitive enough to return response, response to agonists is controlled by the actual efficacy of the agonist. Bias simply reflects the relative strength of stimulus given to the respective signaling systems once the agonist engages the receptor.

7 Biased Signaling and Therapeutic Expectations

With the availability of new functional assays to allow the determination of the diversity in signaling controlled by agonist-GPCR interaction has come the realization that ligands impart different qualities of efficacy to cells and that this may be important to the pharmacology of agonism to therapeutics. Given this, the idea that agonist bias may be manipulated through structure-activity modification leads to the notion that better agonist therapy may be achieved in this manner. Thus, elements of a complex signaling pattern could be diminished if they are debilitating. For example, there are data to show that analgesia is linked to Gαi activation, whereas respiratory depression, gastrointestinal dysfunction, and tolerance may be linked to β-arrestin2 recruitment (Bohn et al. 1999, 2003; Ikeda et al. 2002; Raehal et al. 2005; Li et al. 2009; Yang et al. 2011; DeWire et al. 2013). These concepts have led to the development of TRV130 (N-[(3-methoxythiophe-2-yl)methyl]-2-(9-pyridin-2-yll-6-oxaspiro[4,5]decan-9-yl) ethanamine), a μ-opioid receptor agonist for postoperative pain (Chen et al. 2013; Violin et al. 2014). Interestingly, chronic treatment with this agonist does not produce tolerance seen with morphine (Altarifi et al. 2017). Studies in this vein are ongoing with the development of TRV734 (White et al. 2015). This application can be extended to allow the prosecution of drug targets mediating debilitating signals, which should not be pursued for therapy. For example, κ-opioid receptors theoretically could be useful in the treatment of depression and schizophrenia, but agonism at this receptor type produces serious hallucinations limiting their application. However, K-opioid agonists biased away from the pathway mediating these effects, namely β-arrestin, offer the possibility of exploiting these new targets for therapeutic advantage (White et al. 2014; Brust et al. 2016). A variant of this approach is to limit, through receptor antagonism, the natural system from producing a debilitating signal in pathophysiology. For instance, the natural reflex vasoconstriction by release of angiotensin to elevate perfusion pressure in conditions of failing cardiac output can be harmful to a failing heart. The current treatment is through blockade of angiotensin receptors but a better approach is the blockade of these receptors with concomitant beneficial β-arrestin signaling produced by biased molecules such as TRV120 (Violin et al. 2006, 2010). The converse to reducing harmful signaling in an agonist is to augment beneficial signaling. For example, knockout studies suggest that the useful effects of parathyroid hormone in osteoporosis treatment are due to the PTH-receptor mediated β-arrestin signaling therefore β-arrestin biased PTH agonists would be a better fit for this therapy (Gesty-Palmer and Luttrell 2011; Gesty-Palmer et al. 2013).

Finally, the assessment of therapeutic improvements produced by biased ligands is a complex issue because of the interface of differential signal activation in single cells and the varying stoichiometry of signaling components in different cell types found in vivo (Kenakin 2024). This is because bias can be context-dependent and thus vary, an example being the varying biases for dopamine receptor agonists when viewed at different points in the cellular stimulus-response cascade(s) (Klein Herenbrink et al. 2016). The routing of receptor stimulus to different signaling proteins also can be affected by GRKs (G protein receptor kinases), the levels of which vary in different cell types (Latorraca et al. 2020; He et al. 2021; Zidar et al. 2009; Duan et al. 2023). These effects can produce variation in relative agonist potency with cell type (Christmanson et al. 1994; Peters and Scott 2009), relative signaling components (Watson et al. 2005; Singleton et al. 2021), and receptor stoichiometry (Luscombe et al. 2023). Cell background has been shown to affect receptor internalization and, in light of evidence that GCRs can continue signaling from within the cytosol (Viladarga et al. 2014; Sutkeviciute et al. 2019; Molden et al. 2015), this can produce further cell-type effects on agonism.

In addition, the testing of biased ligands must specifically be tailored to the therapeutic application for which the bias is designed. For example, the biased ligand for heart failure TRV120027 did not show superior efficacy over conventional therapy, but this may have been due to the fact that it was tested incorrectly. Specifically, this molecule was tested in an acute randomized double-blind placebo-controlled Phase IIB dose-ranging trial (BLAST-AHF; 24–28 h infusion of TRV 120027 followed by a 30-day endpoint of symptoms and survival) when actually it was designed to enhance beneficial cardiac remodeling in heart failure over many months. Thus, the trial design was a short-term trial design that would not detect the possible beneficial effects of this molecule (shortcomings in study design and duration of treatment, Pang et al. 2017; Sugihara and Burnett 2017).

8 Implications of Biased Signaling Beyond Direct Agonism

The probe-dependent allostery of GPCR-signaling is operative in all facets of GPCR function. The principles governing the quantification of biased signaling, namely the correction for assay sensitivity and comparison to a common reference ligand, are useful in other realms of agonist function such as assessing receptor selectivity. In addition, the consideration of maximal responses as well as potencies with EC_{50}'s adds another layer of accuracy on selectivity measurements. Thus these techniques can be applied to determining the therapeutic index for an agonist vs secondary receptor side effects, i.e., the exact same procedure for quantifying biased signaling can be used to assess receptor selectivity. Figure 5 shows muscarinic agonist selectivity on two types of muscarinic receptor, m1 and m2. Considering the agonist 8d, the comparison of potency on the m1 cell line vs the m2 cell line indicates a 60-fold difference ostensibly showing a 60-fold selectivity of m2 over m1 receptors (Wakeham et al. 2022). However, this number is affected by the differences in the m1 and m2 receptor assays with differing sensitivities and receptor expression levels and thus cannot be taken as a true measure of selectivity. The bias procedure accounts for this, and when the higher sensitivity of the m2 receptor cell line is

M1											M2
Agonist	max	EC_{50} (nM)	Log(M/E)	Δlog(M/E)	ΔΔLog(M/E)	BIAS	Δlog(M/E)	Log(M/E)	EC_{50} (nM)	max	Agonist
Iperoxo	1	0.30	9.52	0.00	0.00	1.00	0.00	10.15	0.07	1	Iperoxo
8c	0.87	13.50	7.81	-1.71	-0.67	4.64	-1.05	9.11	0.78	1	8c
8d	0.95	37.20	7.41	-2.12	-1.18	15.23	-0.93	9.22	0.60	1	8d
8e	0.87	56.20	7.19	-2.33	-0.80	6.28	-1.54	8.62	2.40	1	8e

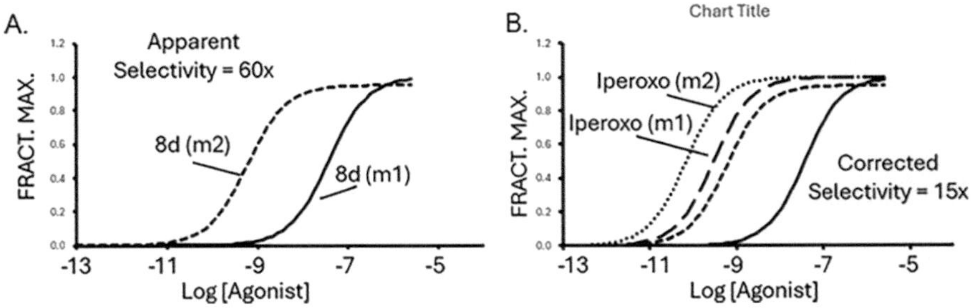

Fig. 5 Potencies of muscarinic agonists for m1 and m2 muscarinic receptors. The table shows the relative selectivity of the agonists for m2 receptors. With iperoxo as the standard, it can be seen that agonist 8d is 15-fold more selective for m2 receptors. Concentration-response curves show the relative activity of compound 8d on the two receptor types in the separate assays (panel A); the difference is 60-fold. Panel B shows the corrected selectivity by showing how the sensitivity of the assay for m2 receptors is fourfold greater than the sensitivity of the assay for m1 receptors (note the difference for iperoxo). When this assay correction is made, the true selectivity for agonist 8d is shown to be 15-fold. (Data from Wakeham et al. 2022)

taken into account by comparing potencies to a reference agonist iperoxo in both assays, the true selectivity of 8d (which is 15-fold) is revealed.

These procedures also have the capability of identifying unique agonist activity in various assays and cell lines. For example, label free analysis of dopamine agonist activity through bias plots for DHX, dopamine, SKF38393, and SKF83859 indicate a similar trajectory (system bias) but a striking departure for the agonist A77636; this reveals that A77636 has a uniquely enhanced activity in U2 cells over SK -N-MC cells U-2 cells (Peters and Scott 2009). Such identification of cell-specific agonism could be relevant in the comparison of agonist activity in normal vs cancer cell lines.

9 Conclusions

Advances in assay technology have led to the discovery of and exploitation of the natural GPCR probe-dependent routing of receptor stimulus to various cytosolic signaling pathways. This is a natural pharmacological property of agonists and GPCRs and should not be ignored in agonist drug discovery programs. The ability to tailor complex signals to cells through GPCR agonists has tremendous potential for drug therapy with tangible benefits for drug therapy. In addition, pursuing bias for GPCRs extends the possible value of these drug targets.

References

Altarifi AA, David B, Muchhala KH, Blough BE, Akbarali H, Negus SS (2017) Effects of acute and repeated treatment with the biased mu opioid receptor agonist TRV130 (oliceridine) on measures of antinociception, gastrointestinal function, and abuse liability in rodents. J Psychopharmacol 31:730–739

Bohn LM, Lefkowitz RJ, Gainetdinov RR, Peppel K, Caron MG, Lin FT (1999) Enhanced morphine analgesia in mice lacking beta-arrestin 2. Science 286:2495–2498

Bohn LM, Gainetdinov RR, Sotnikova TD, Medvedev IO, Lefkowitz RJ, Dykstra LA, Caron MG (2003) Enhanced rewarding properties of morphine, but not cocaine, in beta(arrestin)-2 knock-out mice. J Neurosci 23:10265–10273

Brunton S (2014) GLP-1 receptor agonists vs. DPP-4 inhibitors for type 2 diabetes: is one approach more successful or preferable than the other? Int J Clin Pract 68:557–567

Brust TF, Morgenweck J, Kim SA, Rose JH, Locke JL, Schmid CL, Zhou L, Stahl EL, Cameron MD, Scarry SM et al (2016) Biased agonists of the kappa opioid receptor suppress pain and itch without causing sedation or dysphoria. Sci Signal 9:ra117

Chen XT, Pitis P, Liu G, Yuan C, Gotchev D, Cowan CL, Rominger DH, Koblish M, Dewire SM, Crombie AL et al (2013) Structure-activity relationships and discovery of a G protein biased m opioid receptor ligand, [(3-methoxythiophen-2-yl)methyl] (2-[(9R)-9-(pyridin-2-yl)-6-oxaspiro-[4.5]decan-9-yl]ethyl)amine (TRV130), for the treatment of acute severe pain. J Med Chem 56:8019–8031

Chidiac P, Nout S, Bouvier M (1996) Agonist-induced modulation of inverse agonist efficacy at the β2-adrenergic receptor. Mol Pharmacol 50:662–669

Christmanson L, Westermark P, Betsholtz C (1994) Islet amyloid polypeptide stimulates cyclic AMP accumulation via the porcine calcitonin receptor. Biochem Biophys Res Commun 205: 1226–1235

Cui J, Anquan Shang A, Weiwei Wang W, Chen W (2020) Rational design of a GLP-1/GIP/Gcg receptor triagonist to correct hyperglycemia, obesity and diabetic nephropathy in rodent animals. Life Sci 260:118339

DeWire SM, Yamashita DS, Rominger DH, Liu G, Cowan CL, Graczyk TM, Chen XT, Pitis PM, Gotchev D, Yuan C et al (2013) A G protein-biased ligand at the m-opioid receptor is potently analgesic with reduced gastrointestinal and respiratory dysfunction compared with morphine. J Pharmacol Exp Ther 344:708–717

Dror RO, Jensen MO, Borhani DW, Shaw DE (2010) Exploring atomic resolution physiology on a femtosecond to millisecond timescale using molecular dynamics simulations. J Gen Physiol 135:555–562

Dror RO, Green HF, Valant C, Borhani DW, Valcourt JR, Pan AC, Arlow DH, Canals M, Lane JR, Rahmani R et al (2013) Structural basis for modulation of a G-protein-coupled receptor by allosteric drugs. Nature 503:295–299

Duan J, Liu H, Zhao F, Yuan Q, Ji Y, Cai X, He X et al (2023) GPCR activation and GRK2 assembly by a biased intracellular agonist. Nature 620. https://doi.org/10.1038/s41586-023-06395-9

Filippatos TD, Panagiotopoulou TV, Elisaf MS (2014) Adverse effects of GLP-1 receptor agonists. Rev Diabet Stud 11:202–230

Frauenfelder H, Petsko GA, Tsernoglou D (1979) Temperature dependent X-ray diffraction as a probe of protein structural dynamics. Nature 280:558–563

Gesty-Palmer D, Luttrell LM (2011) 'Biasing' the parathyroid hormone receptor: a novel anabolic approach to increasing bone mass? Br J Pharmacol 164:59–67

Gesty-Palmer D, Yuan L, Martin B, Wood WH 3rd, Lee MH, Janech MG, Tsoi LC, Zheng WJ, Luttrell LM, Maudsley S (2013) B-arrestin-selective G protein coupled receptor agonists engender unique biological efficacy in vivo. Mol Endocrinol 27:296–314

Gray JA, Roth BL (2001) Paradoxical trafficking and regulation of 5-HT(2A) receptors by agonists and antagonists. Brain Res Bull 56:441–451

Hager MV, Clydesdale L, Gellman SH, Sexton PM, Wootten D (2017) Characterization of signal bias at the GLP-1 receptor induced by backbone modification of GLP-1. Biochem Pharmacol 136:99–108

He QT, Xiao P, Huang SM, Jia YL, Zhu ZL, Lin JY et al (2021) Structural studies of phosphorylation-dependent interactions between the V2R receptor and arrestin-2. Nat Commun 12:2396

Hejnova L, Tucek S, El-Fakahany EE (1995) Positive and negative allosteric interactions on muscarinic receptors. Eur J Pharmacol 291:427–430

Ikeda K, Kobayashi T, Kumanishi T, Yano R, Sora I, Niki H (2002) Molecular mechanisms of analgesia induced by opioids and ethanol: is the GIRK channel one of the keys? Neurosci Res 44:121–131

Kenakin T (1995) Agonist-receptor efficacy. II. Agonist trafficking of receptor signals. Trends Pharmacol Sci 16(7):232–238

Kenakin T (1997a) Differences between natural and recombinant G protein-coupled receptor systems with varying receptor/G protein stoichiometry. Trends Pharmacol Sci 18:456–464

Kenakin T (1997b) Protean agonists. Keys to receptor active states? Ann N Y Acad Sci 812:116–125

Kenakin T (2005) New concepts in drug discovery: collateral efficacy and permissive antagonism. Nat Rev Drug Discov 4:919–927

Kenakin T (2015) New lives for seven transmembrane receptors as drug targets. Trends Pharmacol Sci 36(11):705–706

Kenakin T (2016) The mass action equation in pharmacology. Br J Clin Pharmacol 81:41–51

Kenakin T (2017) A scale of agonism and allosteric modulation for assessment of selectivity, bias, and receptor mutation. Mol Pharmacol 92:414–424

Kenakin T (2019) Biased receptor signaling in drug discovery. Pharmacol Rev 7:267–315

Kenakin TP (2024) Bias translation: the final frontier? Br J Pharmacol 181:1345–1360

Kenakin TP, Morgan PH (1989) Theoretical effects of single and multiple transducer receptor coupling proteins on estimates of the relative potency of agonists. Mol Pharmacol 35:214–222

Kenakin T, Onaran O (2002) The ligand paradox between affinity and efficacy: can you be there and not make a difference? Trends Pharmacol Sci 23:275–280. https://doi.org/10.1016/s0165-6147(02)02036-9

Kenakin T, Watson C, Muniz-Medina V, Christopoulos A, Novick S (2012) A simple method for quantifying functional selectivity and agonist bias. ACS ChemNeurosci 3:193–203

Klein Herenbrink C, Sykes DA, Donthamsetti P, Canals M, Coudrat T, Shonberg J, Scammells PJ, Capuano B, Sexton PM, Charlton SJ et al (2016) The role of kinetic context in apparent biased agonism at GPCRs. Nat Commun 7:10842

Latorraca NR, Masureel M, Hollingsworth SA, Heydenreich FM, Suomivuori CM, Brinton C et al (2020) How GPCR phosphorylation patterns orchestrate arrestin-mediated signaling. Cell 183: 1813–1825. e1818

Li Y, Liu X, Liu C, Kang J, Yang J, Pei G, Wu C (2009) Improvement of morphine-mediated analgesia by inhibition of b-arrestin2 expression in mice periaqueductal gray matter. Int J Mol Sci 10:954–963

Liapakis G, Cordomí A, Pardo L (2012) The G-protein coupled receptor family: actors with many faces [published correction appears in Curr Pharm Des (2012) 18: 4583]. Curr Pharm Des 18: 175–185

Luscombe VB, Baena-Lopez L, Bataille CJR, Russell AJ, Greaves DR (2023) Kinetic insights into agonist-dependent signalling bias at the pro-inflammatory G-protein coupled receptor GPR84. Eur Pharmacol 0014-2999

Manglik A, Kobilka B (2014) The role of protein dynamics in GPCR function: insights from the b2AR and rhodopsin. Curr Opin Cell Biol 27:136–143

Manglik A, Kim TH, Masureel M, Altenbach C, Yang Z, Hilger D, Lerch MT, Kobilka TS, Thian FS, Hubbell WL et al (2015) Structural insights into the dynamic process of b2-adrenergic receptor signaling [published correction appears in Cell (2015) 162:1431]. Cell 161:1101–1111

Molden BM, Cooney KA, West K, Van Der Ploeg LHT, Baldini G (2015) Temporal cAMP signaling selectivity by natural and synthetic MC4R agonists. Mol Endocrinol 29(11): 1619–1633

Morissette A, Mulvihill EE (2024) Obesity management for the treatment of type 2 diabetes: emerging evidence and therapeutic approaches. J Pharm Pharm Sci 27:13065

Motlagh HN, Wrabl JO, Li J, Hilser VJ (2014) The ensemble nature of allostery. Nature 508:331–339

Nygaard R, Zou Y, Dror RO, Mildorf TJ, Arlow DH, Manglik A, Pan AC, Liu CW, Fung JJ, Bokoch MP et al (2013) The dynamic process of b(2)-adrenergic receptor activation. Cell 152: 532–542

Onaran HO, Ambrosio C, Ugur Ö, Madaras Koncz E, Grò MC, Vezzi V, Rajagopal S, Costa T (2017) Systematic errors in detecting biased agonism: analysis of current methods and development of a new model-free approach. Sci Rep 7:44247

Pang PS, Butler J, Collins SP, Cotter G, Davison BA, Ezekowitz JA, Filippatos G, Levy PD, Metra M, Ponikowski P et al (2017) Biased ligand of the angiotensin II type 1 receptor in patients with acute heart failure: a randomized, double-blind, placebo-controlled, phase IIB, dose ranging trial (BLAST-AHF). Eur Heart J 38:2364–2373

Park PS (2012) Ensemble of G protein-coupled receptor active states. Curr Med Chem 19:1146–1154

Peters MF, Scott CW (2009) Evaluating cellular impedance assays for detection of GPCR pleiotropic signaling and functional selectivity. J Biomol Screen 14:246–255

Peters MF, Vaillancourt F, Heroux M, Valiquette M, Scott CW (2007) Comparing label-free biosensors for pharmacological screening with cell-based functional assays. J Biomol Screen 12:312–319

Raehal KM, Walker JK, Bohn LM (2005) Morphine side effects in b-arrestin 2 knockout mice. J Pharmacol Exp Ther 314:1195–1201

Roettger BF, Ghanekar D, Rao R, Toledo C, Yingling J, Pinon D et al (1997) Antagonist-stimulated internalization of the G protein-coupled cholecystokinin receptor. Mol Pharmacol 51:357–362
Roth BL, Chuang DM (1987) Multiple mechanisms of serotonergic signal transduction. Life Sci 41: 1051–1064
Singleton S, Baptista-Hon DT, Edelstein E, McCaughey KS, Camplisson E, Hales TG (2021) TRV130 partial agonism and capacity to induce anti-nociceptive tolerance revealed through reducing available μ-opioid receptor number. Br J Pharmacol 178:1855–1868
Skerrit JH, MacDonald RL (1984) Benzodiazepine receptor ligand actions on responses, Benzodiazepines, CL218872, zoplicone. Eur J Pharmacol 101:127
Sugihara S, Burnett JC (2017) BAST-AHF: insights into biased AT1 ligands and heart failure: beginning of the end or end of the beginning? Eur Heart J 38:2374–2376
Sutkeviciute I, Clark LJ, White AD, Gardella TJ, Jean-Pierre Vilardaga J-P (2019) PTH/PTHrP receptor signaling, allostery, and structures. Trends Endocrinol Metab 30(11):860–874
Tang KES, Dill KA (1998) Native protein fluctuations: the conformational-motion temperature and the inverse correlation of protein flexibility with protein stability. J Biomol Struct Dyn 16:397–411
Vardy E, Roth BL (2013) Conformational ensembles in GPCR activation. Cell 152:385–388
Viladarga J-P, Jean-Alphonse FG, Gardella TJ (2014) Endosomal generation of cAMP in GPCR signaling. Nat Chem Biol 10(9):700–706
Violin JD, Dewire SM, Barnes WG, Lefkowitz RJ (2006) G protein-coupled receptor kinase and beta-arrestin-mediated desensitization of the angiotensin II type1A receptor elucidated by diacylglycerol dynamics. J Biol Chem 281:36411–36419
Violin JD, DeWire SM, Yamashita D, Rominger DH, Nguyen L, Schiller K, Whalen EJ, Gowen M, Lark MW (2010) Selectively engaging β-arrestins at the angiotensin II type 1 receptor reduces blood pressure and increases cardiac performance. Pharmacol Exp Ther 335:572–579
Violin JD, Crombie AL, Soergel DG, Lark MW (2014) Biased ligands at G-protein-coupled receptors: promise and progress. Trends Pharmacol Sci 35:308–316
Wakeham MCL, Davie BJ, Chalmers DK, Christopoulos A, Capuano B, Valant C, Scammells PJ (2022) Structural features of Iperoxo–BQCA muscarinic acetylcholine receptor hybrid ligands determining subtype selectivity and efficacy. ACS Chem Neurosci 13:97–111
Watson C, Jenkinson S, Kazmierski W, Kenakin T (2005) The CCR5 receptor based mechanism of action of 873140, a potent allosteric noncompetitive HIV entry inhibitor. Mol Pharmacol 67: 1268–1282
White KL, Scopton AP, Rives ML, Bikbulatov RV, Polepally PR, Brown PJ, Kenakin T, Javitch JA, Zjawiony JK, Roth BL (2014) Identification of novel functionally selective k-opioid receptor scaffolds. Mol Pharmacol 85:83–90
White KL, Robinson JE, Zhu H, DiBerto JF, Polepally PR, Zjawiony JK, Nichols DE, Malanga CJ, Roth BL (2015) The G protein-biased k-opioid receptor agonist RB-64 is analgesic with a unique spectrum of activities in vivo. J Pharmacol Exp Ther 352:98–109
Williams PD, Pollock DD, Goldstein RA (2007) Functionality and the evolution of marginal stability in proteins: inferences from lattice simulations. Evol Bioinformatics Online 2:91–101
Yang CH, Huang HW, Chen KH, Chen YS, Sheen-Chen SM, Lin CR (2011) Antinociceptive potentiation and attenuation of tolerance by intrathecal b-arrestin 2 small interfering RNA in rats. Br J Anaesth 107:774–781
Zidar DA, Violin JD, Whalen EJ, Lefkowitz RJ (2009) Selective engagement of G protein receptor kinases (GRKs) encodes distinct functions of biased ligands. Proc Natl Acad Sci USA 106: 9649–9654

Biased Allosteric Modulation in GPCR Drug Discovery

Jingzhi-Christina Zhou, Michelle Z. Li, Alan Long, and Alem W. Kahsai

Contents

J.-C. Zhou
Department of Chemistry, Duke University, Durham, NC, USA

Department of Medicine, Duke University Medical Center, Durham, NC, USA

M. Z. Li
Department of Medicine, Duke University Medical Center, Durham, NC, USA

Department of Biology, Duke University, Durham, NC, USA

A. Long
Department of Medicine, Duke University Medical Center, Durham, NC, USA

Department of Neuroscience, Duke University, Durham, NC, USA

A. W. Kahsai (✉)
Department of Medicine, Duke University Medical Center, Durham, NC, USA
e-mail: alem.kahsai@duke.edu

© The Author(s), under exclusive license to Springer Nature Switzerland AG 2025

Z. Li, K. Xiao (eds.), *Pharmacology of GPCRs Biased Signaling and Agonists*,
Handbook of Experimental Pharmacology 290, https://doi.org/10.1007/164_2025_771

Abstract

Allosteric modulation of G protein-coupled receptors (GPCRs) is emerging as a powerful approach in drug discovery, offering enhanced subtype selectivity and the ability to bias signaling toward therapeutically preferred pathways, thereby reducing off-target effects. While most approved GPCR drugs act via the orthosteric site, this approach often lacks subtype specificity and induces pleiotropic signaling that can compromise therapeutic efficacy. Orthosteric biased ligands have provided proof of concept for functional selectivity, yet their development has been limited by site homology and challenges in fine-tuning pathway specificity. In contrast, allosteric modulators (AMs) bind to spatially and structurally distinct, less conserved sites located across extracellular, transmembrane, and intracellular receptor domains. By stabilizing discrete receptor conformations, AMs can fine-tune transducer engagement and preferentially direct signaling toward either G protein or β-arrestin (βarr) pathway. Recent structural and biophysical studies have provided insights into how diverse AMs lock GPCRs in specific conformations and modulate signaling across receptor families. Taken together, these findings reflect a shift in GPCR pharmacology, driven by the convergence of biased signaling and allosteric modulation. Biased allosteric modulators (BAMs) represent a promising class of ligands that bind at allosteric sites and selectively tune signaling pathways by biasing orthosteric ligand-induced responses. This review outlines the principles of biased signaling and allosteric modulation and highlights strategies for designing BAMs for GPCRs. Identifying BAMs could revolutionize GPCR drug discovery by enabling pathway-specific precision therapeutics with improved efficacy and fewer side effects.

Keywords

Allosteric modulation · Drug discovery · Functional selectivity · G protein-coupled receptor (GPCR) · Signaling bias · Therapeutic development

Abbreviations

A_1AR	Adenosine A_1 receptor
ADHD	Attention-deficit/hyperactivity disorder
ADMET	Absorption, distribution, metabolism, excretion, and toxicity
Ago-BAM	Biased allosteric agonist
Ago-PAM	Allosteric agonist
AI	Artificial intelligence
AKT	Protein kinase B
AM	Allosteric modulator
ARB	Angiotensin receptor blocker
AT_1R	Angiotensin II receptor type 1
BAM	Biased allosteric modulator
BRET	Bioluminescence resonance energy transfer

cAMP	Cyclic adenosine monophosphate
CaSR	Calcium-sensing receptor
CB_1	Cannabinoid receptor 1
Cryo-EM	Cryogenic electronic microscopy
CXCR	CXC chemokine receptor
D_1R	Dopamine receptor 1
D_2R	Dopamine receptor 2
DEER	Double electron-electron resonance
DEL	DNA-encoded small molecule library
DFPQ	Difluorophenyl quinazoline
ERK	Extracellular signal-regulated kinases
FDA	U.S. Food and Drug Administration
$FFAR_1$	Free fatty acid receptor 1
GDP	Guanosine diphosphate
GFP	Green fluorescent protein
$GHSR_{1a}$	Growth hormone secretagogue receptor 1a
GLP-1R	Glucagon-like peptide-1 receptor
GPCR	G protein-coupled receptor
GRK	G protein-coupled receptor kinase
GTP	Guanosine triphosphate
GTPγS	Guanosine 5'-O-[gamma-thio]triphosphate
HTS	High-throughput screening
IP3/IP1	Inositol trisphosphate 3/1
JNK	C-Jun N-terminal kinases
MAPK	Mitogen-activated protein kinases
NAM	Negative allosteric modulator
NMR	Nuclear magnetic resonance
$NTSR_1$	Neurotensin receptor type 1
OCD	Obsessive-compulsive disorder
PAM	Positive allosteric modulator
PD	Pharmacodynamics
PI3K	Phosphoinositide 3-kinase
PK	Pharmacokinetics
PTH_1R	Parathyroid hormone 1 receptor
Raf	Rapidly accelerated fibrosarcoma
RAMP	Receptor-activity modifying protein
SAR	Structure-activity relationship
sm-FRET	Single-molecule Förster (or fluorescence) resonance energy transfer
$5\text{-}HT_{2A}R$	5-hydroxytryptamine 2A receptor
α_2AR	α_2-adrenergic receptor
β blocker	β-adrenergic receptor blocker
β_1AR	β_1-adrenergic receptor
β_2AR	β_2-adrenergic receptor
βarr	β-arrestin
μOR	μ-opioid receptor

1 Introduction

G protein-coupled receptors (GPCRs) are a large family of seven-transmembrane proteins that play critical roles in cellular communication (Lefkowitz 2013a, b; Lorente et al. 2025). They do so by receiving diverse external stimuli such as light, hormones, ions, and neurotransmitters (Pierce et al. 2002). These ligands induce conformational changes that activate intracellular signaling pathways, primarily via the transducers G proteins and β-arrestins (βarrs) (Pierce et al. 2002; Lefkowitz 2013a, b). The human genome encodes over 800 GPCRs, of which approximately 360 are non-sensory and considered pharmacologically tractable (Pierce et al. 2002; Lorente et al. 2025). To date, roughly one-third of all approved drugs act through GPCRs, with 516 approved compounds targeting 121 distinct receptors across this superfamily (Lorente et al. 2025). This broad clinical footprint underscores the central role of GPCRs in regulating physiological processes such as cognition, immune responses, metabolic control, and homeostasis.

Historically, GPCR-targeting drugs have focused on orthosteric sites, where endogenous ligands initiate receptor activation. However, the high sequence conservation of these pockets across receptor subtypes renders subtype selectivity an intractable challenge, increasing the risk of off-target effects and adverse outcomes (Goupil et al. 2012; Khoury et al. 2014; Shen et al. 2023). Moreover, prolonged orthosteric engagement can drive receptor desensitization and downregulation, ultimately diminishing therapeutic efficacy (Smith et al. 2018), shedding light on the need for alternative strategies. Over the past two decades, our understanding of GPCR signaling has expanded beyond the classical two-state model of receptor activation. Evidence now suggests that GPCRs have multiple conformational states (Kobilka and Deupi 2007; Kahsai et al. 2011; Wingler et al. 2019; Wingler and Lefkowitz 2020), distinguished not only by activation or inactivation of the receptor, but by the degree of transducer activity. This concept underlies biased signaling or functional selectivity, where ligands preferentially activate either G protein- or βarr-mediated pathways (Goupil et al. 2012; Slosky et al. 2021).

Although G proteins were historically considered the primary mediators of GPCR signaling, βarrs are now appreciated not only for their role in receptor desensitization and internalization (Benovic et al. 1987; Lohse et al. 1990; Lefkowitz 2013a, b), but also for their ability to scaffold signaling complexes and mediate βarr-dependent pathways (Peterson and Luttrell 2017). This dual signaling capacity creates opportunities to develop therapeutic ligands that selectively activate beneficial pathways while minimizing adverse effects (Rajagopal et al. 2010, Whalen et al. 2011, Violin et al. 2014, Smith et al. 2018). These pharmacological insights are complemented by structural studies that illuminate both orthosteric and allosteric ligand binding mechanisms across diverse GPCR states (Thal et al. 2018; Persechino et al. 2022).

As the limitations of orthosteric ligands become increasingly evident, interest has grown in allosteric modulators (AMs), which bind to sites topographically distinct from the orthosteric pocket (Wootten et al. 2013). These ligands offer a powerful alternative for modulating GPCR function. By engaging less conserved regions,

AMs can achieve subtype-specific effects and potentially improve drug therapeutic indices (Thal et al. 2018; Lorente et al. 2025). This topographical divergence expands the druggable landscape, enabling access to previously intractable targets and introducing new opportunities for functional selectivity. AMs can stabilize distinct receptor conformations, fine-tune endogenous ligand responses, and bias signaling pathways (Shen et al. 2023). Unlike orthosteric ligands, they do not directly compete with endogenous agonists. Instead, their saturable and cooperative mechanisms help preserve the spatial and temporal fidelity of physiological signaling.

Building on these advances, biased AMs (BAMs) are emerging as a novel class of GPCR pharmacological agents with the ability to preferentially direct signaling toward G protein or βarr pathways (Slosky et al. 2021). Several BAMs are advancing through late-stage preclinical and early-stage clinical development (Slosky et al. 2020; Guo et al. 2025; Sun et al. 2025), reflecting their increasing feasibility in drug discovery. Understanding the complex pharmacology of BAMs, including their mechanisms, conformational effects, and functional outcomes, is essential for advancing this therapeutic approach.

This chapter outlines the fundamental principles of GPCR allosteric modulation and highlights how ligands targeting structurally distinct allosteric sites can reshape receptor pharmacology. It summarizes recent discoveries in allosteric regulation, including examples of modulators acting at extracellular, transmembrane, and intracellular domains. Particular attention is given to how these ligands stabilize receptor conformations to favor either the G protein or βarr pathway, a strategy that holds therapeutic promise across a range of GPCRs and disease contexts. This chapter also explores how AMs provide mechanistic insights that can guide the rational design of more selective and effective therapeutics. Building on these insights, it examines the emerging class of BAMs and presents conceptual strategies for their discovery and design, including how biased allosteric ligands can direct receptor output and offer novel opportunities for drug specificity.

2 Mechanisms of GPCR and Biased Signaling

2.1 GPCR Signaling Paradigm and Canonical Signal Transduction

GPCRs are transmembrane proteins that transduce extracellular signals into intracellular responses. Generally, GPCRs share two common features: seven transmembrane domains and the ability to couple with G proteins (Pierce et al. 2002; Lefkowitz 2013a, b). Building on their conserved architecture, the discovery of diverse regulatory and signaling profiles has cemented GPCRs as adaptable and highly druggable targets. When an agonist binds to a GPCR's orthosteric pocket, atomic interactions with key residues trigger conformational changes that propagate to the receptor's intracellular region. This "active" conformation facilitates the recruitment of downstream transducers, including G proteins and βarrs. The coupling of a heterotrimeric G protein to the receptor causes the G protein to release its bound guanosine diphosphate (GDP) molecule in exchange for a guanosine triphosphate (GTP). This triggers the dissociation of the G protein into its alpha (Gα) and beta-gamma subunits (Gβγ), enabling their interaction with downstream signaling effectors within cells (Rasmussen et al. 2011). Gβγ also acts as a key signaling molecule to recruit G protein-coupled receptor kinases (GRKs) to the plasma membrane. These GRKs then phosphorylate the cytoplasmic tail of the activated receptor, generating a recognition site for βarr proteins (Reiter and Lefkowitz 2006). βarr recruitment sterically hinders G protein coupling, blocking downstream signal transduction while initiating the internalization of the receptor (Lefkowitz and Shenoy 2005; Reiter and Lefkowitz 2006).

In contrast, orthosteric antagonists stabilize an "inactive" receptor conformation that obstructs transducer binding. For many years, GPCR signaling was framed by a two-state model, where receptors were thought to only exist in inactive or fully active conformations. However, functional studies first revealed that GPCRs are capable of pathway-selective signaling, and subsequent structural analyses showed that orthosteric ligands can stabilize distinct ligand-specific receptor conformations, highlighting the conformational flexibility of GPCRs (Kobilka and Deupi 2007; Kahsai et al. 2011; Wingler et al. 2019; Wingler and Lefkowitz 2020). These findings provided a mechanistic foundation for biased signaling, also known as functional selectivity.

2.2 Biased Signaling: Functional Selectivity and Therapeutic Rationale

Signaling bias refers to the phenomenon where a signal input preferentially activates one specific signaling pathway over another. There are many layers of meanings to this concept: (1) the preferential activation of βarr-mediated signaling over G protein-mediated signaling, or vice versa, and (2) the selective activation of a G protein subtype within the broader G protein family (Kenakin and Christopoulos 2013; Slosky et al. 2021). This concept is clinically relevant because G protein and βarr signaling do not necessarily contribute equally to therapeutic outcomes across different GPCR systems. Thus, depending on the specific GPCR involved, one pathway may be therapeutic while the other may lead to adverse outcomes.

G protein activation elicits distinct cellular responses based on the particular type of G protein a GPCR is coupled to, such as $G_{\alpha s}$, $G_{\alpha i/o}$, $G_{\alpha q/11}$, and $G_{\alpha 12/13}$ (Kamato et al. 2015). Similarly, βarr can activate distinct downstream signaling cascades, including the Raf-MEK-ERK pathway, the JNK pathway, the p38-MAPK pathway, and the PI3K-AKT pathway (Kovacs et al. 2009; Kahsai et al. 2023). In the context of different diseases, each of these signaling functions can lead to either therapeutic or detrimental outcomes. For example, angiotensin II receptor type 1 (AT_1R) and β_1-adrenergic receptor (β_1AR) elicit cardioprotective effects through βarr-mediated signaling (Patel et al. 2010; Noor et al. 2011; Wisler et al. 2018). However, chronic G protein signaling can lead to vasoconstriction, which is undesirable in the treatment of hypertension and heart failure. Traditional medicines for heart failure, such as angiotensin receptor blockers (ARBs) and β-adrenergic receptor blockers (β blockers), inhibit both G protein and βarr signaling to the same degree (Patel et al. 2010). In contrast, biased ligands enable more selective therapeutic modulation by preferentially engaging beneficial signaling pathways while minimizing activation of those linked to adverse effects.

Different mechanisms leading to biased signaling patterns have been discovered, including ligand bias (a ligand induces a unique receptor conformation resulting in a biased response), receptor bias (biased signaling generated from the receptor itself), system bias (differential transducer expression levels), and location bias (differential signaling of a receptor across various cellular locations or microdomains) (Smith et al. 2018). An increasing number of biased ligands targeting GPCRs have been identified, offering opportunities to fine-tune receptor signaling with greater therapeutic precision. Among the most well-characterized are G protein-biased agonists for the μ-opioid receptor (μOR), a key target in pain management. TRV130 (oliceridine) and PZM21 are notable examples that preferentially activate $G_{\alpha i}$ signaling while minimizing βarr recruitment, leading to potent analgesia and reduced respiratory depression (Manglik et al. 2016; Fossler et al. 2018; Lambert and Calo 2020). Similarly, VCP746, a G protein-biased agonist for the adenosine A_1 receptor (A_1AR), has demonstrated cardioprotective effects without causing the bradycardia and hypotension typically associated with this target (Valant et al. 2014; Baltos et al. 2016; Chuo et al. 2016; Wall et al. 2022). Additional G-biased ligands for A_1AR have demonstrated potential in cardioprotection and reducing inflammation (Franco et al. 2020; McNeill et al. 2021; Meng et al. 2025).

AT_1R, long studied as a classical G protein-coupled vasoconstrictor target, has become a prototypical model for βarr-biased signaling. TRV027 and TRV023, βarr-biased ligands for AT_1R, dissociate vasoconstriction from cardioprotective signaling (Monasky et al. 2013; Soergel et al. 2013; Wingler et al. 2019; Kashihara et al. 2020). TRV027 has notably progressed into clinical trials for acute heart failure and severe COVID-19 (Manglik et al. 2020), emphasizing its translational potential. ML314, a βarr-biased agonist of the neurotensin receptor type 1 ($NTSR_1$), showed therapeutic potential for methamphetamine addiction with reduced off-target activity (Peddibhotla et al. 2013; Barak et al. 2016). ORG27569, an AM of cannabinoid receptor 1 (CB_1), enhances orthosteric ligand binding while inhibiting G protein signaling and promoting βarr2-dependent responses, resulting in attenuated drug-seeking behavior in preclinical models (Gamage et al. 2016; Scicluna et al. 2024a, b). These diverse examples underscore the pharmacological versatility of biased ligands and support the potential development of pathway-selective therapeutics across multiple disease indications.

2.3 Limitations in Orthosteric Biased Agonism

Traditional orthosteric regulation has proven insufficient for achieving target-specific modulation in GPCRs. Key challenges of these orthosteric drugs include: (1) The binding of orthosteric ligands to highly conserved orthosteric sites across receptor subtypes, resulting in significant off-target effects; for example, dopamine can bind to not only all five subtypes of the dopamine receptor, but also the 5-hydroxytryptamine 2A receptor (5-HT_{2A}R) (Howell and Cunningham 2015). (2) Orthosteric ligands tend to promote balanced signaling, which may not align with therapeutic goals. These limitations highlight the need for alternative strategies, such as allosteric modulation.

3 Biased Allosteric Modulation of GPCRs

3.1 Foundations of Allostery and Pharmacological Advantages

Allosteric modulation centers around cooperativity and conformational ensemble theories (Kenakin and Miller 2010). Allostery was originally discovered through hemoglobin-oxygen binding studies (Ackers and Holt 2006), and its extension to GPCRs has emerged with modern insights (Gentry et al. 2015). In GPCRs, AMs bind to sites that are distinct from the orthosteric pocket, inducing conformational changes that either potentiate (positive allosteric modulators, PAMs) or dampen (negative allosteric modulators, NAMs) receptor activity, indirectly modulating the behavior of orthosteric ligands. The intrinsic existence of allosteric modulation allows AMs to fine-tune and subtly change receptor conformation to optimize functional consequences. From a thermodynamic perspective, AMs shift the conformational equilibria to enrich specific signaling states.

AMs offer several key advantages in the context of GPCR drug discovery and pharmacological targeting. First, because allosteric sites are typically less conserved across receptor subtypes, AMs often confer greater selectivity and reduce off-target effects (Khoury et al. 2014; Shen et al. 2023). Second, the saturable nature of allosteric binding imparts a ceiling effect, which helps prevent excessive receptor activation or inhibition and enhances safety (Wold and Zhou 2018). Third, AMs also have the ability to modulate receptor activity independent of orthosteric ligand binding, enabling control over constitutive signaling (Shen et al. 2023). Finally, some AMs can bias receptor signaling toward specific downstream pathways, offering a route to functionally selective pharmacology (Smith et al. 2018; Slosky et al. 2021).

3.2 BAMs and Translational Outlook

BAMs harness both the spatial flexibility of allosteric binding and the therapeutic precision of biased signaling. These compounds engage allosteric sites, stabilizing conformations that preferentially direct signaling toward either G protein or βarr pathways (Whalen et al. 2011; Khoury et al. 2014; Hauser et al. 2017; Smith et al. 2018; Slosky et al. 2021). BAMs may originate from endogenous sources, including ions (Katritch et al. 2014; Zarzycka et al. 2019), lipids (Dawaliby et al. 2016), and receptor-activity modifying proteins (RAMPs) (Pioszak and Hay 2020). They can also be synthetically engineered to mimic intracellular receptor interfaces, such as pepducins (Carr 3rd et al. 2014), or to selectively recognize receptor conformations, as in the case of nanobodies (Staus et al. 2016), aptamers (Kahsai et al. 2016), and intracellularly targeted bitopic ligands (Keov et al. 2014).

Despite their promise, only four GPCR-targeted allosteric drugs are currently FDA-approved: cinacalcet (Nagano and Tsutsui 2016), maraviroc (Ray 2009), avacopan (Liu et al. 2018), and ticagrelor (Khalil et al. 2024), according to the Allosteric Database (Huang et al. 2011) and FDA Drug Database (FDA 2025). These agents, while not necessarily biased, validate the feasibility of exploiting allosteric mechanisms for therapeutic benefits. BAMs build on this foundation, offering a path to even greater signaling precision.

Biased allosteric modulators (BAMs) offer distinct pharmacological advantages over orthosteric ligands by enabling more selective and tunable receptor modulation. Structural studies have now resolved over 120 GPCR–modulator complexes (Kooistra et al. 2021; Zhuang et al. 2021), though these correspond to approximately half as many unique GPCRs. Notably, these include the μOR (Kaneko et al. 2022), β_2-adrenergic receptor (β_2AR) (Liu et al. 2017, 2019), and an intracellular allosteric agonist (ago-PAM) for the human parathyroid hormone type 1 receptor (PTH_1R) (Kobayashi et al. 2023). These examples reveal a rich diversity of binding sites across extracellular loops, transmembrane domains, and lipid-facing interfaces. These insights were primarily enabled by cryogenic electronic microscopy (cryo-EM), with some structures solved by X-ray crystallography, revealing that GPCRs can have multiple allosteric sites depending on their conformational state. At the same time, computational approaches have become essential for predicting and characterizing allosteric sites, guiding the identification of druggable pockets, and informing ligand design. Together, structural and in silico data have demonstrated that both experimentally resolved and modeled allosteric sites can be exploited to shape receptor signaling (Liu et al. 2020). This integrated strategy supports the development of BAMs as tunable chemotypes capable of producing pathway-selective therapeutic responses.

Key Terms

- PAMs: enhance orthosteric ligand activity
- NAMs: attenuate orthosteric ligand activity
- Ago-PAMs: can act as agonists on their own while enhancing orthosteric ligand activity
- BAMs: direct signaling through preferred transducers
- Ago-BAMs: direct signaling through preferred transducers, even without orthosteric ligands

Here, we present Table 1 that summarizes representative GPCRs with therapeutic potentials in biased signaling. Beyond these GPCRs, examples of BAMs for other receptors in preclinical and clinical pipelines continue to emerge, reinforcing their growing relevance as a next-generation modality in GPCR-targeted drug discovery. Some currently well-studied BAM examples include βarr-biased PAM SBI-553 and

Table 1 Representative examples of GPCR targets with biased agonism and associated therapeutic relevance

GPCR	Desirable pathway	Mediated physiology	References
β_2AR	G_s	Airway smooth muscle cell relaxation and bronchial dilation; concurrent blockade of β-arrestin-mediated inflammation and desensitization; potential treatment for asthma	Torphy (1994), Walker et al. (2003, 2011), Walker and DeFea (2014), Kim et al. (2020), Ahn et al. (2023)
β_1AR	β-arrestin	Provides cardioprotective effect; concurrent blockade of Gs-mediated overactivation of heart; potential treatment for hypertension and heart failure	Noma et al. (2007), Wang et al. (2018, 2021), Wisler et al. (2018)
AT_1R	β-arrestin	Provides cardioprotective effect, which can be applied in acute heart failure and COVID-19; concurrent blockade of G_q-mediated vasoconstriction	Patel et al. (2010), Boerrigter et al. (2011), Kim et al. (2012), Wisler et al. (2018), Manglik et al. (2020)
A_1AR	$G_{i/o}$	Provides cardioprotective effect and reduced inflammatory responses; potential applications in pain relief	Franco et al. (2020), McNeill et al. (2021), Meng et al. (2025)
GLP-1R	G_s	Enhanced antidiabetic and antihyperglycemic effect through sustained insulin production	Zhang et al. (2015), Wootten et al. (2016), Jones et al. (2021), Jones (2022), Douros et al. (2024), Zhu et al. (2024), Douros et al. (2025)
GPR40/FFAR1	$G_{q/11}$	Potentially enhanced antidiabetic and antihyperglycemic effect through insulinotropic activity	Mancini et al. (2015), Chen et al. (2016a), Hamdouchi et al. (2016, 2018), Guan and Xiong (2022)
CaSR	$G_{q/11}$	Potential treatment for hyperparathyroidism, hypercalcemia, colon cancer, and cardiovascular-related diseases	Davey et al. (2012), Leach et al. (2013, 2014, 2015)
PTH_1R	β-arrestin	Promotes anabolic bone formation and reduces bone resorption; potential treatment for osteoporosis	Gesty-Palmer et al. (2009), Gesty-Palmer and Luttrell (2011)
μOR	$G_{i/o}$	Analgesic; concurrent blockade of β-arrestin signaling provides resistance to development of chronic morphine-induced tolerance, respiratory suppression, and constipation	Che et al. (2021), Kelly et al. (2023), Kise and Inoue (2024)
D_2R	β-arrestin	Antidepressant and antipsychotic; potential treatment for schizophrenia and related disorders	Allen et al. (2011), Chen et al. (2012), Urs et al. (2015), Chen et al. (2016b), Park et al. (2016), Urs et al. (2017)

(continued)

Table 1 (continued)

GPCR	Desirable pathway	Mediated physiology	References
CB_1	G_i	Analgesic; concurrent blockade of β-arrestin signaling provides resistance to tolerance development	Laprairie et al. (2017), Mallipeddi et al. (2017), Milligan et al. (2020)
$NTSR_1$	β-arrestin	Blockade of G_q-mediated hypothermia and motor impairment; potential treatment for psychiatric disorders, addictive behavior, and pain management	Barak et al. (2016), Pinkerton et al. (2019), Singhal et al. (2023), Gereau et al. (2024), Guo et al. (2025)
5-$HT_{2A}R$	G_q	Anti-hallucination; potential treatment for schizophrenia, neurodegenerative diseases (e.g. Parkinson's disease), depression, OCD, and attention deficit	Marti-Solano et al. (2015), Zhang and Stackman Jr. (2015)
$GHSR_{1a}$	G_q	Blockade of β-arrestin signaling provides resistance to addiction development; potential treatment for metabolic disorders and neurodegenerative diseases	Gross et al. (2023)

SBI-810 for $NTSR_1$ (Slosky et al. 2020; Guo et al. 2025; Sun et al. 2025), G protein-ago-BAM PCO371 for PTH_1R (Tamura et al. 2016; Zhao et al. 2023), βarr-biased NAM difluorophenyl quinazoline (DFPQ) derivative for β_2AR (Ippolito et al. 2023), and G protein-ago-BAM CB-05 for CB_1 (Shen et al. 2024). Targeting these receptors has a wide range of pathophysiological indications, including cardiovascular, pulmonary, neurological, immunological, and osteological benefits (Slosky et al. 2021; Wang et al. 2021; Meng et al. 2025) (Table 1).

4 Strategies for Identifying Allosteric and Biased Allosteric Modulators of GPCRs

4.1 Functional and Affinity-Based Strategies

Many currently known AMs and BAMs were identified through high-throughput screening (HTS) of large compound libraries, some of which are specifically designed for GPCR targeting and are commercially available. Notable GPCR AMs or ligands identified through library HTS include Compound-15 and Compound-6 from DNA-encoded small molecule library (DEL) screening, an affinity-based method (Ahn et al. 2017, 2018). To assess functionality, a series of screening methods can be utilized to measure the activity of GPCRs modulated by AMs, either in the presence or absence of orthosteric ligands. HTS methods can be categorized as either drug affinity-based or cellular function-based (Yasi et al. 2020). Functional assays that measure downstream effects of G protein activation include GTPγS binding, G protein dissociation, cyclic adenosine monophosphate (cAMP) detection, calcium influx and inositol trisphosphate-3/1 (IP3/IP1) detection, and reporter assays (Berridge 1995; Milligan 2003; Zhang and Xie 2012; Vasudevan 2017; Woszczek et al. 2021).

Functional assays for βarr function include bioluminescence resonance energy transfer (BRET) assays, split luciferase assays, and reporter assays, measuring both βarr recruitment and βarr-mediated receptor internalization (Asher et al. 2021, 2022; Hauge Pedersen et al. 2021; Perry-Hauser et al. 2021). Imaging of green fluorescent protein (GFP)-tagged βarr under the microscope can also qualitatively and quantitatively visualize βarr recruitment (Ferguson and Caron 2004). BAM function is usually tested by evaluating potency and efficacy shifts in the dose response curves of these two transducers in in vitro systems (Kolb et al. 2022).

The choice of assay system should consider signal-to-noise ratio and the possibility of false positives. To ensure reliable results, it is important to conduct primary and secondary assays that are conceptually orthogonal, enabling the effects of the compounds to be validated and eliminating artifacts from the assay system. One challenge in quantitatively determining signal bias is effectively comparing signals from amplified secondary messengers vs. linear signals. This complexity underscores the need for in vitro characterization before proceeding to evaluate candidate molecules' efficacy in animal models. Factors that need to be accounted for and thoroughly tested include bias profile through primary and secondary assay panels, PK/PD, ADMET, compound stability, and optimization SAR (Caldwell et al. 2009; Tuntland et al. 2014; Sun et al. 2022). These methods are costly and time-consuming, but such characterizations would allow for comprehensive and accurate information to be obtained from the subsequent animal experiments. Therefore, the complexity of GPCR signaling requires detailed pharmacological characterization, in vivo/ex vivo testing, and data analysis on candidate molecules to determine their therapeutic potential.

4.2 Structure-Guided and in Silico Strategies

With the development of computational and simulation methods, structure-guided virtual screening has become a cornerstone of AM and BAM discovery. High-throughput docking of large chemical libraries—ranging from hundreds of thousands to over 100 million compounds—into experimentally determined GPCR structures or homology models facilitates efficient identification of promising ligand candidates. Molecular docking can predict ligand binding affinity and suggest conformational compatibility, providing a rational starting point for iterative compound optimization (Katritch et al. 2014). This approach is typically complemented by in vitro and in vivo validation to assess pharmacological efficacy and bias. The recent explosion in GPCR structures has revealed diverse allosteric binding pockets and conformational states across Class A, B, and C GPCRs (Chun et al. 2012;

Wootten et al. 2017; Egyed et al. 2022). Structural insights into receptor ligand interactions—including Dopamine Receptor 1 (D_1R), CB_1, calcium-sensing receptor (CaSR), and β_2AR—have illuminated how specific modulator contact can stabilize a given receptor conformation (Huang et al. 2020; Ling et al. 2021; Zhuang et al. 2021).

Structure-activity relationship (SAR) studies and medicinal chemistry efforts further enable the fine-tuning of ligand efficacy, receptor selectivity, and signaling bias. Scaffold-based ligand design and combinatorial synthesis from parent chemotypes can explore the pharmacophore space systematically. Mutagenesis experiments help validate predicted ligand-receptor interactions and inform refinements. This comprehensive approach not only accelerates BAM discovery, but also deepens our understanding of receptor activation and modulation. Several BAMs identified via this strategy have demonstrated functional selectivity by stabilizing receptor states favoring G protein or βarr signaling. For instance, structure-guided optimization of ligands targeting the κ-opioid receptor yielded compound 81, a potent G protein-biased agonist with significantly reduced βarr2 recruitment (Schmidhammer et al. 2020). Similarly, the structural elucidation of PAM binding at the CaSR and the glucagon-like peptide-1 receptor (GLP-1R) has guided the development of subtype-specific, biased modulators (Chen et al. 2021; Cong et al. 2021). These examples demonstrate how structural biology and computational screening, when integrated with functional and medicinal chemistry workflows, can expedite the rational design of BAMs with precise pharmacological profiles.

Biophysical and structural tools provide an additional layer of information: the specific set of receptor conformations stabilized by the addition of BAMs. Such methods include double electron-electron resonance (DEER) spectroscopy (Manglik et al. 2015; Wingler et al. 2019; Lerch et al. 2020), single-molecule Förster (or fluorescence) resonance energy transfer (sm-FRET) assay (Asher et al. 2021), nuclear magnetic resonance (NMR) spectroscopy (Manglik et al. 2015), and hydrogen-deuterium exchange (Li et al. 2015). While these methods do not yield atomic-resolution structures, they offer critical insights into receptor dynamics, conformational landscapes, and allosteric transitions. Together, such data can inform and refine structure-based drug design strategies, particularly in the context of flexible or transient receptor states.

5 Conclusion and Future Perspectives

Over the past decade, biased signaling has reshaped the landscape of GPCR pharmacology, revealing new opportunities to selectively direct receptor activity toward therapeutically desirable pathways. This shift has emphasized the need for more precise allosteric modulation strategies. By targeting sites outside the orthosteric pocket, allosteric ligands influence receptor behavior in context-dependent ways, amplifying, silencing, or enhancing the precision of bias signaling. At the intersection of these principles lies biased allosteric modulation, a young but promising approach with the potential to fine-tune receptor responses while minimizing unwanted effects. Despite its potential, the discovery and optimization of BAMs remain a complex and gradual progress—hindered by dynamic receptor conformations, elusive binding sites, and steep SARs. Advances in structural biology, such as cryo-EM and NMR, are beginning to shed light on receptor states linked to biased allosteric modulation, but many remain unclear. Concurrently, artificial intelligence (AI) holds predictive potential in BAM design. From identifying allosteric pockets to modeling biased conformations and guiding lead optimization, AI tools offer valuable support but remain limited by early-stage development and dependence on high-quality data. For now, AI's role is best viewed as complementary to experimental approaches, not a replacement.

Looking forward, the future of BAMs will depend on the integration of disciplines—structural insights, pharmacological expertise, and computational innovation. As tools improve and our understanding deepens, GPCR-biased allosteric modulation may evolve from concept to clinic, offering more refined therapies for complex diseases.

Acknowledgments We are grateful for the mentorship and support of Dr. Robert J. Lefkowitz. This work was supported in part by the U.S. National Institutes of Health (Grants T32HL007101 and HL16037-45S1 to A.W.K.). A.W.K. is also supported by the Mandel Foundation SEED Award through the Duke Cardiology Research Center, the St. Jude Children's Research Hospital Collaborative Research Consortium on GPCRs, and the Headley Foundation. A.L. is supported by the Biological and Brain Sciences Summer Undergraduate Research Fellowship from Duke University.

Declaration of Competing Interest The authors declare no competing financial or personal interests related to this work.

References

Ackers GK, Holt JM (2006) Asymmetric cooperativity in a symmetric tetramer: human hemoglobin. J Biol Chem 281(17):11441–11443

Ahn S, Kahsai AW, Pani B, Wang QT, Zhao S, Wall AL, Strachan RT, Staus DP, Wingler LM, Sun LD, Sinnaeve J, Choi M, Cho T, Xu TT, Hansen GM, Burnett MB, Lamerdin JE, Bassoni DL, Gavino BJ, Husemoen G, Olsen EK, Franch T, Costanzi S, Chen X, Lefkowitz RJ (2017) Allosteric "beta-blocker" isolated from a DNA-encoded small molecule library. Proc Natl Acad Sci USA 114(7):1708–1713

Ahn S, Pani B, Kahsai AW, Olsen EK, Husemoen G, Vestergaard M, Jin L, Zhao S, Wingler LM, Rambarat PK, Simhal RK, Xu TT, Sun LD, Shim PJ, Staus DP, Huang LY, Franch T, Chen X, Lefkowitz RJ (2018) Small-molecule positive allosteric modulators of the beta(2)-Adrenoceptor isolated from DNA-encoded libraries. Mol Pharmacol 94(2):850–861

Ahn S, Maarsingh H, Walker JK, Liu S, Hegde A, Sumajit HC, Kahsai AW, Lefkowitz RJ (2023) Allosteric modulator potentiates beta2AR agonist-promoted bronchoprotection in asthma models. J Clin Invest 133(18):e167337

Allen JA, Yost JM, Setola V, Chen X, Sassano MF, Chen M, Peterson S, Yadav PN, Huang XP, Feng B, Jensen NH, Che X, Bai X, Frye SV, Wetsel WC, Caron MG, Javitch JA, Roth BL, Jin J (2011) Discovery of beta-arrestin-biased dopamine D2 ligands for probing signal transduction pathways essential for antipsychotic efficacy. Proc Natl Acad Sci USA 108(45):18488–18493

Asher WB, Geggier P, Holsey MD, Gilmore GT, Pati AK, Meszaros J, Terry DS, Mathiasen S, Kaliszewski MJ, McCauley MD, Govindaraju A, Zhou Z, Harikumar KG, Jaqaman K, Miller LJ, Smith AW, Blanchard SC, Javitch JA (2021) Single-molecule FRET imaging of GPCR dimers in living cells. Nat Methods 18(4):397–405

Asher WB, Terry DS, Gregorio GGA, Kahsai AW, Borgia A, Xie B, Modak A, Zhu Y, Jang W, Govindaraju A, Huang LY, Inoue A, Lambert NA, Gurevich VV, Shi L, Lefkowitz RJ, Blanchard SC, Javitch JA (2022) GPCR-mediated beta-arrestin activation deconvoluted with single-molecule precision. Cell 185(10):1661–1675 e1616

Baltos JA, Gregory KJ, White PJ, Sexton PM, Christopoulos A, May LT (2016) Quantification of adenosine a(1) receptor biased agonism: implications for drug discovery. Biochem Pharmacol 99:101–112

Barak LS, Bai Y, Peterson S, Evron T, Urs NM, Peddibhotla S, Hedrick MP, Hershberger P, Maloney PR, Chung TD, Rodriguiz RM, Wetsel WC, Thomas JB, Hanson GR, Pinkerton AB, Caron MG (2016) ML314: a biased Neurotensin receptor ligand for methamphetamine abuse. ACS Chem Biol 11(7):1880–1890

Benovic JL, Kuhn H, Weyand I, Codina J, Caron MG, Lefkowitz RJ (1987) Functional desensitization of the isolated beta-adrenergic receptor by the beta-adrenergic receptor kinase: potential role of an analog of the retinal protein arrestin (48-kDa protein). Proc Natl Acad Sci USA 84(24):8879–8882

Berridge MJ (1995) Inositol trisphosphate and calcium signaling. Ann N Y Acad Sci 766:31–43

Boerrigter G, Lark MW, Whalen EJ, Soergel DG, Violin JD, Burnett JC Jr (2011) Cardiorenal actions of TRV120027, a novel ss-arrestin-biased ligand at the angiotensin II type I receptor, in healthy and heart failure canines: a novel therapeutic strategy for acute heart failure. Circ Heart Fail 4(6):770–778

Caldwell GW, Yan Z, Tang W, Dasgupta M, Hasting B (2009) ADME optimization and toxicity assessment in early- and late-phase drug discovery. Curr Top Med Chem 9(11):965–980

Carr R 3rd, Du Y, Quoyer J, Panettieri RA Jr, Janz JM, Bouvier M, Kobilka BK, Benovic JL (2014) Development and characterization of pepducins as Gs-biased allosteric agonists. J Biol Chem 289(52):35668–35684

Che T, Dwivedi-Agnihotri H, Shukla AK, Roth BL (2021) Biased ligands at opioid receptors: current status and future directions. Sci Signal 14(677)

Chen X, Sassano MF, Zheng L, Setola V, Chen M, Bai X, Frye SV, Wetsel WC, Roth BL, Jin J (2012) Structure-functional selectivity relationship studies of beta-arrestin-biased dopamine D (2) receptor agonists. J Med Chem 55(16):7141–7153

Chen X, McCorvy JD, Fischer MG, Butler KV, Shen Y, Roth BL, Jin J (2016a) Discovery of G protein-biased D2 dopamine receptor partial agonists. J Med Chem 59(23):10601–10618

Chen Y, Song M, Riley JP, Hu CC, Peng X, Scheuner D, Bokvist K, Maiti P, Kahl SD, Montrose-Rafizadeh C, Hamdouchi C, Miller AR (2016b) A selective GPR40 (FFAR1) agonist LY2881835 provides immediate and durable glucose control in rodent models of type 2 diabetes. Pharmacol Res Perspect 4(6):e00278

Chen X, Wang L, Cui Q, Ding Z, Han L, Kou Y, Zhang W, Wang H, Jia X, Dai M, Shi Z, Li Y, Li X, Geng Y (2021) Structural insights into the activation of human calcium-sensing receptor. elife 10:e68578

Chun L, Zhang WH, Liu JF (2012) Structure and ligand recognition of class C GPCRs. Acta Pharmacol Sin 33(3):312–323

Chuo CH, Devine SM, Scammells PJ, Krum H, Christopoulos A, May LT, White PJ, Wang BH (2016) VCP746, a novel A1 adenosine receptor biased agonist, reduces hypertrophy in a rat neonatal cardiac myocyte model. Clin Exp Pharmacol Physiol 43(10):976–982

Cong Z, Chen LN, Ma H, Zhou Q, Zou X, Ye C, Dai A, Liu Q, Huang W, Sun X, Wang X, Xu P, Zhao L, Xia T, Zhong W, Yang D, Eric Xu H, Zhang Y, Wang MW (2021) Molecular insights into ago-allosteric modulation of the human glucagon-like peptide-1 receptor. Nat Commun 12(1):3763

Davey AE, Leach K, Valant C, Conigrave AD, Sexton PM, Christopoulos A (2012) Positive and negative allosteric modulators promote biased signaling at the calcium-sensing receptor. Endocrinology 153(3):1232–1241

Dawaliby R, Trubbia C, Delporte C, Masureel M, Van Antwerpen P, Kobilka BK, Govaerts C (2016) Allosteric regulation of G protein-coupled receptor activity by phospholipids. Nat Chem Biol 12(1):35–39

Douros JD, Mokrosinski J, Finan B (2024) The GLP-1R as a model for understanding and exploiting biased agonism in next-generation medicines. J Endocrinol 261(2):e230226

Douros JD, Novikoff A, DuBois B, Rohlfs R, Mokrosinski J, Hogendorf WFJ, Augustin R, Merkestein M, Egaa Martini LB, Linderoth L, Gerrard E, Kodra JT, Norlin J, Roed NK, Oldenburger A, Mowery SA, Waldhoer M, Perez-Tilve D, Finan B, Reedtz-Runge S, Muller TD, Knerr PJ (2025) A GLP-1 analogue optimized for cAMP-biased signaling improves weight loss in obese mice. Mol Metab 102124:102124

Egyed A, Kiss DJ, Keseru GM (2022) The impact of the secondary binding pocket on the pharmacology of class A GPCRs. Front Pharmacol 13:847788

FDA (2025) Drugs@FDA: FDA-Approved Drugs. Retrieved June, 2025, from https://www.accessdata.fda.gov/scripts/cder/daf/index.cfm?event=reportsSearch.process

Ferguson SS, Caron MG (2004) Green fluorescent protein-tagged beta-arrestin translocation as a measure of G protein-coupled receptor activation. Methods Mol Biol 237:121–126

Fossler MJ, Sadler BM, Farrell C, Burt DA, Pitsiu M, Skobieranda F, Soergel DG (2018) Oliceridine, a novel G protein-biased ligand at the mu-opioid receptor, demonstrates a predictable relationship between plasma concentrations and pain relief. II: simulation of potential phase 3 study designs using a pharmacokinetic/Pharmacodynamic model. J Clin Pharmacol 58(6): 762–770

Franco R, Rivas-Santisteban R, Reyes-Resina I, Navarro G (2020) The old and new visions of biased Agonism through the prism of adenosine receptor signaling and receptor/receptor and receptor/protein interactions. Front Pharmacol 11:628601

Gamage TF, Anderson JC, Abood ME (2016) 2 Correction to: CB(1) Allosteric Modulator Org27569 Is an Antagonist/Inverse Agonist of ERK1/2 Signaling. Cannabis Cannabinoid Res 1(1):272–280. https://doi.org/10.1089/can.2016.0028. Cannabis Cannabinoid Res 4(4): 285–286

Gentry PR, Sexton PM, Christopoulos A (2015) Novel allosteric modulators of G protein-coupled receptors. J Biol Chem 290(32):19478–19488

Gereau GB, Zhou D, Van Voorhies K, Tyler RE, Campbell J, Murray JG, Alvarez-Pamir A, Wykoff LA, Companion MA, Jackson MR, Olson SH, Barak LS, Slosky LM, Vetreno RP, Besheer J, McElligott ZA (2024) beta-arrestin-biased Allosteric Modulator of Neurotensin Receptor 1 Reduces Ethanol Drinking and Responses to Ethanol Administration in Rodents. bioRxiv

Gesty-Palmer D, Luttrell LM (2011) 'Biasing' the parathyroid hormone receptor: a novel anabolic approach to increasing bone mass? Br J Pharmacol 164(1):59–67

Gesty-Palmer D, Flannery P, Yuan L, Corsino L, Spurney R, Lefkowitz RJ, Luttrell LM (2009) A beta-arrestin-biased agonist of the parathyroid hormone receptor (PTH1R) promotes bone formation independent of G protein activation. Sci Transl Med 1(1):1ra1

Goupil E, Laporte SA, Hebert TE (2012) Functional selectivity in GPCR signaling: understanding the full spectrum of receptor conformations. Mini Rev Med Chem 12(9):817–830

Gross JD, Zhou Y, Barak LS, Caron MG (2023) Ghrelin receptor signaling in health and disease: a biased view. Trends Endocrinol Metab 34(2):106–118

Guan HP, Xiong Y (2022) Learn from failures and stay hopeful to GPR40, a GPCR target with robust efficacy, for therapy of metabolic disorders. Front Pharmacol 13:1043828

Guo R, Chen O, Zhou Y, Bang S, Chandra S, Li Y, Chen G, Xie RG, He W, Xu J, Zhou R, Song S, Person KL, Moore MN, Alwin AR, Spasojevic I, Jackson MR, Olson SH, Caron MG, Slosky LM, Wetsel WC, Barak LS, Ji RR (2025) Arrestin-biased allosteric modulator of neurotensin receptor 1 alleviates acute and chronic pain. Cell 188:4332

Hamdouchi C, Kahl SD, Patel Lewis A, Cardona GR, Zink RW, Chen K, Eessalu TE, Ficorilli JV, Marcelo MC, Otto KA, Wilbur KL, Lineswala JP, Piper JL, Coffey DS, Sweetana SA, Haas JV, Brooks DA, Pratt EJ, Belin RM, Deeg MA, Ma X, Cannady EA, Johnson JT, Yumibe NP, Chen Q, Maiti P, Montrose-Rafizadeh C, Chen Y, Reifel Miller A (2016) The discovery, preclinical, and early clinical development of potent and selective GPR40 agonists for the treatment of type 2 diabetes mellitus (LY2881835, LY2922083, and LY2922470). J Med Chem 59(24):10891–10916

Hamdouchi C, Maiti P, Warshawsky AM, DeBaillie AC, Otto KA, Wilbur KL, Kahl SD, Patel Lewis A, Cardona GR, Zink RW, Chen K, Cr S, Lineswala JP, Neathery GL, Bouaichi C, Diseroad BA, Campbell AN, Sweetana SA, Adams LA, Cabrera O, Ma X, Yumibe NP, Montrose-Rafizadeh C, Chen Y, Miller AR (2018) Discovery of LY3104607: a potent and selective G protein-coupled receptor 40 (GPR40) agonist with optimized pharmacokinetic properties to support once daily Oral treatment in patients with type 2 diabetes mellitus. J Med Chem 61(3):934–945

Hauge Pedersen M, Pham J, Mancebo H, Inoue A, Asher WB, Javitch JA (2021) A novel luminescence-based beta-arrestin recruitment assay for unmodified receptors. J Biol Chem 296:100503

Hauser AS, Attwood MM, Rask-Andersen M, Schioth HB, Gloriam DE (2017) Trends in GPCR drug discovery: new agents, targets and indications. Nat Rev Drug Discov 16(12):829–842

Howell LL, Cunningham KA (2015) Serotonin 5-HT2 receptor interactions with dopamine function: implications for therapeutics in cocaine use disorder. Pharmacol Rev 67(1):176–197

Huang Z, Zhu L, Cao Y, Wu G, Liu X, Chen Y, Wang Q, Shi T, Zhao Y, Wang Y, Li W, Li Y, Chen H, Chen G, Zhang J (2011) ASD: a comprehensive database of allosteric proteins and modulators. Nucleic Acids Res 39(Database issue):D663–D669

Huang S, Xiao P, Sun J (2020) Structural basis of signaling of cannabinoids receptors: paving a way for rational drug design in controling mutiple neurological and immune diseases. Signal Transduct Target Ther 5(1):127

Ippolito M, De Pascali F, Hopfinger N, Komolov KE, Laurinavichyute D, Reddy PAN, Sakkal LA, Rajkowski KZ, Nayak AP, Lee J, Lee J, Cao G, Donover PS, Reichman M, An SS, Salvino JM, Penn RB, Armen RS, Scott CP, Benovic JL (2023) Identification of a beta-arrestin-biased negative allosteric modulator for the beta(2)-adrenergic receptor. Proc Natl Acad Sci USA 120(31):e2302668120

Jones B (2022) The therapeutic potential of GLP-1 receptor biased agonism. Br J Pharmacol 179(4): 492–510

Jones B, McGlone ER, Fang Z, Pickford P, Correa IR Jr, Oishi A, Jockers R, Inoue A, Kumar S, Gorlitz F, Dunsby C, French PMW, Rutter GA, Tan T, Tomas A, Bloom SR (2021) Genetic and biased agonist-mediated reductions in beta-arrestin recruitment prolong cAMP signaling at glucagon family receptors. J Biol Chem 296:100133

Kahsai AW, Xiao K, Rajagopal S, Ahn S, Shukla AK, Sun J, Oas TG, Lefkowitz RJ (2011) Multiple ligand-specific conformations of the β2-adrenergic receptor. Nat Chem Biol 7(10): 692–700

Kahsai AW, Wisler JW, Lee J, Ahn S, Cahill Iii TJ, Dennison SM, Staus DP, Thomsen AR, Anasti KM, Pani B, Wingler LM, Desai H, Bompiani KM, Strachan RT, Qin X, Alam SM, Sullenger BA, Lefkowitz RJ (2016) Conformationally selective RNA aptamers allosterically modulate the beta2-adrenoceptor. Nat Chem Biol 12(9):709–716

Kahsai AW, Shah KS, Shim PJ, Lee MA, Shreiber BN, Schwalb AM, Zhang X, Kwon HY, Huang LY, Soderblom EJ, Ahn S, Lefkowitz RJ (2023) Signal transduction at GPCRs: allosteric activation of the ERK MAPK by beta-arrestin. Proc Natl Acad Sci USA 120(43):e2303794120

Kamato D, Thach L, Bernard R, Chan V, Zheng W, Kaur H, Brimble M, Osman N, Little PJ (2015) Structure, function, pharmacology, and therapeutic potential of the G protein, Galpha/q,11. Front Cardiovasc Med 2:14

Kaneko S, Imai S, Asao N, Kofuku Y, Ueda T, Shimada I (2022) Activation mechanism of the mu-opioid receptor by an allosteric modulator. Proc Natl Acad Sci USA 119(16):e2121918119

Kashihara T, Kawagishi H, Nakada T, Numaga-Tomita T, Kadota S, Wolf EE, Du CK, Shiba Y, Morimoto S, Yamada M (2020) Beta-Arrestin-biased AT(1) agonist TRV027 causes a neonatal-specific sustained positive inotropic effect without increasing heart rate. JACC Basic Transl Sci 5(11):1057–1069

Katritch V, Fenalti G, Abola EE, Roth BL, Cherezov V, Stevens RC (2014) Allosteric sodium in class a GPCR signaling. Trends Biochem Sci 39(5):233–244

Kelly E, Conibear A, Henderson G (2023) Biased Agonism: lessons from studies of opioid receptor agonists. Annu Rev Pharmacol Toxicol 63:491–515

Kenakin T, Christopoulos A (2013) Signalling bias in new drug discovery: detection, quantification and therapeutic impact. Nat Rev Drug Discov 12(3):205–216

Kenakin T, Miller LJ (2010) Seven transmembrane receptors as shapeshifting proteins: the impact of allosteric modulation and functional selectivity on new drug discovery. Pharmacol Rev 62(2): 265–304

Keov P, Lopez L, Devine SM, Valant C, Lane JR, Scammells PJ, Sexton PM, Christopoulos A (2014) Molecular mechanisms of bitopic ligand engagement with the M1 muscarinic acetylcholine receptor. J Biol Chem 289(34):23817–23837

Khalil J, Dimofte T, Roberts T, Keith M, Amaradasa K, Hindle MS, Bancroft S, Hutchinson JL, Naseem K, Johnson T, Mundell SJ (2024) Ticagrelor inverse agonist activity at the P2Y (12) receptor is non-reversible versus its endogenous agonist adenosine 5 -diphosphate. Br J Pharmacol 181(1):21–35

Khoury E, Clement S, Laporte SA (2014) Allosteric and biased g protein-coupled receptor signaling regulation: potentials for new therapeutics. Front Endocrinol (Lausanne) 5:68

Kim KS, Abraham D, Williams B, Violin JD, Mao L, Rockman HA (2012) Beta-Arrestin-biased AT1R stimulation promotes cell survival during acute cardiac injury. Am J Physiol Heart Circ Physiol 303(8):H1001–H1010

Kim J, Grotegut CA, Wisler JW, Mao L, Rosenberg PB, Rockman HA, Lefkowitz RJ (2020) The beta-arrestin-biased beta-adrenergic receptor blocker carvedilol enhances skeletal muscle contractility. Proc Natl Acad Sci USA 117(22):12435–12443

Kise R, Inoue A (2024) GPCR signaling bias: an emerging framework for opioid drug development. J Biochem 175(4):367–376

Kobayashi K, Kawakami K, Kusakizako T, Tomita A, Nishimura M, Sawada K, Okamoto HH, Hiratsuka S, Nakamura G, Kuwabara R, Noda H, Muramatsu H, Shimizu M, Taguchi T, Inoue A, Murata T, Nureki O (2023) Class B1 GPCR activation by an intracellular agonist. Nature 618(7967):1085–1093

Kobilka BK, Deupi X (2007) Conformational complexity of G-protein-coupled receptors. Trends Pharmacol Sci 28(8):397–406

Kolb P, Kenakin T, Alexander SPH, Bermudez M, Bohn LM, Breinholt CS, Bouvier M, Hill SJ, Kostenis E, Martemyanov KA, Neubig RR, Onaran HO, Rajagopal S, Roth BL, Selent J, Shukla AK, Sommer ME, Gloriam DE (2022) Community guidelines for GPCR ligand bias: IUPHAR review 32. Br J Pharmacol 179(14):3651–3674

Kooistra AJ, Mordalski S, Pandy-Szekeres G, Esguerra M, Mamyrbekov A, Munk C, Keseru GM, Gloriam DE (2021) GPCRdb in 2021: integrating GPCR sequence, structure and function. Nucleic Acids Res 49(D1):D335–D343

Kovacs JJ, Hara MR, Davenport CL, Kim J, Lefkowitz RJ (2009) Arrestin development: emerging roles for beta-arrestins in developmental signaling pathways. Dev Cell 17(4):443–458

Lambert D, Calo G (2020) Approval of oliceridine (TRV130) for intravenous use in moderate to severe pain in adults. Br J Anaesth 125(6):e473–e474

Laprairie RB, Bagher AM, Denovan-Wright EM (2017) Cannabinoid receptor ligand bias: implications in the central nervous system. Curr Opin Pharmacol 32:32–43

Leach K, Wen A, Cook AE, Sexton PM, Conigrave AD, Christopoulos A (2013) Impact of clinically relevant mutations on the pharmacoregulation and signaling bias of the calcium-sensing receptor by positive and negative allosteric modulators. Endocrinology 154(3): 1105–1116

Leach K, Sexton PM, Christopoulos A, Conigrave AD (2014) Engendering biased signalling from the calcium-sensing receptor for the pharmacotherapy of diverse disorders. Br J Pharmacol 171(5):1142–1155

Leach K, Conigrave AD, Sexton PM, Christopoulos A (2015) Towards tissue-specific pharmacology: insights from the calcium-sensing receptor as a paradigm for GPCR (patho)physiological bias. Trends Pharmacol Sci 36(4):215–225

Lefkowitz RJ (2013a) Arrestins come of age: a personal historical perspective. Prog Mol Biol Transl Sci 118:3–18

Lefkowitz RJ (2013b) A brief history of G-protein coupled receptors (Nobel lecture). Angew Chem Int Ed Engl 52(25):6366–6378

Lefkowitz RJ, Shenoy SK (2005) Transduction of receptor signals by beta-arrestins. Science 308(5721):512–517

Lerch MT, Matt RA, Masureel M, Elgeti M, Kumar KK, Hilger D, Foys B, Kobilka BK, Hubbell WL (2020) Viewing rare conformations of the beta(2) adrenergic receptor with pressure-resolved DEER spectroscopy. Proc Natl Acad Sci USA 117(50):31824–31831

Li S, Lee SY, Chung KY (2015) Conformational analysis of g protein-coupled receptor signaling by hydrogen/deuterium exchange mass spectrometry. Methods Enzymol 557:261–278

Ling S, Shi P, Liu S, Meng X, Zhou Y, Sun W, Chang S, Zhang X, Zhang L, Shi C, Sun D, Liu L, Tian C (2021) Structural mechanism of cooperative activation of the human calcium-sensing receptor by Ca(2+) ions and L-tryptophan. Cell Res 31(4):383–394

Liu X, Ahn S, Kahsai AW, Meng KC, Latorraca NR, Pani B, Venkatakrishnan AJ, Masoudi A, Weis WI, Dror RO, Chen X, Lefkowitz RJ, Kobilka BK (2017) Mechanism of intracellular allosteric beta(2)AR antagonist revealed by X-ray crystal structure. Nature 548(7668):480–484

Liu H, Kim HR, Deepak R, Wang L, Chung KY, Fan H, Wei Z, Zhang C (2018) Orthosteric and allosteric action of the C5a receptor antagonists. Nat Struct Mol Biol 25(6):472–481

Liu X, Masoudi A, Kahsai AW, Huang LY, Pani B, Staus DP, Shim PJ, Hirata K, Simhal RK, Schwalb AM, Rambarat PK, Ahn S, Lefkowitz RJ, Kobilka B (2019) Mechanism of beta(2)AR regulation by an intracellular positive allosteric modulator. Science 364(6447):1283–1287

Liu X, Kaindl J, Korczynska M, Stossel A, Dengler D, Stanek M, Hubner H, Clark MJ, Mahoney J, Matt RA, Xu X, Hirata K, Shoichet BK, Sunahara RK, Kobilka BK, Gmeiner P (2020) An allosteric modulator binds to a conformational hub in the beta(2) adrenergic receptor. Nat Chem Biol 16(7):749–755

Lohse MJ, Benovic JL, Codina J, Caron MG, Lefkowitz RJ (1990) Beta-Arrestin: a protein that regulates beta-adrenergic receptor function. Science 248(4962):1547–1550

Lorente JS, Sokolov AV, Ferguson G, Schioth HB, Hauser AS, Gloriam DE (2025) GPCR drug discovery: new agents, targets and indications. Nat Rev Drug Discov 24:458

Mallipeddi S, Janero DR, Zvonok N, Makriyannis A (2017) Functional selectivity at G-protein coupled receptors: advancing cannabinoid receptors as drug targets. Biochem Pharmacol 128:1–11

Mancini AD, Bertrand G, Vivot K, Carpentier E, Tremblay C, Ghislain J, Bouvier M, Poitout V (2015) Beta-Arrestin recruitment and biased Agonism at free fatty acid receptor 1. J Biol Chem 290(34):21131–21140

Manglik A, Kim TH, Masureel M, Altenbach C, Yang Z, Hilger D, Lerch MT, Kobilka TS, Thian FS, Hubbell WL, Prosser RS, Kobilka BK (2015) Structural insights into the dynamic process of beta2-adrenergic receptor signaling. Cell 161(5):1101–1111

Manglik A, Lin H, Aryal DK, McCorvy JD, Dengler D, Corder G, Levit A, Kling RC, Bernat V, Hubner H, Huang XP, Sassano MF, Giguere PM, Lober S, Da D, Scherrer G, Kobilka BK, Gmeiner P, Roth BL, Shoichet BK (2016) Structure-based discovery of opioid analgesics with reduced side effects. Nature 537(7619):185–190

Manglik A, Wingler LM, Rockman HA, Lefkowitz RJ (2020) Beta-Arrestin-biased angiotensin II receptor agonists for COVID-19. Circulation 142(4):318–320

Marti-Solano M, Iglesias A, de Fabritiis G, Sanz F, Brea J, Loza MI, Pastor M, Selent J (2015) Detection of new biased agonists for the serotonin 5-HT2A receptor: modeling and experimental validation. Mol Pharmacol 87(4):740–746

McNeill SM, Baltos JA, White PJ, May LT (2021) Biased agonism at adenosine receptors. Cell Signal 82:109954

Meng X, Qin L, Wang X (2025) Biased agonism of G protein-coupled receptors as a novel strategy for osteoarthritis therapy. Bone Res 13(1):52

Milligan G (2003) Principles: extending the utility of [35S]GTP gamma S binding assays. Trends Pharmacol Sci 24(2):87–90

Milligan AL, Szabo-Pardi TA, Burton MD (2020) Cannabinoid receptor type 1 and its role as an analgesic: An opioid alternative? J Dual Diagn 16(1):106–119

Monasky MM, Taglieri DM, Henze M, Warren CM, Utter MS, Soergel DG, Violin JD, Solaro RJ (2013) The beta-arrestin-biased ligand TRV120023 inhibits angiotensin II-induced cardiac hypertrophy while preserving enhanced myofilament response to calcium. Am J Physiol Heart Circ Physiol 305(6):H856–H866

Nagano N, Tsutsui T (2016) Pharmacological characteristics of drugs targeted on calcium-sensing receptor.-properties of cinacalcet hydrochloride as allosteric modulator. Clin Calcium 26(6): 839–850

Noma T, Lemaire A, Naga Prasad SV, Barki-Harrington L, Tilley DG, Chen J, Le Corvoisier P, Violin JD, Wei H, Lefkowitz RJ, Rockman HA (2007) Beta-arrestin-mediated beta1-adrenergic receptor transactivation of the EGFR confers cardioprotection. J Clin Invest 117(9):2445–2458

Noor N, Patel CB, Rockman HA (2011) Beta-arrestin: a signaling molecule and potential therapeutic target for heart failure. J Mol Cell Cardiol 51(4):534–541

Park SM, Chen M, Schmerberg CM, Dulman RS, Rodriguiz RM, Caron MG, Jin J, Wetsel WC (2016) Effects of beta-Arrestin-biased dopamine D2 receptor ligands on schizophrenia-like behavior in Hypoglutamatergic mice. Neuropsychopharmacology 41(3):704–715

Patel CB, Noor N, Rockman HA (2010) Functional selectivity in adrenergic and angiotensin signaling systems. Mol Pharmacol 78(6):983–992

Peddibhotla S, Hedrick MP, Hershberger P, Maloney PR, Li Y, Milewski M, Gosalia P, Gray W, Mehta A, Sugarman E, Hood B, Suyama E, Nguyen K, Heynen-Genel S, Vasile S, Salaniwal S, Stonich D, Su Y, Mangravita-Novo A, Vicchiarelli M, Roth GP, Smith LH, Chung TD, Hanson GR, Thomas JB, Caron MG, Barak LS, Pinkerton AB (2013) Discovery of ML314, a brain penetrant non-Peptidic beta-Arrestin biased agonist of the Neurotensin NTR1 receptor. ACS Med Chem Lett 4(9):846–851

Perry-Hauser NA, Asher WB, Hauge Pedersen M, Javitch JA (2021) Assays for detecting arrestin interaction with GPCRs. Methods Cell Biol 166:43–65

Persechino M, Hedderich JB, Kolb P, Hilger D (2022) Allosteric modulation of GPCRs: from structural insights to in silico drug discovery. Pharmacol Ther 237:108242

Peterson YK, Luttrell LM (2017) The diverse roles of Arrestin scaffolds in G protein-coupled receptor signaling. Pharmacol Rev 69(3):256–297

Pierce KL, Premont RT, Lefkowitz RJ (2002) Seven-transmembrane receptors. Nat Rev Mol Cell Biol 3(9):639–650

Pinkerton AB, Peddibhotla S, Yamamoto F, Slosky LM, Bai Y, Maloney P, Hershberger P, Hedrick MP, Falter B, Ardecky RJ, Smith LH, Chung TDY, Jackson MR, Caron MG, Barak LS (2019) Discovery of beta-Arrestin biased, orally bioavailable, and CNS penetrant Neurotensin receptor 1 (NTR1) allosteric modulators. J Med Chem 62(17):8357–8363

Pioszak AA, Hay DL (2020) RAMPs as allosteric modulators of the calcitonin and calcitonin-like class B G protein-coupled receptors. Adv Pharmacol 88:115–141

Rajagopal S, Rajagopal K, Lefkowitz RJ (2010) Teaching old receptors new tricks: biasing seven-transmembrane receptors. Nat Rev Drug Discov 9(5):373–386

Rasmussen SG, DeVree BT, Zou Y, Kruse AC, Chung KY, Kobilka TS, Thian FS, Chae PS, Pardon E, Calinski D, Mathiesen JM, Shah ST, Lyons JA, Caffrey M, Gellman SH, Steyaert J,

Skiniotis G, Weis WI, Sunahara RK, Kobilka BK (2011) Crystal structure of the beta2 adrenergic receptor-Gs protein complex. Nature 477(7366):549–555

Ray N (2009) Maraviroc in the treatment of HIV infection. Drug Des Devel Ther 2:151–161

Reiter E, Lefkowitz RJ (2006) GRKs and beta-arrestins: roles in receptor silencing, trafficking and signaling. Trends Endocrinol Metab 17(4):159–165

Schmidhammer H, Erli F, Guerrieri E, Spetea M (2020) Development of Diphenethylamines as selective kappa opioid receptor ligands and their pharmacological activities. Molecules 25(21): 5092

Scicluna RL, Everett NA, Badolato CJ, Wilson BB, Bowen MT (2024a) Correction to: effects of CB1 receptor negative allosteric modulator Org27569 on oxycodone withdrawal symptoms in mice. Psychopharmacology 241(8):1719

Scicluna RL, Everett NA, Badolato CJ, Wilson BB, Bowen MT (2024b) Effects of CB1 receptor negative allosteric modulator Org27569 on oxycodone withdrawal symptoms in mice. Psychopharmacology 241(8):1705–1717

Shen S, Zhao C, Wu C, Sun S, Li Z, Yan W, Shao Z (2023) Allosteric modulation of G protein-coupled receptor signaling. Front Endocrinol 14:1137604

Shen S, Wu C, Lin G, Yang X, Zhou Y, Zhao C, Miao Z, Tian X, Wang K, Yang Z, Liu Z, Guo N, Li Y, Xia A, Zhou P, Liu J, Yan W, Ke B, Yang S, Shao Z (2024) Structure-based identification of a G protein-biased allosteric modulator of cannabinoid receptor CB1. Proc Natl Acad Sci USA 121(24):e2321532121

Singhal SM, Zell V, Faget L, Slosky LM, Barak LS, Caron MG, Pinkerton AB, Hnasko TS (2023) Neurotensin receptor 1-biased ligand attenuates neurotensin-mediated excitation of ventral tegmental area dopamine neurons and dopamine release in the nucleus accumbens. Neuropharmacology 234:109544

Slosky LM, Bai Y, Toth K, Ray C, Rochelle LK, Badea A, Chandrasekhar R, Pogorelov VM, Abraham DM, Atluri N, Peddibhotla S, Hedrick MP, Hershberger P, Maloney P, Yuan H, Li Z, Wetsel WC, Pinkerton AB, Barak LS, Caron MG (2020) Beta-arrestin-biased allosteric modulator of NTSR1 selectively attenuates addictive behaviors. Cell 181(6):1364–1379 e1314

Slosky LM, Caron MG, Barak LS (2021) Biased allosteric modulators: new Frontiers in GPCR drug discovery. Trends Pharmacol Sci 42(4):283–299

Smith JS, Lefkowitz RJ, Rajagopal S (2018) Biased signalling: from simple switches to allosteric microprocessors. Nat Rev Drug Discov 17(4):243–260

Soergel DG, Subach RA, Cowan CL, Violin JD, Lark MW (2013) First clinical experience with TRV027: pharmacokinetics and pharmacodynamics in healthy volunteers. J Clin Pharmacol 53(9):892–899

Staus DP, Strachan RT, Manglik A, Pani B, Kahsai AW, Kim TH, Wingler LM, Ahn S, Chatterjee A, Masoudi A, Kruse AC, Pardon E, Steyaert J, Weis WI, Prosser RS, Kobilka BK, Costa T, Lefkowitz RJ (2016) Allosteric nanobodies reveal the dynamic range and diverse mechanisms of G-protein-coupled receptor activation. Nature 535(7612):448–452

Sun D, Gao W, Hu H, Zhou S (2022) Why 90% of clinical drug development fails and how to improve it? Acta Pharm Sin B 12(7):3049–3062

Sun D, Li X, Yuan Q, Wang Y, Shi P, Zhang H, Wang T, Sun W, Ling S, Liu Y, Lai J, Xie W, Yin W, Liu L, Xu HE, Tian C (2025) Molecular mechanism of the arrestin-biased agonism of neurotensin receptor 1 by an intracellular allosteric modulator. Cell Res 35(4):284–295

Tamura T, Noda H, Joyashiki E, Hoshino M, Watanabe T, Kinosaki M, Nishimura Y, Esaki T, Ogawa K, Miyake T, Arai S, Shimizu M, Kitamura H, Sato H, Kawabe Y (2016) Identification of an orally active small-molecule PTHR1 agonist for the treatment of hypoparathyroidism. Nat Commun 7:13384

Thal DM, Glukhova A, Sexton PM, Christopoulos A (2018) Structural insights into G-protein-coupled receptor allostery. Nature 559(7712):45–53

Torphy TJ (1994) Beta-adrenoceptors, cAMP and airway smooth muscle relaxation: challenges to the dogma. Trends Pharmacol Sci 15(10):370–374

Tuntland T, Ethell B, Kosaka T, Blasco F, Zang RX, Jain M, Gould T, Hoffmaster K (2014) Implementation of pharmacokinetic and pharmacodynamic strategies in early research phases of drug discovery and development at Novartis Institute of Biomedical Research. Front Pharmacol 5:174

Urs NM, Bido S, Peterson SM, Daigle TL, Bass CE, Gainetdinov RR, Bezard E, Caron MG (2015) Targeting beta-arrestin2 in the treatment of L-DOPA-induced dyskinesia in Parkinson's disease. Proc Natl Acad Sci USA 112(19):E2517–E2526

Urs NM, Peterson SM, Caron MG (2017) New concepts in dopamine D(2) receptor biased signaling and implications for schizophrenia therapy. Biol Psychiatry 81(1):78–85

Valant C, May LT, Aurelio L, Chuo CH, White PJ, Baltos JA, Sexton PM, Scammells PJ, Christopoulos A (2014) Separation of on-target efficacy from adverse effects through rational design of a bitopic adenosine receptor agonist. Proc Natl Acad Sci USA 111(12):4614–4619

Vasudevan NT (2017) cAMP assays in GPCR drug discovery. Methods Cell Biol 142:51–57

Violin JD, Crombie AL, Soergel DG, Lark MW (2014) Biased ligands at G-protein-coupled receptors: promise and progress. Trends Pharmacol Sci 35(7):308–316

Walker JK, DeFea KA (2014) Role for beta-arrestin in mediating paradoxical beta2AR and PAR2 signaling in asthma. Curr Opin Pharmacol 16:142–147

Walker JK, Fong AM, Lawson BL, Savov JD, Patel DD, Schwartz DA, Lefkowitz RJ (2003) Beta-arrestin-2 regulates the development of allergic asthma. J Clin Invest 112(4):566–574

Walker JK, Penn RB, Hanania NA, Dickey BF, Bond RA (2011) New perspectives regarding beta (2) -adrenoceptor ligands in the treatment of asthma. Br J Pharmacol 163(1):18–28

Wall MJ, Hill E, Huckstepp R, Barkan K, Deganutti G, Leuenberger M, Preti B, Winfield I, Carvalho S, Suchankova A, Wei H, Safitri D, Huang X, Imlach W, La Mache C, Dean E, Hume C, Hayward S, Oliver J, Zhao FY, Spanswick D, Reynolds CA, Lochner M, Ladds G, Frenguelli BG (2022) Selective activation of Galphaob by an adenosine a(1) receptor agonist elicits analgesia without cardiorespiratory depression. Nat Commun 13(1):4150

Wang J, Gareri C, Rockman HA (2018) G-protein-coupled receptors in heart disease. Circ Res 123(6):716–735

Wang J, Pani B, Gokhan I, Xiong X, Kahsai AW, Jiang H, Ahn S, Lefkowitz RJ, Rockman HA (2021) Beta-Arrestin-biased allosteric modulator potentiates carvedilol-stimulated beta adrenergic receptor Cardioprotection. Mol Pharmacol 100(6):568–579

Whalen EJ, Rajagopal S, Lefkowitz RJ (2011) Therapeutic potential of beta-arrestin- and G protein-biased agonists. Trends Mol Med 17(3):126–139

Wingler LM, Lefkowitz RJ (2020) Conformational basis of G protein-coupled receptor signaling versatility. Trends Cell Biol 30(9):736–747

Wingler LM, Elgeti M, Hilger D, Latorraca NR, Lerch MT, Staus DP, Dror RO, Kobilka BK, Hubbell WL, Lefkowitz RJ (2019) Angiotensin analogs with divergent bias stabilize distinct receptor conformations. Cell 176(3):468–478 e411

Wisler JW, Rockman HA, Lefkowitz RJ (2018) Biased G protein-coupled receptor signaling: changing the paradigm of drug discovery. Circulation 137(22):2315–2317

Wold EA, Zhou J (2018) GPCR allosteric modulators: mechanistic advantages and therapeutic applications. Curr Top Med Chem 18(23):2002–2006

Wootten D, Christopoulos A, Sexton PM (2013) Emerging paradigms in GPCR allostery: implications for drug discovery. Nat Rev Drug Discov 12(8):630–644

Wootten D, Reynolds CA, Smith KJ, Mobarec JC, Koole C, Savage EE, Pabreja K, Simms J, Sridhar R, Furness SGB, Liu M, Thompson PE, Miller LJ, Christopoulos A, Sexton PM (2016) The extracellular surface of the GLP-1 receptor is a molecular trigger for biased Agonism. Cell 165(7):1632–1643

Wootten D, Miller LJ, Koole C, Christopoulos A, Sexton PM (2017) Allostery and biased Agonism at class B G protein-coupled receptors. Chem Rev 117(1):111–138

Woszczek G, Fuerst E, Maguire TJA (2021) FLIPR calcium mobilization assays in GPCR drug discovery. Methods Mol Biol 2268:193–205

Yasi EA, Kruyer NS, Peralta-Yahya P (2020) Advances in G protein-coupled receptor high-throughput screening. Curr Opin Biotechnol 64:210–217

Zarzycka B, Zaidi SA, Roth BL, Katritch V (2019) Harnessing ion-binding sites for GPCR pharmacology. Pharmacol Rev 71(4):571–595

Zhang G, Stackman RW Jr (2015) The role of serotonin 5-HT2A receptors in memory and cognition. Front Pharmacol 6:225

Zhang R, Xie X (2012) Tools for GPCR drug discovery. Acta Pharmacol Sin 33(3):372–384

Zhang H, Sturchler E, Zhu J, Nieto A, Cistrone PA, Xie J, He L, Yea K, Jones T, Turn R, Di Stefano PS, Griffin PR, Dawson PE, McDonald PH, Lerner RA (2015) Autocrine selection of a GLP-1R G-protein biased agonist with potent antidiabetic effects. Nat Commun 6:8918

Zhao LH, He Q, Yuan Q, Gu Y, He X, Shan H, Li J, Wang K, Li Y, Hu W, Wu K, Shen J, Xu HE (2023) Conserved class B GPCR activation by a biased intracellular agonist. Nature 621(7979): 635–641

Zhu D, Wang W, Tong G, Ma G, Ma J, Han J, Zhang X, Liu Y, Gan S, Qin H, Zheng Q, Ning J, Zhu Z, Guo M, Bu Y, Li Y, Jones CL, Fenaux M, Junaidi MK, Xu S, Pan H (2024) Efficacy and safety of GLP-1 analog ecnoglutide in adults with type 2 diabetes: a randomized, double-blind, placebo-controlled phase 2 trial. Nat Commun 15(1):8408

Zhuang Y, Xu P, Mao C, Wang L, Krumm B, Zhou XE, Huang S, Liu H, Cheng X, Huang XP, Shen DD, Xu T, Liu YF, Wang Y, Guo J, Jiang Y, Jiang H, Melcher K, Roth BL, Zhang Y, Zhang C, Xu HE (2021) Structural insights into the human D1 and D2 dopamine receptor signaling complexes. Cell 184(4):931–942 e918

Structure-Bias Relationship of μ-Opioid Receptor Agonists

Guodong He and Xiangyu Liu

Contents

Abstract

The μ-opioid receptor (μOR) is the primary drug target of opioid analgesics such as morphine and fentanyl. Activation of μORs in the central nervous system inhibits ascending pain signaling to the cortex, thereby producing analgesic effects. However, the clinical use of opioid analgesics is severely limited by adverse side effects, including respiratory depression, constipation, addiction, and the development of tolerance. μOR-mediated signaling involves both the $G_{i/o/z}$ protein pathway and the β-arrestin1/2 pathway. Recent research has indicated that G protein-biased agonists, which preferentially activate the $G_{i/o/z}$ pathway over the β-arrestin1/2 pathway, may provide effective analgesia with reduced side effects, thus offering improved therapeutic potential. In this chapter, we review the molecular basis of μOR-biased agonism. By integrating findings from structural and dynamic studies, we summarize the structure–bias relationships of various μOR agonists, aiming to provide valuable insights for the development of next-generation μOR-biased agonists.

G. He · X. Liu (✉)
Tsinghua University, Beijing, China
e-mail: liu_xy@mail.tsinghua.edu.cn

© The Author(s), under exclusive license to Springer Nature Switzerland AG 2025

Z. Li, K. Xiao (eds.), *Pharmacology of GPCRs Biased Signaling and Agonists*,
Handbook of Experimental Pharmacology 290, https://doi.org/10.1007/164_2025_772

Keywords

Biased signaling · Cryo-EM · Drug development · G Protein-Coupled Receptors (GPCRs) · GPCR dynamics · Opioid analgesics · μ-opioid receptors (μORs)

The μ-opioid receptor (μOR) is widely recognized as a paramount drug target for the development of central nervous system analgesics. To date, approximately 40 different drugs that target the μOR have been approved by FDA for analgesic or other related clinical applications. These drugs include the well-known substances such as morphine, tramadol, sufentanil, and buprenorphine. However, the clinical use of these analgesics is subject to strict supervision due to the significant risks associated with opioid medications, which can cause severe side effects like respiratory depression, constipation, sedation, dizziness, nausea, and vomiting. Additionally, these drugs can lead to the development of tolerance and addiction, thereby escalating the risk of opioid misuse and overdose (Walsh 1990).

The μOR belongs to Family A GPCRs (G protein-coupled receptors). Activation of μOR triggers the G protein signaling pathway, resulting in cellular cAMP inhibition, GIRK channel (G protein-coupled inwardly-rectifying potassium channel) activation, and VGCC (Voltage-gated calcium channel) inhibition (Weiss and Zamponi 2021). In addition to the G protein-dependent signaling pathway, activated μOR can also be phosphorylated by GRK (G protein-coupled receptor kinase), which in turn recruits β-arrestin1/2 to induce receptor endocytosis, a process that is part of the G protein-independent signaling pathway (Kelly et al. 2008; Williams et al. 2013).

Previous studies on the μOR signaling have revealed that the analgesic effect is primarily mediated by the G protein signaling pathway, while drug tolerance and overdose are largely attributed to β-arrestin-induced receptor endocytosis (Bohn et al. 2000; Corder et al. 2018). However, the detailed mechanisms of other side effects of opioid analgesics, such as respiratory depression, constipation, and sedation, remain subjects of ongoing debate. Previous gene knockout (KO) studies suggested that β-arrestin 2 KO could significantly reduce respiratory depression induced by morphine (Raehal et al. 2005). However, recent research has cast doubt on this conclusion, as β-arrestin 2 KO mice showed similar respiratory depression as the wild-type (WT) mice after morphine treatment (Bachmutsky et al. 2021). Even though the mechanisms underlying these lethal side effects remain unclear, decoupling the β-arrestin signaling pathway from the G protein signaling pathway of the μOR still holds significant promise for reducing the risk of opioid overdose and, consequently, enhancing the safety of drug usage. Based on this theory, G protein-biased agonists, which preferentially activate the μOR G protein signaling pathway over the β-arrestin signaling pathway, are believed to have better therapeutic value. TRV130, also known as Oliceridine, is the first μOR-biased agonist approved by FDA in 2020 for pain management (Chen et al. 2013). To date, various types of biased agonists targeting the μOR have been developed through medicinal chemistry modification (TRV130 (Chen et al. 2013), SR-17018

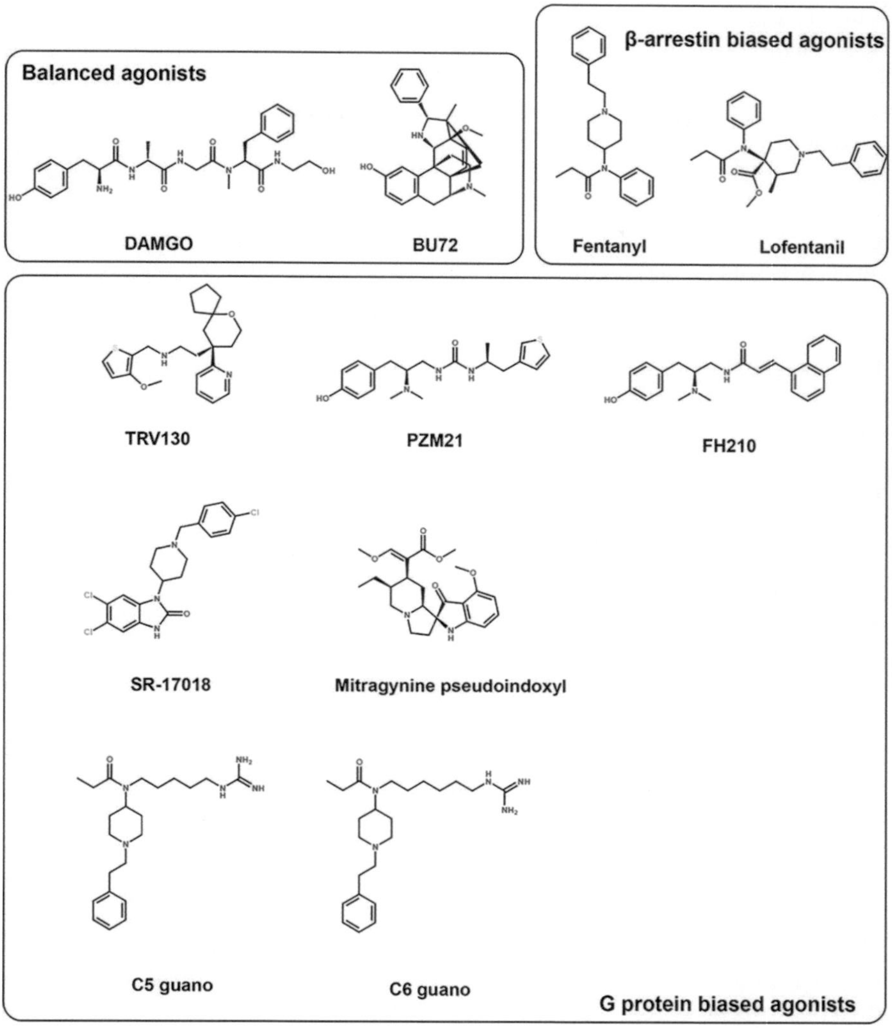

Fig. 1 Gallery of different opioid agonists

(Schmid et al. 2017), C5 guano and C6 guano (Faouzi et al. 2022)), high-throughput virtual screening and optimization (PZM21 (Manglik et al. 2016) and FH210 (Gmeiner et al. 2022)), and natural product optimization (mitragynine pseudoindoxyl (Kruegel et al. 2019)) (Fig. 1). However, the detailed structural mechanisms by which these compounds bind to the same pocket of μOR yet exhibit distinct signaling profiles remain elusive. This gap in understanding significantly hampers the development of biased agonists for GPCRs. With advancements in cryo-electron microscopy (cryo-EM), the complex structures of μOR-G_i with various balanced and biased agonists have been elucidated. These studies seek to unravel the structural mechanisms underlying μOR-biased agonism, with the hope that this detailed structural information will guide the development of novel-biased drugs. Additionally, given that GPCRs perform their physiological functions through a series of dynamic conformational changes (Deupi and Kobilka 2010; Hilger 2021), which cannot be fully captured by structural determination alone, molecular dynamics simulations (MD simulations) and spectroscopy methods such as nuclear magnetic resonance (NMR) are employed to explore the intrinsic dynamic behaviors of the μOR and its association with biased agonism. Collectively, these studies aid researchers in understanding the distinct conformational changes elicited by biased versus balanced agonists of μOR. They aim to elucidate the structure-bias relationship, demonstrating how different chemical structures of compounds ultimately lead to either balanced or biased downstream signaling. This knowledge helps inspire the development of more biased agonists for GPCRs, considering the potential to reduce on-target side effects and achieve a broader therapeutic window.

1 Structural Determination of μOR with Balanced and Biased Agonists

Structure information of the μOR in complex with its ligands and transducers provides a snapshot of the binding state, aiding researchers in understanding crucial interactions and conformational changes. The first structure of μOR was determined using X-ray crystallography in 2012 by Ashish Manglik et al. (2012). This structure revealed how the covalent morphinan antagonist β-FNA binds to the orthosteric pocket of the receptor. This binding mode is conserved among all μOR ligands and includes the formation of a salt bridge with $D^{3.32}$ (superscript refers to the Ballesteros-Weinstein numbering (Ballesteros and Weinstein 1995)), a water-mediated hydrogen bond with $H^{6.52}$ and some hydrophobic interactions. To understand the receptor activation mechanism, Weijiao Huang et al. reported the first high-resolution crystal structure of active μOR bound to the high-affinity agonist BU72 and a nanobody in 2015 (Huang et al. 2015). Additionally, Antoine Koehl et al. solved the first cryo-EM structure of the μOR-G_i complex with DAMGO in 2018 (Koehl et al. 2018). These structures indicated that μOR bound to G protein in a conserved manner as other Family A GPCRs, such as β_2AR-G_s (Rasmussen et al. 2011), with its TM6 undergoing an outward movement to facilitate G protein binding, while the orthosteric pocket of the receptor slightly shrinks.

The resolution revolution of Cryo-EM has facilitated the structure determination of GPCR-G protein complexes with various ligands, especially for biased agonists, whose efficacy is often limited (Fig. 2). In 2022, the first complex structure of μOR with a biased agonist, PZM21, was reported (Gmeiner et al. 2022). Compared to other reported active structures of μOR, PZM21 binds to the receptor's orthosteric pocket in a similar manner, including the polar interaction network with $D^{3.32}$-$Y^{7.43}$, the conserved water-mediated hydrogen bond with $H^{6.52}$ and $K^{5.39}$ (as confirmed by MD simulations), and several hydrophobic contacts. High-resolution structure is also available for μOR-G_i in complex with FH210, a derivative of PZM21 that shows even lower β-arrestin recruitment ability than PZM21. Structure analysis

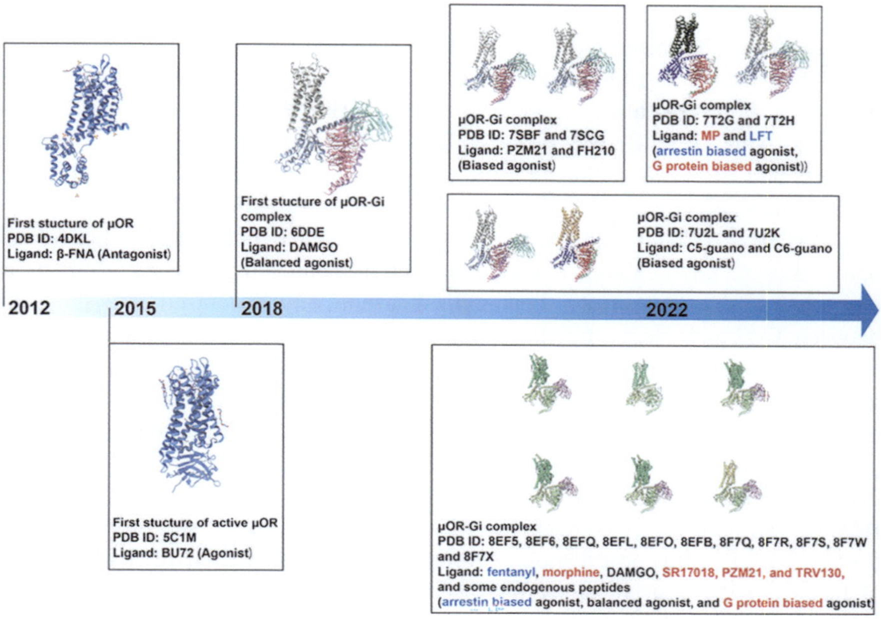

Fig. 2 Structure gallery of μOR with different ligands

revealed that, compared to PZM21, FH210 forms stronger hydrophobic contacts with TM2, TM3, ECL2, and ECL3 through a naphthyl substitution. These additional interactions may contribute to decreased β-arrestin recruitment ability (Gmeiner et al. 2022).

In addition to PZM21 and its derivatives, which were identified through in-silico docking and optimization (Manglik et al. 2016; Gmeiner et al. 2022), Mitragynine pseudoindoxyl (MP), reported by Kruegel, A. C. et al., was optimized from mitragynine, the primary alkaloid found in the kratom plant (Kruegel et al. 2019). MP has a unique chemical scaffold compared to other opioid ligands and exhibits minimal β-arrestin recruitment ability (undetectable in BRET assay and slightly different from mock in NanoBiT assay). Qianhui Qu et al. reported the complex structures of μOR-G_i-MP and μOR-G_i-lofentanil (LFT) (Qu et al. 2022) to investigate the structural differences between a G protein-biased agonist and a β-arrestin-biased agonist, and to understand how these differences result in distinct signaling behaviors of the two ligands. The structural information revealed that, although MP and LFT bind to the same pocket in μOR, their interaction modes are significantly different. Unlike FH210, which was discussed earlier, the β-arrestin-biased agonist LFT also shows stronger hydrophobic contacts with the extracellular vestibule surrounded by TM2, TM3, and ECL1–2 compared to MP. This difference may be associated with the enhanced β-arrestin recruitment ability for LFT. In contrast, MP occupies a new sub-pocket surrounded by TM1, TM2, and TM7, suggesting that MP can directly influence the conformation of TM7 in a specific way, which may result in its decreased β-arrestin recruitment (Qu et al. 2022).

To understand how μOR recognizes ligands with different scaffolds and signaling behaviors, Youwen Zhuang et al. also reported a series structures of μOR-Gi in complex with six different ligands: DAMGO, morphine, fentanyl, TRV130, PZM21, and SR-17018 (Zhuang et al. 2022). Morphine, which has the elliptical morphinan scaffold, occupies a limited space in the orthosteric pocket and primarily binds to the receptor through TM3 and TM5. Compared to morphine, the more lethal opioid drug fentanyl exhibits a unique interaction mode with the receptor due to its elongated Y-shaped scaffold. Fentanyl's benzene ring can insert into the cleft between TM2 and TM3, while the propionyl group and the n-aniline ring maintain common contacts with TM6 and TM7. These interactions were confirmed by mutagenesis studies and may provide clues to fentanyl's enhanced β-arrestin recruitment levels. Further comparison of all these structures confirmed the relationship between β-arrestin recruitment levels and ligands' interaction with TM6/7. Compared to fentanyl and DAMGO, the three biased agonists—SR-17018, TRV130, and PZM21—showed fewer contacts with TM6 and TM7 in the orthosteric binding pocket. Based on this observation, Youwen Zhuang et al. designed two derivatives of fentanyl with reduced interactions with TM6/7. These new compounds indeed exhibited less β-arrestin recruitment levels. Since MP, as mentioned earlier, also shows strong contact with TM7 (Qu et al. 2022), the structure-bias relationship may vary among ligands with different chemotypes.

Allosteric modulation represents a novel approach to modulate the receptor's function and signaling profile (Jeffrey Conn et al. 2009; Wold et al. 2019). The sodium ion is a conserved negative allosteric modulator for Family A GPCRs, favoring the receptor's inactive state and potentially biasing the receptor's signaling toward either G protein signaling or β-arrestin signaling (Pert et al. 1973; Shang et al. 2014). Abdelfattah Faouzi et al. designed a series of bitopic ligands for μOR, targeting both the orthosteric binding pocket and the sodium pocket, based on the scaffold of fentanyl (Faouzi et al. 2022). They validated two bitopic agonists, C5 guano and C6 guano, which exhibited G protein-biased signaling and promising therapeutic value in mice. For these two bitopic agonists, the fentanyl moiety occupied the orthosteric pocket of μOR, while the positively charged guano group was directed toward the sodium pocket ($D^{2.50}$) and connected to the fentanyl moiety via an aliphatic chain linker. Unlike other biased agonists, which primarily achieve their biased signaling behavior through different interaction patterns in the orthosteric pocket, C5 guano and C6 guano utilize allosteric modulation. This represents a new strategy for the rational design of biased agonists for GPCRs.

2 Spectroscopy Study of μOR with Different Agonists

All solved complex structures of μOR with different ligands provide snapshots of the receptor in both its inactive and active state, as well as insights into how balanced and biased agonists interact with it. As an allosteric protein, conformational changes in GPCRs are typically initiated by ligand binding to the orthosteric pocket and ultimately propagate to the intracellular domain, a process that cannot be fully captured by structural determination methods. To complement these findings, NMR spectroscopy offers the ability to observe the receptor's dynamic conformational changes with high temporal and spatial resolution (Shimada et al. 2019). For μOR's biased signaling, understanding how these biased agonists trigger distinct conformational changes and how these changes propagate from the ligand-binding pocket to the intracellular pocket is crucial for elucidating the mechanisms of biased signaling and guiding the development of novel biased agonists.

The first NMR dynamic study for μOR was reported by Rémy Sounier et al. in 2015, using lysine as a probe (Sounier et al. 2015). This study not only provided spectroscopic evidence for the outward movement of transmembrane segment 6 (TM6) but also observed conformational changes in Helix 8 and the intracellular loop 1 (ICL1), suggesting their potential involvement in G-protein signaling specificity.

Junya Okude et al. were among the first to use NMR methods to study the mechanism of μOR-biased signaling (Okude et al. 2015). They correlated the signaling behavior of ligands with the intracellular conformational states of the receptor. Both balanced agonists and biased agonists can stabilize the intracellular portion of the receptor into distinct conformational states compared to the inactive state. These different conformational states exist in equilibrium, and their varying distributions determine whether the receptor signals through G protein or β-arrestin. This study presented a new perspective on understanding μOR's biased signaling. However, the lack of connection between the ligands' scaffolds or interaction modes makes it insufficient to fully comprehend the detailed structure-bias relationship.

Xiaojing Cong et al. collected NMR data for multiple μOR agonists to investigate the continuous conformational changes from ligand-binding pocket through the transmembrane connector region to the intracellular pocket, using both lysine and methionine as probes (Cong et al. 2021). They observed slightly varied NMR signals originating from the ligand-binding pocket for different agonists (DAMGO, BU72, PZM21, TRV130, and buprenorphine). These differences were further amplified through the connector region, as reflected by the signal from $M^{5.49}$, which is close to the PIF motif, to the intracellular pocket, as reflected by the signals from $K100^{12.51}$ and $K^{8.51}/K98^{12.49}$. This suggests that distinct conformational states of Helix 8 and ICL1 may be associated with the ligand's biased signaling and are initiated from ligand binding.

Beyond NMR, other spectroscopic techniques including double electron–electron resonance (DEER) and single-molecule fluorescence resonance energy transfer (smFRET) have also been utilized to investigate the dynamic properties of μOR, particularly the relationship between ligand efficacy and receptor conformations. By measuring the distance distribution between TM6 and TM4 after receptor is stimulated by different agonists, Jiawei Zhao et al. identified the different behaviors of μOR after the receptor was stimulated by G protein-biased agonists (PZM21, TRV130 and MP) and other agonists (DAMGO, BU72 and lofentanil). Specifically, biased agonists with low efficacy tended to stabilize a shorter distance between TM6

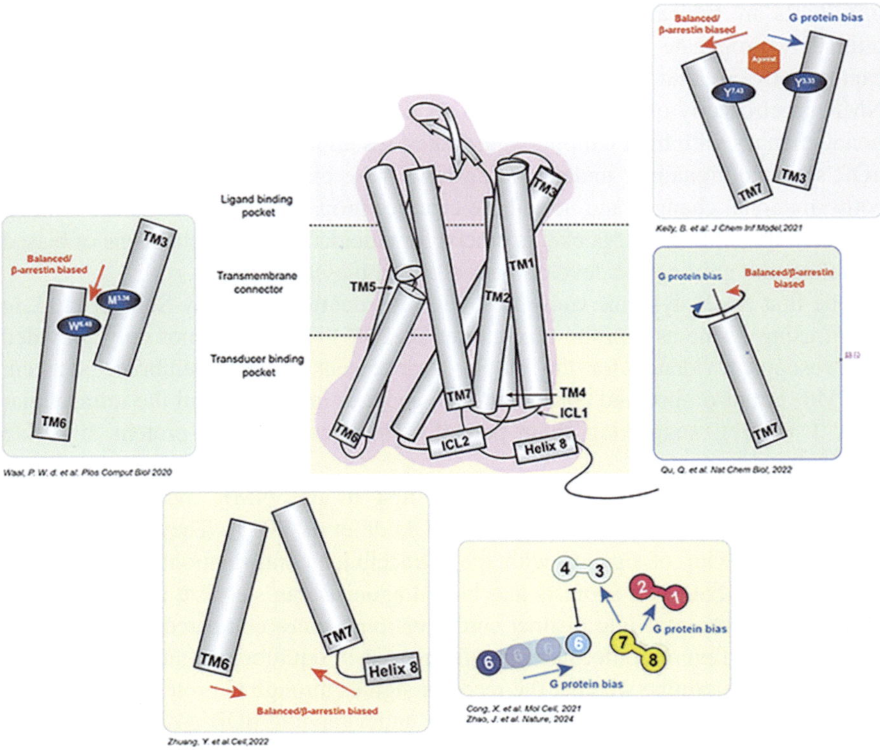

Fig. 3 Dynamics investigations on the μOR biased signaling

and TM4, resulting in a smaller intracellular pocket for transducers whereas other agonists exhibited the opposite effect. Furthermore, for the same agonists, the presence of β-arrestin1 also stabilize a longer distance compared to G_i (Zhao et al. 2024). (Fig. 3).

3 MD Simulations of μOR Conformational Change

Compared to structure determination and spectroscopy methods, computational molecular dynamics (MD) simulations can offer more detailed information about atomic interactions, motion, energy landscapes, and protein dynamics, which are often not fully accessible through experimental methods (Latorraca et al. 2017). To understand the mechanism of μOR's biased signaling, Parker W. de Waal et al. used MD simulations to investigate how the β-arrestin-biased agonist fentanyl interacts with μOR. Their results provided new evidence about the role of residue $M^{3.36}$ in β-arrestin signaling (de Waal et al. 2020). $M^{3.36}$ is located between the ligand binding pocket and the toggle switch. The residue thus can sense ligand binding and further displace $W^{6.48}$. The study found that, compared to DAMGO, fentanyl induced a greater downward movement of $M^{3.36}$, leading to more significant conformational changes in $W^{6.48}$. This results in enhanced β-arrestin signaling by fentanyl.

In order to distinguish the G protein signaling pathway from the β-arrestin signaling pathway, Brendan Kelly et al. used MD simulations to determine how different residues contribute to either G protein signaling or β-arrestin signaling (Kelly et al. 2021). They simulated the R- and S-enantiomers of the same compound, previously validated by *Pfizer,* which exhibit distinct biased signaling profiles despite having only chirality differences. They found that these two enantiomers bind to the receptor in different ways after simulation. The R-enantiomer (the G protein-biased one) formed a T-π interaction with $Y^{3.33}$ (TM3), while the S-enantiomer formed a π-π stacking interaction with $Y^{7.43}$ (TM7). These findings suggest that the interactions with TM3 or TM7 contribute differently to μOR's β-arrestin signaling. Additionally, they observed that a strong salt bridge with $D^{3.32}$ favored β-arrestin signaling.

MD simulations can also help researchers gain deeper insights based on their experimental results. To further interpret the NMR data, Xiaojing Cong et al. integrated MD simulations to explore the propagation of conformational changes from the ligand binding pocket to the intracellular pocket (Cong et al. 2021). They observed that, for biased agonists, the lower half of TM7 shifted toward TM3, while Helix 8 moved closer to ICL1. This specific phenomenon was not observed with balanced agonists. The differences were primarily attributed to distinct conformational changes in residues within the transmembrane connector region, including the sodium pocket, the NPxxY motif, and the toggle switch.

Qianhui Qu et al. and Youwen Zhuang et al. also used MD simulations to further understand the mechanism of biased agonism after solving a series of new structures (Qu et al. 2022; Zhuang et al. 2022). Qianhui Qu et al. ran MD simulations without G proteins to observe the relaxation of the receptor. They proposed that the different signaling behaviors of MP and LFT were due to these two ligands stabilizing the receptor in distinct conformational states, as reflected by the rotation of TM7. Specifically, MP stabilized the canonical conformation of μOR, while LFT stabilized an alternative state where TM7 rotated counterclockwise (when viewed from the extracellular side) and moved inward towards TM3. This resulted in a narrower intracellular pocket that favored β-arrestin binding. The different rotation of TM7 in the intracellular part was due to changes in the hydrogen-bond network around the sodium pocket (Qu et al. 2022).

Youwen Zhuang et al. also ran MD simulations based on the structures they solved. Similar to other studies, they focused on the conformational changes in TM7 and Helix 8. They observed that, compared to SR-17018, TRV130, and PZM21, ligands like DAMGO and fentanyl caused TM7 to move inward toward the receptor's core, particularly at the junction of TM7 and Helix 8, resulting in a narrow intracellular pocket (Zhuang et al. 2022). This finding is consistent with Qianhui Qu et al.'s theory but differs from Xiaojing Cong et al.'s observations. To further elucidate the relationship between the volume of the intracellular pocket and transducer coupling, Youwen Zhuang et al. built atomic models of μOR with β-arrestin and different ligands. They calculated the solvent accessible surface area

(SASA) stabilized by balanced agonists and biased agonists, and their results further supported the theory that the inward movement of TM7 leads to enhanced β-arrestin signaling (Fig. 3).

4 Discussion

As the target for central nervous system opioid analgesics, μOR plays an irreplaceable role in blocking pain signals from ascending to the cerebral cortex from peripheral tissues. Opioids like morphine remain among the most important analgesics for managing severe pain. However, the lethal side effects induced by opioid overdose significantly restrict the use of these drugs. How to safely use opioid drugs or how to discover novel opioids with reduced side effects has been a critical scientific question for several decades. Previous functional studies of μOR have indicated that the drug tolerance and other side effects of opioid drugs are primarily caused by the β-arrestin signaling pathway of μOR, driving efforts to find biased agonists that do not recruit β-arrestin. However, recent research on the role of β-arrestin has shown that morphine-induced respiratory depression can still be observed in β-arrestin knockout mice, suggesting that the mechanisms of opioid side effects are more complex than initially thought. Despite this, β-arrestin-induced receptor endocytosis remains a major contributor to opioid tolerance and abuse. Decoupling μOR's arrestin signaling from its G protein signaling by identifying novel biased agonists is still beneficial for safer opioid clinical use. To date, several-biased agonists of μOR with different scaffolds have been developed, but the detailed relationship between ligands' chemical scaffolds and their biased behavior remains complex and unclear. This complexity restricts the rational design of novel biased agonists for μOR and other GPCRs.

In this chapter, we summarize recent efforts on understanding the structure-bias relationship of μOR, including structure determination, NMR spectroscopy, and MD simulations. Determining the complex structures of μOR with balanced agonists or biased agonists provide clear insights into the interactions between ligands and the receptor. These interactions are mostly conserved and include the interactions with $D^{3.32}/Y^{7.43}$, the water-mediated hydrogen bond network around $H^{6.52}$, and some hydrophobic contacts with the transmembrane domains and extracellular loops (Manglik et al. 2012). The exact binding positions of different ligands may slightly vary within the orthosteric binding pocket, leading to enhanced or reduced interactions with nearby residues (such as $D^{3.32}$ and $M^{3.36}$) (de Waal et al. 2020; Kelly et al. 2021) or with the transmembrane helices (such as TM2/3 and TM7) (Qu et al. 2022; Zhuang et al. 2022). These variations ultimately result in different conformational changes and signaling behaviors. However, these relationships are highly dependent on the ligand's entire chemical scaffold, meaning that distinct types of ligands may follow different rules. While TM6 is considered the hallmark of GPCR activation, TM7 (along with Helix 8) has been described as the "macro-switch" for biased versus balanced signaling. The conformational changes in TM7 induced by ligands differ between balanced agonists and biased agonists for GPCRs.

Several studies using NMR spectroscopy or MD simulations have reported that TM7 behaves differently when the receptor is activated by balanced agonists versus biased agonists, primarily involving differences in the movement or rotation of TM7 (Cong et al. 2021; Qu et al. 2022). Although these studies about TM7's behavior in biased agonism are not entirely consistent with each other, they collectively confirm the crucial role of TM7 as the link of ligand binding and biased signaling. It remains unknown which residues are most important for sensing and propagating the conformational changes to the intracellular part.

However, the precise mechanisms underlying the side effects of opioid analgesics remain insufficiently understood, and further research is required to accelerate the development of safer and more effective opioid analgesics. For instance, it is unclear how the six different subtypes of $G_{i/o/z}$ proteins contribute to the analgesic effects and adverse side effects of opioid analgesics. Dissecting the specific roles of these G protein subtypes in both pain relief and side effect profiles could greatly inform the rational design of more selective and safer μOR-targeted drugs.

Additionally, there is an urgent need to elucidate how to reverse the opioid analgesics-activated reward circuitry in the central nervous system, which underlies their addictive potential. Understanding the molecular and cellular mechanisms that link μOR activation to reward pathways will be crucial for designing opioid analgesics that retain therapeutic efficacy while minimizing the risk of addiction. Future research efforts aimed at disentangling these complex signaling networks will be pivotal for guiding the development of next-generation opioid analgesics with improved safety and efficacy profiles.

The development of cryo-EM has accelerated the structure determination of μOR with different ligands, and this structural information and comparative analysis further supplement our understanding of the structure-bias relationship. There is a great need to identify more biased agonists with diverse chemotypes and scaffolds to provide additional data for analysis. Additionally, the advancement of deep learning and AI has provided new tools to extract more information from structural studies, bringing new insights that can guide the rational design and de novo design of biased agonists for μOR, as well as for other GPCRs like angiotensin receptors and chemokine receptors, where biased signaling is crucial for improved therapeutic value.

References

Bachmutsky I, Wei XP, Durand A, Yackle K (2021) ß-arrestin 2 germline knockout does not attenuate opioid respiratory depression. elife 10:e62552

Ballesteros JA, Weinstein H (1995) [19] Integrated methods for the construction of three-dimensional models and computational probing of structure-function relations in G protein-coupled receptors. Methods Neurosci 25:366–428

Bohn LM, Gainetdinov RR, Lin F-T, Lefkowitz RJ, Caron MG (2000) μ-Opioid receptor desensitization by β-arrestin-2 determines morphine tolerance but not dependence. Nature 408(6813): 720–723

Chen X-T, Pitis P, Liu G, Yuan C, Gotchev D, Cowan CL, Rominger DH, Koblish M, DeWire SM, Crombie AL, Violin JD, Yamashita DS (2013) Structure–activity relationships and discovery of a G protein biased μ opioid receptor ligand, [(3-Methoxythiophen-2-yl)methyl]({2-[(9R)-9-(pyridin-2-yl)-6-oxaspiro-[4.5]decan-9-yl]ethyl})amine (TRV130), for the Treatment of Acute Severe Pain. J Med Chem 56(20):8019–8031

Cong X, Maurel D, Déméné H, Vasiliauskaité-Brooks I, Hagelberger J, Peysson F, Saint-Paul J, Golebiowski J, Granier S, Sounier R (2021) Molecular insights into the biased signaling mechanism of the μ-opioid receptor. Mol Cell 81(20):4165–4175.e4166

Corder G, Castro DC, Bruchas MR, Scherrer G (2018) Endogenous and exogenous opioids in pain. Annu Rev Neurosci 41(1):1–21

de Waal PW, Shi J, You E, Wang X, Melcher K, Jiang Y, Xu HE, Dickson BM (2020) Molecular mechanisms of fentanyl mediated β-arrestin biased signaling. PLoS Comput Biol 16(4): e1007394

Deupi X, Kobilka BK (2010) Energy landscapes as a tool to integrate GPCR structure, dynamics, and function. Physiology 25(5):293–303

Faouzi A, Wang H, Zaidi SA, DiBerto JF, Che T, Qu Q, Robertson MJ, Madasu MK, Daibani AE, Varga BR, Zhang T, Ruiz C, Liu S, Xu J, Appourchaux K, Slocum ST, Eans SO, Cameron MD, Al-Hasani R, Pan YX, Roth BL, McLaughlin JP, Skiniotis G, Katritch V, Kobilka BK, Majumdar S (2022) Structure-based design of bitopic ligands for the μ-opioid receptor. Nature:1–3. https://doi.org/10.1016/j.drudis.2024.103950

Gmeiner P, Wang H, Hetzer F, Huang W, Qu Q, Meyerowitz J, Kaindl J, Hübner H, Skiniotis G, Kobilka BK (2022) Structure-based evolution of G protein-biased μ-opioid receptor agonists. Angew Chem Int Ed 61:e202200269

Hilger D (2021) The role of structural dynamics in GPCR-mediated signaling. FEBS J 288(8): 2461–2489

Huang W, Manglik A, Venkatakrishnan AJ, Laeremans T, Feinberg EN, Sanborn AL, Kato HE, Livingston KE, Thorsen TS, Kling R, Granier S, Gmeiner P, Husbands SM, Traynor JR, Weis WI, Steyaert J, Dror RO, Kobilka BK (2015) Structural insights into μ-opioid receptor activation. Nature 524(7565):315–321

Jeffrey Conn P, Christopoulos A, Lindsley CW (2009) Allosteric modulators of GPCRs: a novel approach for the treatment of CNS disorders. Nat Rev Drug Discov 8(1):41–54

Kelly E, Bailey CP, Henderson G (2008) Agonist-selective mechanisms of GPCR desensitization. Br J Pharmacol 153(Suppl 1):S379–S388

Kelly B, Hollingsworth SA, Blakemore DC, Owen RM, Storer RI, Swain NA, Aydin D, Torella R, Warmus JS, Dror RO (2021) Delineating the ligand–receptor interactions that lead to biased signaling at the μ-opioid receptor. J Chem Inf Model 61(7):3696–3707

Koehl A, Hu H, Maeda S, Zhang Y, Qu Q, Paggi JM, Latorraca NR, Hilger D, Dawson R, Matile H, Schertler GFX, Granier S, Weis WI, Dror RO, Manglik A, Skiniotis G, Kobilka BK (2018) Structure of the μ opioid receptor-Gi protein complex. Nature 558(7711):547–552

Kruegel AC, Uprety R, Grinnell SG, Langreck C, Pekarskaya EA, Rouzic VL, Ansonoff M, Gassaway MM, Pintar JE, Pasternak GW, Javitch JA, Majumdar S, Sames D (2019) 7-Hydroxymitragynine is an active metabolite of Mitragynine and a key mediator of its analgesic effects. ACS Central Sci 5(6):992–1001

Latorraca NR, Venkatakrishnan AJ, Dror RO (2017) GPCR dynamics: structures in motion. Chem Rev 117(1):139–155

Manglik A, Kruse AC, Kobilka TS, Thian FS, Mathiesen JM, Sunahara RK, Pardo L, Weis WI, Kobilka BK, Granier S (2012) Crystal structure of the μ-opioid receptor bound to a morphinan antagonist. Nature 485(7398):321–326

Manglik A, Lin H, Aryal DK, McCorvy JD, Dengler D, Corder G, Levit A, Kling RC, Bernat V, Hübner H, Huang X-P, Sassano MF, Giguère PM, Löber S, Duan D, Scherrer G, Kobilka BK, Gmeiner P, Roth BL, Shoichet BK (2016) Structure-based discovery of opioid analgesics with reduced side effects. Nature 537(7619):185–190

Okude J, Ueda T, Kofuku Y, Sato M, Nobuyama N, Kondo K, Shiraishi Y, Mizumura T, Onishi K, Natsume M, Maeda M, Tsujishita H, Kuranaga T, Inoue M, Shimada I (2015) Identification of a conformational equilibrium that determines the efficacy and functional selectivity of the μ-opioid receptor. Angew Chem Int Ed 54(52):15771–15776

Pert CB, Pasternak G, Snyder SH (1973) Opiate agonists and antagonists discriminated by receptor binding in brain. Science 182(4119):1359–1361

Qu Q, Huang W, Aydin D, Paggi JM, Seven AB, Wang H, Chakraborty S, Che T, DiBerto JF, Robertson MJ, Inoue A, Suomivuori C-M, Roth BL, Majumdar S, Dror RO, Kobilka BK, Skiniotis G (2022) Insights into distinct signaling profiles of the μOR activated by diverse agonists. Nat Chem Biol 19:1–8

Raehal KM, Walker JKL, Bohn LM (2005) Morphine side effects in β-Arrestin 2 knockout mice. J Pharmacol Exp Ther 314(3):1195–1201

Rasmussen SGF, DeVree BT, Zou Y, Kruse AC, Chung KY, Kobilka TS, Thian FS, Chae PS, Pardon E, Calinski D, Mathiesen JM, Shah STA, Lyons JA, Caffrey M, Gellman SH, Steyaert J, Skiniotis G, Weis WI, Sunahara RK, Kobilka BK (2011) Crystal structure of the β2Adrenergic receptor-Gs protein complex. Nature 477(7366):549–555

Schmid CL, Kennedy NM, Ross NC, Lovell KM, Yue Z, Morgenweck J, Cameron MD, Bannister TD, Bohn LM (2017) Bias factor and therapeutic window correlate to predict safer opioid analgesics. Cell 171(5):1165–1175.e1113

Shang Y, LeRouzic V, Schneider S, Bisignano P, Pasternak GW, Filizola M (2014) Mechanistic insights into the allosteric modulation of opioid receptors by sodium ions. Biochemistry 53(31): 5140–5149

Shimada I, Ueda T, Kofuku Y, Eddy MT, Wüthrich K (2019) GPCR drug discovery: integrating solution NMR data with crystal and cryo-EM structures. Nat Rev Drug Discov 18(1):59–82

Sounier R, Mas C, Steyaert J, Laeremans T, Manglik A, Huang W, Kobilka BK, Déméné H, Granier S (2015) Propagation of conformational changes during μ-opioid receptor activation. Nature 524(7565):375–378

Walsh TD (1990) Prevention of opioid side effects. J Pain Symptom Manag 5(6):362–367

Weiss N, Zamponi GW (2021) Opioid receptor regulation of neuronal voltage-gated calcium channels. Cell Mol Neurobiol 41(5):839–847

Williams JT, Ingram SL, Henderson G, Chavkin C, Zastrow v M, Schulz S, Koch T, Evans CJ, Christie MJ (2013) Regulation of μ-opioid receptors: desensitization, phosphorylation, internalization, and tolerance. Pharmacol Rev 65(1):223–254

Wold EA, Chen J, Cunningham KA, Zhou J (2019) Allosteric modulation of class A GPCRs: targets, agents, and emerging concepts. J Med Chem 62(1):88–127

Zhao J, Elgeti M, O'Brien ES, Sár CP, Daibani AEI, Heng J, Sun X, White E, Che T, Hubbell WL, Kobilka BK, Chen C (2024) Ligand efficacy modulates conformational dynamics of the μ-opioid receptor. Nature 629:1–7

Zhuang Y, Wang Y, He B, He X, Zhou XE, Guo S, Rao Q, Yang J, Liu J, Zhou Q, Wang X, Liu M, Liu W, Jiang X, Yang D, Jiang H, Shen J, Melcher K, Chen H, Jiang Y, Cheng X, Wang M-W, Xie X, Xu HE (2022) Molecular recognition of morphine and fentanyl by the human μ-opioid receptor. Cell 185(23):4361–4375.e4319

Part IV

Therapeutic Applications of GPCR Biased Signaling

GPCR Biased Signaling in Cancer

Ariella C. Avigad, Melody Zhou, Chengyu Sun, Levin Ma, Xue Li, Rosie J. Blodgett, Vera S. Donnenberg, Albert D. Donnenberg, Patrick L. Wagner, David L. Bartlett, and Kunhong Xiao

Contents

Authors Ariella C. Avigad, Melody Zhou and Chengyu Sun have equally contributed to this chapter.

A. C. Avigad · M. Zhou · C. Sun · L. Ma · X. Li · R. J. Blodgett
Allegheny Health Network Cancer Institute, Allegheny Health Network, Pittsburgh, PA, USA

Allegheny Health Network Research Institute, Allegheny Health Network, Pittsburgh, PA, USA

Centers for Proteomics & Artificial Intelligence and Clinical Mass Spectrometry, Allegheny Health Network Cancer Institute, Allegheny Health Network, Pittsburgh, PA, USA

V. S. Donnenberg
Department of Cardiothoracic Surgery, University of Pittsburgh School of Medicine, Pittsburgh, PA, USA

A. D. Donnenberg · P. L. Wagner · D. L. Bartlett
Allegheny Health Network Cancer Institute, Allegheny Health Network, Pittsburgh, PA, USA

Allegheny Health Network Research Institute, Allegheny Health Network, Pittsburgh, PA, USA

K. Xiao (✉)
Allegheny Health Network Cancer Institute, Allegheny Health Network, Pittsburgh, PA, USA

Allegheny Health Network Research Institute, Allegheny Health Network, Pittsburgh, PA, USA

Centers for Proteomics & Artificial Intelligence and Clinical Mass Spectrometry, Allegheny Health Network Cancer Institute, Allegheny Health Network, Pittsburgh, PA, USA

Department of Biomedical Engineering, College of Engineering, Carnegie Mellon University, Pittsburgh, PA, USA
e-mail: kunhongkevin.xiao@ahn.org; kxiao2@andrew.cmu.edu

© The Author(s), under exclusive license to Springer Nature Switzerland AG 2025

Z. Li, K. Xiao (eds.), *Pharmacology of GPCRs Biased Signaling and Agonists*, Handbook of Experimental Pharmacology 290, https://doi.org/10.1007/164_2025_773

Abstract

G protein–coupled receptors (GPCRs) represent the largest family of cell surface receptors. They orchestrate various signaling pathways, playing a central role in regulating various physiological and pathophysiological processes. Dysregulation of GPCR signaling has been intricately linked to cancer pathogenesis, including tumor growth, angiogenesis, metastasis, and immune modulation. Biased GPCR signaling occurs when a ligand preferentially activates one signaling pathway over another, leading to distinct cellular outcomes. In cancer, biased GPCR signaling represents a complex, dynamic phenomenon, significantly influencing cancer development, progression, and treatment resistance. This chapter reviews recent advances in our understanding of GPCR biased signaling in various aspects of cancer biology and explores its therapeutic potential. Given the fragmented nature of existing evidence, we integrate available literature with findings from our own proteomics studies on GPCR and β-arrestin function to provide a preliminary framework for understanding β-arrestin–mediated signaling in cancer. While this overview may capture only a limited snapshot of the broader landscape, it provides a valuable foundation for generating new hypotheses and guiding future research and drug discovery efforts in oncology.

Keywords

Cancer · GPCR · GPCR biased signaling · β-arrestin · β-arrestin-mediated signaling

Abbreviations

APC	activated protein C
ARF-GAP21	ADP-ribosylation factor GTPase-activating protein 21
BAD	Bcl-2-associated death promoter
BiP	binding immunoglobulin protein
BMPR-II	type II bone morphogenetic protein receptor
CAMKII	calcium/calmodulin-dependent protein kinase II
cAMP	cyclic AMP
COX-2	cyclooxygenase 2
CTLs	cytotoxic T lymphocytes
CXCL12	C-X-C motif chemokine ligand 12
CXCR4	C-X-C chemokine receptor type 4
DAG	diacylglycerol
DCs	dendritic cells
DEN	diethylnitrosamine
Dvl	dishevelled
ECM	extracellular matrix
ECs	endothelial cells
EMT	ERK-mediated epithelial–mesenchymal transition
eNOS	endothelial nitric oxide synthase
EOC	epithelial ovarian cancer
ER	endoplasmic reticulum
ERK	extracellular signal-regulated kinases
ET-1	endothelin-1
ETAR	endothelin A receptor
FDA	Food and Drug Administration
FFAs	adipocyte-derived free fatty acids
FLS	fibroblast-like synoviocytes
GAPDH	glyceraldehyde-3-phosphate dehydrogenase
GEF	guanine nucleotide exchange factor
GENC	glomerular endothelial cell
GLUT1	glucose transporter 1
GPCRs	G protein–coupled receptors
GPR3	G-protein–coupled receptor 3
GRKs	G protein–coupled receptor kinases
HATs	histone acetyltransferases
HCC	hepatocellular carcinoma
HIF-1α	hypoxia-inducible factor-1α
HMGB1	high-mobility group box 1
IBD	inflammatory bowel disease
IP3	inositol trisphosphate
IQGAP	IQ motif–containing GTPase-activating protein
IRG1	immune responsive gene 1

JNK	c-Jun N-terminal kinase
LDHA	lactate dehydrogenase A
LPA	lysophosphatidic acid
LPARs	lysophosphatidic acid receptors
MAPK	mitogen-activated protein kinase
MASH	metabolic dysfunction-associated steatohepatitis
MCT4	monocarboxylate transporter 4
MDSCs	myeloid-derived suppressor cells
MMPs	matrix metalloproteinases
MPC1	mitochondrial pyruvate carrier
NEC	necrotizing enterocolitis
NF-κB	nuclear factor kappa B
NK1R	neurokinin-1 receptor
NO	nitric oxide
NSCLC	non-small cell lung cancer
p70S6K	p70 ribosomal S6 kinase
PAK	p21-activated kinases
PAR1	protease-activated receptor 1
PAR2	protease-activated receptor
PcG	polycomb group
PGE2	prostaglandin E2
PGE2Rs	prostaglandin E2 receptors
PI3K	phosphoinositide 3-kinase
PIP2	phosphatidylinositol 4,5-bisphosphate
PKA	protein kinase A
PKC	protein kinase C
PKM2	pyruvate kinase M2
PLCβ	phospholipase Cβ
PPARγ	peroxisome proliferator-activated receptor gamma
PUMA	p53-upregulated modulator of apoptosis
RalA	Ras-related protein Ral-A
RalGDS	Ral guanine nucleotide dissociation stimulator
RhoGEFs	Rho guanine nucleotide exchange factors
ROS	reactive oxygen species
RXRα	retinoid X receptor alpha
S1PR	sphingosine-1-phosphate receptor
SDF1	stromal cell-derived factor-1α
SIP	sphingosine-1-phosphate
STATs	signal transducer and activator of transcription proteins
TAMs	tumor-associated macrophages
TGCT	tenosynovial giant cell tumor
TME	tumor microenvironment
TNBC	triple-negative breast cancer
Tregs	regulatory T cells
VE	vascular endothelial

VEGF	vascular endothelial growth factor
YAP	yes-associated protein
ZEB1	zinc finger E-box-binding homeobox 1
ZEB2	zinc finger E-box-binding homeobox 2

1 Introduction: GPCR Signaling in Cancer

G protein–coupled receptors (GPCRs) are the largest and most diverse family of cell surface receptors, responsible for converting extracellular signals into intracellular responses and accounting for approximately 30–40% of all Food and Drug Administration (FDA)-approved drugs (Lefkowitz 2007, 2013; Liu et al. 2024b; Pierce et al. 2002; Hauser et al. 2017; Lorente et al. 2025). With over 800 GPCRs encoded in the human genome, GPCRs regulate a wide range of cellular functions, including cell growth, directed migration, and programmed cell death. Dysregulation of GPCR signaling often plays a pivotal role in various aspects of cancer biology, such as tumor initiation, progression, metastasis, immune response, metabolic regulation, and modulation of the tumor microenvironment (TME) (Chaudhary and Kim 2021; de Visser and Joyce 2023; Yang et al. 2025). An overview of selected cancer-related GPCRs is provided in Table 1. For example, C-X-C chemokine receptor type 4 (CXCR4) is frequently upregulated in malignancies such as breast, lung, and prostate cancers. Its interaction with C-X-C motif chemokine ligand 12 (CXCL12, also known as stromal cell-derived factor 1, or SDF-1), promotes tumor cell migration and metastasis (Mukherjee and Zhao 2013; Chatterjee et al. 2014; Rueda et al. 2025; Burger and Kipps 2006; Domanska et al. 2013; Zielinska and Katanaev 2020; Singh et al. 2004; Liu and Sun 2025; Sarvaiya et al. 2013; Tanaka et al. 2005; Mortezaee 2020; Bianchi and Mezzapelle 2020). Likewise, lysophosphatidic acid receptors (LPARs) enhance cancer cell survival and invasion, contributing to aggressive tumor phenotypes (Yu et al. 2008; Panupinthu et al. 2010; Geraldo et al. 2021; Balijepalli et al. 2021; Lin et al. 2021; Yamamoto et al. 2025; Tamura et al. 2025; Yun 2019; Qi et al. 2024). The ability of GPCRs to integrate multiple signaling inputs highlights their central role in cancer development and progression.

GPCRs significantly influence the TME, which is comprised of immune cells, stromal cells, and extracellular matrix (ECM) components that support tumor growth and immune evasion (Dickinson et al. 2024; Wu et al. 2023; Korbecki et al. 2023; Wang et al. 2022; Zhou et al. 2009). Some GPCRs, such as adenosine receptors (e.g., A2ARs) and prostaglandin E2 receptors (PGE2Rs, or EP receptors), modulate immune responses by suppressing cytotoxic T-cell activity and promoting immunosuppressive cell populations like regulatory T cells and myeloid-derived suppressor cells (Nataraj et al. 2001; Yang et al. 2020; Su et al. 2008; Whiteside and Jackson 2013; Cekic et al. 2014). Many GPCRs also regulate stromal cell behavior, including

Table 1 Representative GPCRs involved in cancer

GPCR Class	Example receptors	Example ligands	Cancer types involved	Key role	References
Chemokine	CXCR4, CCR7	CXCL12, CCL19, CCL21	Breast, lung, prostate, gastric, colorectal	Metastasis, migration	Singh et al. (2011), Bocchi et al. (2023), Mortezaee (2020), Zhou et al. (2018), Zielinska and Katanaev (2020), Zhang et al. (2020b), Salem et al. (2021) and Hughes and Nibbs (2018)
Protease-activated	PAR1, PAR2	Thrombin, trypsin, APC	Breast, colon, melanoma, prostate, esophageal squamous cell carcinoma	Invasion, inflammation	Jaber et al. (2014, 2017), Lv et al. (2023), Versteeg et al. (2008), Adams et al. (2018), Sedda et al. (2014), Wojtukiewicz et al. (2015), Han et al. (2011), Patnaik et al. (2025) and Kennedy et al. (2020)
Lysophos-pholipid	LPARs, S1PRs	LPA, S1P	Ovarian, colon, hematologic	Angiogenesis, proliferation	Xu (2018), Rolin and Maghazachi (2011) and Aiello and Casiraghi (2021)
Frizzled	FZD7, FZD10	Wnt3a, Wnt5a	Liver, colorectal, sarcoma	Wnt signaling, stemness	Wong et al. (2013), Pourreyron et al. (2012), Zeng et al. (2018) and Xia et al. (2024)
Orphan	GPR56, GPR161	TG2, HCC	Melanoma, glioblastoma, breast	Varies by cancer	Yang et al. (2014), Luo et al. (2024) and Jin et al. (2017)
Secretin family	VIPR1, GLP-1R	VIP, GLP-1	Colon, pancreatic, prostate, Gastrointestinal	Hormonal regulation	Klussmeier et al. (2022), Poyner and Hay (2012)
Rhodopsin-like	ADRB2, HRH1	Epinephrine, Histamine	Breast, various	Stress, immune modulation	Kulik (2019), Xu et al. (2022), Li et al. (2022), Ding et al. (2025) and Salmeron et al. (2025)

fibroblast activation and ECM remodeling, creating a tumor-supportive niche (Lappano and Maggiolini 2023; Dwivedi et al. 2023). Endothelin receptors, such as ETAR, contribute to the development of tumors through vascular restructuring and promotion of endothelial cell growth, ensuring that enough oxygen and nutrients are sent to the tumor (Bagnato and Spinella 2003; Wang and Dashwood 2011; Harrison et al. 2024; Kandalaft et al. 2009; Arndt et al. 2024; Tocci et al. 2021). The multifaceted role of GPCRs in shaping the TME underscores their contribution to cancer progression and resistance to therapies, as they facilitate cross-talk between tumor cells and their surrounding environment.

Given their significant role in cancer biology, GPCRs are promising therapeutic targets for developing novel cancer drugs. Therapeutic agents such as antagonists, agonists, biased agonists, and allosteric modulators targeting specific GPCRs are being explored as a means to disrupt oncogenic signaling and modulate the TME (Chaudhary and Kim 2021; Cornwell and Feigin 2020; Jayakody et al. 2025; Usman et al. 2020; O'Hayre et al. 2014). For example, CXCR4 antagonists like Plerixafor (Mozobil), which block the interaction between CXCR4 and its natural ligand CXCL12 (also known as stromal cell-derived factor-1α or SDF-1α), are being investigated for their potential to inhibit metastasis in cancers such as multiple myeloma, sarcoma, and breast cancer, as well as various hematologic malignancies (Berning et al. 2018; Martino et al. 2024; Chen et al. 2019). Similarly, targeting sphingosine-1-phosphate (S1P) receptors or lysophosphatidic acid (LPA) receptors has shown potential to reduce tumor growth, invasion, angiogenesis, and progression in preclinical models (Visentin et al. 2006; Murph and Mills 2007; Limbu et al. 2024). Despite this potential, challenges remain, including the need for more selective and efficacious ligands with minimal on-target off-tumor (or off-TME) toxicities. The discovery that different ligands interacting with the same receptro can preferentially activate different downstream pathways has important implications for both normal and malignant cell behavior. In this regard, the development of biased or pathway-selective ligands for specific GPCRs offers a novel strategy to develop innovative cancer therapies with enhanced therapeutic precision and improved patient outcomes. The concept of biased signaling, where ligands selectively activate either G protein–mediated or G protein–independent, β-arrestin–mediated pathways, has opened new avenues for drug development in cancer. Although biased ligands have been developed and approved for non-cancer indications, such as Oliceridine (Olinvyk™) for pain (Lambert and Calo 2020), there are currently no β-arrestin–biased GPCR drugs specifically approved for cancer treatment. Oliceridine, a recently approved μ-opioid receptor agonist, exemplifies the concept of biased GPCR signaling by preferentially activating G protein pathways while minimizing β-arrestin recruitment. This selective signaling bias is associated with effective analgesia and a reduced risk of respiratory depression—a common and potentially life-threatening side effect of conventional opioids. The clinical success of Oliceridine highlights the therapeutic potential of biased GPCR ligands, not only in pain management, but also as a promising strategy in oncology, where selective modulation of GPCR signaling could enhance anticancer efficacy while minimizing adverse effects. This chapter will focus specifically on β-arrestin–mediated GPCR biased signaling in the context of cancer.

2 Contributions of GPCR Biased Signaling to Cancer Hallmarks

Researchers originally thought that GPCR activation and signaling followed a linear process, in which G proteins mediated acute intracellular signaling, while β-arrestins regulated the signal via receptor desensitization and internalization (Lefkowitz and Shenoy 2005; Liu et al. 2024b; Rockman and Lefkowitz 2024; Shukla et al. 2011). Research over the past three decades has fundamentally reshaped this concept, revealing that GPCRs can initiate two parallel and distinct intracellular signaling pathways: one mediated by G proteins and the other by β-arrestins (Fig. 1, top) (Lefkowitz 2007, 2013; Shukla et al. 2011; Xiao et al. 2007, 2010; Wisler et al. 2014; Lefkowitz and Shenoy 2005). G protein–mediated signaling represents the classical pathway activated by GPCRs upon ligand binding (Wettschureck and Offermanns 2005; Hauser et al. 2017, 2018; Schioth and Fredriksson 2005; Yang et al. 2021; Carman and Benovic 1998). When a ligand, such as a hormone, neurotransmitter, or chemokine, binds to a GPCR, the receptor undergoes a conformational change that activates an associated heterotrimeric G protein, composed of α, β, and γ subunits. This activation promotes the exchange of GDP for GTP on the Gα subunit, resulting in the dissociation of Gα from the Gβγ dimer. Both Gα and Gβγ can then interact with distinct downstream effectors to propagate intracellular signaling. The specific response depends on the type of Gα subunit involved. For example, Gαs stimulates adenylyl cyclase, leading to increased levels of cyclic AMP (cAMP) and activation of protein kinase A (PKA). In contrast, Gαi/o inhibits adenylyl cyclase, thereby reducing cAMP levels. Gαq/11 activates phospholipase Cβ (PLCβ), which hydrolyzes phosphatidylinositol 4,5-bisphosphate (PIP2) to produce inositol trisphosphate (IP3) and diacylglycerol (DAG). Consequently, intracellular calcium ions (Ca^{2+}) are elevated, activating of protein kinase C (PKC). Gα12/13 plays a key role in modulating actin cytoskeleton dynamics through its interaction with Rho guanine nucleotide exchange factors (RhoGEFs). G protein–mediated GPCR signaling, through these pathways, regulates a wide range of cellular processes and functions, including metabolism, gene expression, cell growth, differentiation, and migration.

β-arrestin–mediated signaling represents a distinct and versatile branch of GPCR signaling that extends beyond the traditional role of β-arrestins in receptor desensitization and internalization (Jean-Charles et al. 2017; Lefkowitz 2000, 2007, 2013; Whalen et al. 2011; Lefkowitz and Shenoy 2005; Shukla et al. 2011; Xiao et al. 2007; Xiao and Sun 2018). Ligand binding activates GPCRs, triggering phosphorylation by G protein–coupled receptor kinases (GRKs) and recruitment of β-arrestins. β-arrestins not only terminate G protein signaling but also initiate distinct G protein–independent signaling cascades. They act as scaffolding proteins by facilitating the assembly of multi-protein signaling complexes. These complexes activate key pathways such as ERK1/2, JNK, p38 MAPK, and AKT. Such activation leads to a variety of cellular responses including proliferation, survival, apoptosis, migration, and inflammation (Xiao et al. 2007; Xiao and Sun 2018; Zhao and Xiao 2019). This signaling arm is spatially and temporally distinct from G protein signaling, often

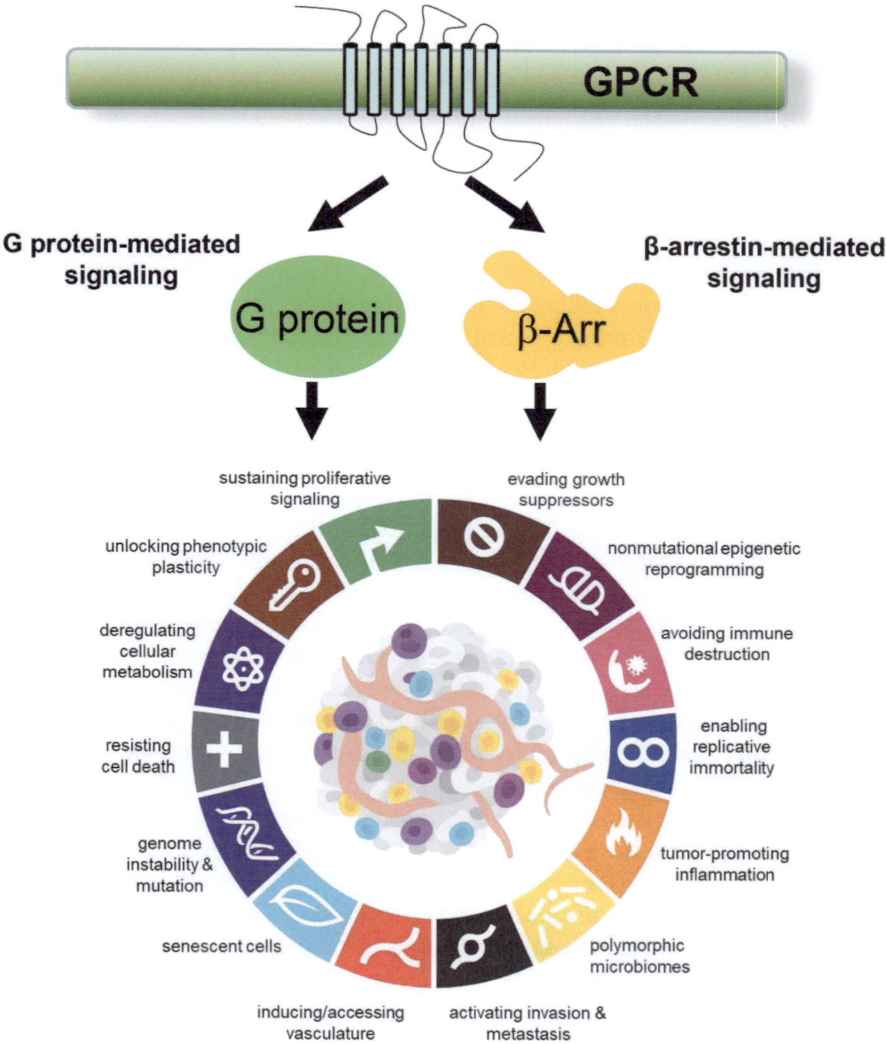

Fig. 1 GPCR biased signaling in cancer. The top section illustrates that GPCRs can activate two parallel mechanistically distinct intracellular signaling pathways: one mediated by heterotrimeric G proteins and the other by β-arrestins (Wisler et al. 2014; Lefkowitz and Shenoy 2005). These pathways can differentially regulate cellular responses and contribute to cancer initiation growth, progression, and metastasis. The bottom section presents the current framework of cancer hallmarks, incorporating both the original and emerging hallmarks. This illustration is adapted from the 2022 update (Hanahan 2022) to the cancer hallmark model, which expands upon the foundational concepts introduced in 2000 and revised in 2011, incorporating new insights gained through advances in cancer biology

occurring at endosomes rather than at the plasma membrane (Gidon et al. 2016). The discovery of β-arrestin–biased ligands, which preferentially activate β-arrestin–mediated pathways while minimizing G protein activation, has opened new avenues for targeted drug development, particularly in diseases such as cancer, cardiovascular disorders, and neurological conditions. β-arrestin–mediated signaling has been implicated in processes such as tumor growth, metastasis, angiogenesis, and therapy resistance in cancer, highlighting its significance as both a biomarker and a therapeutic target.

It is now well established that GPCRs can signal through either pathway independently, a phenomenon referred to as biased agonism, biased signaling, or functional selectivity. In G protein–biased signaling, the receptor selectively engages certain G protein subtypes, triggering second messenger pathways. For example, Gαs stimulates cAMP production, Gαi/o inhibits cAMP production, and Gαq/11 stimulates IP3 formation. In contrast, β-arrestin–biased signaling is characterized by β-arrestins functioning as scaffold proteins that bind to activated, phosphorylated receptors and facilitate the recruitment and organization of signaling complexes, including ERK1/2, JNK, AKT, and c-Src. This pathway-selective engagement allows for fine-tuned regulation of diverse cellular responses, such as proliferation, apoptosis, migration, and inflammation, depending on the signaling context. As a result, biased GPCR ligands that selectively activate G protein- or β-arrestin-mediated pathways are being actively investigated as next-generation therapeutics, offering the potential to enhance efficacy while minimizing adverse effects.

Cancer hallmarks refer to the fundamental biological traits that cancer cells acquire during their development and progression. The concept was originally introduced in a landmark paper published in 2000 that proposed six “hallmarks of cancer”: enabling replicative immortality, evading growth suppressors, sustaining proliferative signaling, resisting cell death, inducing angiogenesis and activating invasion and metastasis (Hanahan and Weinberg 2000). Updates in 2011 and 2022 expanded the original hallmarks of cancer to include additional ones, enabling characteristics and emerging concepts, such as reprogramming of energy metabolism, evasion of immune destruction, unlocking phenotypic plasticity (e.g., epithelial-mesenchymal transition, acquisition of stem-like traits), nonmutational epigenetic reprogramming, polymorphic microbiomes, senescent cells, tumor-promoting inflammation, and genomic instability (Fig. 1, bottom) (Hanahan 2022; Hanahan and Weinberg 2011). Together, these features define the common capabilities that cells acquire to become malignant and provide a unifying framework to understand cancer biology and guide therapeutic development.

Recent discoveries in GPCR biased signaling, in which receptors selectively activate either G protein-dependent or β-arrestin-dependent pathways, have revealed distinct and nuanced contributions to specific cancer hallmarks (Fig. 1). For example, it was reported that, in uveal melanoma, the Gαq-mediated signaling activates the guanine nucleotide exchange factor (GEF), Trio, and its regulated Rho GTPase signaling facilitates tumorigenesis through the activation of mitogen-activated protein kinase (MAPK) and the transcriptional co-activator yes-associated protein (YAP) pathways, rather than depending solely on the stimulation of the better known PLC-β and PKC pathway (O'Hayre et al. 2014; Vaque et al. 2013). In solid tumors such as prostate cancer, breast cancer, and glioblastoma, Gα12/13-mediated signaling was found to enhance invasion and metastasis via Rho GTPase activation (Rasheed et al. 2022). Additionally, Gαi/o-coupled GPCRs contribute to tumor progression in prostate and ovarian cancers through activation of the PI3K/AKT and other pro-survival pathways (Arang and Gutkind 2020). These pathways not only support tumor cell-intrinsic functions, but also shape the tumor microenvironment to facilitate immune evasion and angiogenesis. Similarly, β-arrestin-mediated signaling is widely reported to drive oncogenic processes, including cell proliferation, survival, migration, and angiogenesis. In addition, signaling through β-arrestins has been shown to influence immune evasion, chronic inflammation, and metabolic reprogramming within the tumor microenvironment. These findings emphasize the central role of GPCRs in cancer development and progression. Biased signaling offers a promising strategy for selectively targeting key hallmark pathways in cancer therapy, potentially enhancing therapeutic precision and reducing side effects.

3 Cell Type–Specific Roles of β-arrestin Biased Signaling in Cancer

In cancer, β-arrestin biased signaling plays multifaceted roles within malignant cells and across diverse stromal and immune cell populations that constitute the TME (Table 2). In this section, we will discuss the roles of β-arrestin biased signaling in different cell types involved in cancer.

3.1 Cancer Cells

In malignant cells, β-arrestin-mediated signaling contributes to several hallmark features of cancer. Many tumors exhibit upregulation or constitutive activation of GPCRs and their downstream effectors, including β-arrestins and GRKs (Bagnato and Rosano 2019; Shukla and Dwivedi-Agnihotri 2020; Sobolesky and Moussa 2013a; Song et al. 2018; Yu et al. 2018; Sun et al. 2018; Jiang et al. 2018; Gao et al.

Table 2 The roles β-arrestin-biased signaling by cell type

Cell type	Key GPCR functions in cancer
Cancer cells	Proliferation, EMT, metastasis, metabolism, drug resistance
T cells	Immune suppression (A2AR), trafficking (CCR7, CXCR3)
Tregs	Recruitment (CCR4), suppression enhancement
Myeloid cells	Infiltration (CCR2, CXCR2), M2 polarization, T cell suppression
Fibroblasts (CAFs)	Activation (LPA, endothelin receptors), ECM remodeling
Endothelial cells	Angiogenesis (S1P1, CXCR2), vascular remodeling
Neurons/glia	Tumor innervation, neurotransmitter effects (β-adrenergic, muscarinic)
Adipose/endocrine	Hormonal influence (GPER, TSHR), metabolic support

2025). These pathways drive cancer cell proliferation by activating key oncogenic signaling cascades, such as MAPK, PI3K/AKT, and YAP/TAZ pathways. Some GPCRs, such as LPAR, protease-activated receptor 1 (PAR1), and sphingosine-1-phosphate receptor (S1PR), contribute to cancer progression by facilitating epithelial–mesenchymal transition, enhancing cell migration, and promoting invasive behavior. Similarly, chemokine receptors, such as CXCR4 and CCR7, play key roles in guiding metastatic dissemination to distant organs. β-arrestin-mediated biased signaling is an increasingly recognized modulator of these processes, functioning independently of classical G protein pathways. In addition, β-arrestin-mediated biased signaling also modulates cancer cell metabolism and confers resistance to chemotherapy by activating anti-apoptotic and stress adaptation programs (Yu et al. 2022; Song et al. 2018; Ryu et al. 2023; Ahn et al. 2009; Zhan et al. 2016).

3.2 T Cells and Regulatory T Cells (Tregs)

T cells, including cytotoxic and helper subsets, are essential components of the adaptive immune system, responsible for recognizing and eliminating cancerous cells (Ahmed et al. 2023; Chen et al. 2023). In cancer, Tregs can suppress anti-tumor immune responses, allowing tumors to evade the immune surveillance and proliferate unchecked (Chaudhary and Elkord 2016; Ge et al. 2019). Chemokine receptors such as CXCR3 and CCR7, together with β-arrestins, regulate T cell trafficking and localization within the TME (Wang et al. 2022; Hahn et al. 2025; Strazza and Mor 2017; Moreno Ayala et al. 2023; Maekawa et al. 2008). β-arrestin 2 has been shown to mediate the chemotactic responses of T cells to chemokines like CXCL12, influencing their ability to home to and infiltrate tumors (Jiang et al. 2013). While β-arrestins may be involved in regulating T cell activation, their precise function may vary depending on the inflammatory context (Fan 2014). β-arrestin 1 has been reported to epigenetically regulate the expression of *BCL2*, a protein crucial for CD4+ T cell survival and homeostasis (Shi et al. 2007). Overexpression of β-arrestin 1 promotes T cell proliferation and interferon production, while concurrently suppressing NF-κB and AP-1 activity. This is accompanied by modulation of histone H4 acetylation, promoting acetylation at the promoter regions of CD40L, LIGHT, IL-17, and interferon-γ, and reducing acetylation at the promoters of TRAIL, Apo2, and HDAC7A, thereby regulating the expression of these immune-related genes (Hu et al. 2011). β-arrestins can furthermore enhance Tregs function and contribute to Treg-mediated immunosuppression within the TME, thereby promoting cancer progression (Song et al. 2018; Scott et al. 2021; Nakai et al. 2019). Tregs are recruited through CCR4–CCL22 interactions and can be functionally potentiated by β-arrestin-dependent signaling, further facilitating immune evasion by the tumor (Rapp et al. 2019; Zhang et al. 2024a; Ajram et al. 2014; Gobert et al. 2009).

3.3 Myeloid Cells (Macrophages, Myeloid-Derived Suppressor Cells (MDSCs), Neutrophils)

β-arrestin-mediated signaling also plays an important role in regulating the recruitment, polarization, and function of tumor-associated myeloid cells, including macrophages, MDSCs, and neutrophils (Fan 2014). For example, chemokine CCL2 (also known as MCP-1) binds to CCR2 on monocytes and macrophages, forming a CCR2/β-arrestin/GRK2 signaling complex that promotes chemotaxis (Adams et al. 2018; Jiang et al. 2013). Similarly, CCL4 binding to CCR5 induces membrane translocation of β-arrestins together with phosphoinositide 3-kinase (PI3K) and Pyk2, forming a multi-kinase signaling complex essential for macrophage migration (Cheung et al. 2009). Activation of protease-activated receptor 2 (PAR2) enhances β-arrestin- and ERK1/2-dependent regulation of actin cytoskeleton reorganization in macrophages. This process facilitates the extension of polarized pseudopodia, thereby promoting directed macrophage chemotaxis (Jiang et al. 2013; Ge et al. 2003; Xu et al. 2024). In neutrophils, β-arrestins, together with CXCR2, regulate IL-8-induced immune cell signaling and migration, contributing to their recruitment and functional responses in the TME (Barlic et al. 1999; Su et al. 2005; Fan 2014).

3.4 Cancer-Associated Fibroblasts (CAFs)

Overexpression of β-arrestin in CAFs is associated with tumor progression and poor prognosis in certain cancers, underscoring their role in tumorigenesis (Rosano and Bagnato 2016; Asif et al. 2021; Yan et al. 2015; Yin et al. 2024; Zhang et al. 2022). β-arrestin 1 promotes CAF migration and invasion by being activated by chemokines such as CXCL12 and CXCL14 (Suvarna et al. 2018). This pro-invasive effect is mediated through the interaction between β-arrestin 1 and cofilin, an actin filament-serving protein, facilitating the formation of membrane protrusions required for cellular invasion (Suvarna et al. 2018; Lovgren et al. 2011). β-arrestin 1 also bolsters CAF-dependent invadosome activity and increases the metastatic potential of cancer cells through the endothelin-1 (ET-1) signaling pathway (Del Rio et al. 2024; Tocci et al. 2021). β-arrestin 2 may have inhibitory effects by promoting degradation of unstimulated receptors, thereby potentially attenuating CAF activity and limiting tumor progression (Suleymanova et al. 2017). β-arrestins have also been implicated in regulating ECM remodeling by CAFs, further influencing tumor cell behavior and metastasis (Shah et al. 2022).

3.5 Endothelial Cells

β-arrestin-mediated signaling plays a critical role in endothelial cell function, regulating multiple key processes. Such processes include nitric oxide (NO) production, cell adhesion, and responses to various stimuli like shear stress and bacterial infection, collectively influencing vascular biology and angiogenesis (Romagnani et al. 2001; Lee and Blobe 2007; Zhang and He 2019; Lee et al. 2020). β-arrestins modulate signaling cascades of a number of GPCRs essential for endothelial cell function, such as chemokine receptors and receptors for vasoactive molecules such as endothelin-1, angiotensin II, and prostaglandins, thereby influencing vasodilation, cell migration, and immune responses (Lee et al. 2020). Tumor-associated endothelial cells (TECs), while not malignant themselves, are integral to cancer progression by facilitating tumor growth and metastasis. TECs exploit chemokine receptors, particularly ACKR1, CXCR4, CXCR7, and CCR2, to promote angiogenesis and tumor advancement (Salazar and Zabel 2019). Consequently, β-arrestin-mediated signaling represents a promising therapeutic target to disrupt tumor vascular support and inhibit cancer progression. Additionally, elevated expression of the orphan adhesion GPCR ADGRL4/ELTD1 enhances endothelial sprouting angiogenesis without activating canonical GPCR pathways, suggesting it regulates the endothelial tip-cell phenotype via non-canonical and yet-to-be-elucidated mechanisms (Favara et al. 2021). GPCRs broadly mediate tumor-induced angiogenesis by transducing signals from pro-angiogenic factors, like thrombin, prostaglandins, S1P, and chemokines. These factors stimulate endothelial proliferation, migration, and sprouting, as well as recruit immune cells that further potentiate vascular growth through secretion of VEGF and other signaling molecules (Wu et al. 2019). Endothelial cell-derived S1P promotes colorectal cancer cell migration and stemness by binding to GPR63 and activating the Src-JAK2/STAT3 signaling axis, revealing a novel mechanism driving metastasis (Zeng et al. 2022). Inflammatory cytokines, chemokines, and vasoactive factors activate endothelial cells through pathways including NFκB, JAK/STAT, and MAPK, leading to endothelial barrier disruption, immune cell recruitment, and tissue repair (Birch et al. 2021). These processes are often mediated via GPCRs, indicating that β-arrestin-mediated signaling likely plays an important role. Moreover, β-arrestins are essential for shear stress-induced NO production through their interaction with AKT and endothelial nitric oxide synthase (eNOS) in human vascular endothelial cells (Carneiro et al. 2017).

3.6 Neurons and Glia

Recent studies have underscored the crucial role of the neuro-immune–tumor axis in cancer development, progression, and treatment response (Pu et al. 2025; Huang et al. 2025; Yaman et al. 2022). This neuroimmune-tumor axis is comprised of a complex network of interactions among the nervous system, the immune system, and cancer cells with the TME. β-arrestin-mediated signaling downstream of neurotransmitter receptors, such as β-adrenergic and muscarinic GPCRs, has been implicated in modulating tumor cell growth and metastasis, especially in breast, pancreatic, and prostate cancers (Song et al. 2018). For instance, β-adrenergic signaling has been linked to the progression of pancreatic adenocarcinoma, and evidence suggests that beta-blockers may offer therapeutic benefits in managing this cancer type (Upadhyaya et al. 2020; Renz et al. 2018). Activation of β-adrenergic receptor, likely through β-arrestin-mediated pathways, can stimulate proliferation and migration in pancreatic cancer cells. Moreover, stress-induced activation of β-adrenergic receptors on both tumor and immune cells may exacerbate immune suppression and facilitate disease dissemination (Cole and Sood 2012; Zhang et al. 2020a).

3.7 Adipocytes and Endocrine Cells

β-arrestin-mediated signaling via GPCRs may play a pivotal role in integrating hormonal and metabolic cues that influence cancer development and progression (Oliveira de Souza et al. 2021; Husted et al. 2017). In epithelial ovarian cancer (EOC), adipocyte-derived free fatty acids (FFAs) promote tumor growth by serving as a key metabolic fuel to meet the heightened energy demands of cancer cells (Munkarah et al. 2016). This effect may be partially mediated through the free fatty acid receptor FFAR1 (also known as GPR40). In addition, receptors for endocrine hormones, such as GPER for estrogen and TSHR for thyroid-stimulating hormone, serve as key links between energy metabolism, hormonal regulation, and the development and progression of cancer (Belfiore and Perks 2013; Molina Calistro et al. 2025; Chu and Yeh 2020; Tirado-Garibay et al. 2023; Xu et al. 2025). Together, these GPCRs represent a mechanistic interface between metabolic and hormonal signaling pathways that drive cancer biology and offer promising targets for therapeutic intervention.

4 Roles of β-arrestin–Mediated Signaling in Cancer Initiation, Progression, and Metastasis

Recent studies have highlighted the pivotal role of β-arrestin-mediated signaling in virtually all stage of cancer development, including initiation, progression, and metastasis (Bagnato and Rosano 2019; Crudden et al. 2019; Sobolesky and Moussa 2013b; Tocci et al. 2019; Shukla and Dwivedi-Agnihotri 2020; Kaparianos et al. 2012; Wang et al. 2012). In addition to their traditional functions in GPCR desensitization and trafficking, β-arrestins participate in key cellular processes such as cell cycle regulation, migration, and apoptotic signaling. In vitro studies suggest that β-arrestins promote cancer cell proliferation, motility, and survival by acting as scaffolds for cytoplasmic signaling complexes, and, in some cases, by translocating to the nucleus to regulate gene transcription directly. In vivo, altered β-arrestin expression has been shown to influence tumor initiation, growth kinetics, angiogenesis, hypoxic survival, invasiveness, and metastatic potential. Data from patients with various tumors, such as breast, lung, prostate, brain, and hematologic cancers, have shown that abnormal β-arrestin expression, localization, or phosphorylation is associated with increased tumor aggressiveness and poorer clinical outcomes (Sobolesky and Moussa 2013a). With advance in our understanding of β-arrestin–mediated signaling, it has become evident that these pathways are pleotropic, activating specific downstream effectors in a tumor type- and context-specific manner. β-arrestin expression is tightly regulated at both transcriptional and post-transcriptional levels, many of which are frequently altered in cancer. As β-arrestins are increasingly recognized as central modulators of oncologic signaling, the development of context-specific approaches to target β-arrestin-mediated pathways is emerging as a new strategy to improve therapeutic outcomes in various cancers. Notably, the ability of β-arrestins to recruit multiple signaling proteins enables the formation of distinct β-arrestin–dependent signaling complexes or "signalosomes," which triggers unique downstream signaling cascades and networks (Fig. 2). The following sections will explore how β-arrestin-mediated signaling contributes to several major hallmarks of cancer.

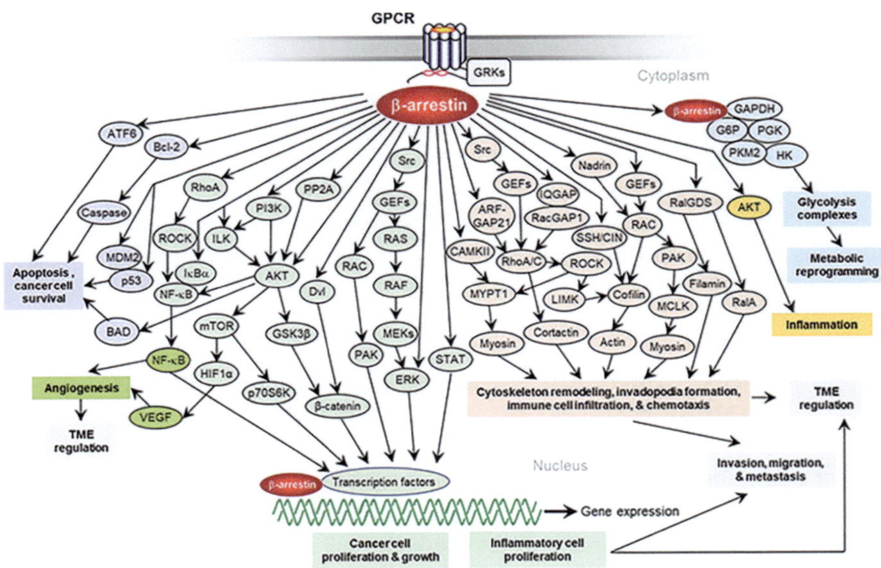

Fig. 2 The role of β-arrestin–mediated signaling in cancer growth, progression, invasion, and metastasis. In β-arrestin–mediated signaling, β-arrestins act as scaffolding proteins that recruit various signaling molecules to form multi-protein complexes, often referred to as "signalsomes." These complexes initiate distinct intracellular signaling cascades independent of G protein activation. In the context of cancer, β-arrestin–mediated pathways play critical roles in regulating multiple biological processes that contribute to tumor development and progression. These include promoting the proliferation of cancer and inflammatory cells (light green), remodeling the cytoskeleton, invadopodia formation, immune cell infiltration, and chemotaxis (light pink), regulating apoptosis and enhancing cancer cell survival (light purple), driving angiogenesis (bright green), modulating inflammatory responses (yellow), and altering cellular metabolism through metabolic reprogramming (light blue). Together, these β-arrestin–dependent mechanisms contribute to the hallmarks of cancer, including sustained proliferation, invasion, metastasis, immune evasion, and tumor-promoting inflammation

4.1 β-arrestin–Mediated Cytoskeletal Rearrangement, Cell Migration, Invasion, and Metastasis

One of the most well-established roles of β-arrestin–mediated signaling in cancer is its ability to regulate cytoskeletal dynamics and reorganization, promoting cell migration, invasion, and metastasis (Bagnato and Rosano 2019; Song et al. 2018; Rosano and Bagnato 2016; Rosanò and Bagnato 2019; Xiao et al. 2010; Barnes et al. 2005; Hunton et al. 2005; Fong et al. 2002; DeFea 2007; McGovern and DeFea 2014). β-arrestin–driven cytoskeletal reorganization is a central mechanism underlying the migratory and invasive behaviors of both cancer and immune cells (Table 3). β-arrestin–mediated signaling promotes invasive growth and metastasis in cancer cells. In immune cells, this biased GPCR signaling modulates chemotaxis and contributes to anti-tumor immune responses within the TME. β-arrestin–mediated signaling serves a dual role by regulating tumor cell migration and invasion, along with modulating immune cell function. Targeting β-arrestin–dependent pathways may offer novel strategies for controlling cancer progression and enhancing immune surveillance and anti-tumor immunity.

In particular, β-arrestin–mediated signaling, independent of G protein activation, plays a central role in orchestrating these cytoskeletal rearrangements by serving as scaffolds for various intracellular signaling molecules (Xiao et al. 2007, 2010). These include Src family kinases, guanine nucleotide exchange factors (GEFs), Ral guanine nucleotide dissociation stimulator (RalGDS), IQ motif–containing GTPase-activating protein (IQGAP), ADP-ribosylation factor GTPase-activating protein 21 (ARF-GAP21), Calcium/calmodulin-dependent protein kinase II (CAMKII), and Nadrin. Together, these molecules modulate signaling pathways that govern actin dynamics (Fig. 2, light pink section) (Xiao et al. 2007, 2010; Bhattacharya et al. 2002; Szenasi et al. 2023; Rosanò and Bagnato 2019; Bagnato and Rosano 2019). Through these interactions, β-arrestins assemble unique signalosomes, which facilitates the activation or inhibition of downstream effectors that regulate the organization and remodeling of cytoskeletal components such as myosin, actin, cortactin, and Ras-related protein Ral-A (RalA). This leads to β-arrestin–dependent cytoskeletal rearrangements that are essential for the formation of dynamic cellular protrusions, such as lamellipodia, filopodia, invadopodia, and

Table 3 β-arrestin–mediated cytoskeletal reorganization in cancer vs. immune cells

Cell type	Role in cancer	Key chemoattractants
Cancer Cells	Migrate toward *growth factors (EGF, HGF)* Escape hypoxia via *CXCL12/CXCR4* Metastasize to lymph nodes (CCL21)	EGF, HGF, CXCL12, CCL2, Lysophosphatidic acid (LPA)
Immune Cells	*T cells/NK cells* track CCL5, CXCL9/10 (from tumors) *Macrophages* follow CSF-1, CCL2 (tumor-recruited TAMs) *Neutrophils* respond to IL-8, CXCL1/2	CXCL9/10/11 (T cell attractants), CSF-1, CCL2, IL-8

Table 4 Immune vs. cancer cell protrusions & chemotaxis

Feature	Cancer cells	Immune cells
Lamellipodia	Motility & invasion	T cell migration, DC scanning
Filopodia	ECM sensing, metastasis	Immune synapse (CTLs), neutrophil navigation
Invadopodia	ECM degradation (MMPs)	Macrophage podosomes (rare)

podosomes, which enable cancer cell motility and invasion (Table 4) (Pratiwi et al. 2024; Machesky 2008; Yamaguchi and Condeelis 2007; Alblazi and Siar 2015). For instance, in non-small cell lung cancer (NSCLC) cell lines, β-arrestin 1 promotes the expression of mesenchymal markers vimentin and fibronectin, as well as EMT regulators zinc finger E-box-binding homeobox 1 (ZEB1) and zinc finger E-box-binding homeobox 2 (ZEB2), thereby modulating NSCLC growth and metastasis (Pillai et al. 2015). In hepatocellular carcinoma (HCC), β-arrestin 2 expression is significantly reduced in malignant cells compared to normal tissues, while β-arrestin 1 levels remain largely unchanged. Overexpression of β-arrestin 2 in HCC cell lines upregulates E-cadherin, downregulates vimentin, and inhibits AKT activation, ultimately suppressing cell migration and invasion (Sun et al. 2016a, b). Meanwhile, β-arrestin 1 contributes to HCC metastasis through ERK-mediated epithelial–mesenchymal transition (EMT), suggesting that modulating β-arrestin signaling could be a promising therapeutic approach for HCC (Xu et al. 2020). In breast cancer, the recruitment of β-arrestins to PAR2 directly activates ERK at the pseudopodia of migrating cells and promotes cancer cell migration through the cofilin pathway. The cofilin pathway is a key regulator of actin remodeling and cytoskeleton reorganization (Ge et al. 2004; Zoudilova et al. 2007; Ruf et al. 2010). In addition, PAR2-mediated chemotaxis in MDA-MB 231 breast cancer cell line is impaired in the absence of both β-arrestins 1 and 2, highlighting their essential roles in the chemotactic response of non-immune cells with implications in cancer progression (Ge et al. 2004). In colorectal cancer, β-arrestin 1 has been shown to regulate the migration of colorectal carcinoma cells in vitro and to promote liver metastasis in vivo (Buchanan et al. 2006). Mechanistically, this involves the formation of β-arrestin 1-dependent signalosomes with prostaglandin E receptor 4 and c-Src, leading to EGFR transactivation and activation of downstream AKT signaling pathways.

Lamellipodia are broad, sheet-like, actin-rich protrusions at the leading edge of migrating cells that push the plasma membrane forward, driving migration and enabling cancer cells to infiltrate surrounding tissues (Machesky 2008). Filopodia are slender, finger-like projections that extend from the lamellipodium or cell body and serve as sensory structures to probe the ECM and guide directional movement, both of which are critical steps in metastasis. In contrast, invadopodia and podosomes are dot-like, actin-rich structures that form on the ventral surface of invasive cells (Alblazi and Siar 2015). Unlike lamellipodia and filopodia, which are primarily involved in motility, invadopodia and podosomes are enriched with matrix metalloproteinases (MMPs), including MMP-2, MMP-9, and MT1-MMP, all of which facilitate ECM degradation. The formation of invadopodia and podosomes enables cancer cells to breach basement membranes and invade adjacent tissues, key events in local invasion and metastasis.

β-arrestin–mediated cytoskeletal remodeling also plays a vital role in immune cell function within the TME (Jiang et al. 2013; Sharma and Parameswaran 2015; Fan 2014; Nguyen et al. 2020; Sobolesky and Moussa 2013a). Immune cell migration and infiltration rely on similar mechanisms of actin reorganization. In response to chemotactic cues, β-arrestins promote lamellipodia formation in T cells, NK cells, dendritic cells (DCs), and macrophages, enhancing their motility and tissue surveillance. Extended lamellipodia enable T cells and natural killer (NK) cells to chase and infiltrate tumors, while DCs use them to migrate toward lymph nodes for antigen presentation. Tumor-associated macrophages (TAMs) modulate their lamellipodial activity to adopt either pro-tumor (M2) or anti-tumor (M1) phenotypes, depending on environmental cues. Filopodia in immune cells act as fine-tuned environmental sensory structures. Cytotoxic T lymphocytes (CTLs), for instance, use filopodia to establish immune synapses with cancer cells, guiding precise and targeted cytotoxic responses. Neutrophils extend filopodia to migrate toward hypoxic tumor regions, while Tregs use filopodia to engage with and suppress effector immune responses in tumors. Although invadopodia and podosomes are more commonly associated with cancer cells, certain immune cells can form similar structures for ECM degradation and tissue infiltration. For example, macrophages generate podosomes to breach tissue barriers and infiltrate tumors, and neutrophils may form invadopodia-like structures to traverse basement membranes during inflammatory responses or metastasis facilitation.

Cyclooxygenase 2 (COX-2) and COX-2 product prostaglandin E2 (PGE2) have been implicated in all stages of tumorigenesis (Luttrell et al. 1999; Krysan et al. 2005; Zhang et al. 2009; Alaa et al. 2009; Zhu et al. 2008). PGE2 promotes lung cancer cell migration by activating the EP4 receptor, which engages β-arrestin 1 and c-Src to drive downstream signaling. Knockdown of EP4 or β-arrestin 1 significantly impairs PGE2-induced c-Src activation and cell migration in A549 lung cancer cells (Kim et al. 2010). These findings highlight the EP4–β-arrestin 1–c-Src signaling axis as a potential therapeutic target for managing advanced lung cancer.

4.2 β-arrestin–Mediated Transcriptional Regulation, Uncontrolled Proliferation, Tumor Initiation, and Progression ("Growth Turned On")

In normal tissues, transcription and cell proliferation are tightly regulated by growth factors, cell cycle checkpoints, and contact inhibition (Zhang et al. 2024b; Dhanasekaran et al. 2022; Feitelson et al. 2015). β-arrestin–mediated signaling plays a pivotal role in modulating these processes in a manner that is both cell type- and receptor context-dependent (Ma and Pei 2007; Jean-Charles et al. 2017). Upon ligand binding and receptor activation, GPCRs are phosphorylated by GRKs, which promotes the recruitment of β-arrestins to the activated and phosphorylated receptors. Once engaged, β-arrestins act as multifunctional scaffolding proteins, interacting with multiple intracellular signaling molecules to assemble distinct signalosomes that initiate non-canonical signaling cascades. This ultimately leads to transcriptional activation and cell proliferation (Fig. 2, light green section). These signaling cascades vary depending on the cellular and receptor context and can involve the activation of non-canonical effectors such as Src family kinases, PI3K, RhoA, and Dishevelled (Dvl). Through these pathways, β-arrestins can activate or inhibit downstream effectors, such as extracellular signal-regulated kinases (ERK), p21-activated kinases (PAK), nuclear factor kappa B (NF-κB), p70 ribosomal S6 kinase (p70S6K), β-catenin, and signal transducer and activator of transcription proteins (STATs) (Ma and Pei 2007; Xiao et al. 2007; Xiao et al. 2010; Kim et al. 2023). These downstream events collectively influence cell proliferation, survival, and differentiation.

In certain contexts, β-arrestins, particularly β-arrestin 1, can translocate into the nucleus and directly bind to various transcriptional regulators and epigenetic modulation enzymes to modulate gene expression (Ma and Pei 2007; Kang et al. 2005; Beaulieu and Caron 2005; Xiao et al. 2007). Within the nucleus, β-arrestin 1 binds to histone acetyltransferases (HATs) such as p300 and the polycomb group (PcG) protein EZH2, promoting local histone H4 acetylation and chromatin remodeling (Kang et al. 2005; Beaulieu and Caron 2005). β-arrestin 1 also interacts with peroxisome proliferator-activated receptor gamma (PPARγ), inhibiting PPARγ–retinoid X receptor alpha (RXRα)-dependent gene transcription (Zhuang et al. 2011; Wang et al. 2016). Additionally, β-arrestin 1 sequesters the transcriptional repressor Yin Yang 1 (YY1), alleviating PcG-mediated repression of cdx4-hox gene transcription (Yue et al. 2009). It associates with β-catenin to enhance TCF/LEF-dependent transcription and acts as a scaffold for TC45-mediated dephosphorylation of STAT1, ultimately suppressing interferon-γ signaling (Mo et al. 2008; Sun et al. 2016a, b; Pelzel et al. 2013). β-arrestin 1 also binds to E2F1 to enhance its transcriptional activity and promote transcription of genes such as *p27*, *c-fos*, and *BCL2*, further supporting cell proliferation (Pillai et al. 2015; Abballe et al. 2023).

In cancer, regulation of transcription and proliferation is often disrupted due to mutations in oncogenes (e.g., *KRAS*, *MYC*) or loss of tumor suppressor genes (e.g., *TP53*, *RB1*), resulting in uncontrolled proliferation and tumor formation. β-arrestin–mediated signaling can significantly contribute to this dysregulation and oncogenic transformation by hijacking transcriptional machinery to modulate gene expression and promote oncogenic cellular behaviors. Aberrant β-arrestin activity has been implicated in various malignancies, correlating with uncontrolled proliferation, tumor initiation, and disease progression (Hu et al. 2013; Bostanabad et al. 2021; Aamna et al. 2022; Eishingdrelo et al. 2014). As such, therapeutic strategies aimed at correcting or selectively targeting these aberrant β-arrestin–mediated pathways represent promising approaches for suppressing tumorigenesis and improving treatment outcomes.

For example, glioblastoma, the most common malignant brain tumor, often overexpresses the neurokinin-1 receptor (NK1R, a member of the tachykinin receptor family), making it a promising therapeutic target (Zhang et al. 2017). β-arrestin 1-mediated signaling is critical for NK1R-mediated glioblastoma cell proliferation by facilitating sustained ERK1/2 and AKT activation, which regulates CDC25C/CDK1/cyclin B1 activity and induces G2/M phase cell cycle arrest. In addition, β-arrestin 1 modulates the transcriptional activity of NF-κB and AP-1, both of which contribute to cyclin B1 expression. The knockdown of β-arrestin 1 disrupts these pathways, highlighting β-arrestin 1–mediated signaling as a potential therapeutic target in glioblastoma. In triple-negative breast cancer (TNBC) cell lines MDA-MB-231 and MDA-MB-468, both β-arrestin 1 and β-arrestin 2 are involved in regulating the cell cycle and proliferation through interactions with HER3, IGF-1R, and Snail (Bostanabad et al. 2021). Reducing β-arrestin 1 and β-arrestin 2 promotes TNBC cell proliferation and motility, while overexpression of β-arrestins suppresses these functions. Clinically, low β-arrestin 1 expression correlates with elevated levels of *CDC45*, *BUB1*, *CCNB1*, and *CCNB2*, and is associated with poor prognosis in breast cancer. This suggests that β-arrestins play a tumor-suppressive role by modulating cell cycle and proliferation.

As mentioned above, β-arrestin 1 can translocate to the nucleus, where it directly regulates gene expression by interacting with transcriptional regulators and epigenetic modulators. In gastric cancer, nuclear β-arrestin 1 binds to transcription factor E2F1, triggering the up-regulation of proliferative genes (Yu et al. 2022). In prostate cancer cells, nuclear β-arrestin1 promotes cancer cell growth by inhibiting the transcriptional activity and expression of FOXO3a both in vitro and in vivo (Kong et al. 2018; Habrowska-Gorczynska et al. 2021). In epithelial ovarian cancer cells, endothelin-1 (ET-1) activates NF-κB signaling through the endothelin A receptor (ETAR) in a β-arrestin 1–dependent manner. β-arrestin 1 is essential for ET-1–induced phosphorylation of NF-κB components and their transcriptional activity, acting as a scaffold and interacting with p65 in the nucleus and indicating a nuclear function of β-arrestin 1 in ETAR-driven NF-κB transcriptional activity in ovarian cancer (Cianfrocca et al. 2014). These findings underscore the dual role of β-arrestins as cytoplasmic signaling scaffolds and nuclear transcriptional regulators, highlighting their broad impact on gene expression programs that support tumor initiation and growth.

4.3 β-arrestin–Mediated Signaling in Regulating Apoptosis and Resisting Cell Death in Cancer (Death Turned Off)

Apoptosis, or programmed cell death, is a vital mechanism for eliminating damaged or unwanted cells. Cancer cells, however, often develop strategies to evade this process. β-arrestin–mediated GPCR signaling plays an important role in regulating apoptosis by converging on multiple apoptotic checkpoints, including Bcl-2-associated death promoter (BAD) inactivation, BCL2 stabilization, caspase inhibition, endoplasmic reticulum (ER) stress response via ATF6, NF-κB activation, and modulation of mitochondrial dynamics, collectively promoting cell survival (Fig. 2, light purple section) (Kook et al. 2014). Their role thus depends on the specific upstream trigger and cellular environment, making them either pro- or anti-apoptotic regulators. For example, β-arrestin 2 has been implicated in mediating anti-apoptotic signals through the activation of the ERK1/2-p90RSK and PI3K-AKT signaling pathways (Ahn et al. 2009). These pathways converge on the pro-apoptotic protein Bcl-2-associated death promoter (BAD), leading to its phosphorylation, inactivation, and sequestration in the cytosol by 14-3-3 proteins. BAD is a pro-apoptotic member of the Bcl-2 family, and its phosphorylation by survival factors can prevent its translocation to the mitochondria and interaction with anti-apoptotic proteins like Bcl-xL and Bcl-2, thereby inhibiting the mitochondrial pathway of apoptosis (Saddam et al. 2024). In this context, β-arrestin 2–dependent signaling is anti-apoptotic and acts cytoprotectively. However, in intestinal epithelial cells, β-arrestin 2 triggers apoptosis in response to endoplasmic reticulum stress and induces necrotizing enterocolitis (NEC) development by binding immunoglobulin protein (BiP) and promoting its polyubiquitination and degradation (Fu et al. 2019). In the glomerular endothelial cell (GENC), silencing of β-arrestin 2 prevents GENC apoptosis by inhibiting ATF6-mediated ER stress in vivo and in vitro (Liu et al. 2024a). During apoptosis triggered by various stimuli, caspases cleave β-arrestin 1 to generate a fragment, β-arrestin 1 (1–380), which translocates to the mitochondria and enhances cytochrome C release induced by tBID (a caspase-cleaved BID product (Kook et al. 2014). This β-arrestin 1 fragment selectively promotes the death of BID-expressing cells by facilitating mitochondrial cytochrome C release. More investigation is needed to elucidate the molecular mechanisms of β-arrestin–mediated GPCR signaling in cancer cells. However, current research in other cell types has revealed key aspects of this signaling pathway that may also operate in cancer cells.

For example, β-arrestin–mediated signaling has been shown to promote apoptosis in breast cancer (Wu et al. 2014). Specifically, β-arrestins facilitate c-Jun N-terminal kinase (JNK)-mediated apoptosis via recruiting JNK to the $GABA_B$ receptors and inducing its activation, as demonstrated in MCF-7 and T-47D breast cancer cells. Notably, β-arrestin expression is decreased in breast cancer cells compared to controls. However, increased expression of β-arrestin enhances the phosphorylation of JNK and induces apoptosis in cancer cells, suggesting that β-arrestin promotes JNK-mediated apoptosis via a $GABA_B$R-β-arrestin-JNK signaling module. In contrast, in diffuse-type tenosynovial giant cell tumor (TGCT), β-arrestin 2 is significantly upregulated and plays a key role in suppressing apoptosis of fibroblast-like synoviocytes (FLS). Functional studies revealed that β-arrestin 2 inhibits caspase-3–mediated apoptosis while promoting FLS proliferation by activating the PI3K-AKT survival pathway, highlighting its potential as a therapeutic target for limiting TGCT progression (Cao et al. 2021). Additionally, in inflammatory bowel disease, β-Arrestin2 has been implicated in promoting inflammation-induced epithelial apoptosis through activation of the endoplasmic reticulum stress/p53-upregulated modulator of apoptosis (PUMA) pathway (Zeng et al. 2015).

4.4 β-arrestin–Mediated Signaling in Tumor Angiogenesis

Angiogenesis is the formation of new blood vessels. It is tightly regulated by signaling pathways that modulate endothelial cell migration, growth, and differentiation (Haibe et al. 2020; Vasudev and Reynolds 2014; Nishida et al. 2006; Liu et al. 2023). As a hallmark of cancer, angiogenesis supplies tumors with nutrients and oxygen, supporting their growth and survival (Liu et al. 2023; Lugano et al. 2020; Olejarz et al. 2020). Tumor-driven angiogenesis also facilitates metastasis by creating vascular pathways, allowing cancer cells to enter the circulation. β-arrestins play a significant role in angiogenesis by functioning as scaffolding proteins that initiate noncanonical signaling cascades involved in vascular remodeling and endothelial cell function (Song et al. 2018; Bagnato and Rosano 2019). Through these pathways, β-arrestin–mediated signaling regulates the expression and activity of key pro-angiogenic factors such as vascular endothelial growth factor (VEGF) (Ghalehbandi et al. 2023), matrix metalloproteinases (MMPs) (Quintero-Fabian et al. 2019), and angiopoietins (Fagiani and Christofori 2013), thereby modulating endothelial cell proliferation, migration, and tube formation (Fig. 2, bright green section).

In vivo studies using β-arrestin 1 transgenic mice subcutaneously inoculated with liver cancer Hepa1-6 cells or lymphoma EL4 cells demonstrated accelerated tumor onset and growth compared to wild-type and β-arrestin 2 transgenic mice (Zou et al. 2008). These effects were linked to increased MMP9 activity, elevated VEGF concentration in plasma, and enhanced tumor angiogenesis. Pharmacologic inhibition of MMP9 or PI3K signaling abrogated these changes, underscoring their functional importance. Mechanistic studies further revealed that the C-terminal region of β-arrestin 1 (amino acids 181–418) mediates MMP9 activation and contributes to a tumor-promoting microenvironment. β-arrestin 1 has also been shown to interact with hypoxia-inducible factor-1α (HIF-1α), enhancing HIF-1-dependent transcription of the pro-angiogenic factor VEGF under hypoxic conditions commonly found in breast cancer (Shenoy et al. 2012). This β-arrestin 1- HIF-1α complex promotes breast cancer colonization and angiogenesis in nude mouse models, with elevated β-arrestin 1 levels correlating with increased VEGF expression. In breast carcinoma cells, anti-angiogenic agent thalidomide disrupts HIF-1-dependent VEGF transcription by inducing perinuclear mislocalization of HIF-1α and promoting the nuclear export of β-arrestin 1. Likewise, the tyrosine kinase inhibitor imatinib mesylate, known to inhibit VEGF release, also facilitates nuclear export of the β-arrestin1–HIF-1α complexes from the nucleus. These findings suggest that enhancing β-arrestin1 nuclear export may serve as a novel anti-angiogenic strategy, and targeting β-arrestin–mediated signaling could improve the efficacy of existing anti-angiogenic and immunotherapeutic treatments.

β-arrestin 2 has also been implicated in modulating lung cancer tumorigenesis by regulating angiogenesis through CXCR2 and NF-κB signaling pathways (Raghuwanshi et al. 2008). In a murine model of lung cancer, the loss of β-arrestin 2 resulted in enhanced NF-κB activity, reduced HIF-1α expression, and significantly greater tumor growth and metastasis of Lewis lung cancer compared to control mice.

These effects were associated with a decrease in tumor-infiltrating lymphocytes and an increase in ELR (+) chemokines (CXCL1/keratinocyte-derived chemokine and CXCL2/MIP-2), VEGF expression, and microvessel density, indicating enhanced tumor angiogenesis and immune evasion.

Beyond its roles in cancer, β-arrestin2 has also been reported to promote angiogenesis in liver sinusoidal endothelial cells through the VEGF/VEGFR2 pathway, contributing to the progression of cirrhosis (Gao et al. 2024a). In addition, β-arrestin 2-mediated signaling downstream of protease-activated receptor 1 (PAR-1) has been shown to play a pivotal role in activated protein C (APC)-induced angiogenesis and endothelial function in stroke models, acting through the β-arrestin 2-MAPK-PDGF-β signaling pathway (Kanki et al. 2019). The potential roles of these β-arrestin 2–mediated pathways in cancer-associated angiogenesis merits further investigation.

4.5 β-arrestin–Mediated Signaling in Metabolic Reprogramming

Metabolic reprogramming is a hallmark of cancer that enables tumor cells to alter their energy production and biosynthetic pathways to support rapid growth and metastatic plasticity (Ahn and Kaipparettu 2025; Navarro et al. 2022; Lin et al. 2022). This complex process involves increased aerobic glycolysis even in the presence of oxygen (the Warburg effect), enhanced lipid biosynthesis, and dysregulation in glutaminolysis and autophagy (Halbrook and Lyssiotis 2017). Many aggressive tumors adopt a hybrid metabolic phenotype, using both glycolysis and mitochondrial respiration to maximize metabolic flexibility.

β-arrestins have emerged as important regulators of metabolic processes (Zhao and Pei 2013). Studies using mouse models with selective deletion of β-arrestin 1 and/or 2 in metabolically relevant cell types have revealed their essential roles in maintaining key metabolic processes including whole-body glucose and energy homeostasis (Pydi et al. 2021; Wess 2022). β-arrestin-mediated signaling in cancer is increasingly acknowledged for its significant role in metabolic reprogramming by modulating energy production and nutrient utilization. In our previously β-arrestin interactome analyses, we identified over a dozen metabolic enzymes that interact with β-arrestins, suggesting a role in recruiting glycolytic enzymes to promote glycolysis under conditions of high energy demand (Fig. 2, light blue section) (Xiao et al. 2007). Recent studies have begun to substantiate this hypothesis. For example, pyruvate kinase M2 isoform (PKM2) and glyceraldehyde-3-phosphate dehydrogenase (GAPDH) were identified as β-arrestin binding partners (Xiao et al. 2007). Activation of G-protein coupled receptor 3 (GPR3) stimulates glycolytic activity through the formation of GPR3-β-arrestin2-GAPDH-PKM2 enzymatic super-complex in Kupffer cells (macrophages in liver), thereby protecting mice from obesity and fatty liver disease (Dong et al. 2024). In gastric cancer, cytoplasmic β-arrestin 1 was found to play a pivotal role in metabolic reprogramming by binding to PKM2 and inhibiting its tetramerization, suppressing its enzymatic activity and shifting cellular metabolism from oxidative phosphorylation to aerobic glycolysis (Yu et al. 2022). Notably, overexpression of β-arrestin 1 in gastric cancer tissues was associated with poor prognosis, suggesting that the β-arrestin 1–PKM2 axis represents a potential therapeutic target for exploiting metabolic vulnerabilities in gastric cancer.

In stem cell-like bladder cancer cells, β-arrestin 1 acts as a metabolic switch, promoting metabolic reprogramming toward glycolysis by downregulating mitochondrial pyruvate carrier 1 (MPC1) and upregulating glucose transporter 1 (GLUT1), thereby enhancing glucose uptake (Mamouni et al. 2021). Loss of β-arrestin 1 led to reduced glycolytic activity and induced a shift toward oxidative phosphorylation, while its reintroduction restored the glycolytic phenotype. These findings underscore the critical role of β-arrestin 1 in modulating cancer cell metabolism and highlight β-arrestin 1-mediated signaling as a therapeutic target for bladder cancer.

Beyond glycolysis, β-arrestin 1-mediated signaling has also been implicated in lactate metabolism (Dong et al. 2017). In astrocyte-derived U251 cells, β-arrestin 1 forms a ternary complex with phosphorylated mitogen-activated protein kinase (MAPK) and HIF-1α to upregulate the expression of monocarboxylate transporter 4 (MCT4) and lactate dehydrogenase A (LDHA), promoting lactate production. In liver macrophages of patients with metabolic dysfunction-associated steatohepatitis (MASH), β-arrestin 2 plays a key role in metabolic programming by promoting the ubiquitination and degradation of immune responsive gene 1 (IRG1) (Wei et al. 2024). This reduces itaconate production, enhances succinate dehydrogenase activity, and increases mitochondrial reactive oxygen species (ROS), thereby driving M1 macrophage polarization. Myeloid-specific deletion of β-arrestin 2 alleviates MASH in mice, revealing its potential as a therapeutic target through modulation of macrophage metabolism. Collectively, these findings underscore the emerging role of β-arrestins in orchestrating cell metabolism and immune metabolic responses. Further investigation is warranted to fully understand their potential as therapeutic targets in cancer-associated metabolic reprogramming.

4.6 β-arrestin–Mediated Signaling in Inflammation in Cancer

Tumor-promoting inflammation is a paradoxical process in which a protective immune response inadvertently nurtures cancer instead of eliminating it (Hanahan and Weinberg 2011; Hanahan 2022). Emerging evidence highlights the critical role of β-arrestins in regulating inflammatory responses, particularly through biased agonism at GPCRs (Fan 2014; Sharma and Parameswaran 2015; Li et al. 2011; Vroon et al. 2006; Gao et al. 2024b). β-arrestin-mediated signaling contributes to the recruitment of immune cells, like macrophages and neutrophils, the modulation of inflammatory factor release, the promotion of immune cell proliferation, and infiltration. By interacting with inflammation-associated GPCRs, such as CXCR2 and CXCR4, β-arrestins scaffold key inflammatory signaling pathways like MAPK, JAK/STAT, and NF-κB, leading to sustained production of pro-inflammatory cytokines (e.g., TNF-α, IL-6, IL-8), chemokines, and adhesion molecules (Crecelius et al. 2024).

β-arrestin–mediated signaling in cancer contributes to a tumor-supportive inflammatory milieu that favors tumorigenesis (Fig. 2, yellow section). For instance, β-arrestin 1 is upregulated in both inflammation-associated hepatocellular carcinoma (HCC) and adjacent tissues in humans (Yang et al. 2015). In a mouse model, exposure to the genotoxic carcinogen diethylnitrosamine (DEN) triggers hepatic inflammation, TNF-α production, and selective induction of β-arrestin 1. In addition, β-arrestin 1 deficiency suppresses DEN-induced hepatocellular tumorigenesis by inhibiting malignant proliferation in mice. Mechanistically, TNF-α upregulates hepatic β-arrestin 1 expression and promotes its interaction with AKT, enhancing AKT phosphorylation. These findings signal that β-arrestin 1 enhances hepatocellular tumorigenesis through inflammation-driven AKT signaling, making it a potential therapeutic target for HCC.

β-arrestin–mediated inflammation has been extensively studied in non-cancer disease models, offering mechanistic insights potentially translatable to oncology. For instance, metoprolol, a β-blocker, exerts anti-inflammatory effects in human cardiomyocytes via β-arrestin 2–biased agonism, suppressing TNF-α–induced NF-κB activation and downstream cytokines such as IL-1β and IL-6 (Ricci et al. 2023). This anti-inflammatory effect is lost in β-arrestin 2–silenced cells, underscoring the protein's regulatory role independent of classical β1-adrenergic blockade. Similarly, β-arrestin 2 promotes antiviral inflammation by enhancing cGAS–STING signaling and IFN-β production through increased dsDNA binding to cGAS, a process facilitated by Lys171 deacetylation (Zhang et al. 2020c). Viral degradation of β-arrestin 2 represents an immune evasion strategy, which can be counteracted by β-blockers like carvedilol, offering a potential avenue for anti-inflammatory or antiviral therapy. β-arrestin 2 also negatively regulates skin inflammation by limiting neutrophil-attracting chemokines such as CXCL1/KC in keratinocytes during contact hypersensitivity, as its deficiency leads to exaggerated neutrophilic inflammation (Gaffal et al. 2014). These studies suggest that β-arrestin–mediated inflammatory pathways may be relevant to tumor-promoting inflammation, though further research is needed to confirm their roles in cancer progression. For example, in inflammatory bowel disease (IBD), CCR5 expression is elevated and positively correlates with lymphocyte infiltration, while inversely correlating with β-arrestin 2 expression. Enhancing the interaction between β-arrestin 2 and CCR5 could reduce inflammatory cell recruitment, indicating a broader regulatory role for β-arrestin 2 in chemokine receptor signaling via biased agonism (Ye et al. 2017). Whether similar strategies can be used to modulate the tumor immune microenvironment remains to be determined.

β-arrestin 1 has also been implicated in T cell–mediated inflammation. It promotes CD4+ T cell survival by increasing Bcl2 expression via histone H4 acetylation and is associated with heightened autoimmunity when overexpressed (Shi et al. 2007). In autoreactive T cells, β-arrestin 1 enhances proliferation, IFN production, and histone modifications at inflammatory gene loci (Hu et al. 2011). Additionally, the CXCL12/high-mobility group box 1 (HMGB1) heterocomplex has emerged as a key player in sterile inflammation models, acting through CXCR4 in a β-arrestin-dependent manner (Schiraldi et al. 2012; D'Agostino et al. 2020). These findings highlight the therapeutic potential of targeting CXCR4-biased signaling to modulate inflammation. Notably, β-arrestin isoforms can exert opposing effects. In microglia, β-arrestin 1 promotes, while β-arrestin 2 suppresses, STAT1 and NF-κB pathway activation via differential regulation of Nprl3 (Fang et al. 2021). These contrasting roles underscore the complexity of β-arrestin–mediated signaling in inflammation. It remains an open question whether these pathways contribute to immune evasion in cancer, and further investigation is needed.

5 Future Prospects

The landscape of GPCR signaling is rapidly evolving, with biased signaling, particularly β-arrestin–biased signaling, emerging as a transformative concept in cancer biology. Once appreciated solely as terminators of GPCR activity through desensitization and internalization, β-arrestins (β-arrestin 1 and β-arrestin 2) are now recognized as dynamic scaffold proteins that orchestrate a wide range of intracellular signaling cascades. This scaffolding function has profound implications for how cells interpret extracellular cues and respond through proliferation, migration, survival, and immune modulation.

While accumulating evidence implicates β-arrestins in key oncogenic pathways, their functions appear highly context-dependent and occasionally contradictory. This duality underscores the complexity of β-arrestin–mediated signaling and highlights the need for deeper mechanistic studies. Their ability to regulate kinase activity, intracellular trafficking, and gene transcription positions β-arrestins as both potential biomarkers and therapeutic targets in oncology.

One of the major challenges in cancer drug development remains the management of unwanted side effects, including cardiotoxicity, neurotoxicity, gastrointestinal toxicity, immunosuppression, and off-target effects that can limit dosing, reduce patient quality of life, and compromise treatment efficacy (Lustberg et al. 2023; Kourek et al. 2022; Dietrich 2020; Brahmer et al. 2018). In this context, the emergence of biased GPCR ligands that selectively engage β-arrestin pathways offers a promising strategy to fine-tune receptor signaling in a receptor- and tissue-specific manner. Such ligands may minimize adverse effects linked to broad GPCR activation while harnessing the anti-tumor potential of β-arrestin–mediated signaling. Additionally, β-arrestin modulators, including small-molecule inhibitors or activators that selectively influence β-arrestin function, represent a novel and expanding frontier in cancer therapy (Kahsai et al. 2025).

Looking ahead, integrative approaches that combine proteomics, phosphoproteomics, and single-cell signaling analyses will be essential for unraveling the context-specific roles of β-arrestins across diverse cancer types and stages. These technologies will enable a more precise understanding of β-arrestin–driven signaling dynamics, ultimately guiding the development of more effective, targeted cancer therapeutics.

6 Conclusion

GPCR biased signaling, particularly through β-arrestins, has emerged as a pivotal modulator of cancer-related processes, influencing tumor behavior, the microenvironment, and immune dynamics. This chapter has explored the multifaceted and context-dependent roles of β-arrestin–mediated signaling across various cancer hallmarks and cell types. While the current understanding remains incomplete, mounting evidence supports the therapeutic potential of targeting β-arrestin–biased pathways. Continued research into their molecular mechanisms and cell-specific, temporally-specificoutcomes will be essential to fully harness this promising avenue for cancer diagnosis, prognosis, and therapy.

Acknowledgments This work was performed as part of the AHNCI Moonshot Biomarker Program and supported in part by Highmark Health. In addition, this study is partially supported by Prostate Cancer Foundation Challenge Award (to K.X., grant number 2023CHAL4223), the PA State Formula Grant (to K.X., SAP #: 4100095527), and funding from the Pittsburgh Foundation (to K.X., cc#45126409), Claude-Worthington Benedum Foundation and NIH 1R21OD034476-01.

Declaration of Competing Interest The authors declare no competing financial or personal interests related to this work.

References

Aamna B, Dan AK, Sahu R, Behera SK, Parida S (2022) Deciphering the signaling mechanisms of β-arrestin1 and β-arrestin2 in regulation of cancer cell cycle and metastasis. J Cell Physiol 237: 3717–3733

Abballe L, Alfano V, Antonacci C, Cefalo MG, Cacchione A, Del Baldo G, Pezzullo M, Po A, Moretti M, Mastronuzzi A, De Smaele E, Ferretti E, Locatelli F, Miele E (2023) β-arrestin1-E2F1-ac axis regulates physiological apoptosis and cell cycle exit in cellular models of early postnatal cerebellum. Front Cell Dev Biol. https://doi.org/10.3389/fcell.2023.990711

Adams GN, Sharma BK, Rosenfeldt L, Frederick M, Flick MJ, Witte DP, Mosnier LO, Harmel-Laws E, Steinbrecher KA, Palumbo JS (2018) Protease-activated receptor-1 impedes prostate and intestinal tumor progression in mice. J Thromb Haemost 16:2258–2269

Ahmed H, Mahmud AR, Siddiquee MF, Shahriar A, Biswas P, Shimul MEK, Ahmed SZ, Ema TI, Rahman N, Khan MA, Mizan MFR, Emran TB (2023) Role of T cells in cancer immunotherapy: opportunities and challenges. Cancer Pathog Ther 1:116–126

Ahn S, Kaipparettu BA (2025) G-protein coupled receptors in metabolic reprogramming and cancer. Pharmacol Ther 270:108849

Ahn S, Kim J, Hara MR, Ren XR, Lefkowitz RJ (2009) Beta-Arrestin-2 mediates anti-apoptotic signaling through regulation of BAD phosphorylation. J Biol Chem 284:8855–8865

Aiello S, Casiraghi F (2021) Lysophosphatidic acid: promoter of Cancer progression and of tumor microenvironment development. A promising target for anticancer therapies? Cells 10:1390

Ajram L, Begg M, Slack R, Cryan J, Hall D, Hodgson S, Ford A, Barnes A, Swieboda D, Mousnier A, Solari R (2014) Internalization of the chemokine receptor CCR4 can be evoked by orthosteric and allosteric receptor antagonists. Eur J Pharmacol 729:75–85

Alaa M, Suzuki M, Yoshino M, Tian L, Suzuki H, Nagato K, Fujiwara T, Wada H, Moriya Y, Hoshino H, Motohashi S, Yoshida S, Shibuya K, Hiroshima K, Nakatani Y, Abdrabou A, Elkholy M, Mahfouz T, Yoshino I (2009) Prostaglandin E2 receptor 2 overexpression in

squamous cell carcinoma of the lung correlates with p16INK4A methylation and an unfavorable prognosis. Int J Oncol 34:805–812
Alblazi KM, Siar CH (2015) Cellular protrusions–lamellipodia, filopodia, invadopodia and podosomes–and their roles in progression of orofacial tumours: current understanding. Asian Pac J Cancer Prev 16:2187–2191
Arang N, Gutkind JS (2020) G protein-coupled receptors and heterotrimeric G proteins as cancer drivers. FEBS Lett 594:4201–4232
Arndt PF, Turkowski K, Cekay MJ, Eul B, Grimminger F, Savai R (2024) Endothelin and the tumor microenvironment: a finger in every pie. Clin Sci (Lond) 138:617–634
Asif PJ, Longobardi C, Hahne M, Medema JP (2021) The role of Cancer-associated fibroblasts in Cancer invasion and metastasis. Cancers (Basel) 13:13
Bagnato A, Rosano L (2019) New routes in GPCR/beta-Arrestin-driven signaling in Cancer progression and metastasis. Front Pharmacol 10:114
Bagnato A, Spinella F (2003) Emerging role of endothelin-1 in tumor angiogenesis. Trends Endocrinol Metab 14:44–50
Balijepalli P, Sitton CC, Meier KE (2021) Lysophosphatidic acid signaling in Cancer cells: what makes LPA so special? Cells 10
Barlic J, Khandaker MH, Mahon E, Andrews J, DeVries ME, Mitchell GB, Rahimpour R, Tan CM, Ferguson SS, Kelvin DJ (1999) Beta-arrestins regulate interleukin-8-induced CXCR1 internalization. J Biol Chem 274:16287–16294
Barnes WG, Reiter E, Violin JD, Ren XR, Milligan Lefkowitz RJ (2005) beta-Arrestin 1 and Galphaq/11 coordinately activate RhoA and stress fiber formation following receptor stimulation. J Biol Chem. https://doi.org/10.1074/jbc.M412924200
Beaulieu JM, Caron MG (2005) Beta-arrestin goes nuclear. Cell 123:755–757
Belfiore A, Perks CM (2013) Grand challenges in cancer endocrinology: endocrine related cancers, an expanding concept. Front Endocrinol (Lausanne) 4:141
Berning P, Schaefer C, Clemens D, Korsching E, Dirksen U, Potratz J (2018) The CXCR4 antagonist plerixafor (AMD3100) promotes proliferation of Ewing sarcoma cell lines in vitro and activates receptor tyrosine kinase signaling. Cell Commun Signal 16:21
Bhattacharya M, Anborgh PH, Babwah AV, Dale LB, Dobransky T, Benovic JL, Feldman RD, Verdi JM, Rylett RJ, Ferguson SS (2002) Beta-arrestins regulate a Ral-GDS Ral effector pathway that mediates cytoskeletal reorganization. Nat Cell Biol 4:547–555
Bianchi ME, Mezzapelle R (2020) The chemokine receptor CXCR4 in cell proliferation and tissue regeneration. Front Immunol 11:2109
Birch CA, Molinar-Inglis O, Trejo J (2021) Subcellular hot spots of GPCR signaling promote vascular inflammation. Curr Opin Endocr Metab Res 16:37–42
Bocchi M, de Sousa Pereira N, de Oliveira KB, Amarante MK (2023) Involvement of CXCL12/CXCR4 axis in colorectal cancer: a mini-review. Mol Biol Rep 50:6233–6239
Bostanabad SY, Noyan S, Dedeoglu BG, Gurdal H (2021) Overexpression of beta-Arrestins inhibits proliferation and motility in triple negative breast cancer cells. Sci Rep 11:1539
Brahmer JR, Lacchetti C, Schneider BJ, Atkins MB, Brassil KJ, Caterino JM, Chau I, Ernstoff MS, Gardner JM, Ginex P, Hallmeyer S, Holter Chakrabarty J, Leighl NB, Mammen JS, McDermott DF, Naing A, Nastoupil LJ, Phillips T, Porter LD, Puzanov I, Reichner CA, Santomasso BD, Seigel C, Spira A, Suarez-Almazor ME, Wang Y, Weber JS, Wolchok JD, Thompson JA, Network National Comprehensive Cancer (2018) Management of Immune-Related Adverse Events in patients treated with immune checkpoint inhibitor therapy: American Society of Clinical Oncology clinical practice guideline. J Clin Oncol 36:1714–1768
Buchanan FG, Gorden DL, Matta P, Shi Q, Matrisian LM, DuBois RN (2006) Role of beta-arrestin 1 in the metastatic progression of colorectal cancer. Proc Natl Acad Sci USA 103:1492–1497
Burger JA, Kipps TJ (2006) CXCR4: a key receptor in the crosstalk between tumor cells and their microenvironment. Blood 107:1761–1767
Cao C, Zhang Y, Cheng J, Wu F, Niu X, Hu X, Duan X, Fu X, Zhang J, Zhang X, Ao Y (2021) Beta-Arrestin2 inhibits the apoptosis and facilitates the proliferation of fibroblast-like

Synoviocytes in diffuse-type Tenosynovial Giant cell tumor. Cancer Genomics Proteomics 18: 461–470

Carman CV, Benovic JL (1998) G-protein-coupled receptors: turn-ons and turn-offs. Curr Opin Neurobiol 8:335–344

Carneiro AP, Fonseca-Alaniz MH, Dallan LAO, Miyakawa AA, Krieger JE (2017) Beta-arrestin is critical for early shear stress-induced Akt/eNOS activation in human vascular endothelial cells. Biochem Biophys Res Commun 483:75–81

Cekic C, Day YJ, Sag D, Linden J (2014) Myeloid expression of adenosine A2A receptor suppresses T and NK cell responses in the solid tumor microenvironment. Cancer Res 74: 7250–7259

Chatterjee S, Behnam Azad B, Nimmagadda S (2014) The intricate role of CXCR4 in cancer. Adv Cancer Res 124:31–82

Chaudhary B, Elkord E (2016) Regulatory T cells in the tumor microenvironment and Cancer progression: role and therapeutic targeting. Vaccines (Basel) 4:28

Chaudhary PK, Kim S (2021) An insight into GPCR and G-proteins as Cancer drivers. Cells 10: 3288

Chen IX, Chauhan VP, Posada J, Ng MR, Wu MW, Adstamongkonkul P, Huang P, Lindeman N, Langer R, Jain RK (2019) Blocking CXCR4 alleviates desmoplasia, increases T-lymphocyte infiltration, and improves immunotherapy in metastatic breast cancer. Proc Natl Acad Sci USA 116:4558–4566

Chen C, Liu X, Chang CY, Wang HY, Wang RF (2023) The interplay between T cells and Cancer: the basis of immunotherapy. Genes (Basel) 14:1008

Cheung R, Malik M, Ravyn V, Tomkowicz B, Ptasznik A, Collman RG (2009) An arrestin-dependent multi-kinase signaling complex mediates MIP-1beta/CCL4 signaling and chemotaxis of primary human macrophages. J Leukoc Biol 86:833–845

Chu YD, Yeh CT (2020) The molecular function and clinical role of thyroid stimulating hormone receptor in Cancer cells. Cells 9

Cianfrocca R, Tocci P, Semprucci E, Spinella F, Di Castro V, Bagnato A, Rosano L (2014) Beta-Arrestin 1 is required for endothelin-1-induced NF-kappaB activation in ovarian cancer cells. Life Sci 118:179–184

Cole SW, Sood AK (2012) Molecular pathways: beta-adrenergic signaling in cancer. Clin Cancer Res 18:1201–1206

Cornwell AC, Feigin ME (2020) Unintended effects of GPCR-targeted drugs on the Cancer phenotype. Trends Pharmacol Sci 41:1006–1022

Crecelius JM, Manz AR, Benzow S, Marchese A (2024) Receptor determinants for beta-Arrestin functional specificity at C-X-C chemokine receptor 5. Mol Pharmacol 106:287–297

Crudden C, Song D, Cismas S, Trocme E, Pasca S, Calin GA, Girnita A, Girnita L (2019) Below the surface: IGF-1R therapeutic targeting and its endocytic journey. Cells 8

D'Agostino G, Artinger M, Locati M, Perez L, Legler DF, Bianchi ME, Ruegg C, Thelen M, Marchese A, Rocchi MBL, Cecchinato V, Uguccioni M (2020) Beta-Arrestin1 and beta-Arrestin2 are required to support the activity of the CXCL12/HMGB1 Heterocomplex on CXCR4. Front Immunol 11:550824

de Visser KE, Joyce JA (2023) The evolving tumor microenvironment: from cancer initiation to metastatic outgrowth. Cancer Cell 41:374–403

DeFea KA (2007) Stop that cell! Beta-arrestin-dependent chemotaxis: a tale of localized actin assembly and receptor desensitization. Annu Rev Physiol 69:535–560

Del Rio D, Masi I, Caprara V, Ottavi F, Albertini Petroni G, Salvati E, Trisciuoglio D, Giannitelli SM, Bagnato A, Mauri E, Spadaro F, Rosano L (2024) The beta-arrestin1/endothelin axis bolsters ovarian fibroblast-dependent invadosome activity and cancer cell metastatic potential. Cell Death Dis 15:358

Dhanasekaran R, Auid-Orcid Deutzmann A, Mahauad-Fernandez WD, Auid-Orcid Hansen AS, Gouw AM, Felsher DW (2022) The MYC oncogene – the grand orchestrator of cancer growth and immune evasion. Nat Rev Clin Oncol 19:23–36

Dickinson K, Yee EJ, Vigil I, Schulick RD, Zhu Y (2024) GPCRs: emerging targets for novel T cell immune checkpoint therapy. Cancer Immunol Immunother 73:253

Dietrich J (2020) Neurotoxicity of Cancer therapies. Continuum (Minneap Minn) 26:1646–1672

Ding YF, Ho KH, Lee WJ, Chen LH, Hsieh FK, Tung MC, Lin SH, Hsiao M, Yang SF, Yang YC, Chien MH (2025) Cyclic increase in the histamine receptor H1-ADAM9-snail/slug axis as a potential therapeutic target for EMT-mediated progression of oral squamous cell carcinoma. Cell Death Dis 16:191

Domanska UM, Kruizinga RC, Nagengast WB, Timmer-Bosscha H, Huls G, de Vries EG, Walenkamp AM (2013) A review on CXCR4/CXCL12 axis in oncology: no place to hide. Eur J Cancer 49:219–230

Dong JH, Wang YJ, Cui M, Wang XJ, Zheng WS, Ma ML, Yang F, He DF, Hu QX, Zhang DL, Ning SL, Liu CH, Wang C, Wang Y, Li XY, Yi F, Lin A, Kahsai AW, Cahill TJ 3rd, Chen ZY, Yu X, Sun JP (2017) Adaptive activation of a stress response pathway improves learning and memory through Gs and beta-Arrestin-1-regulated lactate metabolism. Biol Psychiatry 81:654–670

Dong T, Hu G, Fan Z, Wang H, Gao Y, Wang S, Xu H, Yaffe MB, Vander Heiden MG, Lv G, Chen J (2024) Activation of GPR3-beta-arrestin2-PKM2 pathway in Kupffer cells stimulates glycolysis and inhibits obesity and liver pathogenesis. Nat Commun 15:807

Dwivedi NV, Datta S, El-Kersh K, Sadikot RT, Ganti AK, Batra SK, Jain M (2023) GPCRs and fibroblast heterogeneity in fibroblast-associated diseases. FASEB J 37:e23101

Eishingdrelo H, Sun W, Li H, Wang L, Eishingdrelo A, Dai S, McKew JC, Zheng W (2014) ERK and β-Arrestin interaction: a converging point of signaling pathways for multiple types of cell surface receptors. J Biomol Screen 20:341–349

Fagiani E, Christofori G (2013) Angiopoietins in angiogenesis. Cancer Lett 328(1):18–26. https://doi.org/10.1016/j.canlet.2012.08.018

Fan H (2014) Beta-Arrestins 1 and 2 are critical regulators of inflammation. Innate Immun 20:451–460

Fang Y, Jiang Q, Li S, Zhu H, Rong X, Song N, Ding X, Liu J, Chen M, Song M, Ding J, Ming L, Guangyu W, Gang H (2021) Opposing functions of β-arrestin 1 and 2 in Parkinson's disease via microglia inflammation and Nprl3. Cell Death Differ 28:1822–1836

Favara DM, Liebscher I, Jazayeri A, Nambiar M, Sheldon H, Banham AH, Harris AL (2021) Elevated expression of the adhesion GPCR ADGRL4/ELTD1 promotes endothelial sprouting angiogenesis without activating canonical GPCR signalling. Sci Rep 11:8870

Feitelson MA, Arzumanyan A, Kulathinal RJ, Blain SW, Holcombe RF, Mahajna J, Marino M, Martinez-Chantar ML, Nawroth R, Sanchez-Garcia I, Sharma D, Saxena NK, Singh N, Vlachostergios PJ, Guo S, Honoki K, Fujii H, Georgakilas AG, Bilsland A, Amedei A, Niccolai E, Amin A, Ashraf SS, Boosani CS, Guha G, Ciriolo MR, Aquilano K, Chen S, Mohammed SI, Azmi AS, Bhakta D, Halicka D, Keith WN, Nowsheen S (2015) Sustained proliferation in cancer: mechanisms and novel therapeutic targets. Semin Cancer Biol. https://doi.org/10.1016/j.semcancer.2015.02.006

Fong AM, Premont RT, Richardson RM, Yu Y-RA, Lefkowitz RJ, Patel DD (2002) Defective lymphocyte chemotaxis in β-arrestin2- and GRK6-deficient mice. Proc Natl Acad Sci 99:7478–7483

Fu D, Li P, Sheng Q, Lv Z (2019) Beta-arrestin-2 enhances intestinal epithelial apoptosis in necrotizing enterocolitis. Aging (Albany NY) 11:8294–8312

Gaffal E, Jakobs M, Glodde N, Schröder R, Kostenis E, Tüting T (2014) β-Arrestin 2 inhibits Proinflammatory chemokine production and attenuates contact allergic inflammation in the skin. J Invest Dermatol 134:2131–2137

Gao F, Mu W, Fan J, Shen J (2024a) Beta-arrestin2 promotes angiogenesis of liver sinusoidal endothelial cells through the VEGF/VEGFR2 pathway to aggravate cirrhosis. Toxicol Lett 401: 1–12

Gao PP, Li L, Chen TT, Li N, Li MQ, Zhang HJ, Chen YN, Zhang SH, Wei W, Sun WY (2024b) Beta-arrestin2: an emerging player and potential therapeutic target in inflammatory immune diseases. Acta Pharmacol Sin. https://doi.org/10.1038/s41401-024-01390-w
Gao X, Jing D, Zhang Y, Zhu F, Yang Y, Zhou G (2025) Unveiling the role of GRK2: from immune regulation to Cancer therapeutics. Mediat Inflamm 2025:8837640
Ge L, Ly Y, Hollenberg M, DeFea K (2003) A beta-arrestin-dependent scaffold is associated with prolonged MAPK activation in pseudopodia during protease-activated receptor-2-induced chemotaxis. J Biol Chem 278:34418–34426
Ge L, Shenoy SK, Lefkowitz RJ, DeFea K (2004) Constitutive protease-activated receptor-2-mediated migration of MDA MB-231 breast cancer cells requires both beta-arrestin-1 and -2. J Biol Chem 279:55419–55424
Ge Y, Bohm HH, Rathinasamy A, Xydia M, Hu X, Pincha M, Umansky L, Breyer C, Hillier M, Bonertz A, Sevko A, Domschke C, Schuetz F, Frebel H, Dettling S, Herold-Mende C, Reissfelder C, Weitz J, Umansky V, Beckhove P (2019) Tumor-specific regulatory T cells from the bone marrow orchestrate antitumor immunity in breast Cancer. Cancer Immunol Res 7: 1998–2012
Geraldo LHM, Tcls Spohr RFD, Amaral AF, Garcia C, Mendes FA, Freitas C, dosSantos MF, Lima FRS (2021) Role of lysophosphatidic acid and its receptors in health and disease: novel therapeutic strategies. Signal Transduct Target Ther 6:45
Ghalehbandi S, Yuzugulen J, Pranjol MZI, Pourgholami MH (2023) The role of VEGF in cancer-induced angiogenesis and research progress of drugs targeting VEGF. Eur J Pharmacol 949: 175586
Gidon A, Feinstein TN, Xiao K, Vilardaga JP (2016) Studying the regulation of endosomal cAMP production in GPCR signaling. Methods Cell Biol 132:109–126
Gobert M, Treilleux I, Bendriss-Vermare N, Bachelot T, Goddard-Leon S, Arfi V, Biota C, Doffin AC, Durand I, Olive D, Perez S, Pasqual N, Faure C, Ray-Coquard I, Puisieux A, Caux C, Blay JY, Menetrier-Caux C (2009) Regulatory T cells recruited through CCL22/CCR4 are selectively activated in lymphoid infiltrates surrounding primary breast tumors and lead to an adverse clinical outcome. Cancer Res 69:2000–2009
Habrowska-Gorczynska DE, Koziel MJ, Kowalska K, Piastowska-Ciesielska AW (2021) FOXO3a and its regulators in prostate Cancer. Int J Mol Sci 22
Hahn H, Daly C, Little J 4th, Perry-Hauser NA, Flores-Espinoza E, Inoue A, Plouffe B, Thomsen ARB (2025) Endosomal chemokine receptor signalosomes regulate central mechanisms underlying cell migration. elife 13:RP99373
Haibe Y, Kreidieh M, El Hajj H, Khalifeh I, Mukherji D, Temraz S, Shamseddine A (2020) Resistance mechanisms to anti-angiogenic therapies in Cancer. Front Oncol 10:221
Halbrook CJ, Lyssiotis CA (2017) Employing metabolism to improve the diagnosis and treatment of pancreatic Cancer. Cancer Cell 31:5–19
Han N, Jin K, He K, Cao J, Teng L (2011) Protease-activated receptors in cancer: A systematic review. Oncol Lett 2:599–608
Hanahan D (2022) Hallmarks of Cancer: new dimensions. Cancer Discov 12:31–46
Hanahan D, Weinberg RA (2000) The hallmarks of cancer. Cell 100:57–70
Hanahan D, Weinberg RA (2011) Hallmarks of cancer: the next generation. Cell 144:646–674
Harrison M, Zinovkin D, Pranjol MZI (2024) Endothelin-1 and its role in Cancer and potential therapeutic opportunities. Biomedicine 12
Hauser AS, Attwood MM, Rask-Andersen M, Schioth HB, Gloriam DE (2017) Trends in GPCR drug discovery: new agents, targets and indications. Nat Rev Drug Discov 16:829–842
Hauser AS, Chavali S, Masuho I, Jahn LJ, Martemyanov KA, Gloriam DE, Babu MM (2018) Pharmacogenomics of GPCR drug targets. Cell 172(41–54):e19
Hu Z, Huang Y, Liu Y, Sun Y, Zhou Y, Gu M, Chen Y, Xia R, Chen S, Deng A, Zhong R (2011) beta-Arrestin 1 modulates functions of autoimmune T cells from primary biliary cirrhosis patients. J Clin Immunol 31:346–355

Hu S, Wang D, Wu J, Jin J, Wei W, Sun W (2013) Involvement of β-arrestins in cancer progression. Mol Biol Rep. https://doi.org/10.1007/s11033-012-2148-0

Huang S, Zhu J, Yu L, Huang Y, Hu Y (2025) Cancer-nervous system crosstalk: from biological mechanism to therapeutic opportunities. Mol Cancer 24:133

Hughes CE, Nibbs RJB (2018) A guide to chemokines and their receptors. FEBS J 285:2944–2971

Hunton DL, Barnes WG, Kim J, Ren X-R, Violin JD, Reiter E, Milligan G, Patel DD, Lefkowitz RJ (2005) β-arrestin 2-dependent angiotensin II type 1A receptor-mediated pathway of chemotaxis. Mol Pharmacol 67:1229–1236

Husted AS, Trauelsen M, Rudenko O, Hjorth SA, Schwartz TW (2017) GPCR-mediated signaling of metabolites. Cell Metab 25:777–796

Jaber M, Maoz M, Kancharla A, Agranovich D, Peretz T, Grisaru-Granovsky S, Uziely B, Bar-Shavit R (2014) Protease-activated-receptor-2 affects protease-activated-receptor-1-driven breast cancer. Cell Mol Life Sci 71:2517–2533

Jaber M, Maoz M, Kancharla A, Agranovich D, Peretz T, Grisaru-Granovsky S, Uziely B, Bar-Shavit R (2017) Erratum to: protease-activated-receptor-2 affects protease-activated-receptor-1-driven breast cancer. Cell Mol Life Sci 74:571–577

Jayakody T, Budagoda DK, Mendis K, Dilshan WD, Bethmage D, Dissasekara R, Dawe GS (2025) Biased agonism in peptide-GPCRs: A structural perspective. Pharmacol Ther 269:108806

Jean-Charles PY, Sudha K, Shenoy SK (2017) G protein-coupled receptor signaling through β-arrestin-dependent mechanisms. J Cardiovasc Pharmacol 70:142–158. https://doi.org/10.1097/FJC.0000000000000482

Jiang D, Xie T, Liang J, Noble PW (2013) Beta-Arrestins in the immune system. Prog Mol Biol Transl Sci 118:359–393

Jiang LP, Fan SQ, Xiong QX, Zhou YC, Yang ZZ, Li GF, Huang YC, Wu MG, Shen QS, Liu K, Yang CP, Chen YB (2018) GRK5 functions as an oncogenic factor in non-small-cell lung cancer. Cell Death Dis 9:295

Jin G, Sakitani K, Wang H, Jin Y, Dubeykovskiy A, Worthley DL, Tailor Y, Wang TC (2017) The G-protein coupled receptor 56, expressed in colonic stem and cancer cells, binds progastrin to promote proliferation and carcinogenesis. Oncotarget 8:40606–40619

Kahsai AW, Pakharukova N, Kwon HY, Shah KS, Liang-Lin JG, Del Real CT, Shim PJ, Lee MA, Ngo VA, Shreiber BN, Liu S, Schwalb AM, Espinoza EF, Thomas BN, Kunzle CA, Smith JS, Wang J, Kim J, Zhang X, Rockman HA, Thomsen ARB, Rein LAM, Shi L, Ahn S, Masoudi A, Lefkowitz RJ (2025) Small-molecule modulation of beta-arrestins. bioRxiv

Kallifatidis G, Mamouni K, Lokeshwar BL (2020) The role of β-Arrestins in regulating stem cell phenotypes in Normal and tumorigenic cells. Int J Mol Sci. https://doi.org/10.3390/ijms21239310

Kandalaft LE, Facciabene A, Buckanovich RJ, Coukos G (2009) Endothelin B receptor, a new target in cancer immune therapy. Clin Cancer Res 15:4521–4528

Kang J, Shi Y, Xiang B, Qu B, Su W, Zhu M, Zhang M, Bao G, Wang F, Zhang X, Yang R, Fan F, Chen X, Pei G, Ma L (2005) A nuclear function of beta-arrestin1 in GPCR signaling: regulation of histone acetylation and gene transcription. Cell 123:833–847

Kanki H, Sasaki T, Matsumura S, Yokawa S, Yukami T, Shimamura M, Sakaguchi M, Furuno T, Suzuki T, Mochizuki H (2019) Beta-arrestin-2 in PAR-1-biased signaling has a crucial role in endothelial function via PDGF-beta in stroke. Cell Death Dis 10:100

Kaparianos A, Argyropoulou E, Spiropoulos K (2012) The role of Beta-arrestins in respiratory pathophysiology and tumorigenesis: going a step beyond the cell surface. Eur Rev Med Pharmacol Sci 16:1781–1794

Kennedy AJ, Sundstrom L, Geschwindner S, Poon EKY, Jiang Y, Chen R, Cooke R, Johnstone S, Madin A, Lim J, Liu Q, Lohman RJ, Nordqvist A, Friden-Saxin M, Yang W, Brown DG, Fairlie DP, Dekker N (2020) Protease-activated receptor-2 ligands reveal orthosteric and allosteric mechanisms of receptor inhibition. Commun Biol 3:782

Kim JI, Lakshmikanthan V, Frilot N, Daaka Y (2010) Prostaglandin E2 promotes lung cancer cell migration via EP4-betaArrestin1-c-Src signalsome. Mol Cancer Res 8:569–577

Kim JY, Shin JH, Kim MJ, Kang Y, Lee JS, Son J, Jeong SK, Kim D, Kim DH, Chun E, Lee KY (2023) Beta-arrestin 2 negatively regulates lung cancer progression by inhibiting the TRAF6 signaling axis for NF-kappaB activation and autophagy induced by TLR3 and TLR4. Cell Death Dis 14:422

Klussmeier A, Aurich S, Niederstadt L, Wiedenmann B, Grotzinger C (2022) Secretin receptor as a target in gastrointestinal Cancer: expression analysis and ligand development. Biomedicine 10

Kong Z, Deng T, Zhang M, Zhao Z, Liu Y, Luo L, Cai C, Wu W, Duan X (2018) Beta-arrestin1-medieated inhibition of FOXO3a contributes to prostate cancer cell growth in vitro and in vivo. Cancer Sci 109:1834–1842

Kook S, Gurevich VV, Gurevich EV (2014) Arrestins in apoptosis. Handb Exp Pharmacol 219: 309–339

Korbecki J, Kupnicka P, Barczak K, Bosiacki M, Zietek P, Chlubek D, Baranowska-Bosiacka I (2023) The role of CXCR1, CXCR2, CXCR3, CXCR5, and CXCR6 ligands in molecular cancer processes and clinical aspects of acute myeloid leukemia (AML). Cancers (Basel) 15

Kourek C, Touloupaki M, Rempakos A, Loritis K, Tsougkos E, Paraskevaidis I, Briasoulis A (2022) Cardioprotective strategies from cardiotoxicity in Cancer patients: a comprehensive review. J Cardiovasc Dev Dis 9:259

Krysan K, Reckamp KL, Dalwadi H, Sharma S, Rozengurt E, Dohadwala M, Dubinett SM (2005) Prostaglandin E2 activates mitogen-activated protein kinase/Erk pathway signaling and cell proliferation in non-small cell lung cancer cells in an epidermal growth factor receptor-independent manner. Cancer Res 65:6275–6281

Kulik G (2019) ADRB2-targeting therapies for prostate Cancer. Cancers (Basel) 11

Lambert D, Calo G (2020) Approval of oliceridine (TRV130) for intravenous use in moderate to severe pain in adults. Br J Anaesth 125:e473–ee74

Lappano R, Maggiolini M (2023) Role of the G protein-coupled receptors in Cancer and stromal cells: from functions to novel therapeutic perspectives. Cells 12

Lee NY, Blobe GC (2007) The interaction of endoglin with beta-arrestin2 regulates transforming growth factor-beta-mediated ERK activation and migration in endothelial cells. J Biol Chem 282:21507–21517

Lee C, Viswanathan G, Choi I, Jassal C, Kohlmann T, Rajagopal S (2020) Beta-Arrestins and receptor signaling in the vascular endothelium. Biomolecules 11:9

Lefkowitz RJ (2000) The superfamily of heptahelical receptors. Nat Cell Biol 2:E133–E136

Lefkowitz RJ (2007) Seven transmembrane receptors: something old, something new. Acta Physiol (Oxf) 190:9–19

Lefkowitz RJ (2013) A brief history of G-protein coupled receptors (Nobel Lecture). Angew Chem Int Ed Engl 52:6366–6378

Lefkowitz RJ, Shenoy SK (2005) Transduction of receptor signals by beta-arrestins. Science 308: 512–517

Li P, Cook JA, Gilkeson GS, Luttrell LM, Wang L, Borg KT, Halushka PV, Fan H (2011) Increased expression of beta-arrestin 1 and 2 in murine models of rheumatoid arthritis: isoform specific regulation of inflammation. Mol Immunol 49:64–74

Li H, Xiao Y, Li Q, Yao J, Yuan X, Zhang Y, Yin X, Saito Y, Fan H, Li P, Kuo WL, Halpin A, Gibbons DL, Yagita H, Zhao Z, Pang D, Ren G, Yee C, Lee JJ, Yu D (2022) The allergy mediator histamine confers resistance to immunotherapy in cancer patients via activation of the macrophage histamine receptor H1. Cancer Cell 40(36–52):e9

Limbu KR, Chhetri RB, Kim S, Shrestha J, Oh YS, Baek DJ, Park EY (2024) Targeting sphingosine 1-phosphate and sphingosine kinases in pancreatic cancer: mechanisms and therapeutic potential. Cancer Cell Int 24:353

Lin YH, Lin YC, Chen CC (2021) Lysophosphatidic acid receptor antagonists and Cancer: the current trends, clinical implications, and trials. Cells 10

Lin Y, Zhou X, Ni Y, Zhao X, Liang X (2022) Metabolic reprogramming of the tumor immune microenvironment in ovarian cancer: a novel orientation for immunotherapy. Front Immunol 13:1030831

Liu P, Sun Z (2025) Chemokines and their receptors in the esophageal carcinoma tumor microenvironment: key factors for metastasis and progression. Front Oncol 15:1523751
Liu ZL, Chen HH, Zheng LL, Sun LP, Shi L (2023) Angiogenic signaling pathways and anti-angiogenic therapy for cancer. Signal Transduct Target Ther 8:198
Liu J, Song XY, Li XT, Yang M, Wang F, Han Y, Jiang Y, Lei YX, Jiang M, Zhang W, Tang DQ (2024a) Beta-Arrestin-2 enhances endoplasmic reticulum stress-induced glomerular endothelial cell injury by activating transcription factor 6 in diabetic nephropathy. World J Diabetes 15: 2322–2337
Liu S, Anderson PJ, Rajagopal S, Lefkowitz RJ, Rockman HA (2024b) G protein-coupled receptors: A century of research and discovery. Circ Res 135:174–197
Lorente JS, Sokolov AV, Ferguson G, Schioth HB, Hauser AS, Gloriam DE (2025) GPCR drug discovery: new agents, targets and indications. Nat Rev Drug Discov 24:458–479
Lovgren AK, Kovacs JJ, Xie T, Potts EN, Li Y, Foster WM, Liang J, Meltzer EB, Jiang D, Lefkowitz RJ, Noble PW (2011) Beta-arrestin deficiency protects against pulmonary fibrosis in mice and prevents fibroblast invasion of extracellular matrix. Sci Transl Med 3:74ra23
Lugano R, Ramachandran M, Dimberg A (2020) Tumor angiogenesis: causes, consequences, challenges and opportunities. Cell Mol Life Sci 77:1745–1770
Luo Y, Lu J, Lei Z, Rao D, Wang T, Fu C, Zhu H, Zhang Z, Liao Z, Liang H, Huang W (2024) GPR56 facilitates hepatocellular carcinoma metastasis by promoting the TGF-beta signaling pathway. Cell Death Dis 15:715
Lustberg MB, Kuderer NM, Desai A, Bergerot C, Lyman GH (2023) Mitigating long-term and delayed adverse events associated with cancer treatment: implications for survivorship. Nat Rev Clin Oncol 20:527–542
Luttrell LM, Ferguson SS, Daaka Y, Miller WE, Maudsley S, Della Rocca GJ, Lin F, Kawakatsu H, Owada K, Luttrell DK, Caron MG, Lefkowitz RJ (1999) Beta-arrestin-dependent formation of beta2 adrenergic receptor-Src protein kinase complexes. Science 283:655–661
Lv J, Liu J, Chao G, Zhang S (2023) PARs in the inflammation-cancer transformation of CRC. Clin Transl Oncol 25:1242–1251
Ma L, Pei G (2007) Beta-arrestin signaling and regulation of transcription. J Cell Sci 120:213–218. https://doi.org/10.1242/jcs.03338
Machesky LM (2008) Lamellipodia and filopodia in metastasis and invasion. FEBS Lett 582:2102–2111
Maekawa S, Iwasaki A, Shirakusa T, Kawakami T, Yanagisawa J, Tanaka T, Shibaguchi H, Kinugasa T, Kuroki M, Kuroki M (2008) Association between the expression of chemokine receptors CCR7 and CXCR3, and lymph node metastatic potential in lung adenocarcinoma. Oncol Rep 19:1461–1468
Mamouni K, Kim J, Lokeshwar BL, Kallifatidis G (2021) ARRB1 regulates metabolic reprogramming to promote glycolysis in stem cell-like bladder Cancer cells. Cancers (Basel) 13
Martino EA, Bruzzese A, Labanca C, Mendicino F, Lucia E, Olivito V, Stanzione G, Zimbo A, Pozzi S, Neri A, Morabito F, Vigna E, Gentile M (2024) Investigational CXCR4 inhibitors in early phase development for the treatment of hematological malignancies. Expert Opin Investig Drugs 33:915–924
McGovern KW, DeFea KA (2014) Molecular mechanisms underlying beta-arrestin-dependent chemotaxis and actin-cytoskeletal reorganization. Handb Exp Pharmacol 219:341–359
Mo W, Zhang L, Yang G, Zhai J, Hu Z, Chen Y, Chen X, Hui L, Huang R, Hu G (2008) Nuclear beta-arrestin1 functions as a scaffold for the dephosphorylation of STAT1 and moderates the antiviral activity of IFN-gamma. Mol Cell. https://doi.org/10.1016/j.molcel.2008.06.017
Molina Calistro L, Arancibia Y, Olivera MA, Domke S, Torres RF (2025) Interaction of GPER-1 with the endocrine signaling axis in breast cancer. Front Endocrinol (Lausanne) 16:1494411
Moreno Ayala MA, Campbell TF, Zhang C, Dahan N, Bockman A, Prakash V, Feng L, Sher T, DuPage M (2023) CXCR3 expression in regulatory T cells drives interactions with type I dendritic cells in tumors to restrict CD8(+) T cell antitumor immunity. Immunity 56(1613–30): e5

Mortezaee K (2020) CXCL12/CXCR4 axis in the microenvironment of solid tumors: a critical mediator of metastasis. Life Sci 249:117534

Mukherjee D, Zhao J (2013) The role of chemokine receptor CXCR4 in breast cancer metastasis. Am J Cancer Res 3:46–57

Munkarah A, Mert I, Chhina J, Hamid S, Poisson L, Hensley-Alford S, Giri S, Rattan R (2016) Targeting of free fatty acid receptor 1 in EOC: A novel strategy to restrict the adipocyte-EOC dependence. Gynecol Oncol 141:72–79

Murph M, Mills GB (2007) Targeting the lipids LPA and S1P and their signalling pathways to inhibit tumour progression. Expert Rev Mol Med 9:1–18

Nakai A, Fujimoto J, Miyata H, Stumm R, Narazaki M, Schulz S, Baba Y, Kumanogoh A, Suzuki K (2019) The COMMD3/8 complex determines GRK6 specificity for chemoattractant receptors. J Exp Med 216:1630–1647

Nataraj C, Thomas DW, Tilley SL, Nguyen MT, Mannon R, Koller BH, Coffman TM (2001) Receptors for prostaglandin E(2) that regulate cellular immune responses in the mouse. J Clin Invest 108:1229–1235

Navarro C, Ortega A, Santeliz R, Garrido B, Chacin M, Galban N, Vera I, De Sanctis JB, Bermudez V (2022) Metabolic reprogramming in cancer cells: emerging molecular mechanisms and novel therapeutic approaches. Pharmaceutics 14:1303

Nguyen HT, Reyes-Alcaraz A, Yong HJ, Nguyen LP, Park H-K, Inoue A, Lee CS, Seong JY, Hwang J-I (2020) CXCR7: a β-arrestin-biased receptor that potentiates cell migration and recruits β-arrestin2 exclusively through gβγ subunits and GRK2. Cell Biosci 10:134

Nishida N, Yano H, Nishida T, Kamura T, Kojiro M (2006) Angiogenesis in cancer. Vasc Health Risk Manag 2:213–219

O'Hayre M, Degese MS, Gutkind JS (2014) Novel insights into G protein and G protein-coupled receptor signaling in cancer. Curr Opin Cell Biol 27:126–135

Olejarz W, Kubiak-Tomaszewska G, Chrzanowska A, Lorenc T (2020) Exosomes in angiogenesis and anti-angiogenic therapy in cancers. Int J Mol Sci 21

Oliveira de Souza C, Sun X, Oh D (2021) Metabolic functions of G protein-coupled receptors and beta-Arrestin-mediated signaling pathways in the pathophysiology of type 2 diabetes and obesity. Front Endocrinol (Lausanne) 12:715877

Panupinthu N, Lee HY, Mills GB (2010) Lysophosphatidic acid production and action: critical new players in breast cancer initiation and progression. Br J Cancer 102:941–946

Patnaik R, Varghese RL, Banerjee Y (2025) Selective modulation of PAR-2-driven inflammatory pathways by Oleocanthal: attenuation of TNF-alpha and calcium dysregulation in colorectal Cancer models. Int J Mol Sci 26:5521

Pelzel C, Begitt A, Wenta N, Vinkemeier U (2013) Evidence against a role for β-Arrestin1 in STAT1 Dephosphorylation and the inhibition of interferon-γ signaling. Mol Cell 50:149–156

Pierce KL, Premont RT, Lefkowitz RJ (2002) Seven-transmembrane receptors. Nat Rev Mol Cell Biol 3:639–650

Pillai S, Trevino J, Rawal B, Singh S, Kovacs M, Li X, Schell M, Haura E, Bepler G, Chellappan S (2015) Beta-arrestin-1 mediates nicotine-induced metastasis through E2F1 target genes that modulate epithelial-mesenchymal transition. Cancer Res 75:1009–1020

Pourreyron C, Reilly L, Proby C, Panteleyev A, Fleming C, McLean K, South AP, Foerster J (2012) Wnt5a is strongly expressed at the leading edge in non-melanoma skin cancer, forming active gradients, while canonical Wnt signalling is repressed. PLoS One 7:e31827

Poyner DR, Hay DL (2012) Secretin family (class B) G protein-coupled receptors—from molecular to clinical perspectives. Br J Pharmacol 166:1–3

Pratiwi L, Elisa E, Sutanto H (2024) Probing the protrusions: lamellipodia and filopodia in cancer invasion and beyond. Mechanobiol Med 2:100064

Pu T, Sun J, Ren G, Li H (2025) Neuro-immune crosstalk in cancer: mechanisms and therapeutic implications. Signal Transduct Target Ther 10:176

Pydi SP, Barella LF, Meister J, Wess J (2021) Key metabolic functions of beta-Arrestins: studies with novel mouse models. Trends Endocrinol Metab 32:118–129

Qi Y, Wang Y, Yuan J, Xu Y, Pan H (2024) Unveiling the therapeutic promise: exploring lysophosphatidic acid (LPA) signaling in malignant bone tumors for novel cancer treatments. Lipids Health Dis 23:204

Quintero-Fabian S, Arreola R, Becerril-Villanueva E, Torres-Romero JC, Arana-Argaez V, Lara-Riegos J, Ramirez-Camacho MA, Alvarez-Sanchez ME (2019) Role of matrix Metalloproteinases in angiogenesis and cancer. Front Oncol 9:1370

Raghuwanshi SK, Nasser MW, Chen X, Strieter RM, Richardson RM (2008) Depletion of beta-arrestin-2 promotes tumor growth and angiogenesis in a murine model of lung cancer. J Immunol 180:5699–5706

Rapp M, Wintergerst MWM, Kunz WG, Vetter VK, Knott MML, Lisowski D, Haubner S, Moder S, Thaler R, Eiber S, Meyer B, Rohrle N, Piseddu I, Grassmann S, Layritz P, Kuhnemuth B, Stutte S, Bourquin C, von Andrian UH, Endres S, Anz D (2019) CCL22 controls immunity by promoting regulatory T cell communication with dendritic cells in lymph nodes. J Exp Med 216:1170–1181

Rasheed SAK, Subramanyan LV, Lim WK, Udayappan UK, Wang M, Casey PJ (2022) The emerging roles of Galpha12/13 proteins on the hallmarks of cancer in solid tumors. Oncogene 41:147–158

Renz BW, Takahashi R, Tanaka T, Macchini M, Hayakawa Y, Dantes Z, Maurer HC, Chen X, Jiang Z, Westphalen CB, Ilmer M, Valenti G, Mohanta SK, Habenicht AJR, Middelhoff M, Chu T, Nagar K, Tailor Y, Casadei R, Di Marco M, Kleespies A, Friedman RA, Remotti H, Reichert M, Worthley DL, Neumann J, Werner J, Iuga AC, Olive KP, Wang TC (2018) beta2 adrenergic-Neurotrophin feedforward loop promotes pancreatic Cancer. Cancer Cell 33:75–90 e7

Ricci F, Di Credico A, Gaggi G, Iannetti G, Ghinassi B, Gallina S, Olshansky B, Di Baldassarre A (2023) Metoprolol disrupts inflammatory response of human cardiomyocytes via β-arrestin2 biased agonism and NF-κB signaling modulation. Biomed Pharmacother 168:115804

Rockman HA, Lefkowitz RJ (2024) G protein-coupled receptors: from radioligand binding to cellular signaling. J Clin Invest 134:e178109

Rolin J, Maghazachi AA (2011) Effects of lysophospholipids on tumor microenvironment. Cancer Microenviron 4:393–403

Romagnani P, Annunziato F, Lasagni L, Lazzeri E, Beltrame C, Francalanci M, Uguccioni M, Galli G, Cosmi L, Maurenzig L, Baggiolini M, Maggi E, Romagnani S, Serio M (2001) Cell cycle-dependent expression of CXC chemokine receptor 3 by endothelial cells mediates angiostatic activity. J Clin Invest 107:53–63

Rosano L, Bagnato A (2016) Beta-arrestin1 at the cross-road of endothelin-1 signaling in cancer. J Exp Clin Cancer Res 35:121

Rosanò L, Bagnato A (2019) Chapter 4: new insights into the regulation of the actin cytoskeleton dynamics by GPCR/β-arrestin in cancer invasion and metastasis. In: Galluzzi L (ed) International review of cell and molecular biology. Academic

Rueda A, Serna N, Mangues R, Villaverde A, Unzueta U (2025) Targeting the chemokine receptor CXCR4 for cancer therapies. Biomark Res 13:68

Ruf W, Yokota N, Schaffner F (2010) Tissue factor in cancer progression and angiogenesis. Thromb Res 125(Suppl 2):S36–S38

Ryu JW, Shin HY, Kim HS, Han GH, Kim JW, Lee HN, Cho H, Chung JY, Kim JH (2023) Prognostic value of beta-Arrestins in combination with glucocorticoid receptor in epithelial ovarian cancer. Front Oncol 13:1104521

Saddam M, Paul SK, Habib MA, Fahim MA, Mimi A, Islam S, Paul B, Helal MMU (2024) Emerging biomarkers and potential therapeutics of the BCL-2 protein family: the apoptotic and anti-apoptotic context. Egypt J Med Hum Genet 25:12

Salazar N, Zabel BA (2019) Support of tumor endothelial cells by chemokine receptors. Front Immunol 10:147

Salem A, Alotaibi M, Mroueh R, Basheer HA, Afarinkia K (2021) CCR7 as a therapeutic target in Cancer. Biochim Biophys Acta Rev Cancer 1875:188499

Salmeron C, Tomas Bort E, Sriram K, Javadi-Paydar M, Smitham JE, Pham K, Grose RP, McCormick PJ, DiNardo A, Weitz J, Tiriac H, Lowy AM, Insel PA (2025) Histamine H1 receptor: A potential therapeutic target for pancreatic ductal adenocarcinoma. J Pharmacol Exp Ther 392:103573

Sarvaiya PJ, Guo D, Ulasov I, Gabikian P, Lesniak MS (2013) Chemokines in tumor progression and metastasis. Oncotarget 4:2171–2185

Schioth HB, Fredriksson R (2005) The GRAFS classification system of G-protein coupled receptors in comparative perspective. Gen Comp Endocrinol 142:94–101

Schiraldi M, Raucci A, Munoz LM, Livoti E, Celona B, Venereau E, Apuzzo T, De Marchis F, Pedotti M, Bachi A, Thelen M, Varani L, Mellado M, Proudfoot A, Bianchi ME, Uguccioni M (2012) HMGB1 promotes recruitment of inflammatory cells to damaged tissues by forming a complex with CXCL12 and signaling via CXCR4. J Exp Med 209:551–563

Scott EN, Gocher AM, Workman CJ, Vignali DAA (2021) Regulatory T cells: barriers of immune infiltration into the tumor microenvironment. Front Immunol 12:702726

Sedda S, Marafini I, Caruso R, Pallone F, Monteleone G (2014) Proteinase activated-receptors-associated signaling in the control of gastric cancer. World J Gastroenterol 20:11977–11984

Shah K, Mallik SB, Gupta P, Iyer A (2022) Targeting tumour-associated fibroblasts in cancers. Front Oncol 12:908156

Sharma D, Parameswaran N (2015) Multifaceted role of beta-arrestins in inflammation and disease. Genes Immun 16:499–513

Shenoy SK, Han S, Zhao YL, Hara MR, Oliver T, Cao Y, Dewhirst MW (2012) Beta-arrestin1 mediates metastatic growth of breast cancer cells by facilitating HIF-1-dependent VEGF expression. Oncogene 31:282–292

Shi Y, Feng Y, Kang J, Liu C, Li Z, Li D, Cao W, Qiu J, Guo Z, Bi E, Zang L, Lu C, Zhang JZ, Pei G (2007) Critical regulation of CD4+ T cell survival and autoimmunity by beta-arrestin 1. Nat Immunol 8:817–824

Shukla AK, Dwivedi-Agnihotri H (2020) Structure and function of beta-arrestins, their emerging role in breast cancer, and potential opportunities for therapeutic manipulation. Adv Cancer Res 145:139–156

Shukla AK, Xiao K, Lefkowitz RJ (2011) Emerging paradigms of beta-arrestin-dependent seven transmembrane receptor signaling. Trends Biochem Sci 36:457–469

Singh S, Singh UP, Grizzle WE, Lillard JW Jr (2004) CXCL12-CXCR4 interactions modulate prostate cancer cell migration, metalloproteinase expression and invasion. Lab Investig 84: 1666–1676

Singh R, Lillard JW Jr, Singh S (2011) Chemokines: key players in cancer progression and metastasis. Front Biosci (Schol Ed) 3:1569–1582

Sobolesky PM, Moussa O (2013a) The role of beta-arrestins in cancer. Prog Mol Biol Transl Sci 118:395–411

Sobolesky PM, Moussa O (2013b) Chapter 15: The role of β-Arrestins in Cancer. In: Luttrell LM (ed) Progress in molecular biology and translational science. Academic

Song Q, Ji Q, Li Q (2018) The role and mechanism of beta-arrestins in cancer invasion and metastasis (review). Int J Mol Med 41:631–639

Strazza M, Mor A (2017) Consider the chemokines: a review of the interplay between chemokines and T cell subset function. Discov Med 24:31–39

Su Y, Raghuwanshi SK, Yu Y, Nanney LB, Richardson RM, Richmond A (2005) Altered CXCR2 signaling in beta-arrestin-2-deficient mouse models. J Immunol 175:5396–5402

Su Y, Huang X, Raskovalova T, Zacharia L, Lokshin A, Jackson E, Gorelik E (2008) Cooperation of adenosine and prostaglandin E2 (PGE2) in amplification of cAMP-PKA signaling and immunosuppression. Cancer Immunol Immunother 57:1611–1623

Suleymanova N, Crudden C, Shibano T, Worrall C, Oprea I, Tica A, Calin GA, Girnita A, Girnita L (2017) Functional antagonism of beta-arrestin isoforms balance IGF-1R expression and signalling with distinct cancer-related biological outcomes. Oncogene 36:5734–5744

Sun JJ, Yang HT, Niu GJ, Feng XW, Lan JF, Zhao XF, Wang JX (2016a) β-Arrestin 1's Interaction with TC45 Attenuates Stat signaling by dephosphorylating Stat to inhibit antimicrobial peptide expression. Sci Rep 6:35808

Sun W-Y, Shan-Shan H, Jing-Jing W, Huang Q, Ma Y, Wang Q-T, Chen J-Y, Wei W (2016b) Down-regulation of β-arrestin2 promotes tumour invasion and indicates poor prognosis of hepatocellular carcinoma. Sci Rep 6:35609

Sun WY, Wu JJ, Peng WT, Sun JC, Wei W (2018) The role of G protein-coupled receptor kinases in the pathology of malignant tumors. Acta Pharmacol Sin 39:1699–1705

Suvarna K, Honda K, Kondoh Y, Osada H, Watanabe N (2018) Identification of a small-molecule ligand of beta-arrestin1 as an inhibitor of stromal fibroblast cell migration accelerated by cancer cells. Cancer Med 7:883–893

Szenasi T, Turu G, Hunyady L (2023) Interactions between beta-arrestin proteins and the cytoskeletal system, and their relevance to neurodegenerative disorders. Front Endocrinol (Lausanne) 14:957981

Tamura M, Takai M, Yamamoto M, Yashiro N, Taniguchi A, Kusumoto Y, Nagano S, Shimomura N, Tsujiuchi T (2025) Lysophosphatidic acid (LPA) receptor signaling enhances malignant potential in highly migratory lung cancer cells under hypoxic conditions. Acta Histochem 127:152268

Tanaka T, Bai Z, Srinoulprasert Y, Yang BG, Hayasaka H, Miyasaka M (2005) Chemokines in tumor progression and metastasis. Cancer Sci 96:317–322

Tirado-Garibay AC, Falcon-Ruiz EA, Ochoa-Zarzosa A, Lopez-Meza JE (2023) GPER: an estrogen receptor key in metastasis and Tumoral microenvironments. Int J Mol Sci 24:14993

Tocci P, Rosano L, Bagnato A (2019) Targeting Endothelin-1 receptor/beta-Arrestin-1 Axis in ovarian Cancer: from basic research to a therapeutic approach. Front Endocrinol (Lausanne) 10: 609

Tocci P, Blandino G, Bagnato A (2021) YAP and endothelin-1 signaling: an emerging alliance in cancer. J Exp Clin Cancer Res 40:27

Upadhyaya VD, Douedi S, Garcia B, Gonzalez J, Udongwo N, Wei J, Nai Q, Asif A, Sen S (2020) Mechanism and effect of Beta-blockers on pancreatic adenocarcinoma: a literature review. J Clin Med Res 12:753–757

Usman S, Khawer M, Rafique S, Naz Z, Saleem K (2020) The current status of anti-GPCR drugs against different cancers. J Pharm Anal 10:517–521

Vaque JP, Dorsam RT, Feng X, Iglesias-Bartolome R, Forsthoefel DJ, Chen Q, Debant A, Seeger MA, Ksander BR, Teramoto H, Gutkind JS (2013) A genome-wide RNAi screen reveals a trio-regulated rho GTPase circuitry transducing mitogenic signals initiated by G protein-coupled receptors. Mol Cell 49:94–108

Vasudev NS, Reynolds AR (2014) Anti-angiogenic therapy for cancer: current progress, unresolved questions and future directions. Angiogenesis 17:471–494

Versteeg HH, Schaffner F, Kerver M, Ellies LG, Andrade-Gordon P, Mueller BM, Ruf W (2008) Protease-activated receptor (PAR) 2, but not PAR1, signaling promotes the development of mammary adenocarcinoma in polyoma middle T mice. Cancer Res 68:7219–7227

Visentin B, Vekich JA, Sibbald BJ, Cavalli AL, Moreno KM, Matteo RG, Garland WA, Lu Y, Yu S, Hall HS, Kundra V, Mills GB, Sabbadini RA (2006) Validation of an anti-sphingosine-1-phosphate antibody as a potential therapeutic in reducing growth, invasion, and angiogenesis in multiple tumor lineages. Cancer Cell 9:225–238

Vroon A, Heijnen CJ, Kavelaars A (2006) GRKs and arrestins: regulators of migration and inflammation. J Leukoc Biol 80:1214–1221

Wang R, Dashwood RH (2011) Endothelins and their receptors in cancer: identification of therapeutic targets. Pharmacol Res 63:519–524

Wang LG, Su BH, Du JJ (2012) Expression of beta-arrestin 1 in gastric cardiac adenocarcinoma and its relation with progression. Asian Pac J Cancer Prev 13:5671–5675

Wang C, Zeng X, Zhou Z, Zhao J, Pei G (2016) β-arrestin-1 contributes to brown fat function and directly interacts with PPARα and PPARγ. Sci Rep 6:26999

Wang X, Zhang Y, Wang S, Ni H, Zhao P, Chen G, Xu B, Yuan L (2022) The role of CXCR3 and its ligands in cancer. Front Oncol 12:1022688

Wei X, Wu D, Li J, Wu M, Li Q, Che Z, Cheng X, Cheng Q, Yin F, Zhang H, Wang X, Abtahi S, Zuo L, Hang L, Ma L, Kuo WT, Liu X, Turner JR, Wang H, Xiao J, Wang F (2024) Myeloid beta-arrestin 2 depletion attenuates metabolic dysfunction-associated steatohepatitis via the metabolic reprogramming of macrophages. Cell Metab 36(2281–97):e7

Wess J (2022) The two beta-Arrestins regulate distinct metabolic processes: studies with novel mutant mouse models. Int J Mol Sci 23

Wettschureck N, Offermanns S (2005) Mammalian G proteins and their cell type specific functions. Physiol Rev 85:1159–1204

Whalen EJ, Rajagopal S, Lefkowitz RJ (2011) Therapeutic potential of beta-arrestin- and G protein-biased agonists. Trends Mol Med 17:126–139

Whiteside TL, Jackson EK (2013) Adenosine and prostaglandin e2 production by human inducible regulatory T cells in health and disease. Front Immunol 4:212

Wisler JW, Xiao K, Thomsen ARB, Lefkowitz RJ (2014) Recent developments in biased agonism. Curr Opin Cell Biol 27:18–24

Wojtukiewicz MZ, Hempel D, Sierko E, Tucker SC, Honn KV (2015) Protease-activated receptors (PARs)--biology and role in cancer invasion and metastasis. Cancer Metastasis Rev 34:775–796

Wong SC, He CW, Chan CM, Chan AK, Wong HT, Cheung MT, Luk LL, Au TC, Chiu MK, Ma BB, Chan AT (2013) Clinical significance of frizzled homolog 3 protein in colorectal cancer patients. PLoS One 8:e79481

Wu JX, Shan FX, Zheng JN, Pei DS (2014) β-arrestin promotes c-Jun N-terminal kinase mediated apoptosis via a GABA(B)R·β-arrestin·JNK signaling module. Asian Pac J Cancer Prev 15: 1041–1046

Wu V, Yeerna H, Nohata N, Chiou J, Harismendy O, Raimondi F, Inoue A, Russell RB, Tamayo P, Gutkind JS (2019) Illuminating the Onco-GPCRome: novel G protein-coupled receptor-driven oncocrine networks and targets for cancer immunotherapy. J Biol Chem 294:11062–11086

Wu VH, Yung BS, Faraji F, Saddawi-Konefka R, Wang Z, Wenzel AT, Song MJ, Pagadala MS, Clubb LM, Chiou J, Sinha S, Matic M, Raimondi F, Hoang TS, Berdeaux R, Vignali DAA, Iglesias-Bartolome R, Carter H, Ruppin E, Mesirov JP, Gutkind JS (2023) The GPCR-Galpha (s)-PKA signaling axis promotes T cell dysfunction and cancer immunotherapy failure. Nat Immunol 24:1318–1330

Xia Y, Wang S, Sun Y, Wang W, Chang S, Zhang Z, Zhao C (2024) Frizzled class receptor 5 contributes to ovarian cancer chemoresistance through aldehyde dehydrogenase 1A1. Cell Commun Signal 22:194

Xiao K, Sun J (2018) Elucidating structural and molecular mechanisms of beta-arrestin-biased agonism at GPCRs via MS-based proteomics. Cell Signal 41:56–64

Xiao K, McClatchy DB, Shukla AK, Zhao Y, Chen M, Shenoy SK, Yates JR 3rd, Lefkowitz RJ (2007) Functional specialization of beta-arrestin interactions revealed by proteomic analysis. Proc Natl Acad Sci USA 104:12011–12016

Xiao K, Sun J, Kim J, Rajagopal S, Zhai B, Villen J, Haas W, Kovacs JJ, Shukla AK, Hara MR, Hernandez M, Lachmann A, Zhao S, Lin Y, Cheng Y, Mizuno K, Ma'ayan A, Gygi SP, Lefkowitz RJ (2010) Global phosphorylation analysis of beta-arrestin-mediated signaling downstream of a seven transmembrane receptor (7TMR). Proc Natl Acad Sci USA 107: 15299–15304

Xu Y (2018) Lysophospholipid signaling in the epithelial ovarian Cancer tumor microenvironment. Cancers (Basel) 10:227

Xu X, Lei Y, Zhou H, Guo Y, Liu H, Jiang J, Yang Y, Wu B (2020) Beta-Arrestin1 is involved in hepatocellular carcinoma metastasis via extracellular signal-regulated kinase-mediated epithelial-mesenchymal transition. J Gastroenterol Hepatol 35:2229–2240

Xu Y, Wang J, Wang X, Zhou X, Tang J, Jie X, Yang X, Rao X, Xu Y, Xing B, Li Z, Wu G (2022) Targeting ADRB2 enhances sensitivity of non-small cell lung cancer to VEGFR2 tyrosine kinase inhibitors. Cell Death Discov 8:36

Xu K, Wang L, Lin M, He G (2024) Update on protease-activated receptor 2 in inflammatory and autoimmune dermatological diseases. Front Immunol 15:1449126

Xu S, Peng Y, Li X, Li H, Liu T, Li X, Du Y (2025) TSHR in thyroid cancer: bridging biological insights to targeted strategies. Eur Thyroid J 14:e240369

Yamaguchi H, Condeelis J (2007) Regulation of the actin cytoskeleton in cancer cell migration and invasion. Biochim Biophys Acta 1773:642–652

Yamamoto M, Takai M, Yashiro N, Tamura M, Kusumoto Y, Nagano S, Taniguchi A, Shimomura N, Tsujiuchi T (2025) Lysophosphatidic acid (LPA) receptor signaling modulates cellular functions of colon cancer cells under cobalt chloride-induced hypoxic conditions. Adv Biol Regul 96:101098

Yaman I, Agac Cobanoglu D, Xie T, Ye Y, Amit M (2022) Advances in understanding cancer-associated neurogenesis and its implications on the neuroimmune axis in cancer. Pharmacol Ther 239:108199

Yan Y, Wang LF, Wang RF (2015) Role of cancer-associated fibroblasts in invasion and metastasis of gastric cancer. World J Gastroenterol 21:9717–9726

Yang L, Friedland S, Corson N, Xu L (2014) GPR56 inhibits melanoma growth by internalizing and degrading its ligand TG2. Cancer Res 74:1022–1031

Yang Y, Guo Y, Tan S, Ke B, Tao J, Liu H, Jiang J, Chen J, Chen G, Wu B (2015) Beta-Arrestin1 enhances hepatocellular carcinogenesis through inflammation-mediated Akt signalling. Nat Commun 6:7369

Yang Y, Li C, Liu T, Dai X, Bazhin AV (2020) Myeloid-derived suppressor cells in tumors: from mechanisms to antigen specificity and microenvironmental regulation. Front Immunol 11:1371

Yang D, Zhou Q, Labroska V, Qin S, Darbalaei S, Wu Y, Yuliantie E, Xie L, Tao H, Cheng J, Liu Q, Zhao S, Shui W, Jiang Y, Wang MW (2021) G protein-coupled receptors: structure- and function-based drug discovery. Signal Transduct Target Ther 6:7

Yang Y, Ma X, Li Y, Jin L, Zhou X (2025) The evolving tumor-associated adipose tissue microenvironment in breast cancer: from cancer initiation to metastatic outgrowth. Clin Transl Oncol 27:2778–2788

Ye X, Liu S, Hu M, Song Y, Huang H, Zhong Y (2017) CCR5 expression in inflammatory bowel disease and its correlation with inflammatory cells and beta-arrestin2 expression. Scand J Gastroenterol 52:551–557

Yin J, Zhu W, Feng S, Yan P, Qin S (2024) The role of cancer-associated fibroblasts in the invasion and metastasis of colorectal cancer. Front Cell Dev Biol 12:1375543

Yu S, Murph MM, Lu Y, Liu S, Hall HS, Liu J, Stephens C, Fang X, Mills GB (2008) Lysophosphatidic acid receptors determine tumorigenicity and aggressiveness of ovarian cancer cells. J Natl Cancer Inst 100:1630–1642

Yu S, Sun L, Jiao Y, Lee LTO (2018) The role of G protein-coupled receptor kinases in Cancer. Int J Biol Sci 14:189–203

Yu H, Wang M, Zhang T, Cao L, Li Z, Du Y, Hai Y, Gao X, Ji J, Wu J (2022) Dual roles of beta-arrestin 1 in mediating cell metabolism and proliferation in gastric cancer. Proc Natl Acad Sci USA 119:e2123231119

Yue R, Kang J, Zhao C, Hu W, Tang Y, Liu X, Pei G (2009) Beta-arrestin1 regulates zebrafish hematopoiesis through binding to YY1 and relieving polycomb group repression. Cell. https://doi.org/10.1016/j.cell.2009.08.038

Yun CC (2019) Lysophosphatidic acid and Autotaxin-associated effects on the initiation and progression of colorectal cancer. Cancers (Basel) 11:958

Zeng CM, Chen Z, Fu L (2018) Frizzled receptors as potential therapeutic targets in human cancers. Int J Mol Sci 19:1543

Zeng S, Liang Y, Hu H, Wang F, Liang L (2022) Endothelial cell-derived S1P promotes migration and stemness by binding with GPR63 in colorectal cancer. Pathol Res Pract 240:154197

Zhan Y, Xu C, Liu Z, Yang Y, Tan S, Yang Y, Jiang J, Liu H, Chen J, Wu B (2016) Beta-Arrestin1 inhibits chemotherapy-induced intestinal stem cell apoptosis and mucositis. Cell Death Dis 7:e2229

Zhang H, He B (2019) SDF1/CXCR4 axis plays a role in angiogenesis during the degeneration of intervertebral discs. Mol Med Rep 20:1203–1211

Zhang Y, Liu Q, Zhang M, Yu Y, Liu X, Cao X (2009) Fas signal promotes lung cancer growth by recruiting myeloid-derived suppressor cells via cancer cell-derived PGE2. J Immunol 182: 3801–3808

Zhang YX, Li XF, Yuan GQ, Hu H, Song XY, Li JY, Miao XK, Zhou TX, Yang WL, Zhang XW, Mou LY, Wang R (2017) Beta-Arrestin 1 has an essential role in neurokinin-1 receptor-mediated glioblastoma cell proliferation and G(2)/M phase transition. J Biol Chem 292:8933–8947

Zhang L, Pan J, Chen W, Jiang J, Huang J (2020a) Chronic stress-induced immune dysregulation in cancer: implications for initiation, progression, metastasis, and treatment. Am J Cancer Res 10: 1294–1307

Zhang L, Wang F, Yao X, Ma S, Zhang L, Qin Z (2020b) Progress in targeting therapy of cancer metastasis by CCL21/CCR7 axis. Sheng Wu Gong Cheng Xue Bao 36:2741–2754

Zhang Y, Li M, Li L, Qian G, Wang Y, Chen Z, Liu J, Fang C, Huang F, Guo D, Zou Q, Chu Y, Yan D (2020c) Beta-arrestin 2 as an activator of cGAS-STING signaling and target of viral immune evasion. Nat Commun 11:6000

Zhang M, Guan WB, Li JL, Li LX, Wang KZ, Wang RF, Wang LF (2022) Cancer-associated fibroblasts subtypes and role in invasion and metastasis of gastric cancer. Neoplasma 69:1277–1288

Zhang A, Fan T, Liu Y, Yu G, Li C, Jiang Z (2024a) Regulatory T cells in immune checkpoint blockade antitumor therapy. Mol Cancer 23:251

Zhang S, Xiao X, Yi Y, Wang X, Zhu L, Shen Y, Lin D, Chen W (2024b) Tumor initiation and early tumorigenesis: molecular mechanisms and interventional targets. Signal Transduct Target Ther 9:149

Zhao J, Pei G (2013) Arrestins in metabolic regulation. Prog Mol Biol Transl Sci 118:413–427

Zhao Y, Xiao K (2019) Proteomic analysis of the beta-Arrestin Interactomes. Methods Mol Biol 1957:217–232

Zhou P, Zheng X, Zhang H, Liu Y, Zheng P (2009) B7 blockade alters the balance between regulatory T cells and tumor-reactive T cells for immunotherapy of cancer. Clin Cancer Res 15: 960–970

Zhou Y, Cao HB, Li WJ, Zhao L (2018) The CXCL12 (SDF-1)/CXCR4 chemokine axis: oncogenic properties, molecular targeting, and synthetic and natural product CXCR4 inhibitors for cancer therapy. Chin J Nat Med 16:801–810

Zhu YM, Azahri NS, Yu DC, Woll PJ (2008) Effects of COX-2 inhibition on expression of vascular endothelial growth factor and interleukin-8 in lung cancer cells. BMC Cancer 8:218

Zhuang LN, Hu W-x, Xin S-m, Zhao J, Pei G (2011) Beta-arrestin-1 protein represses adipogenesis and inflammatory responses through its interaction with peroxisome proliferator-activated receptor-gamma (PPARgamma). J Biol Chem. https://doi.org/10.1074/jbc.M111.256099

Zielinska KA, Katanaev VL (2020) The signaling duo CXCL12 and CXCR4: chemokine fuel for breast Cancer tumorigenesis. Cancers (Basel) 12

Zou L, Yang R, Chai J, Pei G (2008) Rapid xenograft tumor progression in beta-arrestin1 transgenic mice due to enhanced tumor angiogenesis. FASEB J 22:355–364

Zoudilova M, Kumar P, Ge L, Wang P, Bokoch GM, DeFea KA (2007) Beta-arrestin-dependent regulation of the cofilin pathway downstream of protease-activated receptor-2. J Biol Chem 282: 20634–20646

GPCR Biased Signaling in Metabolism

Zhaoyu Zhang and Zijian Li

Contents

Z. Zhang
Department of Cardiology and Institute of Vascular Medicine, Peking University Third Hospital; Beijing Key Laboratory of Cardiovascular Receptors Research, State Key Laboratory of Vascular Homeostasis and Remodeling, and NHC Key Laboratory of Cardiovascular Molecular Biology and Regulatory Peptides, Peking University; Research Unit of Medical Science Research Management/Basic and Clinical Research of Metabolic Cardiovascular Diseases, Chinese Academy of Medical Sciences, Beijing, China

Z. Li (✉)
Department of Cardiology and Institute of Vascular Medicine, Peking University Third Hospital; Beijing Key Laboratory of Cardiovascular Receptors Research, State Key Laboratory of Vascular Homeostasis and Remodeling, and NHC Key Laboratory of Cardiovascular Molecular Biology and Regulatory Peptides, Peking University; Research Unit of Medical Science Research Management/Basic and Clinical Research of Metabolic Cardiovascular Diseases, Chinese Academy of Medical Sciences, Beijing, China

Department of Pharmacy, Peking University Third Hospital, Beijing, China
e-mail: lizijian@bjmu.edu.cn

© The Author(s), under exclusive license to Springer Nature Switzerland AG 2025

Z. Li, K. Xiao (eds.), *Pharmacology of GPCRs Biased Signaling and Agonists*,
Handbook of Experimental Pharmacology 290, https://doi.org/10.1007/164_2025_774

Abstract

G protein-coupled receptors (GPCRs) are the largest family of transmembrane receptors and the most prominent drug targets. GPCR-biased signaling exerts different functions through distinct downstream signaling pathways of receptor to maintain body homeostasis. Metabolism is the series of biochemical processes that occur within a living organism to maintain life. GPCR-biased signaling and metabolism exhibit bidirectional interplay. On the one hand, metabolites including short-chain fatty acids (SCFAs) and long-chain fatty acids (LCFAs) act as ligands inducing biased GPCRs signaling. On the other hand, activated GPCRs regulate diverse metabolic functions by biased signal sorting (G protein or β-arrestin-mediated). G protein signaling mainly mediates rapid metabolic reaction, and β-arrestin signaling mainly mediates sustained metabolic effects. In clinical drug applications, GPCR-biased drugs can revolutionize metabolic disease therapeutics by enabling pathway-selective drug design to enhance efficacy while reducing side effects. Thus, delving deeper into the relationship between GPCR-biased signaling and metabolism is of great importance in physiology, pathology, and pharmacology. A systematic exploration of biased signaling will enhance insights into GPCRs-metabolism interactions, aiding disease mechanism studies, drug discovery, and clinical treatment strategies.

Keywords

Biased signaling · Drug · GPCR · Metabolism

1 Introduction

G protein-coupled receptors (GPCRs) represent one of the largest and most diverse families of membrane receptors, regulating numerous physiological and pathological processes (Lefkowitz 2013). GPCRs primarily mediate the transmission of signals between cells and external environment by sensing external stimuli and activating downstream signal transduction pathways. The downstream signaling of GPCRs is mediated by effector proteins such as G protein and β-arrestin (Rakesh et al. 2010). Upon receiving external stimuli, GPCRs can simultaneously activate multiple signaling pathways or selectively activate a specific signaling pathway, known as biased activation. Different biased signaling pathways may mediate distinct biological effects to adapt to changes in the body and maintain homeostasis (Lefkowitz 2013).

Metabolism is the most fundamental process of life, such as the growth, development, energy balance, and other aspects of all living organisms. Metabolic homeostasis is crucial, which supports cellular function, adapts to environmental changes, and ensures overall health and survival (Judge and Dodd 2020). Metabolism is broadly categorized into two main processes: catabolism and anabolism. Catabolism involves the breakdown of nutrients and biomolecules to release energy, often in the form of adenosine triphosphate (ATP), while anabolism uses energy to synthesize essential macromolecules such as proteins, lipids, and nucleic acids. Dysregulation of metabolic processes is closely linked to a wide range of diseases, including cardiovascular disease, cancer, obesity, and type 2 diabetes.

G protein-coupled receptors (GPCRs) are critically important regulators of metabolic physiology. First, they are extensively and widely expressed across key metabolic tissues, including pancreas (α and β cells), liver, white and brown adipose tissues, skeletal muscle, gastrointestinal tract, and central nervous system (particularly hypothalamic nuclei controlling appetite). This pervasive presence enables GPCRs to participate fundamentally in orchestrating all aspects of metabolic homeostasis. Second, they could regulate various metabolic processes such as glucose homeostasis, lipid metabolism, energy expenditure, amino acid catabolism, mineral balance, etc. Third, targeting GPCRs has led to significant clinical advances in the treatment of metabolic diseases, as evidenced by the success of glucagon-like peptide-1 receptor (GLP-1R) agonists (liraglutide, semaglutide) for type 2 diabetes and obesity, and β-blockers for energy metabolism in heart failure.

Recently, GPCR-biased signaling has represented a major frontier in metabolic researches. A frontier research direction is to understand how ligands selectively activate either G proteins or β-arrestins and how this selectivity precisely regulates physiological processes and contributes to disease. GPCR-biased signaling also drives the development of novel clinically biased therapeutics designed to target specific pathways for more effective and safer treatment of metabolic diseases.

2 Function of GPCRs in Metabolism

Research in the 1990s significantly advanced our understanding of GPCRs as crucial regulators of metabolism, revealing their important roles in glucose homeostasis and lipid metabolism. Among them, the GLP-1R and glucose-dependent insulinotropic polypeptide receptor (GIPR) emerged as prominent examples (Miyawaki et al. 1999; Scrocchi et al. 1998). Simultaneously, GPCRs like the β-adrenergic receptors (β-AR) were established as central regulators of energy metabolism, influencing processes such as thermogenesis and lipolysis (Borea et al. 1998). The calcium-sensing receptor (CaSR) as GPCR also were revealed to regulate mineral metabolism by maintaining calcium homeostasis and thereby influencing bone metabolism (Chattopadhyay 2000). Moving into the 2000s, the scope of GPCR-mediated metabolic regulation was further expanded. With the rapid advancement of genomics and transcriptomics, GPCRs were found not only to respond to classical neurotransmitters and hormones, but also to sense a wide array of metabolically relevant small molecules, including amino acids, free fatty acids, bile acids, and ketone bodies (Boeckler et al. 2005; Kostenis 2004; Tikhonova et al. 2007). These discoveries laid the foundation for the identification and development of "metabolite-sensing GPCRs," significantly expanding the scope of GPCR function in metabolic physiology. This two-way communication enables GPCRs to act as both metabolic sensors and coordinators, connecting external metabolic signals with the cell's internal responses. Through these key mechanisms, GPCRs play a crucial role in maintaining the dynamic and coordinated regulation of metabolism throughout the body.

First, GPCRs function as molecular sensors that dynamically interface extracellular stimuli with intracellular signaling cascades. Through N-terminal ectodomains and extracellular loops, GPCRs detect diverse ligands such as metabolic hormones and metabolites. GPCRs regulate metabolic functions in two main ways. First, various metabolites can act as ligands to activate GPCRs, thereby triggering intracellular signaling cascades. These activating ligands encompass a broad spectrum, including classical hormones (e.g., glucagon, epinephrine, GLP-1) that bind specific GPCRs to exert metabolic effects. Additionally, numerous metabolites themselves act as direct GPCR ligands. This diverse group of metabolite ligands includes gut microbiota-derived products and host-derived circulating metabolites. Gut microbiota-derived products include short-chain fatty acids (SCFAs) (Tang et al. 2015; Ulven 2012), medium-chain fatty acids (MCFAs) (Wang et al. 2006), long-chain fatty acids (LCFAs) (Hirasawa et al. 2005), and secondary bile acids (de Oliveira et al. 2016; Haussinger and Keitel 2017). Host-derived circulating metabolites includes intermediates of energy metabolism like lactate (Engelstoft et al. 2013; Liu et al. 2012a), ketone bodies (Kimura et al. 2011; Offermanns et al. 2011), and key lipid signaling molecules such as ceramides and metabolites of arachidonic acid (e.g., prostaglandins and leukotrienes) (Catoire et al. 2010; Wang et al. 2018). Remarkably, even metabolites typically confined to intracellular compartments can function extracellularly as GPCR ligands. A key example is succinate, a classical tricarboxylic acid (TCA) cycle intermediate generated within mitochondria, which targets the receptor GPR91 (SUCNR1). (Littlewood-Evans et al. 2016).

Second, GPCRs modulate different metabolic processes. As a superfamily of cell surface receptors, GPCRs are classified into five distinct subfamilies based on structural and functional characteristics, and all GPCR subfamilies are implicated in regulating metabolic processes. Class A GPCRs (rhodopsin-like family), the largest and most extensively studied group (Staubert et al. 2022), primarily mediate rapid metabolic responses through interactions with small molecule hormones such as norepinephrine and dopamine. Key examples include β-Ars, which regulate gluconeogenesis and lipolysis, and dopamine receptors that modulate insulin secretion and energy balance, making them critical targets for metabolic syndrome, obesity, and diabetes therapeutics (Bordicchia et al. 2012; Erraji-Benchekroun et al. 2005; Farino et al. 2020). Class B GPCRs, characterized by large extracellular domains (ECDs), predominantly bind peptide hormones (Wang et al. 2023). For instance, the GLP-1R activated by GLP-1 stimulates insulin secretion, while the glucagon receptor (GCGR) activated by glucagon promotes hepatic glycogenolysis and gluconeogenesis (Barrera et al. 2011; Godfrey et al. 2022). Class C GPCRs commonly function as dimers and are activated by amino acid-derived ligands, thereby bridging neural and metabolic signaling pathways (Lin et al. 2021). Notably, the CaSR regulates indirectly modulating bone metabolism and calcium-phosphate balance (Greer et al. 2008; Hannan et al. 2018). Class F GPCRs, such as Smoothened

(SMO), are implicated in developmental processes and tumor metabolism, driving glycolytic and lipogenic pathways within cancer microenvironments to fuel malignancy progression (Ge et al. 2015; Shi and Long 2017). Adhesion GPCRs, a unique subclass, sense mechanical forces to regulate organ development and metabolic functions (Wilde et al. 2022). ADGRG2/GPR133, for example, governs adipocyte lipolysis and lipid accumulation, thereby influencing lipid metabolism (Suchy et al. 2020).

In addition, GPCRs regulate nearly all metabolic processes. In glucose metabolism, GLP-1R, melanocortin 4 receptor (MC4R), calcitonin receptor (CALCR2), and cannabinoid receptor type 1 (CB1R) help maintain blood glucose levels by controlling insulin secretion, glycolysis, and glucose uptake (Fang et al. 2018; Mosialou et al. 2017; Ruiz de Azua et al. 2017). In lipid metabolism, GPR120, thyroid stimulating hormone receptor (TSHR), β3-AR, etc. regulate lipid breakdown, fatty acid uptake, and lipid synthesis to balance energy storage and use (Ichimura et al. 2012; Larsson et al. 2016; Liu et al. 2019). In amino acid metabolism, AT1R and GLP-1R adjust pathways according to amino acid levels (Kitaura et al. 2021; Samms et al. 2022). In energy metabolism, GPR91, GPR54, and melanin-concentrating hormone receptor 1 (MCHR1) control energy expenditure and thermogenesis (Rabe et al. 2022; Tolson et al. 2014; Zhang et al. 2014). In mineral metabolism, GPR68, GPR4, CaSR etc. regulate calcium and phosphorus balance by influencing mineral dissolution and deposition (Diaz-Tocados et al. 2019; Frick et al. 2009; Imenez Silva et al. 2020).

In summary, GPCRs play a key role in sensing metabolites and regulating essential metabolic processes such as glucose and lipid metabolism, energy balance, and mineral homeostasis. By linking nutrient sensing to downstream signaling, they serve as central integrators of metabolic networks, helping maintain systemic metabolic balance.

3 Function of GPCR-Biased Signaling in Metabolism

GPCRs serve as crucial sensors for metabolites and hormones, orchestrating systemic homeostasis. Meanwhile, GPCR downstream biased signaling—where ligands preferentially activate specific downstream pathways (e.g., G-protein vs. β-arrestin)—enhances metabolic homeostasis through its "pathway decoupling" capability, shifting pharmacology from mere receptor activation to programmable signaling. This also operates via two key mechanisms: first, endogenous metabolite ligands can function as natural biased agonists for GPCRs; second, downstream biased signaling then precisely regulate metabolic functions.

3.1 Metabolites as Biased Ligands of GPCRs

Traditionally, metabolites were seen only as intermediates in biological production or building blocks for biomolecules. Now, many endogenous metabolites were recognized as ligands that target GPCRs. These metabolites can bind to specific cell surface or intracellular receptors to trigger signaling cascades, influencing cell function, metabolism and even behavior. Thus, metabolites are a rapidly growing and exciting area in pharmacology and metabolic disease research. Emerging evidence also shows that metabolite ligands can induce biased signaling at their cognate GPCRs. Metabolite ligands (e.g., bile acids, fatty acids) often exhibit superior signaling pathway bias compared to traditional ligands, owing to their chemical properties (amphipathicity, charge distribution, and molecular flexibility) and receptor binding modes (orthosteric/allosteric pockets). For example, tauroursodeoxycholic acid (TUDCA)—a natural water-soluble bile acid formed by the conjugation of ursodeoxycholic acid (UDCA) with taurine—acts as a key metabolite ligand that modulates TGR5 and nuclear receptors (FXRs) to exert unique biological activities in diabetes and cardiovascular diseases. TUDCA embeds its steroid nucleus hydrophobic face into the transmembrane domain (TM3/5/6) of TGR5, stabilizing the Gs protein-coupled conformation. This results in pronounced G protein-biased signaling, which stimulates GLP-1 secretion and mitigates β-arrestin-mediated side effects (e.g., gallbladder contraction and pruritus) (Thomas et al. 2009; Yanguas-Casas et al. 2017). In addition, some metabolites exhibit biased agonism favoring G protein signaling pathway. For example, noribogaine is the long-lived human metabolite of the anti-addictive substance ibogaine, which biasedly activate the κ-opioid receptor-G protein signaling pathway and exert analgesic or anti-addictive effects (Maillet et al. 2015). Cannabielsoin (CBE) as an oxidation byproduct of cannabidiol (CBD) and a minor mammalian metabolite of CBD also showed a noteworthy bias toward cannabinoid receptor type 1 (CB1)-G-protein activation, thereby contributing to insulin resistance and obesity (Haghdoost et al. 2024; Liu et al. 2012b). Free fatty acid receptor 4 (FFAR4) is activated by medium-to-long chain free fatty acids, including saturated, monounsaturated, and polyunsaturated fats (Offermanns 2014). As endogenous FFAs, eicosapentaenoic acid (EPA), pinolenic acid, and palmitic acid exhibit far greater Gq protein activation and Ca^{2+} mobilization potency than β-arrestin recruitment potency, potentially eliciting enhanced glucose uptake and improved insulin resistance (Briscoe et al. 2006; Burns et al. 2014; Christiansen et al. 2015; Hudson et al. 2014; Yore et al. 2014). There are also endogenous metabolites capable of biased activation toward β-arrestin signaling pathway. For example, prostaglandin E2 (PGE2) can be metabolized into 15-keto-PGE2, which could terminate Gs protein-mediated cAMP/PKA signaling as a biased agonist (Endo et al. 2020). Activation of hydroxycarboxylic acid receptor 3 (HCA3) by 3-hydroxyoctanoic acid also leads to specifical β-arrestin 2 recruitment, which is relevant for cell-cell adhesion (Peters et al. 2020). Endogenous metabolic ligand ceramide activates adipocyte membrane receptor FPR2, inhibiting Gs-cAMP signaling while promoting β-arrestin recruitment, thereby suppressing lipolysis and thermogenesis – revealing a novel therapeutic target for obesity (Lin et al. 2025).

Understanding the potential bias of these endogenous ligands could provide new insights into GPCR-mediated metabolic control and aid in the development of more precise therapeutic strategies targeting metabolic disorders. Further research is needed to determine how these metabolites differentially influence GPCR signaling and their implications for both physiology and disease.

3.2 GPCR-Biased Signaling Regulates Metabolism

GPCRs are fundamental regulators of cellular metabolism, and biased signaling enables GPCR to orchestrate distinct downstream metabolic functions.

3.2.1 Glucose Metabolism

Glucose metabolism is a crucial component in maintaining energy balance and metabolic homeostasis, involving various biochemical reactions and metabolic pathways. Glucose metabolism primarily involves the core processes of glucose synthesis and storage, transport and uptake, and breakdown and oxidation; insulin sensitivity critically regulates these processes.

G protein-biased signaling pathways are primarily involved in the rapid regulation of metabolic functions, such as promoting insulin secretion and lowering blood glucose levels. Signaling bias fundamentally determines metabolic directionality. Gs-, Gq-, or G12-biased signaling generally promotes hypoglycemic effects—characterized by increased insulin secretion and enhanced glucose consumption—whereas Gi-biased signaling conversely inhibits insulin secretion, consequently elevating blood glucose levels. For example, tirzepatide (LY3298176) can target GLP-1R and activate G protein- biased signaling, which enhances insulin secretion, contributing to tirzepatide's efficacy in improving glucose control and body weight regulation in type 2 diabetes mellitus (Sun et al. 2022; Willard et al. 2020; Zaimia et al. 2023). Additionally, other GLP-1R agonists biased toward the Gs protein including LY3502970 and GL0034 can also exert blood glucose-lowering effects (Jones et al. 2022; Kawai et al. 2020). Beyond biased Gs-protein-cAMP signaling pathway, Gq/11 and G12 protein signaling pathways also play a role in decreasing blood glucose. TAK-875, a synthetic GPR40 agonist, exhibits bias toward Gq/11 signaling, resulting in insulin secretion (Mancini et al. 2015). GHSR1a, a rhodopsin-like Class A GPCR and the cognate receptor for ghrelin (Howard et al. 1996; Kojima et al. 1999), is modulated by melanocortin 2 receptor accessory protein (MRAP2). MRAP2 binding suppresses GHSR1a constitutive activity and biases receptor signaling toward Gq over β-arrestin recruitment, mediating the insulinostatic effects associated with ghrelin pathway activation (Rouault et al. 2020; Yin et al. 2020). Engagement of sphingosine-1-phosphate receptor 3 (S1PR3) by ALESIA (Anticancer Ligand Enhancing Starvation-Induced Apoptosis) results in G12 protein-biased signaling, promoting glucose exhaustion. Intraperitoneal administration of ALESIA improves the survival of mice with peritoneally disseminated rhabdomyosarcoma, indicating its potential as a new type of anticancer drug for glucose starvation therapy (Toyomoto et al. 2021). However, biased activation of canonical Gi protein signaling by dopamine (DA) at α2-adrenergic receptors reduces glucose-stimulated insulin secretion (GSIS) in β cells (Aslanoglou et al. 2021). Also, the interaction of insulin peptide insB:9-23 with olfactory receptor Olfr109 diminishes insulin secretion through Gi-cAMP signaling (Cheng et al. 2022), indicating that Gs protein-biased signaling pathway and Gi protein-biased signaling pathway have opposing effects in the regulation of insulin secretion.

In contrast, β-arrestin-biased signaling pathways primarily mediate sustained metabolic effects, such as promoting hepatic glycogen production and stimulating β cell proliferation. β-arrestin 1 promotes GLP-1R-mediated β cell proliferation (Talbot et al. 2012). Also, β-arrestin 2 is essential for maintaining islet insulin content and beta cell mass without affecting glucose-stimulated insulin secretion or GLP-1/acetylcholine amplification in perifused islets (Ravier et al. 2014). Thus, the GLP-1R-G protein-biased signaling pathway stimulates insulin secretion to lower blood glucose levels, while the GLP-1R-β-arrestin-biased signaling pathway promotes β cell proliferation, thereby delaying the progression of diabetes. In addition, hepatic glucagon receptors (GCGRs)-β-arrestin 2 biased pathway could also suppress hepatic glycogen production, indicating that hepatic β-arrestin 2-biased activity could prove useful for suppressing HGP for therapeutic purposes (Zhu et al. 2017).

Beyond G protein- and β-arrestin-biased signaling in GPCRs, the paradigm of biased agonism extends to preferential coupling with GPCR kinases (GRKs). Traditional β2-AR agonists are limited clinically by G protein-mediated cardiac side effects and β-arrestin-dependent desensitization. The novel GRK2-biased agonist ATR-258 overcomes these limitations through selective GRK2 coupling, which promotes β2-AR-mediated glucose uptake while avoiding activation of other pathways. Preclinical studies show that ATR-258 can enhance muscle glucose metabolism and improve glycemic control in models of hyperglycemia and obesity. Notably, it reduces both cardiotoxicity and muscle atrophy risks compared to conventional β2-AR agonists and incretin mimetics. This offers a new strategic direction for GPCR-biased signaling in metabolic disease therapy (Motso et al. 2025).

In the field of glucose metabolism research, GPCR-biased signaling has primarily been investigated in the context of insulin secretion, insulin sensitivity, and glucose production. However, its roles in other critical processes—such as glycolysis and glucose oxidation, as well as glucose uptake and transport—remain unexplored. Further studies are needed to elucidate whether and how GPCR-biased signaling regulates these pathways and function.

3.2.2 Lipid Metabolism

Lipid metabolism refers to the processes involved in the synthesis, breakdown, and utilization of lipid in the body, primarily including lipogenesis and lipolysis. In lipid metabolism, G protein-biased signaling pathways promote lipogenesis, adaptive thermogenesis, and energy expenditure, while β-arrestin-biased signaling suppresses lipid accumulation and exerts anti-inflammatory effects in adipose tissues. Exendin-P5 is a variant engineered through N-terminal modification of the natural hormone Exendin-4 (exenatide), designed to enhance preferential activation of G protein signaling. In diabetic mouse models, chronic administration of Exendin-P5 significantly promotes browning of white adipose tissue (WAT) along with beige adipogenesis (Zhang et al. 2015).

Importantly, β-arrestin-biased signaling mediates multiple functions in lipid metabolism. MC4R is a brain-expressed Gαs-coupled GPCR involved in weight regulation (Fan et al. 1997). Sixty-one variants in the MC4R gene were found in five hundred thousand people, and gain-of-function MC4R variants could preferentially activate β-arrestin signaling and protect against obesity. β-arrestin-biased MC4R signaling may represent an effective strategy for weight loss and the treatment of obesity-related cardiometabolic diseases (Lotta et al. 2019). Upon activation, growth hormone secretagogue receptor 1a (GHSR1a)'s extracellular loop 2 (ECL2) rearranges into a capping structure over the orthosteric pocket, acting as a critical molecular switch for receptor signaling bias. Missense mutations in ECL2 (e.g., Ala204Glu mutation) markedly reduce ghrelin-induced β-arrestin 2 signaling efficacy while leaving G protein signaling largely unaffected (Mokrosinski et al. 2012), which reduced ghrelin-mediated food intake and compromised adaptations in blood glucose homeostasis and growth hormone (GH) release during energetic stress (Pantel et al. 2006). As a key regulator of lipid metabolism, β3-AR exerts lipolytic effects. Studies reveal that adipocyte-specific β-arrestin 2 knockout mice show reduced adiposity and striking metabolic improvements even under caloric excess (Pydi et al. 2019). This demonstrates β-arrestin 2 as a potent in vivo suppressor of β3-AR activity, whose deletion selectively enhances G protein-biased lipolytic signaling. In addition, β-arrestin-biased signaling can also mediate more sustained and chronic metabolic effects, in contrast to the rapid metabolic responses mediated by G protein signaling. For example, GPR120 could attenuated NF-κB activation via downstream β-arrestin 2 signaling pathway, thus exerting anti-inflammatory role in adipose tissues (Anbazhagan et al. 2016).

However, it remains largely unexplored that GPCR-biased signaling's impact on lipid uptake and transport, thermogenic regulation, and adipose tissue remodeling (including browning and beiging). Elucidating these mechanisms is critical for a comprehensive understanding of metabolic GPCR biology and for leveraging pathway-selective ligands therapeutically.

3.2.3 Mineral Metabolism

Mineral metabolism refers to the complex biochemical processes that regulate the absorption, distribution, storage, and excretion of essential minerals including calcium, phosphorus, and magnesium to maintain systemic homeostasis. As a mineral reservoir, bone stores over 99% of body calcium and 85% of phosphorus, dynamically exchanged via bone remodeling. Bone metabolism refers to the continuous process of bone formation and resorption, essential for maintaining bone health and overall skeletal integrity. An imbalance between bone formation and resorption can lead to bone disorders. Parathyroid hormone receptor 1 (PTH1R) is the most important GPCR in regulating mineral metabolism in bone. Activation of Gs protein-cAMP pathway downstream of PTH1R directly stimulates osteoblast activity and bone formation (Portales-Castillo et al. 2023; Sinha et al. 2016). Intermittent PTH(1-34) (teriparatide) treatment effectively treats osteoporosis by activating the

PTH1R-Gs-biased pathway to stimulate osteoblast-mediated bone formation. However, PTH1R- Gq-biased pathway leads to increased bone resorption, partially offsetting the anabolic benefits. Interestingly, PTH1R-biased agonism reveals that selective β-arrestin activation produces bone responses distinct from conventional PTH(1-34) signaling. D-Trp12, Tyr34-bPTH(7-34) is a modified variant of PTH (7-34). Its N-terminal truncation renders it unable to activate G protein signaling, while modifications at the C-terminus enhance its selective recruitment of β-arrestin. Unlike PTH(1-34), PTH-β-arrestin appears to "uncouple" the anabolic effects of PTH1R activation from its catabolic and calcitropic effects (Bohinc and Gesty-Palmer 2012).

3.2.4 Energy Metabolism

Energy metabolism encompasses the complex biochemical pathways responsible for converting nutrients into usable cellular energy, primarily adenosine triphosphate (ATP). GPR4 acts as an environmental pH sensor via protonation of its conserved histidine residue (H167/H165). This protonation induces a conformational change in ECL2, leading to biased activation of the Gs-cAMP signaling pathway. This biased signaling enables the receptor to maintain cellular ATP synthesis efficiency. The mechanism provides a structural basis for energy balance in metabolic acidosis, directly linking pH sensing to biased GPCR signaling in cellular energy regulation (Wen et al. 2025). Additionally, intracellular accessory proteins can mediate GPCR-biased signaling to participate in energy regulation. GHSR1a functions as a critical regulator of energy metabolism by mediating ghrelin's dual role in promoting positive energy balance. This process is finely tuned by melanocortin receptor accessory protein 2 (MRAP2), a metabolic GPCR signal trafficker that suppresses GHSR1a constitutive activity and exhibits biased signaling toward Gq protein over β-arrestin (Rouault et al. 2020). MRAP2-Gq-biased pathway reduces unnecessary energy expenditure during fasting while enhancing ghrelin's orexigenic effects and gastric acid secretion. Also, the brain-penetrant agonist N8279 (NCATS-SM8864) enables direct targeting of central feeding-regulatory circuits. By stabilizing GHSR1a conformations that favor Gq activation, its dual capability of cerebral accessibility and pathway selectivity establishes N8279 as a translational drug candidate for energy metabolism disorders. (Gross et al. 2022).

Above all, GPCR-biased signaling serves as a master regulator of glucose metabolism, lipid metabolism, mineral metabolism, and energy metabolism by biased metabolite ligands, which allows for precise control of metabolic responses, highlighting the importance of GPCR-biased signaling in maintaining metabolic balance and responding to physiological demands (Table 1). Given the critical role of GPCRs in maintaining metabolic homeostasis, investigating biased signaling in a broader range of metabolic processes holds significant potential. Expanding research in this area could lead to novel insights into metabolic regulation and the development of more targeted therapeutic approaches for metabolic disorders.

Table 1 Biased metabolite ligands and metabolic function

Ligands	Receptors	Effectors	Function	References
Tauroursodeoxycholic acid	TGR5	G protein	Promotes GLP-1 secretion	Yanguas-Casas et al. (2017)
Noribogaine	κ-opioid receptor	G protein	Exert analgesic and anti-addictive effect	Maillet et al. (2015)
Cannabielsoin (CBE)	CB1R	G protein	NA	Haghdoost et al. (2024)
Eicosapentaenoic acid (EPA)	FFA4/ GPR120	Gq protein	Enhances glucose uptake	Briscoe et al. (2006), Christiansen et al. (2015)
Pinolenic acid	FFA4/ GPR120	Gq protein	Improves insulin resistance	Christiansen et al. (2015)
Palmitic acid	FFA4/ GPR120	Gq protein	NA	Briscoe et al. (2006), Christiansen et al. (2015)
15-keto-PGE2	EPR	β-arrestin	Terminates Gs protein signaling	Endo et al. (2020)
Ceramides	FPR2	β-arrestin	Inhibits adipocyte thermogenesis	Lin et al. (2025)
3-hydroxyoctanoic acid	HCA3	β-arrestin 2	Promotes cell-cell adhesion	Peters et al. (2020)
Tirzepatide (LY3298176)	GLP-1R	G protein	Enhances insulin secretion	Sun et al. (2022), Willard et al. (2020) and Zaimia et al. (2023)
LY3502970	GLP-1R	G protein	Enhances insulin secretion	Kawai et al. (2020)
Exendin-F1	GLP-1R	G protein	Prolongs insulin secretion and sustains anti-hyperglycaemic efficacy	Marzook et al. (2021)
GL0034	GLP-1R	G protein	Lowers blood glucose and weight loss	Jones et al. (2022)
P5	GLP-1R	G protein	Increases adipogenesis	Zhang et al. (2015)
R485X	PTH1R	Gs protein	Promotes bone formation	Portales-Castillo et al. (2023)
H^+	GPR4	Gs protein	Maintain cellular ATP synthesis efficiency	Wen et al. (2025)
TAK-875	GPR40	Gq/11 protein	Stimulates insulin secretion	Mancini et al. (2015)
	GHSR1a	Gq/11 protein	Promotes energy homeostasis	Rouault et al. (2020)

(continued)

Table 1 (continued)

Ligands	Receptors	Effectors	Function	References
YIL781	GHSR1a	Gq/11 and G12 protein	Increases food intake and decreases gastric emptying	Mende et al. (2018)
	GHSR1a	Gq protein	Exerts insulinostatic effect	Rouault et al. (2020), Yin et al. (2020)
	GHSR1a	Gq protein	Stimulates food intake	Pantel et al. (2006)
N8279	GHSR1a	Gq protein	Maintains energy homeostasis	Gross et al. (2022)
ALESIA	S1PR3	G12 protein	Promotes the exhaustion of glucose	Toyomoto et al. (2021)
Dopamine (DA)	α2-AR	Gi protein	Reduces glucose-stimulated insulin secretion	Aslanoglou et al. (2021)
insB:9–23	Olfr109	Gi protein	Diminishes insulin secretion	Cheng et al. (2022)
Carvedilol	β-AR	β-arrestin	Increases glucose consumption	Guven et al. (2020)
	MC4R	β-arrestin	Lowers BMI and lowers odds of obesity	Lotta et al. (2019)
D-Trp12,Tyr34-bPTH (7–34)	PTH1R	β-arrestin	Induces anabolic bone formation	Bohinc and Gesty-Palmer (2012)
RAMP2	PTH1R	β-arrestin	Induces anabolic bone formation	Nemec et al. (2022)
	β2-AR	β-arrestin 1	Upregulates lactate metabolism	Dong et al. (2017)
	β3-AR	β-arrestin 2	Inhibits adipocyte β3-AR activity	Pydi et al. (2019)
	GPR120	β-arrestin 2	Inhibits adipose tissues inflammatioin	Anbazhagan et al. (2016)
	GLP-1R	β-arrestin 2	Promote β cell proliferation	Ravier et al. (2014)
ATR-258	β2-AR	GRK2	Enhances muscle metabolism and promotes glucose control	Motso et al. (2025)

4 The Application of Biased GPCR-Targeted Drugs in Metabolic Diseases

As the largest family of membrane proteins in humans, GPCRs play a central role in metabolic regulation. Numerous GPCR-targeted drugs have been approved for treating metabolic disorders, with many drug candidates currently in clinical trials. GLP-1R agonists improve glycemia via insulin stimulation and glucagon suppression, while promoting weight loss through delayed gastric emptying. Tirzepatide, a dual agonist simultaneously targeting GLP-1R and GIPR, demonstrates superior efficacy in reducing HbA1c and body weight (22.5% reduction over 72 weeks). The clinical success of these agents not only validates GPCRs as druggable targets for diabetes and obesity, but also catalyzes drug discovery efforts targeting other metabolic GPCRs (Drucker 2025).

Traditional GPCR drugs simultaneously activate both G protein pathways and β-arrestin signaling, which may lead to unintended side effects. To address these limitations, biased ligands are being designed to selectively engage specific downstream pathways. This strategy enables precision metabolic regulation by tailoring signaling outcomes, thereby improving therapeutic efficacy and safety by enhancing drug efficacy and reducing side effects in metabolic diseases.

4.1 Enhancing Drug Efficacy and Duration in Metabolism

It is commonly believed that GPCRs mediate the transduction of extracellular signals on the cell membrane through G protein signaling. β-arrestins play a role in mediating receptor internalization and degradation. Some ligands can preferentially activate G protein signaling pathways or inhibit β-arrestin signaling pathways, thereby reducing receptor internalization. This results in increased receptor activity on the cell membrane and prolongs the effect of the ligands. In diabetes management, GLP-1R-biased agonists P5 and exendin-F1 significantly suppress β-arrestin 2 recruitment and receptor internalization compared to conventional agonists, enabling persistent retention of active receptor-Gs complexes in early endosomes. This mechanism prolongs insulin secretion by 2.3-fold in vitro and sustains glucose-lowering efficacy beyond 12 h in diabetic mice (Marzook et al. 2021). Similarly, GIP/GLP-1/GCG multi-target-biased analogs extend euglycemia duration by 40% through reduced β-arrestin 2-dependent internalization (Jones et al. 2021). For obesity therapeutics, G protein-biased β3-AR agonists (e.g., optimized CL-316243 derivatives) increase thermogenesis duration 3.1-fold and elevate fat consumption by 68% in preclinical models by avoiding β-arrestin-mediated receptor desensitization (Pydi et al. 2019). These approaches enable monthly dosing by extending drug half-life and maintain adipose-specific β3-AR activation with improved cardiovascular safety.

4.2 Reducing Side Effects in the Treatment of Metabolic Diseases

Biased signaling achieves superior therapeutic precision in chronic metabolic diseases by selectively modulating specific GPCR pathways, thereby reducing adverse effects. The brain-penetrant GHSR1a agonist N8279 (NCATS-SM8864) exhibits pronounced disease-modifying effects through Gq-biased pathway. N8279 normalizes dysregulated feeding behavior within 48 h, reducing binge-eating episodes by 62% in hyperdopaminergic mice. Critically, it normalizes dopamine transporter function in the nucleus accumbens, a key neural target in compulsive eating, and avoids β-arrestin-mediated injure (Gross et al. 2022). In addition, traditional β2-AR agonists activate Gs-cAMP pathway to promote glucose uptake but concurrently cause tachycardia and receptor desensitization. In contrast, GRK-biased β2-AR agonists significantly improve hyperglycemia and insulin sensitivity by increasing muscle glucose uptake via the GRK2/mTORC2 pathway, thereby avoiding the cardiovascular risks associated with traditional agonists. Phase I clinical trials have demonstrated favorable tolerability (Motso et al. 2025).

Despite the therapeutic potential for metabolic diseases, biased GPCR ligands remain predominantly in preclinical stages, with limited advancement to clinical trials. Challenges such as target specificity, off-target effects, and incomplete understanding of pathway-biased signaling in complex metabolic networks hinder clinical translation. Additionally, optimizing pharmacokinetics and ensuring long-term safety require further refinement. Future efforts must prioritize translational validation, leveraging advanced tools (e.g., cryo-EM, AI-driven drug design) to engineer ligands with enhanced precision. Collaborative, interdisciplinary approaches will be critical to bridge the gap between preclinical promise and clinical application in metabolic therapeutics.

5 Future Direction

While the fundamental role of GPCRs in metabolic regulation is well-established, the in-depth exploitation of GPCR signaling bias represents a critical and burgeoning frontier essential for the next generation of metabolic therapeutics. Numerous studies have demonstrated that endogenous metabolites can act as ligands to activate GPCRs, playing a crucial role in metabolic regulation. However, whether these metabolite ligands exhibit biased signaling remains largely unexplored. Circulating metabolites, such as gut microbiota-derived metabolites and metabolites produced by cells themselves, represent a significant area of interest for future studies. Investigating their potential-biased signaling effects could provide novel insights into metabolic regulation and disease mechanisms. Additionally, current research on GPCR-biased signaling has primarily focused on glucose homeostasis, lipid metabolism, and mineral metabolism, leaving many other metabolic pathways largely unexplored. Key metabolic processes such as amino acid metabolism and bile acid metabolism have not yet been extensively examined in the context of GPCR-biased signaling. Furthermore, GPCR-biased signaling regulates metabolic functions through downstream effectors. However, research on novel effectors and the specific mechanisms by which they mediate biased metabolic responses remains limited. Future studies should focus on elucidating how different novel effector contribute to metabolic regulation, which could help refine drug targeting strategies and enhance therapeutic specificity in metabolic diseases.

Future research should prioritize deciphering the combinatorial complexity of metabolite-GPCR interactions. Endogenous ligands frequently engage in "many-to-many" relationships, in which single metabolites often target multiple receptors, while individual GPCRs respond to diverse metabolite ensembles. To navigate this network-level crosstalk, a systems pharmacology approach is essential to map how biased signals propagate through metabolite-linked receptor clusters (e.g., SCFA-sensing GPR41/43/109A hubs) and engineer multi-receptor-biased modulators. Successfully programming such metabolic bias networks will overcome single-target limitations and achieve context-integrated homeostasis restoration.

A critical future direction lies in elucidating how metabolism-driven post-translational modifications (PTMs) dynamically rewire GPCR-biased signaling in response to nutrient fluctuations. Pathological metabolic states (e.g., hyperglycemia, ketoacidosis, or mitochondrial dysfunction) induce aberrant PTMs, such as O-GlcNAcylation, succinylation, or lactoylation, that directly alter receptor conformational landscapes and effector coupling preferences. These metabolic PTM switches act as pathology-specific bias tuners, converting receptors into disease-adapted signaling. Future research should map real-time PTM-bias dynamics using metabolite-integrated structural biology and develop PTM-responsive nanotherapeutics. Decoding this metabolite-PTM-bias axis will enable therapies that adapt to metabolic contexts, moving beyond static receptor targeting toward dynamic, pathology-aware signaling correction.

AI-driven platforms represent a transformative frontier for de novo discovery of functionally selective GPCR ligands with tailored signaling profiles. Building on machine learning models generating peptide-based dual GCGR/GLP-1R agonists with significantly enhanced potency and metabolic efficacy (Puszkarska et al. 2024). Future efforts must prioritize three key interconnected areas: (1) scaling generative AI frameworks to systematically explore complex multi-receptor targeting strategies (e.g., GLP-1R/GIPR/GCGR tri-agonists), requiring advanced algorithms capable of navigating the vast chemical and conformational space for simultaneously optimizing receptor engagement, signaling bias, and metabolic outcomes; (2) rigorously coupling *in silico* predictions with high-throughput experimental validation of signaling bias, establishing robust feedback loops to refine AI models and ensure translational relevance; (3) accelerating clinical translation of optimized AI-generated biased and multi-target ligands into preclinical and clinical development for metabolic diseases (obesity, T2D, NASH), ultimately demonstrating superior clinical efficacy and safety profiles.

References

Anbazhagan AN, Priyamvada S, Gujral T, Bhattacharyya S, Alrefai WA, Dudeja PK, Borthakur A (2016) A novel anti-inflammatory role of GPR120 in intestinal epithelial cells. Am J Physiol Cell Physiol 310:C612–C621. https://doi.org/10.1152/ajpcell.00123.2015

Aslanoglou D, Bertera S, Sanchez-Soto M, Benjamin Free R, Lee J, Zong W, Xue X, Shrestha S, Brissova M, Logan RW, Wollheim CB, Trucco M, Yechoor VK, Sibley DR, Bottino R, Freyberg Z (2021) Dopamine regulates pancreatic glucagon and insulin secretion via adrenergic and dopaminergic receptors. Transl Psychiatry 11:59. https://doi.org/10.1038/s41398-020-01171-z

Barrera JG, Sandoval DA, D'Alessio DA, Seeley RJ (2011) GLP-1 and energy balance: an integrated model of short-term and long-term control. Nat Rev Endocrinol 7:507–516. https://doi.org/10.1038/nrendo.2011.77

Boeckler F, Lanig H, Gmeiner P (2005) Modeling the similarity and divergence of dopamine D2-like receptors and identification of validated ligand-receptor complexes. J Med Chem 48: 694–709. https://doi.org/10.1021/jm049612a

Bohinc BN, Gesty-Palmer D (2012) Biased agonism at the parathyroid hormone receptor: a demonstration of functional selectivity in bone metabolism. Mini Rev Med Chem 12:856–865. https://doi.org/10.2174/138955712800959125

Bordicchia M, Liu D, Amri EZ, Ailhaud G, Dessi-Fulgheri P, Zhang C, Takahashi N, Sarzani R, Collins S (2012) Cardiac natriuretic peptides act via p38 MAPK to induce the brown fat thermogenic program in mouse and human adipocytes. J Clin Invest 122:1022–1036. https://doi.org/10.1172/JCI59701

Borea PA, Varani K, Gessi S, Gilli P, Dalpiaz A (1998) Receptor binding thermodynamics as a tool for linking drug efficacy and affinity. Farmaco 53:249–254. https://doi.org/10.1016/s0014-827x(98)00017-2

Briscoe CP, Peat AJ, McKeown SC, Corbett DF, Goetz AS, Littleton TR, McCoy DC, Kenakin TP, Andrews JL, Ammala C, Fornwald JA, Ignar DM, Jenkinson S (2006) Pharmacological regulation of insulin secretion in MIN6 cells through the fatty acid receptor GPR40: identification of agonist and antagonist small molecules. Br J Pharmacol 148:619–628. https://doi.org/10.1038/sj.bjp.0706770

Burns RN, Singh M, Senatorov IS, Moniri NH (2014) Mechanisms of homologous and heterologous phosphorylation of FFA receptor 4 (GPR120): GRK6 and PKC mediate phosphorylation of Thr(3)(4)(7), Ser(3)(5)(0), and Ser(3)(5)(7) in the C-terminal tail. Biochem Pharmacol 87: 650–659. https://doi.org/10.1016/j.bcp.2013.12.016

Catoire LJ, Damian M, Giusti F, Martin A, van Heijenoort C, Popot JL, Guittet E, Baneres JL (2010) Structure of a GPCR ligand in its receptor-bound state: leukotriene B4 adopts a highly constrained conformation when associated to human BLT2. J Am Chem Soc 132:9049–9057. https://doi.org/10.1021/ja101868c

Chattopadhyay N (2000) Biochemistry, physiology and pathophysiology of the extracellular calcium-sensing receptor. Int J Biochem Cell Biol 32:789–804. https://doi.org/10.1016/s1357-2725(00)00031-5

Cheng J, Yang Z, Ge XY, Gao MX, Meng R, Xu X, Zhang YQ, Li RZ, Lin JY, Tian ZM, Wang J, Ning SL, Xu YF, Yang F, Gu JK, Sun JP, Yu X (2022) Autonomous sensing of the insulin peptide by an olfactory G protein-coupled receptor modulates glucose metabolism. Cell Metab 34:240–255 e10. https://doi.org/10.1016/j.cmet.2021.12.022

Christiansen E, Watterson KR, Stocker CJ, Sokol E, Jenkins L, Simon K, Grundmann M, Petersen RK, Wargent ET, Hudson BD, Kostenis E, Ejsing CS, Cawthorne MA, Milligan G, Ulven T (2015) Activity of dietary fatty acids on FFA1 and FFA4 and characterisation of pinolenic acid as a dual FFA1/FFA4 agonist with potential effect against metabolic diseases. Br J Nutr 113: 1677–1688. https://doi.org/10.1017/S000711451500118X

de Oliveira MC, Gilglioni EH, de Boer BA, Runge JH, de Waart DR, Salgueiro CL, Ishii-Iwamoto EL, Oude Elferink RP, Gaemers IC (2016) Bile acid receptor agonists INT747 and INT777 decrease oestrogen deficiency-related postmenopausal obesity and hepatic steatosis in mice. Biochim Biophys Acta 1862:2054–2062. https://doi.org/10.1016/j.bbadis.2016.07.012

Diaz-Tocados JM, Rodriguez-Ortiz ME, Almaden Y, Pineda C, Martinez-Moreno JM, Herencia C, Vergara N, Pendon-Ruiz de Mier MV, Santamaria R, Rodelo-Haad C, Casado-Diaz A, Lorenzo V, Carvalho C, Frazao JM, Felsenfeld AJ, Richards WG, Aguilera-Tejero E, Rodriguez M, Lopez I, Munoz-Castaneda JR (2019) Calcimimetics maintain bone turnover in uremic rats despite the concomitant decrease in parathyroid hormone concentration. Kidney Int 95:1064–1078. https://doi.org/10.1016/j.kint.2018.12.015

Dong JH, Wang YJ, Cui M, Wang XJ, Zheng WS, Ma ML, Yang F, He DF, Hu QX, Zhang DL, Ning SL, Liu CH, Wang C, Wang Y, Li XY, Yi F, Lin A, Kahsai AW, Cahill TJ 3rd, Chen ZY, Yu X, Sun JP (2017) Adaptive activation of a stress response pathway improves learning and memory through Gs and beta-Arrestin-1-regulated lactate metabolism. Biol Psychiatry 81:654–670. https://doi.org/10.1016/j.biopsych.2016.09.025

Drucker DJ (2025) GLP-1-based therapies for diabetes, obesity and beyond. Nat Rev Drug Discov 24. https://doi.org/10.1038/s41573-025-01183-8

Endo S, Suganami A, Fukushima K, Senoo K, Araki Y, Regan JW, Mashimo M, Tamura Y, Fujino H (2020) 15-Keto-PGE(2) acts as a biased/partial agonist to terminate PGE(2)-evoked signaling. J Biol Chem 295:13338–13352. https://doi.org/10.1074/jbc.RA120.013988

Engelstoft MS, Park WM, Sakata I, Kristensen LV, Husted AS, Osborne-Lawrence S, Piper PK, Walker AK, Pedersen MH, Nohr MK, Pan J, Sinz CJ, Carrington PE, Akiyama TE, Jones RM, Tang C, Ahmed K, Offermanns S, Egerod KL, Zigman JM, Schwartz TW (2013) Seven transmembrane G protein-coupled receptor repertoire of gastric ghrelin cells. Mol Metab 2: 376–392. https://doi.org/10.1016/j.molmet.2013.08.006

Erraji-Benchekroun L, Couton D, Postic C, Borde I, Gaston J, Guillet JG, Andre C (2005) Overexpression of beta2-adrenergic receptors in mouse liver alters the expression of gluconeogenic and glycolytic enzymes. Am J Physiol Endocrinol Metab 288:E715–E722. https://doi.org/10.1152/ajpendo.00113.2004

Fan W, Boston BA, Kesterson RA, Hruby VJ, Cone RD (1997) Role of melanocortinergic neurons in feeding and the agouti obesity syndrome. Nature 385:165–168. https://doi.org/10.1038/385165a0

Fang P, He B, Yu M, Shi M, Zhu Y, Zhang Z, Bo P (2018) Central galanin receptor 2 mediates galanin action to promote systemic glucose metabolism of type 2 diabetic rats. Biochem Pharmacol 156:241–247. https://doi.org/10.1016/j.bcp.2018.08.036

Farino ZJ, Morgenstern TJ, Maffei A, Quick M, De Solis AJ, Wiriyasermkul P, Freyberg RJ, Aslanoglou D, Sorisio D, Inbar BP, Free RB, Donthamsetti P, Mosharov EV, Kellendonk C, Schwartz GJ, Sibley DR, Schmauss C, Zeltser LM, Moore H, Harris PE, Javitch JA, Freyberg Z (2020) New roles for dopamine D(2) and D(3) receptors in pancreatic beta cell insulin secretion. Mol Psychiatry 25:2070–2085. https://doi.org/10.1038/s41380-018-0344-6

Frick KK, Krieger NS, Nehrke K, Bushinsky DA (2009) Metabolic acidosis increases intracellular calcium in bone cells through activation of the proton receptor OGR1. J Bone Miner Res 24: 305–313. https://doi.org/10.1359/jbmr.081015

Ge X, Lyu P, Gu Y, Li L, Li J, Wang Y, Zhang L, Fu C, Cao Z (2015) Sonic hedgehog stimulates glycolysis and proliferation of breast cancer cells: modulation of PFKFB3 activation. Biochem Biophys Res Commun 464:862–868. https://doi.org/10.1016/j.bbrc.2015.07.052

Godfrey J, Riscal R, Skuli N, Simon MC (2022) Glucagon signaling via supraphysiologic GCGR can reduce cell viability without stimulating gluconeogenic gene expression in liver cancer cells. Cancer Metab 10:4. https://doi.org/10.1186/s40170-022-00280-1

Greer ER, Perez CL, Van Gilst MR, Lee BH, Ashrafi K (2008) Neural and molecular dissection of a C. elegans sensory circuit that regulates fat and feeding. Cell Metab 8:118–131. https://doi.org/10.1016/j.cmet.2008.06.005

Gross JD, Kim DW, Zhou Y, Jansen D, Slosky LM, Clark NB, Ray CR, Hu X, Southall N, Wang A, Xu X, Barnaeva E, Wetsel WC, Ferrer M, Marugan JJ, Caron MG, Barak LS, Toth K (2022) Discovery of a functionally selective ghrelin receptor (GHSR(1a)) ligand for modulating brain dopamine. Proc Natl Acad Sci USA 119:e2112397119. https://doi.org/10.1073/pnas.2112397119

Guven B, Kara Z, Onay-Besikci A (2020) Metabolic effects of carvedilol through beta-arrestin proteins: investigations in a streptozotocin-induced diabetes rat model and in C2C12 myoblasts. Br J Pharmacol 177:5580–5594. https://doi.org/10.1111/bph.15269

Haghdoost M, Young S, Roberts M, Krebs C, Bonn-Miller MO (2024) Cannabielsoin (CBE), a CBD oxidation product, is a biased CB(1) agonist. Biomedicine 12. https://doi.org/10.3390/biomedicines12071551

Hannan FM, Kallay E, Chang W, Brandi ML, Thakker RV (2018) The calcium-sensing receptor in physiology and in calcitropic and noncalcitropic diseases. Nat Rev Endocrinol 15:33–51. https://doi.org/10.1038/s41574-018-0115-0

Haussinger D, Keitel V (2017) Dual role of the bile acid receptor Takeda G-protein-coupled receptor 5 for hepatic lipid metabolism in feast and famine. Hepatology 65:767–770. https://doi.org/10.1002/hep.29017

Hirasawa A, Tsumaya K, Awaji T, Katsuma S, Adachi T, Yamada M, Sugimoto Y, Miyazaki S, Tsujimoto G (2005) Free fatty acids regulate gut incretin glucagon-like peptide-1 secretion through GPR120. Nat Med 11:90–94. https://doi.org/10.1038/nm1168

Howard AD, Feighner SD, Cully DF, Arena JP, Liberator PA, Rosenblum CI, Hamelin M, Hreniuk DL, Palyha OC, Anderson J, Paress PS, Diaz C, Chou M, Liu KK, McKee KK, Pong SS, Chaung LY, Elbrecht A, Dashkevicz M, Heavens R, Rigby M, Sirinathsinghji DJ, Dean DC, Melillo DG, Patchett AA, Nargund R, Griffin PR, DeMartino JA, Gupta SK, Schaeffer JM, Smith RG, Van der Ploeg LH (1996) A receptor in pituitary and hypothalamus that functions in growth hormone release. Science 273:974–977. https://doi.org/10.1126/science.273.5277.974

Hudson BD, Shimpukade B, Milligan G, Ulven T (2014) The molecular basis of ligand interaction at free fatty acid receptor 4 (FFA4/GPR120). J Biol Chem 289:20345–20358. https://doi.org/10.1074/jbc.M114.561449

Ichimura A, Hirasawa A, Poulain-Godefroy O, Bonnefond A, Hara T, Yengo L, Kimura I, Leloire A, Liu N, Iida K, Choquet H, Besnard P, Lecoeur C, Vivequin S, Ayukawa K, Takeuchi M, Ozawa K, Tauber M, Maffeis C, Morandi A, Buzzetti R, Elliott P, Pouta A, Jarvelin MR, Korner A, Kiess W, Pigeyre M, Caiazzo R, Van Hul W, Van Gaal L, Horber F, Balkau B, Levy-Marchal C, Rouskas K, Kouvatsi A, Hebebrand J, Hinney A, Scherag A, Pattou F, Meyre D, Koshimizu TA, Wolowczuk I, Tsujimoto G, Froguel P (2012) Dysfunction of lipid sensor GPR120 leads to obesity in both mouse and human. Nature 483:350–354. https://doi.org/10.1038/nature10798

Imenez Silva PH, Katamesh-Benabbas C, Chan K, Pastor Arroyo EM, Knopfel T, Bettoni C, Ludwig MG, Gasser JA, Brandao-Burch A, Arnett TR, Bonny O, Seuwen K, Wagner CA (2020) The proton-activated ovarian cancer G protein-coupled receptor 1 (OGR1) is responsible for renal calcium loss during acidosis. Kidney Int 97:920–933. https://doi.org/10.1016/j.kint.2019.12.006

Jones B, McGlone ER, Fang Z, Pickford P, Correa IR Jr, Oishi A, Jockers R, Inoue A, Kumar S, Gorlitz F, Dunsby C, French PMW, Rutter GA, Tan T, Tomas A, Bloom SR (2021) Genetic and biased agonist-mediated reductions in beta-arrestin recruitment prolong cAMP signaling at glucagon family receptors. J Biol Chem 296:100133. https://doi.org/10.1074/jbc.RA120.016334

Jones B, Burade V, Akalestou E, Manchanda Y, Ramchunder Z, Carrat G, Nguyen-Tu MS, Marchetti P, Piemonti L, Leclerc I, Thennati R, Vilsboll T, Thorens B, Tomas A, Rutter GA (2022) In vivo and in vitro characterization of GL0034, a novel long-acting glucagon-like peptide-1 receptor agonist. Diabetes Obes Metab 24:2090–2101. https://doi.org/10.1111/dom.14794

Judge A, Dodd MS (2020) Metabolism. Essays Biochem 64:607–647. https://doi.org/10.1042/EBC20190041

Kawai T, Sun B, Yoshino H, Feng D, Suzuki Y, Fukazawa M, Nagao S, Wainscott DB, Showalter AD, Droz BA, Kobilka TS, Coghlan MP, Willard FS, Kawabe Y, Kobilka BK, Sloop KW

(2020) Structural basis for GLP-1 receptor activation by LY3502970, an orally active nonpeptide agonist. Proc Natl Acad Sci USA 117:29959–29967. https://doi.org/10.1073/pnas.2014879117

Kimura I, Inoue D, Maeda T, Hara T, Ichimura A, Miyauchi S, Kobayashi M, Hirasawa A, Tsujimoto G (2011) Short-chain fatty acids and ketones directly regulate sympathetic nervous system via G protein-coupled receptor 41 (GPR41). Proc Natl Acad Sci USA 108:8030–8035. https://doi.org/10.1073/pnas.1016088108

Kitaura Y, Shindo D, Ogawa T, Sato A, Shimomura Y (2021) Antihypertensive drug valsartan as a novel BDK inhibitor. Pharmacol Res 167:105518. https://doi.org/10.1016/j.phrs.2021.105518

Kojima M, Hosoda H, Date Y, Nakazato M, Matsuo H, Kangawa K (1999) Ghrelin is a growth-hormone-releasing acylated peptide from stomach. Nature 402:656–660. https://doi.org/10.1038/45230

Kostenis E (2004) A glance at G-protein-coupled receptors for lipid mediators: a growing receptor family with remarkably diverse ligands. Pharmacol Ther 102:243–257. https://doi.org/10.1016/j.pharmthera.2004.04.005

Larsson S, Jones HA, Goransson O, Degerman E, Holm C (2016) Parathyroid hormone induces adipocyte lipolysis via PKA-mediated phosphorylation of hormone-sensitive lipase. Cell Signal 28:204–213. https://doi.org/10.1016/j.cellsig.2015.12.012

Lefkowitz RJ (2013) A brief history of G-protein coupled receptors (Nobel Lecture). Angew Chem Int Ed Engl 52:6366–6378. https://doi.org/10.1002/anie.201301924

Lin S, Han S, Cai X, Tan Q, Zhou K, Wang D, Wang X, Du J, Yi C, Chu X, Dai A, Zhou Y, Chen Y, Zhou Y, Liu H, Liu J, Yang D, Wang MW, Zhao Q, Wu B (2021) Structures of G(i)-bound metabotropic glutamate receptors mGlu2 and mGlu4. Nature 594:583–588. https://doi.org/10.1038/s41586-021-03495-2

Lin H, Ma C, Cai K, Guo L, Wang X, Lv L, Zhang C, Lin J, Zhang D, Ye C, Wang T, Huang S, Han J, Zhang Z, Gao J, Zhang M, Pu Z, Li F, Guo Y, Zhou X, Qin C, Yi F, Yu X, Kong W, Jiang C, Sun JP (2025) Metabolic signaling of ceramides through the FPR2 receptor inhibits adipocyte thermogenesis. Science 388:eado4188. https://doi.org/10.1126/science.ado4188

Littlewood-Evans A, Sarret S, Apfel V, Loesle P, Dawson J, Zhang J, Muller A, Tigani B, Kneuer R, Patel S, Valeaux S, Gommermann N, Rubic-Schneider T, Junt T, Carballido JM (2016) GPR91 senses extracellular succinate released from inflammatory macrophages and exacerbates rheumatoid arthritis. J Exp Med 213:1655–1662. https://doi.org/10.1084/jem.20160061

Liu C, Kuei C, Zhu J, Yu J, Zhang L, Shih A, Mirzadegan T, Shelton J, Sutton S, Connelly MA, Lee G, Carruthers N, Wu J, Lovenberg TW (2012a) 3,5-Dihydroxybenzoic acid, a specific agonist for hydroxycarboxylic acid 1, inhibits lipolysis in adipocytes. J Pharmacol Exp Ther 341:794–801. https://doi.org/10.1124/jpet.112.192799

Liu J, Zhou L, Xiong K, Godlewski G, Mukhopadhyay B, Tam J, Yin S, Gao P, Shan X, Pickel J, Bataller R, O'Hare J, Scherer T, Buettner C, Kunos G (2012b) Hepatic cannabinoid receptor-1 mediates diet-induced insulin resistance via inhibition of insulin signaling and clearance in mice. Gastroenterology 142:1218–1228 e1. https://doi.org/10.1053/j.gastro.2012.01.032

Liu P, Huang S, Ling S, Xu S, Wang F, Zhang W, Zhou R, He L, Xia X, Yao Z, Fan Y, Wang N, Hu C, Zhao X, Tucker HO, Wang J, Guo X (2019) Foxp1 controls brown/beige adipocyte differentiation and thermogenesis through regulating beta3-AR desensitization. Nat Commun 10:5070. https://doi.org/10.1038/s41467-019-12988-8

Lotta LA, Mokrosinski J, Mendes de Oliveira E, Li C, Sharp SJ, Luan J, Brouwers B, Ayinampudi V, Bowker N, Kerrison N, Kaimakis V, Hoult D, Stewart ID, Wheeler E, Day FR, Perry JRB, Langenberg C, Wareham NJ, Farooqi IS (2019) Human gain-of-function MC4R variants show signaling bias and protect against obesity. Cell 177(597–607):e9. https://doi.org/10.1016/j.cell.2019.03.044

Maillet EL, Milon N, Heghinian MD, Fishback J, Schurer SC, Garamszegi N, Mash DC (2015) Noribogaine is a G-protein biased kappa-opioid receptor agonist. Neuropharmacology 99:675–688. https://doi.org/10.1016/j.neuropharm.2015.08.032

Mancini AD, Bertrand G, Vivot K, Carpentier E, Tremblay C, Ghislain J, Bouvier M, Poitout V (2015) Beta-Arrestin recruitment and biased Agonism at Free fatty acid receptor 1. J Biol Chem 290:21131–21140. https://doi.org/10.1074/jbc.M115.644450

Marzook A, Chen S, Pickford P, Lucey M, Wang Y, Correa IR Jr, Broichhagen J, Hodson DJ, Salem V, Rutter GA, Tan TM, Bloom SR, Tomas A, Jones B (2021) Evaluation of efficacy-versus affinity-driven agonism with biased GLP-1R ligands P5 and exendin-F1. Biochem Pharmacol 190:114656. https://doi.org/10.1016/j.bcp.2021.114656

Mende F, Hundahl C, Plouffe B, Skov LJ, Sivertsen B, Madsen AN, Luckmann M, Diep TA, Offermanns S, Frimurer TM, Bouvier M, Holst B (2018) Translating biased signaling in the ghrelin receptor system into differential in vivo functions. Proc Natl Acad Sci USA 115: E10255–E10264. https://doi.org/10.1073/pnas.1804003115

Miyawaki K, Yamada Y, Yano H, Niwa H, Ban N, Ihara Y, Kubota A, Fujimoto S, Kajikawa M, Kuroe A, Tsuda K, Hashimoto H, Yamashita T, Jomori T, Tashiro F, Miyazaki J, Seino Y (1999) Glucose intolerance caused by a defect in the entero-insular axis: a study in gastric inhibitory polypeptide receptor knockout mice. Proc Natl Acad Sci USA 96:14843–14847. https://doi.org/10.1073/pnas.96.26.14843

Mokrosinski J, Frimurer TM, Sivertsen B, Schwartz TW, Holst B (2012) Modulation of constitutive activity and signaling bias of the ghrelin receptor by conformational constraint in the second extracellular loop. J Biol Chem 287:33488–33502. https://doi.org/10.1074/jbc.M112.383240

Mosialou I, Shikhel S, Liu JM, Maurizi A, Luo N, He Z, Huang Y, Zong H, Friedman RA, Barasch J, Lanzano P, Deng L, Leibel RL, Rubin M, Nickolas T, Chung W, Zeltser LM, Williams KW, Pessin JE, Kousteni S (2017) MC4R-dependent suppression of appetite by bone-derived lipocalin 2. Nature 543:385–390. https://doi.org/10.1038/nature21697

Motso A, Pelcman B, Kalinovich A, Kahlous NA, Bokhari MH, Dehvari N, Halleskog C, Waara E, de Jong J, Cheesman E, Kallenberg C, Yakala GK, Murad P, Wetterdal E, Andersson P, van Beek S, Sandstrom A, Alleluia DN, Talamonti E, Youhanna S, Sabatier P, Koenig C, Willems S, Kemas AM, Hutchinson DS, Ham S, Gratz L, Voss J, Marchan-Alvarez JG, Priede M, Jaunsleine K, Spura J, Kovada V, Supe L, Stoddart LA, Holliday ND, Newton PT, Pillon NJ, Schulte G, Summers RJ, Mutule I, Suna E, Olsen JV, Molenaar P, Carlsson J, Lauschke VM, Wright SC, Bengtsson T (2025) GRK-biased adrenergic agonists for the treatment of type 2 diabetes and obesity. Cell. https://doi.org/10.1016/j.cell.2025.05.042

Offermanns S (2014) Free fatty acid (FFA) and hydroxy carboxylic acid (HCA) receptors. Annu Rev Pharmacol Toxicol 54:407–434. https://doi.org/10.1146/annurev-pharmtox-011613-135945

Offermanns S, Colletti SL, Lovenberg TW, Semple G, Wise A, IJzerman AP (2011) International Union of Basic and Clinical Pharmacology. LXXXII: Nomenclature and Classification of Hydroxy-carboxylic Acid Receptors (GPR81, GPR109A, and GPR109B). Pharmacol Rev 63: 269–290. https://doi.org/10.1124/pr.110.003301

Pantel J, Legendre M, Cabrol S, Hilal L, Hajaji Y, Morisset S, Nivot S, Vie-Luton MP, Grouselle D, de Kerdanet M, Kadiri A, Epelbaum J, Le Bouc Y, Amselem S (2006) Loss of constitutive activity of the growth hormone secretagogue receptor in familial short stature. J Clin Invest 116: 760–768. https://doi.org/10.1172/JCI25303

Peters A, Rabe P, Krumbholz P, Kalwa H, Kraft R, Schoneberg T, Staubert C (2020) Natural biased signaling of hydroxycarboxylic acid receptor 3 and G protein-coupled receptor 84. Cell Commun Signal 18:31. https://doi.org/10.1186/s12964-020-0516-2

Portales-Castillo I, Dean T, Cheloha RW, Creemer BA, Vilardaga JP, Savransky S, Khatri A, Juppner H, Gardella TJ (2023) Altered signaling and desensitization responses in PTH1R mutants associated with Eiken syndrome. Commun Biol 6:599. https://doi.org/10.1038/s42003-023-04966-0

Puszkarska AM, Taddese B, Revell J, Davies G, Field J, Hornigold DC, Buchanan A, Vaughan TJ, Colwell LJ (2024) Machine learning designs new GCGR/GLP-1R dual agonists with enhanced biological potency. Nat Chem 16:1436–1444. https://doi.org/10.1038/s41557-024-01532-x

Pydi SP, Jain S, Tung W, Cui Y, Zhu L, Sakamoto W, Jain S, Abel BS, Skarulis MC, Liu J, Huynh T, Pacak K, Caron MG, Gavrilova O, Finkel T, Wess J (2019) Adipocyte beta-arrestin-2 is essential for maintaining whole body glucose and energy homeostasis. Nat Commun 10: 2936. https://doi.org/10.1038/s41467-019-11003-4

Rabe P, Liebing AD, Krumbholz P, Kraft R, Staubert C (2022) Succinate receptor 1 inhibits mitochondrial respiration in cancer cells addicted to glutamine. Cancer Lett 526:91–102. https://doi.org/10.1016/j.canlet.2021.11.024

Rakesh K, Yoo B, Kim IM, Salazar N, Kim KS, Rockman HA (2010) Beta-Arrestin-biased agonism of the angiotensin receptor induced by mechanical stress. Sci Signal 3:ra46. https://doi.org/10.1126/scisignal.2000769

Ravier MA, Leduc M, Richard J, Linck N, Varrault A, Pirot N, Roussel MM, Bockaert J, Dalle S, Bertrand G (2014) Beta-Arrestin2 plays a key role in the modulation of the pancreatic beta cell mass in mice. Diabetologia 57:532–541. https://doi.org/10.1007/s00125-013-3130-7

Rouault AAJ, Rosselli-Murai LK, Hernandez CC, Gimenez LE, Tall GG, Sebag JA (2020) The GPCR accessory protein MRAP2 regulates both biased signaling and constitutive activity of the ghrelin receptor GHSR1a. Sci Signal 13. https://doi.org/10.1126/scisignal.aax4569

Ruiz de Azua I, Mancini G, Srivastava RK, Rey AA, Cardinal P, Tedesco L, Zingaretti CM, Sassmann A, Quarta C, Schwitter C, Conrad A, Wettschureck N, Vemuri VK, Makriyannis A, Hartwig J, Mendez-Lago M, Bindila L, Monory K, Giordano A, Cinti S, Marsicano G, Offermanns S, Nisoli E, Pagotto U, Cota D, Lutz B (2017) Adipocyte cannabinoid receptor CB1 regulates energy homeostasis and alternatively activated macrophages. J Clin Invest 127: 4148–4162. https://doi.org/10.1172/JCI83626

Samms RJ, Zhang G, He W, Ilkayeva O, Droz BA, Bauer SM, Stutsman C, Pirro V, Collins KA, Furber EC, Coskun T, Sloop KW, Brozinick JT, Newgard CB (2022) Tirzepatide induces a thermogenic-like amino acid signature in brown adipose tissue. Mol Metab 64:101550. https://doi.org/10.1016/j.molmet.2022.101550

Scrocchi LA, Marshall BA, Cook SM, Brubaker PL, Drucker DJ (1998) Identification of glucagon-like peptide 1 (GLP-1) actions essential for glucose homeostasis in mice with disruption of GLP-1 receptor signaling. Diabetes 47:632–639. https://doi.org/10.2337/diabetes.47.4.632

Shi Y, Long F (2017) Hedgehog signaling via Gli2 prevents obesity induced by high-fat diet in adult mice. elife 6. https://doi.org/10.7554/eLife.31649

Sinha P, Aarnisalo P, Chubb R, Poulton IJ, Guo J, Nachtrab G, Kimura T, Swami S, Saeed H, Chen M, Weinstein LS, Schipani E, Sims NA, Kronenberg HM, Wu JY (2016) Loss of Gsalpha in the postnatal skeleton leads to low bone mass and a blunted response to anabolic parathyroid hormone therapy. J Biol Chem 291:1631–1642. https://doi.org/10.1074/jbc.M115.679753

Staubert C, Wozniak M, Dupuis N, Laschet C, Pillaiyar T, Hanson J (2022) Superconserved receptors expressed in the brain: expression, function, motifs and evolution of an orphan receptor family. Pharmacol Ther 240:108217. https://doi.org/10.1016/j.pharmthera.2022.108217

Suchy T, Zieschang C, Popkova Y, Kaczmarek I, Weiner J, Liebing AD, Cakir MV, Landgraf K, Gericke M, Pospisilik JA, Korner A, Heiker JT, Dannenberger D, Schiller J, Schoneberg T, Liebscher I, Thor D (2020) The repertoire of Adhesion G protein-coupled receptors in adipocytes and their functional relevance. Int J Obes 44:2124–2136. https://doi.org/10.1038/s41366-020-0570-2

Sun B, Willard FS, Feng D, Alsina-Fernandez J, Chen Q, Vieth M, Ho JD, Showalter AD, Stutsman C, Ding L, Suter TM, Dunbar JD, Carpenter JW, Mohammed FA, Aihara E, Brown RA, Bueno AB, Emmerson PJ, Moyers JS, Kobilka TS, Coghlan MP, Kobilka BK, Sloop KW (2022) Structural determinants of dual incretin receptor agonism by tirzepatide. Proc Natl Acad Sci USA 119:e2116506119. https://doi.org/10.1073/pnas.2116506119

Talbot J, Joly E, Prentki M, Buteau J (2012) Beta-Arrestin1-mediated recruitment of c-Src underlies the proliferative action of glucagon-like peptide-1 in pancreatic beta INS832/13 cells. Mol Cell Endocrinol 364:65–70. https://doi.org/10.1016/j.mce.2012.08.010

Tang C, Ahmed K, Gille A, Lu S, Grone HJ, Tunaru S, Offermanns S (2015) Loss of FFA2 and FFA3 increases insulin secretion and improves glucose tolerance in type 2 diabetes. Nat Med 21:173–177. https://doi.org/10.1038/nm.3779

Thomas C, Gioiello A, Noriega L, Strehle A, Oury J, Rizzo G, Macchiarulo A, Yamamoto H, Mataki C, Pruzanski M, Pellicciari R, Auwerx J, Schoonjans K (2009) TGR5-mediated bile acid sensing controls glucose homeostasis. Cell Metab 10:167–177. https://doi.org/10.1016/j.cmet.2009.08.001

Tikhonova IG, Sum CS, Neumann S, Thomas CJ, Raaka BM, Costanzi S, Gershengorn MC (2007) Bidirectional, iterative approach to the structural delineation of the functional "chemoprint" in GPR40 for agonist recognition. J Med Chem 50:2981–2989. https://doi.org/10.1021/jm0614782

Tolson KP, Garcia C, Yen S, Simonds S, Stefanidis A, Lawrence A, Smith JT, Kauffman AS (2014) Impaired kisspeptin signaling decreases metabolism and promotes glucose intolerance and obesity. J Clin Invest 124:3075–3079. https://doi.org/10.1172/JCI71075

Toyomoto M, Inoue A, Iida K, Denawa M, Kii I, Ngako Kadji FM, Kishi T, Im D, Shimamura T, Onogi H, Yoshida S, Iwata S, Aoki J, Hosoya T, Hagiwara M (2021) S1PR3-G(12)-biased agonist ALESIA targets cancer metabolism and promotes glucose starvation. Cell Chem Biol 28:1132–1144 e9. https://doi.org/10.1016/j.chembiol.2021.01.004

Ulven T (2012) Short-chain free fatty acid receptors FFA2/GPR43 and FFA3/GPR41 as new potential therapeutic targets. Front Endocrinol (Lausanne) 3:111. https://doi.org/10.3389/fendo.2012.00111

Wang J, Wu X, Simonavicius N, Tian H, Ling L (2006) Medium-chain fatty acids as ligands for orphan G protein-coupled receptor GPR84. J Biol Chem 281:34457–34464. https://doi.org/10.1074/jbc.M608019200

Wang L, Yao D, Deepak R, Liu H, Xiao Q, Fan H, Gong W, Wei Z, Zhang C (2018) Structures of the human PGD(2) receptor CRTH2 reveal novel mechanisms for ligand recognition. Mol Cell 72(48–59):e4. https://doi.org/10.1016/j.molcel.2018.08.009

Wang H, Hu W, Xu T, Yuan Y, Liu D, Wuthrich K (2023) Selective polypeptide ligand binding to the extracellular surface of the transmembrane domains of the class B GPCRs GLP-1R and GCGR. iScience 26:106918. https://doi.org/10.1016/j.isci.2023.106918

Wen X, Shang P, Chen H, Guo L, Rong N, Jiang X, Li X, Liu J, Yang G, Zhang J, Zhu K, Meng Q, He X, Wang Z, Liu Z, Cheng H, Zheng Y, Zhang B, Pang J, Liu Z, Xiao P, Chen Y, Liu L, Luo F, Yu X, Yi F, Zhang P, Yang F, Deng C, Sun JP (2025) Evolutionary study and structural basis of proton sensing by Mus GPR4 and Xenopus GPR4. Cell 188(653–670):e24. https://doi.org/10.1016/j.cell.2024.12.001

Wilde C, Mitgau J, Suchy T, Schoneberg T, Liebscher I (2022) Translating the force-mechano-sensing GPCRs. Am J Physiol Cell Physiol 322:C1047–C1060. https://doi.org/10.1152/ajpcell.00465.2021

Willard FS, Douros JD, Gabe MB, Showalter AD, Wainscott DB, Suter TM, Capozzi ME, van der Velden WJ, Stutsman C, Cardona GR, Urva S, Emmerson PJ, Holst JJ, D'Alessio DA, Coghlan MP, Rosenkilde MM, Campbell JE, Sloop KW (2020) Tirzepatide is an imbalanced and biased dual GIP and GLP-1 receptor agonist. JCI Insight 5. https://doi.org/10.1172/jci.insight.140532

Yanguas-Casas N, Barreda-Manso MA, Nieto-Sampedro M, Romero-Ramirez L (2017) TUDCA: an agonist of the bile acid receptor GPBAR1/TGR5 with anti-inflammatory effects in microglial cells. J Cell Physiol 232:2231–2245. https://doi.org/10.1002/jcp.25742

Yin TC, Bauchle CJ, Rouault AAJ, Stephens SB, Sebag JA (2020) The Insulinostatic effect of ghrelin requires MRAP2 expression in delta cells. iScience 23:101216. https://doi.org/10.1016/j.isci.2020.101216

Yore MM, Syed I, Moraes-Vieira PM, Zhang T, Herman MA, Homan EA, Patel RT, Lee J, Chen S, Peroni OD, Dhaneshwar AS, Hammarstedt A, Smith U, McGraw TE, Saghatelian A, Kahn BB (2014) Discovery of a class of endogenous mammalian lipids with anti-diabetic and anti-inflammatory effects. Cell 159:318–332. https://doi.org/10.1016/j.cell.2014.09.035

Zaimia N, Obeid J, Varrault A, Sabatier J, Broca C, Gilon P, Costes S, Bertrand G, Ravier MA (2023) GLP-1 and GIP receptors signal through distinct beta-arrestin 2-dependent pathways to regulate pancreatic beta cell function. Cell Rep 42:113326. https://doi.org/10.1016/j.celrep.2023.113326

Zhang LN, Sinclair R, Selman C, Mitchell S, Morgan D, Clapham JC, Speakman JR (2014) Effects of a specific MCHR1 antagonist (GW803430) on energy budget and glucose metabolism in diet-induced obese mice. Obesity (Silver Spring) 22:681–690. https://doi.org/10.1002/oby.20418

Zhang H, Sturchler E, Zhu J, Nieto A, Cistrone PA, Xie J, He L, Yea K, Jones T, Turn R, Di Stefano PS, Griffin PR, Dawson PE, McDonald PH, Lerner RA (2015) Autocrine selection of a GLP-1R G-protein biased agonist with potent antidiabetic effects. Nat Commun 6:8918. https://doi.org/10.1038/ncomms9918

Zhu L, Rossi M, Cui Y, Lee RJ, Sakamoto W, Perry NA, Urs NM, Caron MG, Gurevich VV, Godlewski G, Kunos G, Chen M, Chen W, Wess J (2017) Hepatic beta-arrestin 2 is essential for maintaining euglycemia. J Clin Invest 127:2941–2945. https://doi.org/10.1172/JCI92913

Future Directions in GPCR Biased Signaling and Ligand Pharmacology

Dannya Estau and Zijian Li

Contents

D. Estau
Department of Cardiology and Institute of Vascular Medicine, Peking University Third Hospital; Beijing Key Laboratory of Cardiovascular Receptors Research, State Key Laboratory of Vascular Homeostasis and Remodeling, and NHC Key Laboratory of Cardiovascular Molecular Biology and Regulatory Peptides, Peking University; Research Unit of Medical Science Research Management/ Basic and Clinical Research of Metabolic Cardiovascular Diseases, Chinese Academy of Medical Sciences, Peking University, Beijing, China

Z. Li (✉)
Department of Cardiology and Institute of Vascular Medicine, Peking University Third Hospital; Beijing Key Laboratory of Cardiovascular Receptors Research, State Key Laboratory of Vascular Homeostasis and Remodeling, and NHC Key Laboratory of Cardiovascular Molecular Biology and Regulatory Peptides, Peking University; Research Unit of Medical Science Research Management/ Basic and Clinical Research of Metabolic Cardiovascular Diseases, Chinese Academy of Medical Sciences, Peking University, Beijing, China

Department of Pharmacy, Peking University Third Hospital, Beijing, China
e-mail: lizijian@bjmu.edu.cn

© The Author(s), under exclusive license to Springer Nature Switzerland AG 2025

Z. Li, K. Xiao (eds.), *Pharmacology of GPCRs Biased Signaling and Agonists*,
Handbook of Experimental Pharmacology 290, https://doi.org/10.1007/164_2025_775

Abstract

G protein-coupled receptor (GPCR) biased signaling has emerged as a transformative paradigm, reshaping both fundamental understanding of receptor biology and pharmacological intervention. Significant advances have been made in deciphering the mechanisms underlying biased signaling and in the development of ligands that selectively engage specific pathways. Here, we outline key future directions in GPCR biased signaling and ligand pharmacology including the biased signaling theories, structural insights, methodological innovations and ligand pharmacology theories. We hope that these perspectives will contribute to pharmacological research, drug R & D, and clinical drug research and promoting safer and more effective GPCR-targeted treatments for human diseases.

Keywords

Biased signaling · Future directions · G protein-coupled receptor · Ligand pharmacology

1 The Need for New Theories of GPCR-Biased Signaling

Approximately 10 years ago, the adaptor β-arrestins were discovered to initiate parallel G protein-independent signaling pathways (Luttrell et al. 1999; Shenoy and Lefkowitz 2011). GPCRs can activate either G protein-dependent signaling pathways or β-arrestin-dependent signaling pathways, called "biased activation" theory (Lefkowitz 2013). Based on the classical bias activation theory, the broad definition of "bias" will continue to expand theoretically in the future. These advances will deepen our insight into GPCR mechanisms and transform disease treatment strategies.

1.1 Effector-Diverse Biased Theory

Effector proteins are the mediators of GPCR functions. The traditional understanding of biased signaling has largely focused on the binary choice of G proteins and β-arrestins or different subtypes of G proteins. Future research should expand the understanding of effector proteins that can directly interact with GPCRs and reveal more effector proteins that directly mediate GPCR function, such as adaptor proteins, regulatory kinases like GRKs, and other novel protein types. More importantly, the GPCR function mediated by these new effectors will bring us a new understanding of diverse biased theories.

1.2 Spatial and Temporal Biased Theory

In addition to differential effector recruitment, spatial and temporal regulation also significantly contributes to GPCR biased signaling by generating subcellular organelle-dependent signaling and temporally distinct activation modes. Spatially, the same GPCR activates different downstream pathways and elicits distinct physiological outcomes depending on its subcellular localization, such as the Golgi apparatus or endosomes. A systematic characterization of such spatially biased signaling, including its regulatory mechanisms and molecular determinants, represents a critical direction for future research.

Temporally, GPCRs display intrinsic biases toward either transient or sustained activation patterns. For example, G protein-mediated responses are often transient, and β-arrestin-dependent signaling tends to be sustained. The precise molecular switches governing these temporal dynamics and their pathophysiological implications remain incompletely understood. Clarifying spatially and temporally biased GPCR signaling may inform novel therapeutic strategies for context-specific receptor modulation in disease.

1.3 Cell-, Tissue-, and Organ-Specific Biased Theory

GPCR signaling exhibits profound complexity with system-level biased activation across cellular, tissue, and organ scales. At the cellular level, the same ligand-receptor pairs can elicit cell-specific biased signaling outcomes due to differential expression, combinations and post-translational modifications of receptor and effector. At the tissue scale, it is crucial to understand how localized molecular regulators integrate with specialized intercellular communication networks to collectively determine tissue-specific pathway selection.

At the organ level, on the one hand, the ligands/receptors microenvironments of different organs may lead to different signaling pathways. The composition of these ligands/receptors' microenvironments can dynamically change in pathological and physiological conditions, making the signaling processes highly elusive. On the other hand, maintaining whole-body homeostasis necessitates intricate coordination across different organs, which requires more precise, complex, and in-depth regulatory mechanisms. Thus, the composition and regulation of tissue-specific biased ligands/receptors microenvironments have become key to revealing this complex physiological phenomenon. The future development of cell-, tissue-, and organ-specific biased signaling theory will facilitate the translation of in vitro mechanistic studies into the complex in vivo context.

In summary, as research advances, the new theories of GPCR biased signaling will continue to expand to fully capture the sophisticated regulatory mechanisms governing GPCR function and progressively deepen our understanding of GPCRs.

2 Structural Mechanisms of GPCR Biased Signaling

2.1 Structural Biology of GPCR Biased Signaling

GPCR structural biology provides critical insights into biased signaling, where ligand-specific receptor conformations determine pathway selectivity. However, GPCRs present exceptional challenges for structural biology due to their low endogenous expression and intrinsic conformational flexibility. Although protein engineering strategies such as fusion partners and antibody fragment crystallization have enabled the stabilization of specific receptor states, the transient intermediate states and their transition kinetics are still poorly characterized. Most notably, the field still lacks atomic-resolution structures of weak-binding effector proteins and GPCR-effector complexes, such as the GPCR/β-arrestin2 complex.

Importantly, advancing structural techniques to stabilize physiologically relevant lipid-receptor interactions represents a crucial frontier. Cholesterol and phosphoinositides, for instance, have been implicated in stabilizing specific signaling states, yet their structural mechanisms remain elusive.

2.2 Future Directions from Structures to Mechanisms

The future direction of the field is to transform the structural solution into in-depth research on the combination of structure and function/mechanism. Structural biology needs to evolve beyond static images and provide a dynamic, comprehensive understanding of biased signaling networks. This shift is fundamental for advancing GPCR pharmacology from trial-and-error approaches to a predictive and precise science. Three critical advancements will drive this paradigm shift: (i) developing time-resolved structural techniques capable of capturing conformational transitions at physiological timescales; (ii) combining AlphaFold predictions with rigorous experimental validation to resolve elusive GPCRs/effectors complexes; and (iii) establishing quantitative structure-mechanism relationships that predict how atomic-scale receptor dynamics dictate cellular signaling patterns. These breakthroughs will collectively enable the transition from isolated structural observations to a unified, dynamic model of conformation-dependent pathway selection, ultimately paving the way for the precision engineering of function-selective therapeutics.

3 Future Direction of Biased Ligand Pharmacology

3.1 Next-Generation Ligand Design

While traditional drug development was empirical trial-and-error, the emergence of biased signaling provided new theoretical grounds for selectively enhancing efficacy while reducing toxicity (Kenakin 2017; Schulte 2024). Unlike classical ligands that affect multiple downstream pathways without specificity, biased ligands can selectively engage therapeutic signaling under the guidance of precise mechanistic insights.

However, early candidates like TRV130 (μ-opioid receptor) and TRV027 (angiotensin II receptor type 1) demonstrated preclinical promise but have not yet achieved clear clinical efficacy (Bossert et al. 2020; Felker et al. 2015; Manglik et al. 2016; Negus and Freeman 2018; Pang et al. 2017). Moving forward, next-generation ligand design needs to move beyond the initial focus on simple G protein or β-arrestin bias and address signaling specificity across cells, tissues, and organs.

These should integrate three essential dimensions: (i) integrating atomic-level structural insights into ligand-receptor-effector engagement, (ii) mapping systems-biased understanding of signaling networks in cellular-to-organ contexts, and (iii) developing advanced pharmacological models that better replicate human pathophysiology. The field needs to integrate structural biology, systems pharmacology, and clinical trial to transform biased signaling from theory into an actionable blueprint for precision therapeutics.

3.2 Repurposing Existing Drugs with Biased Insights

GPCR-targeting drugs make up nearly 40% of approved medications (Hauser et al. 2017; Lorente et al. 2025), providing a powerful clinical drug library. Although these clinical drugs were not developed based on the bias-ligand theory, some of them may still be potential bias ligands. Therefore, screening for biased drugs among existing clinical drugs will accelerate the development of biased drugs and better guide the clinical application. Moreover, proving that specific signaling pathways cause treatment effects remains challenging and requires validation from laboratory studies to clinical trials. To address these challenges, establishing the "bedside-to-bench-to-bedside" approach is essential, which will accelerate drug development, lower costs, and improve treatment safety and efficacy.

3.3 Receptor Genetics-Based Patient Stratification

GPCR pharmacogenomics is a promising new direction for precision medicine (Hauser et al. 2018). Moving beyond conventional pharmacogenomics focused primarily on pharmacokinetics, future GPCR-targeted therapies should prioritize how genetic variations change biased signaling pathways and cellular responses. While existing studies mainly examine drug response changes caused by GPCR mutations, future work should establish polygenic models incorporating GPCR, effectors, and regulatory variants to systematically quantify signaling bias and optimize therapeutic outcomes. Second, single-cell functional genomics, combining CRISPR-based receptor editing with real-time signaling biosensors, will enable patient-specific biased signaling profiling. Additionally, machine learning models trained on multi-omic datasets could predict personalized biased signatures, transcending static SNP correlations. Ultimately, the field must shift toward evaluating patients not just by genetic markers but also by the dynamic and functional response of cells to therapeutic drugs.

4 Future Novel Methodologies in Biased Signaling Research

4.1 Current Detection of GPCR Biased Signaling Methods

Advances in detecting and quantifying GPCR biased signaling have significantly enhanced both mechanistic understanding and therapeutic development. Current approaches for detecting GPCR biased signaling include BRET and FRET biosensor assays (Malik et al. 2013; Pfleger and Eidne 2006), Tango arrestin recruitment assays, and so on. However, BRET/FRET biosensors face challenges including donor/acceptor saturation, narrow dynamic range, and steric interference that can skew bias measurements. Similarly, Tango arrestin recruitment assays, though widely used, often employ overexpression systems (Saca et al. 2025) that may exaggerate bias compared to physiological conditions. In addition, although the relative intrinsic activity (RA) method, which standardizes ligand efficacy to a reference agonist, reduces false positives compared to traditional techniques, its limited precision in quantifying biased efficacy restricts clinical application. In the future, the field needs to improve these methods and establish standardized measurements of bias.

4.2 Emerging Methodological Frontiers

(i) Improvement to existing assays

The next generation of biosensor technologies must undergo significant improvement to overcome the current limitations in biased signaling detection. First, more sensitive detection methods are needed to exclude confounding factors, making results comparable across different experimental conditions. Second, true compartmentalized signaling resolution should be achieved, particularly in distinguishing GPCR signaling at the plasma membrane from intracellular signaling. Last, developing assay systems that faithfully recapitulate physiological conditions is critical, which enables researchers to study biased signaling in a biological context. This innovation will represent an essential step toward developing truly predictive models of GPCR biased signaling that can reliably inform therapeutic development.

(ii) Novel mechanistic dissection tools

The next frontier in GPCR research demands advances in structural and computational methodologies to fully understand the mechanisms of biased signaling.

Three critical developments will drive this progress: (i) developing higher-resolution cryo-EM and time-resolved spectroscopic techniques to capture the complete spectrum of ligand-stabilized receptor conformations in real time; (ii) creating next-generation AI tools capable of modeling not only static receptor structures but also dynamic changes caused by ligands in their natural membrane environment and connecting detailed structural data with specific cellular responses; (iii) at the cellular level, pioneering single-cell technologies with enhanced sensitivity to map physiologically relevant receptor-effector expression landscapes, resolving low-abundance signaling events.

(iii) Data-driven paradigm shifts

To better understand biased signaling, structural and computational methods must improve. The next decade will see a paradigm shift driven by artificial intelligence and large-scale data integration. First, it is necessary to develop new algorithms that integrate multi-omics data by combining single-cell sequencing, high-throughput structural data, and functional genomics to move from correlation to causation. Second, machine learning-driven drug discovery will transition from retrospective analysis to prospective design, which can screen compound libraries for bias potential, simulate patient-specific signaling, and generate optimized biased ligands. Finally, big-data processing models are needed to classify drug effects in large populations more accurately based on biased signaling theories, thus enabling genuine personalized therapy.

In summary, the future of GPCR biased signaling and ligand pharmacology lies in mastering spatial, temporal, and conformational control. This paradigm shift from simple receptor blockade to biased signaling selection will require converging cutting-edge structural insights, systems pharmacology, and AI-driven design. Ultimately, these advances will enable safer, more effective therapies targeting specific disease mechanisms, ushering in a new era of precision medicine.

References

Bossert JM, Kiyatkin EA, Korah H, Hoots JK, Afzal A, Perekopskiy D, Thomas S, Fredriksson I, Blough BE, Negus SS, Epstein DH, Shaham Y (2020) In a rat model of opioid maintenance, the G protein-biased mu opioid receptor agonist TRV130 decreases relapse to oxycodone seeking and taking and prevents oxycodone-induced brain hypoxia. Biol Psychiatry 88:935–944. https://doi.org/10.1016/j.biopsych.2020.02.014

Felker GM, Butler J, Collins SP, Cotter G, Davison BA, Ezekowitz JA, Filippatos G, Levy PD, Metra M, Ponikowski P, Soergel DG, Teerlink JR, Violin JD, Voors AA, Pang PS (2015) Heart failure therapeutics on the basis of a biased ligand of the angiotensin-2 type 1 receptor. Rationale and design of the BLAST-AHF study (Biased Ligand of the Angiotensin Receptor Study in Acute Heart Failure). JACC Heart Fail 3:193–201. https://doi.org/10.1016/j.jchf.2014.09.008

Hauser AS, Attwood MM, Rask-Andersen M, Schiöth HB, Gloriam DE (2017) Trends in GPCR drug discovery: new agents, targets and indications. Nat Rev Drug Discov 16:829–842. https://doi.org/10.1038/nrd.2017.178

Hauser AS, Chavali S, Masuho I, Jahn LJ, Martemyanov KA, Gloriam DE, Babu MM (2018) Pharmacogenomics of GPCR drug targets. Cell 172:41–54.e19. https://doi.org/10.1016/j.cell.2017.11.033

Kenakin T (2017) Signaling bias in drug discovery. Expert Opin Drug Discov 12:321–333. https://doi.org/10.1080/17460441.2017.1297417

Lefkowitz RJ (2013) A brief history of G-protein coupled receptors (Nobel Lecture). Angew Chem Int Ed Engl 52:6366–6378. https://doi.org/10.1002/anie.201301924

Lorente JS, Sokolov AV, Ferguson G, Schiöth HB, Hauser AS, Gloriam DE (2025) GPCR drug discovery: new agents, targets and indications. Nat Rev Drug Discov 24:458–479. https://doi.org/10.1038/s41573-025-01139-y

Luttrell LM, Ferguson SS, Daaka Y, Miller WE, Maudsley S, Della Rocca GJ, Lin F, Kawakatsu H, Owada K, Luttrell DK, Caron MG, Lefkowitz RJ (1999) Beta-arrestin-dependent formation of beta2 adrenergic receptor-Src protein kinase complexes. Science 283:655–661. https://doi.org/10.1126/science.283.5402.655

Malik RU, Ritt M, DeVree BT, Neubig RR, Sunahara RK, Sivaramakrishnan S (2013) Detection of G protein-selective G protein-coupled receptor (GPCR) conformations in live cells. J Biol Chem 288:17167–17178. https://doi.org/10.1074/jbc.M113.464065

Manglik A, Lin H, Aryal DK, McCorvy JD, Dengler D, Corder G, Levit A, Kling RC, Bernat V, Hübner H, Huang XP, Sassano MF, Giguère PM, Löber S, Da D, Scherrer G, Kobilka BK, Gmeiner P, Roth BL, Shoichet BK (2016) Structure-based discovery of opioid analgesics with reduced side effects. Nature 537:185–190. https://doi.org/10.1038/nature19112

Negus SS, Freeman KB (2018) Abuse potential of biased mu opioid receptor agonists. Trends Pharmacol Sci 39:916–919. https://doi.org/10.1016/j.tips.2018.08.007

Pang PS, Butler J, Collins SP, Cotter G, Davison BA, Ezekowitz JA, Filippatos G, Levy PD, Metra M, Ponikowski P, Teerlink JR, Voors AA, Bharucha D, Goin K, Soergel DG, Felker GM (2017) Biased ligand of the angiotensin II type 1 receptor in patients with acute heart failure: a randomized, double-blind, placebo-controlled, phase IIB, dose ranging trial (BLAST-AHF). Eur Heart J 38:2364–2373. https://doi.org/10.1093/eurheartj/ehx196

Pfleger KD, Eidne KA (2006) Illuminating insights into protein-protein interactions using bioluminescence resonance energy transfer (BRET). Nat Methods 3:165–174. https://doi.org/10.1038/nmeth841

Saca VR, Burdette C, Sakmar TP (2025) GPCR biosensors to study conformational dynamics and signaling in drug discovery. Annu Rev Pharmacol Toxicol 65:7–28. https://doi.org/10.1146/annurev-pharmtox-061724-080836

Schulte G (2024) Seventy-five years of interactions: the Department of Physiology and Pharmacology at Karolinska Institutet and Pharmacological Reviews. Pharmacol Rev 76:972–977. https://doi.org/10.1124/pharmrev.124.001403

Shenoy SK, Lefkowitz RJ (2011) β-Arrestin-mediated receptor trafficking and signal transduction. Trends Pharmacol Sci 32:521–533. https://doi.org/10.1016/j.tips.2011.05.002

MIX
Papier aus verantwortungsvollen Quellen
Paper from responsible sources
FSC® C105338

If you have any concerns about our products,
you can contact us on
ProductSafety@springernature.com

In case Publisher is established outside the EU,
the EU authorized representative is:
Springer Nature Customer Service Center GmbH
Europaplatz 3, 69115 Heidelberg, Germany

Printed by Libri Plureos GmbH
in Hamburg, Germany